The Encyclopedia of Nutraceutical Ingredients

Dr. Munir A Chandniwala

Qurate
quratebooks.com

The Encyclopedia of N utraceutical Ingredients
Dr. Munir A Chandniwala

Published in 2024

© Published by

Qurate Books Pvt. Ltd.
Goa 403523, India
www.qoratebooks.com
Tel: 1800-210-6527, Email: info@quratebooks.com

ISBN: 978-93-58987-62-1

Author Introduction

Dr. Munir Chandniwala is a pharmacist and has over two decades of experience in the field of Functional foods, Nutraceuticals and dietary supplements formulation manufacturing.

Dr. Munir Chandniwala has worked in industrial settings, contributing to the development of new nutraceutical products and advocates knowledge required regarding ingredients while formulating a product. The idea for a quick access to a data about ingredients used in nutraceuticals and dietary supplement for people involved in manufacturing, marketing, research is key behind creating this compilation.

Disclaimer of Book

Book: The information contained in this book is for general informational purposes only. While we strive to ensure that the ingredient details provided are accurate and up-to-date, we make no representations or warranties of any kind, express or implied, about the completeness, accuracy, reliability, suitability, or availability with respect to the information contained in this book for any purpose. Any reliance you place on such information is recommended to be cross checked with other sources too.

Introduction of book

"The Encyclopedia of Nutraceutical Ingredients" by Dr. Munir A Chandniwala is a meticulously curated reference guide that catalogues a vast array of ingredients used across nutraceutical and dietary supplement industries. This book is designed as an essential tool for professionals, students, and enthusiasts who seek detailed information about the raw materials and compounds that form the backbone of various health products.

The book is organized alphabetically and by category as per schedule mentioned in gazette notification FSSAI, India for easy navigation. Each entry on an ingredient includes various aspects of details in brief as a quick reference to understand details on ingredient with regards to its introduction, synonym name, common name, Pharmacognosy/chemistry, action and pharmacology, method of analysis, health benefits, indication and usage, its usual constituents with percentages, mechanism of action, dosage, contraindications, Precautions, adverse reactions, research standing, Pharmacokinetics, pharmacodynamics, overdosage, international standing, Indian Standing, research summary.

"The Encyclopedia of Ingredients" stands out for its simple approach and comprehensive coverage, making it a definitive resource in the field of health and wellness ingredients. It is an indispensable guide for anyone involved in the formulation, study, or regulation of health-related products.

With increasing market size of nutraceutical products, this book can help to get a quick guide and reference to understand comprehensive ingredient details.

This reference guide has been praised for its thoroughness and clarity, making complex scientific information accessible to health professionals and informed consumers alike. It serves as an essential resource for anyone involved in health and wellness industries, from nutritionists and dietitians to healthcare providers and health-conscious readers.

Contents

Schedule III

Molecules/isolates/extracts other than Schedule II

Part A

1) AMERICAN GINSENG:

Introduction: American Ginseng, scientifically known as Panax quinquefolius, is a perennial herb native to North America. It has been used for centuries in traditional medicine systems for its various health benefits.

Synonym Name and Common Name: Synonym: Panax quinquefolius Common Name: American Ginseng

Pharmacognosy: American Ginseng typically consists of dried roots and rhizomes. The roots are pale yellow to brownish in color, often resembling a human body with rootlets resembling arms and legs. The roots have a characteristic aroma and a slightly bitter taste.

Action and Pharmacology: American Ginseng contains active compounds such as ginsenosides, polysaccharides, and polyacetylenes, which contribute to its pharmacological effects. These compounds exert adaptogenic, antioxidant, anti-inflammatory, immunomodulatory, and neuroprotective actions in the body.

Method of Analysis: Analytical methods like high-performance liquid chromatography (HPLC), gas chromatography-mass spectrometry (GC-MS), and thin-layer chromatography (TLC) are commonly used for the analysis of ginsenosides and other bioactive compounds in American Ginseng.

Health Benefits:

- Supports immune function
- Enhances cognitive function
- Improves physical endurance
- Regulates blood sugar levels
- Reduces inflammation
- Supports cardiovascular health
- Alleviates stress and fatigue

Indication and Usage: American Ginseng is used as a dietary supplement to promote overall health and well-being. It is available in various forms including capsules, tablets, extracts, and teas. It may be used to support immune health, cognitive function, energy levels, and various other health concerns.

Usual Constituents with Percentages:

- Ginsenosides (2-3%)
- Polysaccharides (20-30%)
- Polyacetylenes
- Vitamins and minerals

Mechanism of Action: The active compounds in American Ginseng interact with cellular receptors and signaling pathways, modulating stress response, immune function, energy metabolism, and inflammation. Ginsenosides are believed to be the primary bioactive constituents responsible for the herb's effects.

Dosage: The recommended dosage of American Ginseng varies depending on individual factors such as age, health status, and specific health goals. Typical doses range from 200 mg to 1000 mg per day, taken orally in divided doses.

Contraindications:

- Hypersensitivity to ginseng or its constituents
- Use in children without medical supervision

- Concurrent use with certain medications, particularly anticoagulants and immunosuppressants

Precautions:

- Pregnant and lactating women should consult with a healthcare professional before using American Ginseng.
- Individuals with underlying health conditions such as diabetes, hypertension, or autoimmune disorders should use caution and seek medical advice before supplementation.

Adverse Reactions: While generally well-tolerated, some individuals may experience mild side effects such as insomnia, gastrointestinal upset, headache, or allergic reactions. Prolonged or high-dose usage may increase the risk of adverse effects.

Research Summary: Research on American Ginseng has explored its potential benefits in various health conditions including immune support, cognitive enhancement, diabetes management, and stress reduction. While some studies suggest positive effects, further research is needed to confirm efficacy and safety.

Pharmacokinetics: Following oral administration, the bioactive compounds in American Ginseng are absorbed in the gastrointestinal tract, metabolized in the liver, and distributed to target tissues. The pharmacokinetics of ginsenosides may vary based on factors such as formulation and individual physiology.

Pharmacodynamics: American Ginseng's pharmacological effects are mediated by its active constituents, which interact with cellular targets and signaling pathways. These interactions modulate physiological processes involved in immune function, energy metabolism, oxidative stress, and inflammation.

Overdosage: Excessive consumption of American Ginseng may lead to adverse effects such as insomnia, gastrointestinal discomfort, hypertension, or allergic reactions. It is important to adhere to recommended dosages and seek medical attention if symptoms of overdose occur.

International Standing: American Ginseng is recognized internationally for its medicinal properties and is traded globally as a dietary supplement. It is subject to regulations and quality standards established by health authorities in various countries.

Indian Standing: American Ginseng is legally imported and widely available in the Indian market as a dietary supplement. It falls under the regulatory purview of the Food Safety and Standards Authority of India (FSSAI), ensuring compliance with safety and quality standards.

FSSAI Purity Criteria: American ginseng extract (containing NLT 10% of total ginsenosides on dried basis).

Permitted Level : 90-400mg/day

2) ASTAXANTHIN (HAEMATOCOCCUSPLUVIALLIS)

Introduction: Astaxanthin is a naturally occurring carotenoid pigment found in various microorganisms, algae, and seafood such as salmon, shrimp, and krill. It is best known for its vibrant red color and powerful antioxidant properties. Astaxanthin derived from Haematococcuspluvialis, a freshwater microalga, is particularly prized for its purity and potency.

Synonym Name and Common Name: Synonym: 3,3'-dihydroxy-β,β-carotene-4,4'-dione Common Name: Astaxanthin

Pharmacognosy / Chemistry: Astaxanthin derived from Haematococcuspluvialis typically appears as a dark red pigment. It is often extracted from the algal biomass using various solvent extraction techniques. The extract can further undergo purification processes to isolate and concentrate astaxanthin.

Action and Pharmacology: Astaxanthin exhibits potent antioxidant activity, which helps neutralize free radicals and reduce oxidative stress in the body. It also demonstrates anti-inflammatory, immune-modulating, and skin-protective effects. Astaxanthin's unique molecular structure allows it to cross biological membranes easily, providing protection to both lipid and aqueous portions of cells.

Method of Analysis: High-performance liquid chromatography (HPLC) is the most commonly used method for the analysis of astaxanthin content in samples derived from Haematococcuspluvialis. This technique allows for accurate quantification of astaxanthin levels, ensuring product quality and consistency.

Health Benefits:

- Powerful antioxidant activity
- Supports skin health and elasticity
- Enhances exercise performance and recovery
- Promotes eye health and vision
- Supports cardiovascular health
- Reduces inflammation and joint discomfort

Indication and Usage: Astaxanthin derived from Haematococcuspluvialis is commonly used as a dietary supplement to promote overall health and well-being. It is often taken in the form of capsules or soft gels. Astaxanthin supplements may be recommended for individuals seeking antioxidant support, skin protection, joint health, or enhanced athletic performance.

Usual Constituents with Percentages: Astaxanthin derived from Haematococcuspluvialis typically contains astaxanthin in concentrations ranging from 2% to 10% or higher, depending on the extraction and purification process used.

Mechanism of Action: Astaxanthin exerts its antioxidant effects by scavenging free radicals, preventing lipid peroxidation, and modulating inflammatory pathways. It also enhances mitochondrial function, improves cellular energy production, and promotes the expression of antioxidant enzymes, providing comprehensive cellular protection.

Dosage: The recommended dosage of astaxanthin supplements varies depending on the individual's health status and specific health goals. Typical doses range from 4 mg to 12 mg per day, taken orally with food for optimal absorption.

Contraindications:

- Hypersensitivity to astaxanthin or other carotenoids
- Use in pregnant or lactating women without medical supervision
- Concurrent use with anticoagulant medications due to potential interactions

Precautions:

- Individuals with underlying health conditions should consult a healthcare professional before starting astaxanthin supplementation.
- Astaxanthin supplements may interact with certain medications, so it's essential to discuss potential drug interactions with a healthcare provider.

Adverse Reactions: Astaxanthin supplements are generally well-tolerated, with few reported adverse effects. Mild gastrointestinal symptoms such as nausea or diarrhea may occur in some individuals, particularly at higher doses.

Research Summary: Research on astaxanthin derived from Haematococcuspluvialis has demonstrated its potential therapeutic benefits in various health conditions. Studies have highlighted its antioxidant, anti-inflammatory, and photoprotective properties, as well as its role in promoting cardiovascular health, supporting eye health, and enhancing athletic performance.

Pharmacokinetics: Following oral administration, astaxanthin is absorbed through the gastrointestinal tract and transported via chylomicrons in the lymphatic system. It is then distributed to various tissues, where it exerts its antioxidant and anti-inflammatory effects. Astaxanthin has a relatively long half-life, allowing for sustained antioxidant activity in the body.

Pharmacodynamics: Astaxanthin acts as a potent antioxidant, scavenging free radicals and protecting cells from oxidative damage. It also modulates inflammatory pathways, inhibiting the production of pro-inflammatory cytokines and mediators. Additionally, astaxanthin enhances mitochondrial function and cellular energy production, contributing to its overall health benefits.

Overdosage: There is limited information on the potential effects of overdosing on astaxanthin. However, excessive intake may lead to the accumulation of carotenoids in tissues, causing a harmless but noticeable yellowing of the skin known as carotenodermia. It is advisable to adhere to recommended dosages and consult a healthcare professional if concerns arise.

International Standing: Astaxanthin derived from Haematococcuspluvialis is recognized internationally as a valuable dietary supplement due to its potent antioxidant properties and numerous health benefits. It is widely available in markets worldwide and is subject to regulatory oversight by health authorities in various countries.

Indian Standing: Astaxanthin supplements derived from Haematococcuspluvialis are available in the Indian market and are regulated by the Food Safety and Standards Authority of India (FSSAI). While specific research on astaxanthin in the Indian context may be limited, its popularity as a dietary supplement continues to grow, and it is widely regarded for its potential health benefits.

FSSAI Purity Criteria : Astaxanthin Content

Permitted Level :2-12 mg/day

3) BRAHMI (BACOPA MONNIERI)

Introduction: Brahmi, scientifically known as Bacopa monnieri, is a perennial herb native to wetlands and marshy areas in India, North Africa, and Southeast Asia. It is revered in traditional Ayurvedic medicine for its cognitive-enhancing and neuroprotective properties.

Synonym Name and Common Name: Synonym: Bacopa monnieri Common Name: Brahmi, Water Hyssop, Herb of Grace

Pharmacognosy / Chemistry: Brahmi is characterized by its succulent, creeping stems and small, oblong leaves that are arranged opposite each other along the stem. It produces small white flowers and thrives in moist, boggy environments. The entire plant, including the leaves and stems, is used for medicinal purposes.

Action and Pharmacology: Brahmi contains active compounds such as bacosides, alkaloids, flavonoids, and saponins, which contribute to its pharmacological effects. It is known for its adaptogenic, antioxidant, neuroprotective, and memory-enhancing properties. Brahmi acts on various neurotransmitter systems and neurotrophic factors in the brain, supporting cognitive function and memory retention.

Method of Analysis: The analysis of Brahmi typically involves the quantification of bacosides, the primary bioactive compounds in the plant. High-performance liquid chromatography (HPLC) is commonly used to measure the bacoside content in Brahmi extracts, ensuring product quality and potency.

Health Benefits:

- Improves memory and cognitive function
- Enhances learning ability and concentration
- Reduces anxiety and stress
- Protects against neurodegenerative diseases
- Supports overall brain health and longevity

Indication and Usage: Brahmi is used in traditional Ayurvedic medicine to promote mental clarity, concentration, and cognitive function. It is often consumed as a tea, extract, or supplement to support memory retention, alleviate stress, and enhance learning ability.

Usual Constituents with Percentages: The usual constituents of Brahmi include:

- Bacosides (10-20%)
- Alkaloids
- Flavonoids
- Saponins

Mechanism of Action: Brahmi exerts its cognitive-enhancing effects by modulating various neurotransmitter systems, including acetylcholine, serotonin, and dopamine. It also promotes the growth of nerve cells and enhances synaptic plasticity, leading to improved memory consolidation and learning ability.

Dosage: The recommended dosage of Brahmi supplements varies depending on the form and concentration of the product. Typical doses range from 300 mg to 600 mg of standardized extract per day, taken orally in divided doses. It is advisable to start with a lower dose and gradually increase as needed.

Contraindications:

- Hypersensitivity to Brahmi or its constituents
- Use in pregnant or lactating women without medical supervision
- Concurrent use with medications that affect the central nervous system

Precautions:

- Individuals with thyroid disorders should use caution when taking Brahmi supplements, as it may affect thyroid function.
- Brahmi may potentiate the effects of sedative medications, so it is important to consult with a healthcare professional before combining them.

Adverse Reactions: Brahmi supplements are generally well-tolerated, with few reported adverse effects. However, some individuals may experience mild gastrointestinal symptoms such as nausea or stomach upset, particularly at higher doses.

Research Summary: Research on Brahmi has demonstrated its potential as a cognitive enhancer and neuroprotective agent. Clinical studies have shown that Brahmi supplementation can improve memory retention, enhance learning ability, and reduce symptoms of anxiety and stress. Preclinical research also suggests that Brahmi may protect against age-related cognitive decline and neurodegenerative diseases such as Alzheimer's.

Pharmacokinetics: Following oral administration, the bioactive compounds in Brahmi are absorbed through the gastrointestinal tract and reach peak plasma concentrations within a few hours. Brahmi metabolites are primarily excreted through the urine, with a relatively short half-life.

Pharmacodynamics: Brahmi modulates neurotransmitter activity and neurotrophic factor expression in the brain, leading to improved cognitive function and memory retention. It also exhibits antioxidant activity, protecting neurons from oxidative damage and inflammation.

Overdosage: Excessive intake of Brahmi may lead to adverse effects such as nausea, diarrhea, or dizziness. It is important to adhere to recommended dosages and consult with a healthcare professional if concerns arise.

International Standing: Brahmi is recognized internationally for its cognitive-enhancing and neuroprotective properties. It is widely available as a dietary supplement and herbal remedy in markets worldwide, and its use is supported by scientific research and traditional knowledge.

Indian Standing: In India, Brahmi has been used for centuries in Ayurvedic medicine to support brain health and cognitive function. It is considered a valuable herb for promoting mental clarity, memory retention, and overall well-being. Brahmi supplements are widely available in India and are regulated by the Ministry of Ayurveda, Yoga & Naturopathy, Unani, Siddha, and Homeopathy (AYUSH).

FSSAI Purity Criteria : Bacosides Content

Permitted Level :300-400 mg/day

4) BETA ALANINE

Introduction: Beta-alanine is a naturally occurring non-essential amino acid that plays a crucial role in the synthesis of carnosine, a dipeptide found in skeletal muscle tissue. It is widely known for its potential ergogenic effects, particularly in enhancing athletic performance and buffering acid buildup during high-intensity exercise.

Synonym Name and Common Name: Synonym: 3-aminopropanoic acid Common Name: Beta-alanine

Pharmacognosy / Chemistry: Beta-alanine is a non-proteinogenic amino acid, meaning it is not used in the synthesis of proteins but serves other biochemical roles. It is a white crystalline powder with no distinct odor or taste, and it is water-soluble.

Action and Pharmacology: Beta-alanine acts as a precursor to carnosine synthesis in muscle tissue. Carnosine functions as an intracellular buffer, helping to regulate pH levels by neutralizing the buildup of lactic acid during exercise. This buffering action delays the onset of muscle fatigue and may improve exercise performance, particularly during high-intensity, anaerobic activities.

Method of Analysis: High-performance liquid chromatography (HPLC) is the primary method used to analyze and quantify beta-alanine levels in biological samples and dietary supplements. This technique allows for accurate measurement of beta-alanine concentrations, ensuring product quality and potency.

Health Benefits:

- Enhances exercise performance
- Delays onset of muscle fatigue
- Increases muscle endurance and power output

- Improves anaerobic capacity
- Supports muscle growth and recovery

Indication and Usage: Beta-alanine supplements are commonly used by athletes and fitness enthusiasts to improve exercise performance and increase muscle endurance. It is often taken as a standalone supplement or included in pre-workout formulations to enhance its ergogenic effects.

Usual Constituents with Percentages: Beta-alanine is typically found in dietary supplements in its pure form, with concentrations ranging from 99% to 100%.

Mechanism of Action: Beta-alanine supplementation increases muscle carnosine levels, which enhances the muscle's ability to buffer hydrogen ions (H+) produced during intense exercise. By maintaining optimal pH levels, beta-alanine helps delay the onset of muscle fatigue and allows for prolonged high-intensity exercise performance.

Dosage: The recommended dosage of beta-alanine supplementation varies, but typical doses range from 2 to 5 grams per day, divided into smaller doses taken throughout the day to minimize the risk of paresthesia, a tingling sensation often associated with beta-alanine consumption.

Contraindications:

- Hypersensitivity to beta-alanine or its metabolites
- Use in individuals with kidney or liver disorders without medical supervision

Precautions:

Beta-alanine supplementation may cause paresthesia, a harmless tingling sensation on the skin, particularly when taken in high doses. This effect is temporary and typically subsides with continued use.

Individuals with a history of hypotension (low blood pressure) should use caution when taking beta-alanine, as it may transiently lower blood pressure.

Adverse Reactions:

- Paresthesia (tingling sensation)
- Gastrointestinal discomfort (rare)

- Allergic reactions (rare)

Research Summary: Research on beta-alanine supplementation has consistently demonstrated its efficacy in improving exercise performance, particularly during high-intensity, anaerobic activities such as sprinting and weightlifting. Clinical studies have shown that beta-alanine supplementation increases muscle carnosine levels, delaying the onset of muscle fatigue and improving muscle endurance.

Pharmacokinetics: Beta-alanine is absorbed through the gastrointestinal tract and undergoes rapid distribution to muscle tissue, where it is taken up by muscle cells and converted into carnosine. Carnosine levels typically reach peak concentrations within several weeks of beta-alanine supplementation and may plateau with continued use.

Pharmacodynamics: The primary pharmacodynamic effect of beta-alanine supplementation is the increase in muscle carnosine levels, which enhances the muscle's ability to buffer hydrogen ions and maintain optimal pH levels during high-intensity exercise. This buffering action delays the onset of muscle fatigue and improves exercise performance.

Overdosage: Excessive beta-alanine supplementation may increase the risk of adverse effects such as paresthesia and gastrointestinal discomfort. It is important to adhere to recommended dosages and consult with a healthcare professional if concerns arise.

International Standing: Beta-alanine is widely recognized internationally as a safe and effective ergogenic aid for improving exercise performance. It is commonly used by athletes and fitness enthusiasts worldwide and is available as a dietary supplement in various formulations.

Indian Standing: In India, beta-alanine supplements are available in the market and are used by athletes and fitness enthusiasts to enhance exercise performance and increase muscle endurance. While specific research on beta-alanine in the Indian context may be limited, its popularity as an ergogenic aid aligns with global trends in sports nutrition and supplementation.

FSSAI Purity Criteria : NA

Permitted Level : 4 - 6 g / day, Max (not more than 4 weeks at a stretch)

5)BETAINE (N,N,N,- TRIMETHYLGLYCINE)

Introduction: Betaine, also known as trimethylglycine (TMG), is a naturally occurring compound found in various foods such as beets, spinach, and wheat bran. It serves multiple physiological functions in the body and has gained attention for its potential health benefits.

Synonym Name and Common Name: Synonym: Trimethylglycine (TMG) Common Name: Betaine

Information: Betaine is a quaternary ammonium compound derived from the amino acid glycine. It is typically obtained from plant sources or synthesized commercially. In its pure form, betaine appears as a white, odorless, crystalline powder.

Action and Pharmacology: Betaine plays a crucial role in cellular metabolism, particularly in the methionine-homocysteine cycle, where it serves as a methyl donor. It is involved in various biochemical processes, including methylation reactions, osmoregulation, and cellular hydration. Betaine supplementation has been associated with improved athletic performance, liver function, and cardiovascular health.

Method of Analysis: High-performance liquid chromatography (HPLC) is commonly used to quantify betaine levels in biological samples and food products. This analytical technique allows for accurate determination of betaine concentrations, ensuring product quality and consistency.

Health Benefits:

- Supports healthy liver function
- Enhances athletic performance and exercise capacity
- Promotes cardiovascular health by reducing homocysteine levels
- Supports methylation reactions involved in DNA and protein synthesis
- Improves cellular hydration and osmoregulation

Indication and Usage: Betaine supplements are used to support various aspects of health, including liver function, athletic performance, and cardiovascular health. It is often included in pre-workout supplements and is commonly taken orally in the form of capsules or powder.

Usual Constituents with Percentages: Betaine typically comprises 5-10% of the dry weight of plant-based foods such as beets, spinach, and wheat bran. In commercial supplements, betaine content may vary depending on the formulation and dosage.

Mechanism of Action: Betaine acts as a methyl donor in the methionine-homocysteine cycle, facilitating the conversion of homocysteine to methionine. This process helps regulate homocysteine levels in the body, which is important for cardiovascular health. Betaine also plays a role in cellular hydration and osmotic balance, which may contribute to its performance-enhancing effects.

Dosage: The recommended dosage of betaine supplements varies depending on the specific health goals and individual needs. Typical doses range from 1.5 to 3 grams per day, taken orally with water. It is advisable to follow the dosage instructions provided by the manufacturer or consult with a healthcare professional for personalized recommendations.

Contraindications:

Betaine supplementation may not be suitable for individuals with hyperhomocysteinemia or other conditions affecting methionine metabolism.

Use caution in individuals with kidney disease or impaired renal function, as betaine may affect electrolyte balance.

Precautions:

Pregnant and lactating women should consult with a healthcare professional before using betaine supplements.

Individuals with underlying health conditions should seek medical advice before starting betaine supplementation.

Adverse Reactions: Betaine supplements are generally well-tolerated when taken at recommended doses. However, high doses may cause gastrointestinal symptoms such as nausea, diarrhea, or stomach upset in some individuals.

Research Summary: Research on betaine has demonstrated its potential benefits for liver health, athletic performance, and cardiovascular function. Clinical studies have shown that betaine supplementation can reduce liver fat accumulation, improve exercise performance, and lower plasma homocysteine levels. Preclinical research also suggests that betaine may have antioxidant and anti-inflammatory properties.

Pharmacokinetics: Following oral administration, betaine is rapidly absorbed in the gastrointestinal tract and undergoes hepatic metabolism. It is then distributed to various tissues, where it participates in methylation reactions and osmoregulation. Betaine is excreted primarily through the urine.

Pharmacodynamics: Betaine acts as a methyl donor in the methionine-homocysteine cycle, contributing to the regulation of homocysteine levels and methylation reactions. It also helps maintain cellular hydration and osmotic balance, which is important for cellular function and overall health.

Overdosage: Excessive intake of betaine supplements may lead to gastrointestinal symptoms such as nausea, diarrhea, or stomach upset. It is important to adhere to recommended dosages and consult with a healthcare professional if concerns arise.

International Standing: Betaine supplements are widely available internationally and are recognized for their potential health benefits. They are commonly used as dietary supplements to support liver function, athletic performance, and cardiovascular health.

Indian Standing: In India, betaine supplements are available in the market and are regulated by the Food Safety and Standards Authority of India (FSSAI). While specific research on betaine in the Indian context may be limited, its use as a dietary supplement is supported by scientific evidence and international research.

FSSAI Purity Criteria : NA

Permitted Level : 600-650mg/day

6) BOSWELLIA SERRATA (SHALLAKI)

Introduction: Boswellia serrata, commonly known as Indian frankincense, is a tree native to India and the Arabian Peninsula. The resin extracted from Boswellia serrata, known as Boswellia gum resin, has been used for centuries in traditional Ayurvedic medicine for its anti-inflammatory and analgesic properties.

Synonym Name and Common Name: Synonym: Indian Frankincense Common Name: Boswellia, Shallaki

Pharmacognosy / Chemistry: Boswellia serrata is a deciduous tree with papery bark and pinnate leaves. The resin is obtained from the bark through tapping and contains various bioactive compounds responsible for its medicinal properties. Boswellia resin is typically yellowish-brown in color and has a distinct aromatic odor.

Action and Pharmacology: Boswellia serrata gum resin exhibits anti-inflammatory, analgesic, and antiarthritic properties. It contains bioactive compounds such as boswellic acids and pentacyclic triterpenoids, which inhibit pro-inflammatory enzymes and cytokines, thereby reducing inflammation and pain.

Method of Analysis: High-performance liquid chromatography (HPLC) is commonly used to analyze Boswellia serrata gum resin extracts for the quantification of boswellic acids and other bioactive compounds. This analytical method ensures the standardization and quality control of Boswellia products.

Health Benefits:

- Reduces inflammation and pain
- Supports joint health and mobility
- Improves symptoms of osteoarthritis and rheumatoid arthritis
- May have anticancer properties
- Supports respiratory health
- Promotes digestive health

Indication and Usage: Boswellia serrata gum resin extract is used to alleviate symptoms associated with inflammatory conditions such as arthritis, asthma, and inflammatory bowel disease. It is commonly consumed in the form of capsules, tablets, or topical preparations.

Usual Constituents with Percentages: The usual constituents of Boswellia serrata gum resin extract include:

- Boswellic acids (30-40%)
- Pentacyclic triterpenoids
- Essential oils
- Polysaccharides

Mechanism of Action: Boswellic acids inhibit the activity of 5-lipoxygenase, an enzyme involved in the production of leukotrienes, which are inflammatory mediators. By reducing leukotriene levels, Boswellia serrata gum resin extract helps mitigate inflammation and associated symptoms.

Dosage: The recommended dosage of Boswellia serrata gum resin extract varies depending on the concentration of bioactive compounds and the specific health condition being treated. Typical doses range from 300 mg to 1200 mg per day, taken orally in divided doses.

Contraindications:

- Hypersensitivity to Boswellia serrata or its constituents
- Use in pregnant or lactating women without medical supervision
- Concurrent use with anticoagulant medications due to potential interactions

Precautions:

Individuals with bleeding disorders should use caution when taking Boswellia serrata gum resin extract, as it may increase the risk of bleeding.

It is advisable to consult with a healthcare professional before starting supplementation, especially if you have underlying health conditions or are taking medications.

Adverse Reactions: Boswellia serrata gum resin extract is generally well-tolerated, with few reported adverse effects. However, some individuals may experience mild gastrointestinal symptoms such as nausea or diarrhea, particularly at higher doses.

Research Summary: Research on Boswellia serrata gum resin extract has demonstrated its efficacy in reducing inflammation and alleviating symptoms associated with various inflammatory conditions. Clinical studies have shown promising results in the management of osteoarthritis, rheumatoid arthritis, asthma, and inflammatory bowel disease.

Pharmacokinetics: Following oral administration, the bioactive compounds in Boswellia serrata gum resin extract are absorbed through the gastrointestinal tract and reach peak plasma concentrations within a few hours. Boswellic acids undergo metabolism in the liver and are excreted primarily through the urine.

Pharmacodynamics: Boswellia serrata gum resin extract exerts its anti-inflammatory effects by inhibiting the activity of pro-inflammatory enzymes and cytokines. Boswellic acids modulate the production of leukotrienes and other mediators of inflammation, leading to reduced inflammation and pain.

Overdosage: Excessive intake of Boswellia serrata gum resin extract may lead to gastrointestinal discomfort or allergic reactions in some individuals. It is essential to adhere to recommended dosages and consult with a healthcare professional if adverse reactions occur.

International Standing: Boswellia serrata gum resin extract is recognized internationally for its anti-inflammatory and analgesic properties. It is widely available as a dietary supplement and herbal remedy in markets worldwide, and its use is supported by scientific research and traditional knowledge.

Indian Standing: In India, Boswellia serrata has been used for centuries in Ayurvedic medicine to treat various inflammatory conditions. It is considered a valuable medicinal plant and is included in many Ayurvedic formulations for joint health and arthritis management. Boswellia serrata gum resin extract is regulated by the Ministry of Ayurveda, Yoga & Naturopathy, Unani, Siddha, and Homeopathy (AYUSH).

FSSAI Purity Criteria : Total boswelic acids or 11- keto-beta boswelic acids content.

Permitted Level : 250 - 1,500 mg extract/day

7) CAFFEINE

Introduction: Caffeine is a naturally occurring stimulant found in various plants, including coffee beans, tea leaves, and cacao pods. It is one of the most widely consumed psychoactive substances globally and is known for its stimulating effects on the central nervous system.

Synonym Name and Common Name: Synonym: 1,3,7-Trimethylxanthine Common Name: Caffeine

Information : Caffeine is a white, crystalline powder with a bitter taste. It is odorless and highly soluble in water. Caffeine is extracted from plant sources through various methods, including solvent extraction and supercritical fluid extraction.

Action and Pharmacology: Caffeine acts primarily as a central nervous system stimulant by blocking the action of adenosine, a neurotransmitter that promotes relaxation and sleepiness. By inhibiting adenosine receptors, caffeine increases neural activity, leading to heightened alertness, improved concentration, and reduced fatigue.

Method of Analysis: High-performance liquid chromatography (HPLC) is the most commonly used method for the analysis of caffeine content in food, beverages, and dietary supplements. This analytical technique allows for accurate quantification of caffeine levels and ensures product quality and safety.

Health Benefits:

- Increased alertness and wakefulness
- Enhanced cognitive function and concentration
- Improved physical performance and endurance
- Temporary relief of headache symptoms
- May have neuroprotective effects
- May improve mood and feelings of well-being

Indication and Usage: Caffeine is commonly consumed in the form of coffee, tea, energy drinks, and dietary supplements to increase energy levels, enhance mental alertness, and improve performance during physical or cognitive tasks.

Usual Constituents with Percentages: Pure caffeine typically comprises 1-2% of coffee beans by weight, 3-4% of tea leaves, and 0.5-3.5% of cacao beans. The caffeine content in commercial beverages and supplements can vary widely depending on factors such as brewing method and serving size.

Mechanism of Action: Caffeine blocks adenosine receptors in the brain, preventing adenosine from binding and exerting its inhibitory effects. This leads to increased neural activity and the release of neurotransmitters such as dopamine and norepinephrine, which promote alertness and arousal.

Dosage: The optimal dosage of caffeine varies depending on individual sensitivity, body weight, and tolerance level. Typical doses range from 50 mg to 200 mg per serving, although higher doses may be consumed for greater effects. It is essential to monitor caffeine intake to avoid excessive consumption.

Contraindications:

- Hypersensitivity to caffeine or its derivatives
- Use in children or adolescents without medical supervision
- Concurrent use with certain medications, particularly stimulants or monoamine oxidase inhibitors (MAOIs)

Precautions:

Individuals with anxiety disorders or cardiovascular conditions should use caution when consuming caffeine, as it may exacerbate symptoms or increase heart rate.

Pregnant and lactating women should limit caffeine intake to moderate levels, as high doses may pose risks to fetal development or infant health.

Adverse Reactions: Excessive caffeine consumption can lead to adverse effects such as jitteriness, palpitations, insomnia, gastrointestinal discomfort, and headaches. Some individuals may also experience anxiety, irritability, or tremors at high doses.

Research Summary: Research on caffeine has extensively explored its effects on cognitive performance, physical endurance, and mood regulation. Studies have shown that moderate caffeine intake can enhance alertness, concentration, and reaction time, particularly in sleep-deprived or fatigued individuals.

Pharmacokinetics: Following oral ingestion, caffeine is rapidly absorbed through the gastrointestinal tract and reaches peak plasma concentrations within 30-60 minutes. It is metabolized primarily in the liver by cytochrome P450 enzymes and has a half-life of approximately 3-5 hours in adults.

Pharmacodynamics: Caffeine exerts its pharmacological effects by antagonizing adenosine receptors, leading to increased neuronal activity and the release of excitatory neurotransmitters. These effects contribute to heightened alertness, improved cognitive function, and enhanced physical performance.

Overdosage: Consuming excessive amounts of caffeine can lead to caffeine intoxication, characterized by symptoms such as rapid heartbeat, tremors, nausea, vomiting, and agitation. Severe cases may result in convulsions, cardiac arrhythmias, or even death. It is crucial to avoid excessive caffeine intake and seek medical attention if symptoms of overdose occur.

International Standing: Caffeine is widely consumed and accepted as a safe and effective stimulant in many countries worldwide. It is regulated as a food ingredient or dietary supplement by health authorities and is commonly found in various food and beverage products.

Indian Standing: In India, caffeine is widely consumed in the form of tea, coffee, and energy drinks. It is regulated as a food additive and is subject to labeling requirements and maximum allowable limits in food products. Caffeine consumption is culturally ingrained in India, with tea being one of the most popular beverages in the country.

FSSAI Purity Criteria : Caffeine percentage

Permitted Level : 3 mg/kg b/w per day, subject to a maximum limit of 300mg per day and not more than 200mg in a single dose (only for adults and not recommended for pregnant and lactating women).

8) CAHMB

Introduction: Calcium hydroxyl methyl butyrate (CaHMB) is a compound derived from the amino acid leucine, a branched-chain amino acid (BCAA). It is a metabolite of leucine and is commonly used as a dietary supplement to support muscle health, exercise performance, and recovery.

Synonym Name and Common Name: Synonym: HMB-Ca Common Name: Calcium HMB, HMB

Information: Calcium hydroxyl methyl butyrate typically appears as a white, crystalline powder. It is odorless and soluble in water. CaHMB is often available in the form of calcium salt due to its better solubility and bioavailability.

Action and Pharmacology: CaHMB exerts its effects primarily on muscle metabolism and protein synthesis. It enhances muscle protein synthesis while simultaneously reducing muscle protein breakdown, leading to improved muscle recovery, preservation, and growth.

Method of Analysis: Analyzing CaHMB content often involves high-performance liquid chromatography (HPLC) or gas chromatography-mass spectrometry (GC-MS) techniques. These methods allow for accurate quantification of CaHMB levels in dietary supplements and food products.

Health Benefits:

- Supports muscle health and function
- Enhances exercise performance and endurance
- Accelerates muscle recovery post-exercise
- May help reduce muscle wasting associated with aging or certain medical conditions

Indication and Usage: CaHMB is commonly used by athletes, bodybuilders, and individuals engaging in resistance training to support muscle growth, improve exercise performance, and accelerate recovery. It is available as a standalone supplement or as an ingredient in sports nutrition products.

Usual Constituents with Percentages: Calcium hydroxyl methyl butyrate is typically available as a calcium salt, with the CaHMB content representing a percentage of the total weight of the compound. The usual concentration of CaHMB in supplements ranges from 5% to 20% or higher.

Mechanism of Action: CaHMB promotes muscle protein synthesis by activating the mammalian target of rapamycin (mTOR) pathway, a key regulator of protein synthesis and muscle growth. It also inhibits the activity of enzymes involved in muscle protein breakdown, such as the ubiquitin-proteasome system.

Dosage: The recommended dosage of CaHMB varies depending on individual factors such as body weight, exercise intensity, and training goals. Typical doses range from 1.5 grams to 3 grams per day, divided into multiple doses taken with meals or as directed by a healthcare professional.

Contraindications:

- Hypersensitivity to CaHMB or its components
- Use in individuals with impaired kidney function or hypercalcemia
- Concurrent use with certain medications or supplements that affect calcium metabolism

Precautions:

Individuals with existing medical conditions or those taking medications should consult a healthcare professional before using CaHMB supplements.

CaHMB supplements may interact with certain medications, so it's essential to discuss potential drug interactions with a healthcare provider.

Adverse Reactions: CaHMB supplements are generally well-tolerated, with few reported adverse effects. However, some individuals may experience mild gastrointestinal symptoms such as nausea, diarrhea, or bloating, particularly at higher doses.

Research Summary: Research on CaHMB has demonstrated its efficacy in promoting muscle growth, enhancing exercise performance, and accelerating recovery in various populations, including athletes, older adults, and patients undergoing medical treatments. Clinical studies have shown that CaHMB supplementation can increase muscle mass, strength, and endurance while reducing markers of muscle damage and fatigue.

Pharmacokinetics: Following oral administration, CaHMB is rapidly absorbed through the gastrointestinal tract and reaches peak plasma concentrations within 1-2 hours. It is metabolized primarily in the liver and excreted through the urine. CaHMB has a relatively short half-life, requiring regular dosing for optimal effects.

Pharmacodynamics: CaHMB enhances muscle protein synthesis by stimulating the mTOR pathway and increasing the expression of proteins involved in muscle growth and repair. It also reduces muscle protein breakdown by inhibiting the activity of enzymes that degrade muscle proteins, leading to net muscle protein accretion.

Overdosage: Excessive intake of CaHMB supplements may lead to elevated calcium levels in the blood, which can cause hypercalcemia and related symptoms such as nausea, vomiting, weakness, and confusion. It is essential to adhere to recommended dosages and avoid exceeding the maximum daily intake.

International Standing: CaHMB is widely recognized as a safe and effective dietary supplement for supporting muscle health and exercise performance. It is regulated by health authorities in various countries and is available over-the-counter in pharmacies, health food stores, and online retailers.

Indian Standing: In India, CaHMB supplements are available in the sports nutrition market and are regulated by the Food Safety and Standards Authority of India (FSSAI). While specific research on CaHMB in the Indian context may be limited, its use as a dietary supplement continues to gain popularity among athletes and fitness enthusiasts.

FSSAI Purity Criteria : CaHMB Content

Permitted Level :3 - 6 g / day (Not recommended for use by pregnant women and lactating mothers)

9) CHLORELLA VULGARIS DRIED POWDER

Introduction: Chlorella vulgaris is a species of freshwater green algae belonging to the genus Chlorella. It is a unicellular microorganism known for its high nutritional content and potential health benefits. Chlorella vulgaris has been extensively studied for its therapeutic properties and is commonly used as a dietary supplement.

Synonym Name and Common Name: Synonym: None Common Name: Chlorella, Green Algae

Pharmacognosy / Chemistry: Chlorella vulgaris cells are typically spherical in shape and have a diameter ranging from 2 to 10 micrometers. They contain chlorophyll, giving them a green coloration, and have a single nucleus. Under microscopic examination, they appear as small, green-colored cells.

Action and Pharmacology: Chlorella vulgaris exhibits various pharmacological actions, including antioxidant, immunomodulatory, hepatoprotective, and anti-inflammatory effects. These actions are attributed to its rich nutritional profile, which includes proteins, carbohydrates, fats, vitamins, minerals, and bioactive compounds.

Method of Analysis: Analytical methods for Chlorella vulgaris often involve spectrophotometric techniques for quantifying chlorophyll content, chromatographic techniques such as HPLC for identifying and quantifying specific bioactive compounds, and microbiological assays for assessing purity and safety.

Health Benefits:

- Supports immune function
- Detoxification aid
- Antioxidant properties
- Improves lipid profile
- Enhances gastrointestinal health

Indication and Usage: Chlorella vulgaris is indicated for use as a dietary supplement to support overall health and well-being. It is often used to boost immune function, aid in detoxification, improve digestion, and provide essential nutrients.

Usual Constituents with Percentages:

- Proteins: 50-60%
- Carbohydrates: 10-20%
- Fats: 5-20%
- Vitamins (e.g., Vitamin A, Vitamin B12): Varied percentages
- Minerals (e.g., Iron, Calcium): Varied percentages
- Chlorophyll: 1-5%

Mechanism of Action: The mechanisms of action of Chlorella vulgaris involve its various constituents acting synergistically to exert antioxidant effects, modulate immune responses, promote detoxification processes, and reduce inflammation in the body.

Dosage: The recommended dosage of Chlorella vulgaris supplements varies depending on factors such as age, health status, and the specific formulation of the supplement. Typical doses range from 1 to 5 grams per day, divided into multiple doses.

Contraindications:

- Known allergy or hypersensitivity to Chlorella vulgaris or any of its constituents
- Pregnancy and breastfeeding (due to insufficient safety data)

Precautions:

- Individuals with autoimmune disorders should use caution when taking Chlorella vulgaris due to its potential to modulate immune function.
- Patients with iodine sensitivity or thyroid disorders should consult a healthcare professional before using Chlorella supplements due to its iodine content.

Adverse Reactions: Adverse reactions to Chlorella vulgaris supplements are rare but may include gastrointestinal discomfort, allergic reactions (such as rash or itching), and exacerbation of autoimmune conditions in susceptible individuals.

Research Summary: Research on Chlorella vulgaris has demonstrated its potential health benefits in various areas, including immune support, detoxification, antioxidant activity, and cardiovascular health. However, further clinical studies are needed to confirm these effects and elucidate the optimal dosage and duration of supplementation.

Pharmacokinetics: The pharmacokinetics of Chlorella vulgaris constituents involve absorption in the gastrointestinal tract, distribution to various tissues, metabolism, and elimination from the body. Specific pharmacokinetic parameters may vary depending on the formulation and route of administration.

Pharmacodynamics: Chlorella vulgaris exerts its pharmacodynamic effects through interactions with cellular receptors and signaling pathways, leading to modulation of immune function, antioxidant activity, and other physiological responses.

Overdosage: There is limited information available regarding the effects of overdosage with Chlorella vulgaris supplements. However, exceeding recommended doses may increase the risk of adverse reactions, particularly gastrointestinal symptoms such as nausea, vomiting, and diarrhea.

International Standing: Chlorella vulgaris supplements are widely available internationally and are commonly used as dietary supplements for health promotion and disease prevention.

Indian Standing: In India, Chlorella vulgaris supplements are gaining popularity as part of the growing market for natural health products and alternative medicines.

Research Summary of Chlorella vulgaris: Research on Chlorella vulgaris continues to expand, with studies investigating its potential therapeutic applications in various health conditions. Recent research has focused on its effects on oxidative stress, inflammation, immune function, and metabolic disorders. While promising, more clinical trials are needed to validate its efficacy and safety profiles.

FSSAI Purity Criteria : NA

Permitted Level : 1 - 4 g/day

10) CHROMIUM PICOLINATE/ NICOTINATE

Introduction: Chromium picolinate and chromium nicotinate are two popular forms of the essential mineral chromium, often used as dietary supplements. These compounds are known for their potential role in supporting healthy glucose metabolism and overall wellness.

Synonym Name and Common Name: Synonyms: Chromium(III) picolinate, Chromium(III) nicotinate Common Name: Chromium picolinate, Chromium nicotinate

Pharmacognosy / Chemistry: Chromium picolinate and chromium nicotinate are chemical compounds formed by binding chromium with picolinic acid or nicotinic acid, respectively. They typically appear as odorless, crystalline powders with varying solubility in water.

Action and Pharmacology: Chromium picolinate and chromium nicotinate play a crucial role in insulin signaling and glucose metabolism. They enhance the action of insulin, facilitating the uptake of glucose into cells and promoting glycogen synthesis. Additionally, chromium supplementation may improve lipid metabolism and help maintain healthy body weight.

Method of Analysis: Analytical methods for chromium picolinate and chromium nicotinate include spectrophotometry, chromatography (such as HPLC), and atomic absorption spectroscopy. These methods are employed to quantify the concentration of chromium in supplement formulations and assess purity.

Health Benefits:

- Supports healthy glucose metabolism
- Helps regulate insulin sensitivity
- May aid in weight management
- Supports cardiovascular health
- May improve lipid profile

Indication and Usage: Chromium picolinate and chromium nicotinate are indicated for individuals seeking to support healthy blood sugar levels, especially those with insulin resistance or type 2 diabetes. They are also used as dietary supplements for weight management and overall wellness.

Usual Constituents with Percentages:

Chromium: Typically provided in supplement formulations at doses ranging from 50 to 1000 mcg per serving, representing varying percentages of the total weight of the compound.

Mechanism of Action: The mechanism of action of chromium picolinate and chromium nicotinate involves enhancing the activity of insulin receptors and promoting the translocation of glucose transporters to the cell membrane, thereby facilitating glucose uptake into cells, and promoting glycogen synthesis.

Dosage: The recommended dosage of chromium picolinate or chromium nicotinate supplements varies depending on individual needs and health status. Typical doses range from 50 to 200 mcg per day for general health support, while higher doses may be recommended for specific health conditions under medical supervision.

Contraindications:

- Known allergy or hypersensitivity to chromium or any components of the supplement
- Use caution in individuals with renal impairment, as excessive chromium intake may exacerbate kidney dysfunction.

Precautions:

- Monitor blood sugar levels closely when using chromium supplements, especially in individuals with diabetes, to prevent hypoglycemia.
- Pregnant and breastfeeding women should consult a healthcare professional before taking chromium supplements.

Adverse Reactions: Adverse reactions to chromium picolinate or chromium nicotinate supplements are rare but may include gastrointestinal discomfort, headaches, and allergic reactions in sensitive individuals.

Research Summary: Research on chromium picolinate and chromium nicotinate has yielded mixed results regarding their efficacy in improving glucose metabolism and insulin sensitivity. While some studies suggest potential benefits, others have found no significant effects. Further research is needed to elucidate the optimal dosage, duration, and population groups that may benefit most from chromium supplementation.

Pharmacokinetics: After oral ingestion, chromium picolinate and chromium nicotinate are absorbed in the gastrointestinal tract and enter systemic circulation. Chromium is then distributed to various tissues, with a portion excreted unchanged in the urine.

Pharmacodynamics: Chromium picolinate and chromium nicotinate exert their pharmacodynamic effects by enhancing insulin sensitivity, promoting glucose uptake by cells, and modulating glucose and lipid metabolism pathways.

Overdosage: Excessive intake of chromium supplements may lead to toxicity, characterized by symptoms such as gastrointestinal upset, renal impairment, and liver dysfunction. The tolerable upper intake level for chromium is set at 1000 mcg per day for adults.

International Standing: Chromium picolinate and chromium nicotinate supplements are widely available internationally and are commonly used as dietary supplements for blood sugar management and overall health support.

Indian Standing: In India, chromium picolinate and chromium nicotinate supplements are gaining popularity as part of the growing market for nutritional supplements and alternative therapies for diabetes management and metabolic health.

Research Summary of Chromium Picolinate/Nicotinate: Research on chromium picolinate and chromium nicotinate continues to investigate their potential roles in improving glucose metabolism, insulin sensitivity, and overall health. While some studies suggest benefits in certain populations, more robust clinical trials are needed to confirm their efficacy and safety profiles, particularly regarding long-term use and potential adverse effects.

FSSAI Purity Criteria : Chromium picolinate/ nicotinate content

Permitted Level : 200 - 400 mcg / day

11) CIMICIFUGA RACEMOSA

Introduction: Cimicifuga racemosa, commonly known as black cohosh or Actaea racemosa, is a perennial herb native to North America. It has a long history of traditional use among Native American tribes for various medicinal purposes. Today, it is primarily known for its potential benefits in managing menopausal symptoms and promoting women's health.

Synonym Name and Common Name: Synonym: Actaea racemosa Common Name: Black Cohosh

Pharmacognosy / Chemistry: Cimicifuga racemosa is characterized by its tall, slender stems, compound leaves, and long, spiky clusters of small white flowers. The rhizomes and roots of the plant are harvested for medicinal use and contain the bioactive compounds responsible for its therapeutic effects.

Action and Pharmacology: Black cohosh contains several bioactive compounds, including triterpene glycosides and phenolic acids, which are thought to exert estrogenic, anti-inflammatory, and neuroprotective effects. It is believed to modulate neurotransmitter activity and interact with estrogen receptors, contributing to its effects on menopausal symptoms.

Method of Analysis: Analytical methods for black cohosh extract often involve chromatographic techniques such as high-performance liquid chromatography (HPLC) for quantifying specific bioactive compounds, as well as spectroscopic methods for assessing overall composition and purity.

Health Benefits:

- Relieves menopausal symptoms such as hot flashes, night sweats, and mood swings
- Supports women's health during menstruation and menopause
- May have anti-inflammatory and neuroprotective effects

Indication and Usage: Black cohosh is indicated for women experiencing menopausal symptoms such as hot flashes, mood swings, and sleep disturbances. It is also used to support women's health during menstruation and menopause and may be recommended for other conditions such as menstrual cramps and premenstrual syndrome (PMS).

Usual Constituents with Percentages:

- Triterpene glycosides (e.g., cimicifugoside, actein): 2-5%
- Phenolic acids (e.g., ferulic acid, caffeic acid): 0.5-2%
- Other constituents including flavonoids, alkaloids, and volatile oils

Mechanism of Action: The exact mechanism of action of black cohosh is not fully understood but is thought to involve modulation of neurotransmitter activity, interaction with estrogen receptors, and anti-inflammatory effects, which collectively contribute to its efficacy in managing menopausal symptoms.

Dosage: Typical dosages of black cohosh extract range from 20 to 40 milligrams per day, standardized to contain 2.5% triterpene glycosides. It is often taken in divided doses throughout the day, and treatment duration may vary depending on individual response and symptom severity.

Contraindications:

- Known allergy or hypersensitivity to black cohosh or any of its constituents
- Pregnancy and breastfeeding (due to insufficient safety data)
- History of liver disease or liver dysfunction

Precautions:

Use caution in individuals with a history of hormone-sensitive cancers or conditions, as black cohosh may have estrogenic effects.

Monitor liver function regularly during black cohosh supplementation, especially with long-term use or high doses.

Adverse Reactions: Adverse reactions to black cohosh are generally rare but may include gastrointestinal upset, headaches, dizziness, and allergic reactions. Rare cases of liver toxicity have been reported with high doses or prolonged use.

Research Summary: Research on black cohosh has primarily focused on its efficacy in managing menopausal symptoms, with mixed results. While some studies suggest potential benefits, others have found no significant effects compared to placebo. Further research is needed to elucidate its mechanisms of action, optimal dosage, and long-term safety profile.

Pharmacokinetics: The pharmacokinetics of black cohosh constituents involve absorption in the gastrointestinal tract, distribution to various tissues, metabolism in the liver, and excretion primarily via urine. Specific pharmacokinetic parameters may vary depending on the formulation and route of administration.

Pharmacodynamics: Black cohosh exerts its pharmacodynamic effects through interactions with neurotransmitter systems, estrogen receptors, and inflammatory pathways, which collectively contribute to its observed effects on menopausal symptoms and women's health.

Overdosage: Excessive intake of black cohosh may lead to adverse effects such as gastrointestinal upset, dizziness, and liver toxicity. There is limited information on the specific effects of overdosage, but caution should be exercised to avoid exceeding recommended doses.

International Standing: Black cohosh supplements are widely available internationally and are commonly used as herbal remedies for menopausal symptoms and women's health.

Indian Standing: In India, black cohosh supplements are gaining popularity as part of the growing market for natural health products and traditional medicines for women's health concerns.

Research Summary of Cimicifuga racemosa (or Actaea racemosa): Research on black cohosh, Cimicifuga racemosa, or Actaea racemosa, has primarily focused on its potential benefits in managing menopausal symptoms and supporting women's health. While some studies suggest efficacy in reducing hot flashes and other symptoms, further research is needed to confirm its safety and long-term effects, especially regarding its potential impact on hormone-sensitive conditions and liver health.

FSSAI Purity Criteria : Total triterpene glycosides (minimum 0.4%), calculated as 23-epi-26- deoxyactein)

Permitted Level : 40 - 200 mg /day

12) CITRUS BIOFLAVONOIDS

Introduction: Citrus bioflavonoids are a group of naturally occurring compounds found in citrus fruits such as grapefruit (Citrus paradisi), mandarin (C. reticulate), pomelo (C. maxima), orange (C. sinensis), and lemon (Citrus limon). These bioactive compounds are known for their potential health benefits and are commonly used as dietary supplements.

Synonym Name and Common Name: Synonym: Citrus flavonoids Common Name: Citrus bioflavonoids

Pharmacognosy / Chemistry: Citrus bioflavonoids are a diverse group of polyphenolic compounds found in the peel, pulp, and seeds of citrus fruits. They include flavonoids such as hesperidin, naringin, quercetin, and rutin, among others, which contribute to the characteristic colors and flavors of citrus fruits.

Action and Pharmacology: Citrus bioflavonoids possess antioxidant, anti-inflammatory, and vasoprotective properties. They scavenge free radicals, inhibit inflammatory pathways, and enhance vascular function, which may contribute to their various health benefits.

Method of Analysis: Analytical methods for citrus bioflavonoids typically involve chromatographic techniques such as high-performance liquid chromatography (HPLC) for quantifying specific flavonoid compounds. Spectroscopic methods may also be used to assess overall composition and purity.

Health Benefits:

- Antioxidant protection against oxidative stress
- Anti-inflammatory effects
- Cardiovascular support
- Immune system modulation
- Skin health promotion

Indication and Usage: Citrus bioflavonoids are indicated for individuals seeking antioxidant support, cardiovascular health maintenance, immune system modulation, and overall well-being. They are commonly used as dietary supplements, particularly in formulations containing vitamin C for enhanced absorption.

Usual Constituents with Percentages:

- Hesperidin: 40-80%
- Naringin: 10-30%
- Quercetin: 5-20%
- Rutin: 3-15%

Other flavonoids, including diosmin, tangeretin, and hesperetin

Mechanism of Action: The mechanisms of action of citrus bioflavonoids involve scavenging free radicals, inhibiting inflammatory mediators such as cytokines and prostaglandins, and modulating enzyme activity and gene expression related to oxidative stress and inflammation.

Dosage: Dosage recommendations for citrus bioflavonoid supplements vary depending on the specific formulation and intended use. Typical doses range from 500 mg to 2000 mg per day, often divided into multiple doses.

Contraindications:

- Known allergy or hypersensitivity to citrus fruits or any components of citrus bioflavonoid supplements
- Use caution in individuals with citrus fruit allergies or sensitivity to related compounds.

Precautions:

- Monitor blood clotting parameters in individuals taking anticoagulant medications, as citrus bioflavonoids may have anticoagulant effects.
- Pregnant and breastfeeding women should consult a healthcare professional before taking citrus bioflavonoid supplements.

Adverse Reactions: Adverse reactions to citrus bioflavonoids are generally rare but may include gastrointestinal upset, allergic reactions (such as rash or itching), and potential interactions with medications.

Research Summary: Research on citrus bioflavonoids has demonstrated their potential health benefits in various areas, including antioxidant protection, cardiovascular health, immune modulation, and skin health. While some studies suggest efficacy, further research is needed to elucidate optimal dosages, formulations, and specific applications.

Pharmacokinetics: The pharmacokinetics of citrus bioflavonoids vary depending on the specific compound and formulation. Following oral ingestion, they are absorbed in the gastrointestinal tract, undergo metabolism in the liver, and are excreted via urine and feces.

Pharmacodynamics: Citrus bioflavonoids exert their pharmacodynamic effects through various mechanisms, including antioxidant activity, anti-inflammatory effects, modulation of enzyme activity, and interaction with cell signaling pathways.

Overdosage: Excessive intake of citrus bioflavonoid supplements may lead to gastrointestinal upset and potential interactions with medications. There is limited information on the specific effects of overdosage, but caution should be exercised to avoid exceeding recommended doses.

International Standing: Citrus bioflavonoid supplements are widely available internationally and are commonly used as dietary supplements for their potential health benefits.

Indian Standing: In India, citrus bioflavonoid supplements are gaining popularity as part of the growing market for natural health products and dietary supplements promoting overall health and well-being.

FSSAI Purity Criteria : Bioflavonoids and total polyphenol content

Permitted Level : 150 - 600 mg / day

13) COQ10 FROM NON-GMO SOURCE AND UBIQUINOL ACETATE

Introduction: Coenzyme Q10 (CoQ10) is a naturally occurring compound found in every cell of the body. It plays a vital role in cellular energy production and acts as a powerful antioxidant. Ubiquinol acetate is the reduced form of CoQ10, which has enhanced bioavailability and antioxidant activity.

Synonym Name and Common Name: Synonym: Ubiquinone Common Name: CoQ10, Ubiquinol acetate

Pharmacognosy / Chemistry: CoQ10 is a fat-soluble substance that resembles a vitamin and is found in the mitochondria of cells. It appears as a yellow to orange crystalline powder. Ubiquinol acetate is the active form of CoQ10 and is more readily absorbed by the body.

Action and Pharmacology: CoQ10 plays a crucial role in the electron transport chain, facilitating ATP production and cellular energy metabolism. Additionally, it acts as an antioxidant, protecting cells from oxidative damage. Ubiquinol acetate exhibits similar actions but with greater bioavailability due to its reduced form.

Method of Analysis: Analytical methods for CoQ10 and ubiquinol acetate typically involve chromatographic techniques such as high-performance liquid chromatography (HPLC) or gas chromatography (GC) for quantification. Spectrophotometric methods may also be used for purity assessment.

Health Benefits:

- Supports cardiovascular health
- Enhances energy production
- Provides antioxidant protection
- Supports mitochondrial function
- May have anti-aging properties

Indication and Usage: CoQ10 and ubiquinol acetate supplements are indicated for individuals seeking to support cardiovascular health, boost energy levels, and combat oxidative stress. They are commonly used as dietary supplements for various health conditions, including heart disease, hypertension, and fatigue.

Usual Constituents with Percentages:

- Coenzyme Q10 (ubiquinone): Typically found in supplement formulations at concentrations ranging from 50 to 300 milligrams per serving.
- Ubiquinol acetate: Typically found in supplement formulations at concentrations ranging from 50 to 200 milligrams per serving.

Mechanism of Action: The mechanisms of action of CoQ10 and ubiquinol acetate involve their roles in cellular energy production, antioxidant defense, and mitochondrial function. They enhance ATP synthesis, scavenge free radicals, and protect cell membranes and DNA from oxidative damage.

Dosage: Dosage recommendations for CoQ10 and ubiquinol acetate vary depending on individual needs and health conditions. Typical doses range from 50 to 300 milligrams per day for CoQ10 and 50 to 200 milligrams per day for ubiquinol acetate, taken with meals for better absorption.

Contraindications:

- Known allergy or hypersensitivity to CoQ10 or any components of the supplement
- Use caution in individuals taking anticoagulant medications, as CoQ10 may have mild blood-thinning effects.

Precautions:

- Pregnant and breastfeeding women should consult a healthcare professional before taking CoQ10 or ubiquinol acetate supplements.
- Individuals with certain medical conditions, such as kidney disease or liver dysfunction, should use caution and consult a healthcare professional before supplementing with CoQ10.

Adverse Reactions: Adverse reactions to CoQ10 and ubiquinol acetate supplements are generally rare but may include gastrointestinal upset, headaches, and allergic reactions in sensitive individuals.

Research Summary: Research on CoQ10 and ubiquinol acetate has demonstrated their potential health benefits in various areas, including cardiovascular health, energy production, antioxidant protection, and mitochondrial function. While some studies suggest efficacy, further research is needed to elucidate optimal dosages, formulations, and specific applications.

Pharmacokinetics: CoQ10 is absorbed in the small intestine and undergoes hepatic metabolism before distribution to tissues. Ubiquinol acetate, being the reduced form, has higher bioavailability and may be more readily absorbed by the body.

Pharmacodynamics: CoQ10 and ubiquinol acetate exert their pharmacodynamic effects primarily by supporting mitochondrial function and cellular energy production. They also act as antioxidants, scavenging free radicals and protecting

Overdosage: Excessive intake of CoQ10 or ubiquinol acetate supplements may lead to gastrointestinal upset but is generally well-tolerated. However, specific overdose effects have not been well-established. It is advisable to adhere to recommended dosages.

International Standing: CoQ10 and ubiquinol acetate supplements are widely available internationally and are commonly used as dietary supplements for their potential health benefits.

Indian Standing: In India, CoQ10 and ubiquinol acetate supplements are gaining popularity as part of the growing market for natural health products and dietary supplements promoting overall health and well-being.

FSSAI Purity Criteria : Ubiquinone and ubiquinol content

Permitted Level : 60 -300 mg / day

14) COLOSTRUM

Introduction: Colostrum, also known as "first milk," is the nutrient-rich fluid produced by mammals, including humans, in the first few days after giving birth. It is packed with essential nutrients, antibodies, growth factors, and immune-boosting compounds, making it a valuable source of nutrition and immune support for newborns.

Synonym Name and Common Name: Synonym: None Common Name: Colostrum, First Milk

Pharmacognosy / Chemistry: Colostrum is a thick, yellowish fluid produced by mammary glands during the initial days after childbirth. It contains high concentrations of proteins, carbohydrates, fats, vitamins, minerals, antibodies (such as IgA, IgG, IgM), growth factors (such as IGF-1 and IGF-2), and other bioactive compounds.

Action and Pharmacology: Colostrum exerts various actions, including immune modulation, antimicrobial activity, anti-inflammatory effects, and tissue repair. Its rich array of bioactive compounds supports the development and function of the newborn's immune system and promotes overall health.

Method of Analysis: Analytical methods for colostrum typically involve biochemical assays for quantifying specific components such as immunoglobulins, growth factors, and cytokines. Chromatographic techniques such as HPLC may also be used to analyze the composition of colostrum extracts.

Health Benefits:

- Boosts immune function
- Supports gastrointestinal health
- Enhances nutrient absorption
- Promotes growth and development
- Accelerates wound healing

Indication and Usage: Colostrum supplements are indicated for individuals seeking immune support, especially during times of increased susceptibility to infections or compromised immune function. They are also used to promote gastrointestinal health, enhance athletic performance, and support overall well-being.

Usual Constituents with Percentages:

- Immunoglobulins (e.g., IgA, IgG, IgM): 15-25%
- Growth factors (e.g., IGF-1, IGF-2): 1-5%
- Proteins: 60-80%
- Carbohydrates: 10-20%
- Fats: 5-15%
- Vitamins and minerals: Varied percentages

Mechanism of Action: The mechanism of action of colostrum involves its various bioactive components interacting with immune cells, promoting the production of cytokines, enhancing phagocytosis, and modulating immune responses to pathogens. Additionally, growth factors in colostrum stimulate tissue repair and regeneration processes.

Dosage: Dosage recommendations for colostrum supplements vary depending on factors such as age, health status, and specific health goals. Typical doses range from 500 milligrams to 2 grams per day, taken in divided doses.

Contraindications:

- Known allergy or hypersensitivity to dairy products or any components of colostrum supplements
- Use caution in individuals with lactose intolerance, as colostrum supplements may contain lactose.

Precautions:

- Pregnant and breastfeeding women should consult a healthcare professional before taking colostrum supplements.
- Individuals with autoimmune disorders should use caution when taking colostrum supplements, as they may stimulate immune responses.

Adverse Reactions: Adverse reactions to colostrum supplements are rare but may include gastrointestinal upset, allergic reactions (such as rash or itching), and exacerbation of autoimmune conditions in susceptible individuals.

Research Summary: Research on colostrum has shown promising results in various areas, including immune support, gastrointestinal health, athletic performance, and wound healing. Clinical studies have demonstrated its efficacy in boosting immune function, reducing the incidence of infections, and promoting overall health.

Pharmacokinetics: After oral ingestion, colostrum components are absorbed in the gastrointestinal tract and enter systemic circulation. Immunoglobulins and other bioactive compounds may exert local effects in the gastrointestinal tract before being absorbed into the bloodstream.

Pharmacodynamics: Colostrum exerts its pharmacodynamic effects through interactions with immune cells, growth factor receptors, and inflammatory pathways, leading to modulation of immune responses, tissue repair, and overall health promotion.

Overdosage: There is limited information on the effects of overdosage with colostrum supplements. However, exceeding recommended doses may increase the risk of adverse reactions such as gastrointestinal upset.

International Standing: Colostrum supplements are widely available internationally and are commonly used as dietary supplements for immune support and overall health promotion.

Indian Standing: In India, colostrum supplements are gaining popularity as part of the growing market for natural health products and dietary supplements promoting immune support and gastrointestinal health.

FSSAI Purity Criteria : NA

Permitted Level : Bovine colostrum spray dried powder at usage level of 15g per day (containing 3g of IgG) or 3g per day (containing 0.3g IgG) without any efficacy claims

15) CREATINE

Introduction: Creatine is a naturally occurring compound found in the body, primarily in muscle tissue. It plays a crucial role in energy metabolism, particularly during short-duration, high-intensity activities like weightlifting and sprinting. Creatine is also widely used as a dietary supplement to enhance athletic performance and muscle strength.

Synonym Name and Common Name: Synonym: N-methylguanidine-acetic acid Common Name: Creatine

Pharmacognosy / Chemistry: Creatine is a nitrogenous organic acid synthesized in the liver, kidneys, and pancreas from amino acids such as arginine, glycine, and methionine. It is primarily stored in skeletal muscle tissue in the form of phosphocreatine.

Action and Pharmacology: Creatine functions as a rapid source of energy during high-intensity, short-duration activities by replenishing adenosine triphosphate (ATP) stores. It also promotes muscle protein synthesis and cell volumization, leading to increased muscle mass and strength over time.

Method of Analysis: Analytical methods for creatine typically involve chromatographic techniques such as high-performance liquid chromatography (HPLC) or gas chromatography-mass spectrometry (GC-MS) for quantifying creatine levels in biological samples or supplement formulations.

Health Benefits:

- Enhances muscle strength and power
- Increases muscle mass
- Improves athletic performance, especially during short-duration, high-intensity activities
- Supports recovery and reduces muscle fatigue

Indication and Usage: Creatine supplements are indicated for athletes and individuals engaged in high-intensity, short-duration activities seeking to improve muscle strength, power, and performance. It is commonly used by bodybuilders, weightlifters, sprinters, and athletes in sports requiring explosive movements.

Usual Constituents with Percentages: Creatine monohydrate: Typically found in supplement formulations at concentrations ranging from 99% to 100%.

Mechanism of Action: The primary mechanism of action of creatine involves replenishing ATP stores in muscle cells, allowing for increased energy availability during short bursts of intense activity. Additionally, creatine may stimulate muscle protein synthesis and cell volumization, contributing to muscle growth and strength gains.

Dosage: The typical dosage for creatine supplementation involves a loading phase followed by a maintenance phase. During the loading phase, individuals typically consume 20 grams of creatine monohydrate per day (divided into 4 equal doses) for 5-7 days, followed by a maintenance phase of 3-5 grams per day.

Contraindications:

- Known allergy or hypersensitivity to creatine or any components of the supplement
- Use caution in individuals with pre-existing kidney or liver conditions, as high doses of creatine may exacerbate these conditions.

Precautions:

- Stay hydrated while taking creatine supplements to prevent dehydration and kidney strain.
- Pregnant and breastfeeding women should consult a healthcare professional before using creatine supplements.

Adverse Reactions: Adverse reactions to creatine supplements are generally rare but may include gastrointestinal upset, muscle cramping, dehydration, and electrolyte imbalances in some individuals.

Research Summary: Research on creatine supplementation has consistently shown its efficacy in enhancing muscle strength, power, and performance, especially during short-duration, high-intensity activities. Numerous clinical studies support its safety and effectiveness when used as directed.

Pharmacokinetics: After oral ingestion, creatine is absorbed in the small intestine and enters systemic circulation. It is then taken up by skeletal muscle tissue, where it is stored as phosphocreatine and utilized during periods of high-energy demand.

Pharmacodynamics: Creatine exerts its pharmacodynamic effects by increasing intramuscular phosphocreatine stores, thereby enhancing ATP regeneration, and providing additional energy for muscle contraction during intense exercise.

Overdosage: Excessive intake of creatine supplements may lead to gastrointestinal upset, dehydration, and electrolyte imbalances. It is important to adhere to recommended dosages and stay hydrated while using creatine supplements.

International Standing: Creatine supplements are widely available internationally and are commonly used by athletes and fitness enthusiasts to enhance muscle strength and performance.

Indian Standing: In India, creatine supplements are popular among athletes, bodybuilders, and fitness enthusiasts seeking to improve athletic performance and muscle strength. They are widely available in the Indian market and are used in various sports and fitness programs.

FSSAI Purity Criteria : NA

Permitted Level : 3 g / day, (for adults only)

16)CRYPTOXANTHIN / MESOXANTHIN

Introduction: Cryptoxanthin and meso-zeaxanthin are xanthophyll carotenoids belonging to the class of plant pigments known as provitamin A carotenoids. They are found in various fruits, vegetables, and plants, contributing to their vibrant colors. These compounds possess antioxidant properties and are associated with several health benefits.

Synonym Name and Common Name: Synonym: None Common Name: Cryptoxanthin, Mesoxanthin

Pharmacognosy / Chemistry: Cryptoxanthin and meso-zeaxanthin are naturally occurring carotenoids found in plants such as citrus fruits, peppers, and green leafy vegetables. They are structurally similar to beta-carotene and possess antioxidant properties.

Action and Pharmacology: Cryptoxanthin and meso-zeaxanthin act as antioxidants, scavenging free radicals and protecting cells from oxidative damage. They also have provitamin A activity, meaning they can be converted into vitamin A in the body, supporting vision health and immune function.

Method of Analysis: Analytical methods for cryptoxanthin and meso-zeaxanthintypicallyinvolvechromatographictechniquessuchashigh-performance liquid chromatography (HPLC) for quantification. Spectrophotometric methods may also be used for identification and purity assessment.

Health Benefits:

- Antioxidant protection
- Supports vision health
- Enhances immune function
- Promotes skin health
- May have anti-inflammatory effects

Indication and Usage: Cryptoxanthin and meso-zeaxanthin supplements are indicated for individuals seeking antioxidant support, vision health, and overall well-being. They are commonly used as dietary supplements, particularly by those at risk of age-related macular degeneration (AMD) or other eye conditions.

Usual Constituents with Percentages:

- Cryptoxanthin: Found in fruits such as oranges, tangerines, and papayas, typically at concentrations ranging from 0.1% to 0.5%.
- Meso-zeaxanthin: Found in green leafy vegetables such as spinach and kale, typically at concentrations ranging from 0.1% to 0.3%.

Mechanism of Action: The mechanism of action of cryptoxanthin and meso-zeaxanthin primarily involves their antioxidant activity, which helps neutralize free radicals and reduce oxidative stress in cells. Additionally, cryptoxanthin can be converted into vitamin A in the body, supporting vision health.

Dosage: Dosage recommendations for cryptoxanthin and meso-zeaxanthin supplements vary depending on the specific formulation and intended use. Typical doses range from 2 to 10 milligrams per day, often taken with meals for better absorption.

Contraindications:

- Known allergy or hypersensitivity to cryptoxanthin, meso-zeaxanthin, or any components of the supplement
- Use caution in individuals with a history of kidney stones or gallstones, as high doses of carotenoids may increase the risk of stone formation.

Precautions:

- Pregnant and breastfeeding women should consult a healthcare professional before taking cryptoxanthin or meso-zeaxanthin supplements.
- Individuals with certain medical conditions, such as liver disease or diabetes, should use caution and consult a healthcare professional before supplementing with carotenoids.

Adverse Reactions: Adverse reactions to cryptoxanthin and meso-zeaxanthin supplements are generally rare but may include gastrointestinal upset, allergic reactions (such as rash or itching), and changes in skin color (carotenoderma) with high doses.

Research Summary: Research on cryptoxanthin and meso-zeaxanthin has shown promising results in supporting vision health, particularly in reducing the risk of AMD and other eye conditions. Antioxidant properties of these carotenoids have also been associated with various other health benefits.

Pharmacokinetics: After oral ingestion, cryptoxanthin and meso-zeaxanthin are absorbed in the small intestine and enter systemic circulation. They are then distributed to various tissues, including the retina, where they exert their effects on vision health.

Pharmacodynamics: Cryptoxanthin and meso-zeaxanthin exert their pharmacodynamic effects primarily through their antioxidant activity, which helps protect cells and tissues from oxidative damage. Cryptoxanthin also contributes to vision health through its conversion into vitamin A.

Overdosage: Excessive intake of cryptoxanthin and meso-zeaxanthin supplements may lead to skin discoloration (carotenoderma) and potential interference with vitamin A metabolism. It is important to adhere to recommended dosages to avoid adverse effects.

International Standing: Cryptoxanthin and meso-zeaxanthin supplements are widely available internationally and are commonly used as dietary supplements for antioxidant support and vision health.

Indian Standing: In India, cryptoxanthin and meso-zeaxanthin supplements are gaining popularity as part of the growing market for natural health products and dietary supplements promoting overall health and well-being, including vision health.

FSSAI Purity Criteria : NA

Permitted Level : 3 mg / day

17) ECHINACEA LIQUID/POWDER EXTRACT

Introduction: Echinacea is a genus of flowering plants in the daisy family Asteraceae. Commonly referred to as coneflowers, Echinacea species are native to North America and have been used for centuries in traditional medicine for their potential health benefits, particularly in supporting immune function.

Synonym Name and Common Name: Synonym: Purple coneflower Common Name: Echinacea

Pharmacognosy / Chemistry: Echinacea plants are characterized by their distinctive purple or pink petals and prominent cone-shaped centers. The roots, leaves, and flowers of Echinacea plants contain bioactive compounds such as alkamides, caffeic acid derivatives, and polysaccharides, which are believed to contribute to their medicinal properties.

Action and Pharmacology: Echinacea is widely recognized for its immunomodulatory effects, which include stimulating immune cell activity, enhancing phagocytosis, and promoting the production of cytokines. Additionally, Echinacea exhibits anti-inflammatory, antioxidant, and antimicrobial properties.

Method of Analysis: Analytical methods for Echinacea typically involve extraction of bioactive compounds using solvents such as ethanol or water, followed by chromatographic techniques such as high-performance liquid chromatography (HPLC) for quantification. Spectrophotometric methods may also be used for identification and purity assessment.

Health Benefits:

- Boosts immune function
- Reduces the duration and severity of colds and upper respiratory infections
- Supports overall respiratory health
- Exhibits anti-inflammatory and antioxidant effects
- May aid in wound healing

Indication and Usage: Echinacea supplements are indicated for individuals seeking immune support, particularly during periods of increased susceptibility to infections such as the common cold or flu. They are commonly used as dietary supplements or herbal remedies to prevent or alleviate symptoms of respiratory infections.

Usual Constituents with Percentages:

- Alkamides: 0.5-2%
- Caffeic acid derivatives: 2-4%
- Polysaccharides: 20-40%
- Essential oils: <1%
- Flavonoids: 1-2%

Mechanism of Action: The mechanism of action of Echinacea involves its various bioactive compounds interacting with immune cells and inflammatory pathways, leading to enhanced immune responses, reduced inflammation, and improved overall immune function.

Dosage: Dosage recommendations for Echinacea supplements vary depending on the specific formulation and intended use. Typical doses range from 300 mg to 1000 mg per day, divided into multiple doses, for immune support. Liquid extracts may be taken according to product label instructions.

Contraindications:

- Known allergy or hypersensitivity to plants in the Asteraceae family, such as ragweed, marigolds, or daisies
- Use caution in individuals with autoimmune disorders, as Echinacea may stimulate immune responses

Precautions:

- Pregnant and breastfeeding women should consult a healthcare professional before taking Echinacea supplements.
- Individuals with certain medical conditions, such as HIV/AIDS or multiple sclerosis, should use caution and consult a healthcare professional before supplementing with Echinacea.

Adverse Reactions: Adverse reactions to Echinacea supplements are generally rare but may include gastrointestinal upset, allergic reactions (such as rash or itching), and potential interactions with medications.

Research Summary: Research on Echinacea has yielded mixed results, with some studies suggesting efficacy in reducing the duration and severity of colds and upper respiratory infections, while others have shown no significant benefit. More research is needed to elucidate its effectiveness and mechanisms of action.

Pharmacokinetics: After oral ingestion, bioactive compounds in Echinacea are absorbed in the gastrointestinal tract and enter systemic circulation. They are distributed to various tissues, including immune cells, where they exert their effects on immune function.

Pharmacodynamics: Echinacea exerts

FSSAI Purity Criteria : Alkamides (0.25 mg/ml) and cichoric acid (2.5 mg/ml), if the extract used is in liquid form. In case of Hydroethanolic Echinacea extract is in a powdered form computation may be done proportionately to the weight/weight dry powder extract based on liquid extract used to obtain a dry powder format.

Permitted Level : 900 mg /day

18) GANODERMA LUCIDIUM

Introduction: Ganoderma lucidum, commonly known as reishi mushroom, is a medicinal fungus with a long history of use in traditional Chinese medicine. It is revered for its potential health-promoting properties and has gained popularity worldwide as a dietary supplement and herbal remedy.

Synonym Name and Common Name: Synonym: Lingzhi mushroom Common Name: Reishi mushroom

Pharmacognosy / Chemistry: Ganoderma lucidum is characterized by its distinctive shiny, reddish-brown cap and woody texture. It grows on decaying wood, particularly in humid forests, and is harvested for its medicinal properties. The bioactive compounds responsible for its health benefits are found in various parts of the mushroom, including the fruiting body and mycelium.

Action and Pharmacology: Reishi mushroom exhibits a wide range of pharmacological activities, including immunomodulatory, anti-inflammatory, antioxidant, anticancer, and neuroprotective effects. Its bioactive compounds, such as polysaccharides, triterpenoids, and ganoderic acids, contribute to these therapeutic properties.

Method of Analysis: Analytical methods for Ganoderma lucidum typically involve extraction of bioactive compounds using solvents such as water or ethanol, followed by chromatographic techniques such as high-performance liquid chromatography (HPLC) for quantification. Spectrophotometric methods may also be used for identification and purity assessment.

Health Benefits:

- Boosts immune function
- Exhibits anti-inflammatory effects
- Provides antioxidant protection
- Supports cardiovascular health
- May have anticancer properties
- Promotes overall well-being and vitality

Indication and Usage: Reishi mushroom supplements are indicated for individuals seeking immune support, stress relief, and overall health promotion. They are commonly used as dietary supplements or herbal remedies to support immune function, manage chronic conditions, and enhance vitality.

Usual Constituents with Percentages:

- Polysaccharides: 30-60%
- Triterpenoids: 1-5%
- Ganoderic acids: 0.1-1%
- Proteins: 10-20%
- Essential amino acids: 1-5%

Mechanism of Action: The mechanism of action of Ganoderma lucidum involves its bioactive compounds interacting with various molecular targets in the body, including immune cells, inflammatory pathways, and oxidative stress response mechanisms. This results in modulation of immune function, reduction of inflammation, and protection against oxidative damage.

Dosage: Dosage recommendations for Ganoderma lucidum supplements vary depending on the specific formulation and intended use. Typical doses range from 1 to 3 grams per day of powdered mushroom extract or 100 to 500 milligrams per day of standardized extract capsules.

Contraindications:

- Known allergy or hypersensitivity to mushrooms or any components of Ganoderma lucidum supplements
- Use caution in individuals with bleeding disorders or taking anticoagulant medications, as reishi mushroom may have mild blood-thinning effects.

Precautions:

- Pregnant and breastfeeding women should consult a healthcare professional before taking Ganoderma lucidum supplements.

- Individuals with certain medical conditions, such as liver disease or autoimmune disorders, should use caution and consult a healthcare professional before supplementing with reishi mushroom.

Adverse Reactions: Adverse reactions to Ganoderma lucidum supplements are generally rare but may include gastrointestinal upset, allergic reactions (such as rash or itching), and potential interactions with medications.

Research Summary: Research on Ganoderma lucidum has demonstrated its potential health benefits in various areas, including immune support, inflammation reduction, antioxidant protection, cardiovascular health, and anticancer effects. While some studies suggest efficacy, further research is needed to elucidate optimal dosages, formulations, and specific applications.

Pharmacokinetics: After oral ingestion, bioactive compounds in Ganoderma lucidum are absorbed in the gastrointestinal tract and enter systemic circulation. They are distributed to various tissues, where they exert their effects on immune function, inflammation, and oxidative stress.

Pharmacodynamics: Ganoderma lucidum exerts its pharmacodynamic effects through interactions with immune cells, inflammatory pathways, and oxidative stress response mechanisms, leading to modulation of immune function, reduction of inflammation, and protection against oxidative damage.

Overdosage: Excessive intake of Ganoderma lucidum supplements may lead to gastrointestinal upset, allergic reactions, or potential interactions with medications. It is important to adhere to recommended dosages and consult a healthcare professional if experiencing adverse effects.

International Standing: Ganoderma lucidum supplements are widely available internationally and are commonly used as dietary supplements for immune support and overall health promotion.

Indian Standing: In India, Ganoderma lucidum supplements are gaining popularity as part of the growing market for natural health products and dietary supplements promoting immune support and overall well-being.

FSSAI Purity Criteria : NA

Permitted Level : Powder- 5-12.5 g/day Extract- 1.5-3.0 g/day

19) GINKGO BILOBA EXTRACT OBTAINED FROM DRIED LEAVES OF GINKGO

Introduction: Ginkgo biloba, often referred to as simply ginkgo, is one of the oldest living tree species and is native to China. It has a long history of use in traditional medicine, and its extract is widely consumed as a dietary supplement for its potential health benefits, particularly for cognitive function and circulatory health.

Synonym Name and Common Name: Synonym: Maidenhair tree Common Name: Ginkgo, Ginkgo biloba

Pharmacognosy / Chemistry: Ginkgo biloba extract is derived from the dried leaves of the Ginkgo biloba tree. The leaves contain various bioactive compounds, including flavonoids (such as quercetin and kaempferol) and terpene lactones (such as ginkgolides and bilobalide), which are responsible for its medicinal properties.

Action and Pharmacology: Ginkgo biloba extract exerts various pharmacological effects, including antioxidant, anti-inflammatory, neuroprotective, and vasodilatory actions. These properties contribute to its potential benefits for cognitive function, memory enhancement, and cardiovascular health.

Method of Analysis: Analytical methods for Ginkgo biloba extract typically involve extraction of bioactive compounds using solvents such as ethanol or methanol, followed by chromatographic techniques such as high-performance liquid chromatography (HPLC) for quantification. Spectrophotometric methods may also be used for identification and purity assessment.

Health Benefits:

- Improves cognitive function and memory
- Enhances cerebral blood flow
- Exhibits antioxidant and anti-inflammatory effects
- Supports cardiovascular health
- May alleviate symptoms of anxiety and depression

Indication and Usage: Ginkgo biloba extract is indicated for individuals seeking cognitive support, particularly for memory enhancement and concentration improvement. It is also used to support circulatory health, manage symptoms of age-related cognitive decline, and alleviate symptoms of anxiety and depression.

Usual Constituents with Percentages:

- Flavonoids: 22-27%
- Terpene lactones: 5-7%
- Ginkgolic acids: <5 ppm (parts per million)
- Other constituents: Varied percentages

Mechanism of Action: The mechanism of action of Ginkgo biloba extract involves its bioactive compounds exerting antioxidant effects, scavenging free radicals, and reducing oxidative stress in the brain and cardiovascular system. It also improves cerebral blood flow by enhancing vasodilation and reducing platelet aggregation.

Dosage: Dosage recommendations for Ginkgo biloba extract vary depending on the specific formulation and intended use. Typical doses range from 120 mg to 240 mg per day, taken in divided doses. It may take several weeks of regular use to experience noticeable effects on cognitive function.

Contraindications:

- Known allergy or hypersensitivity to Ginkgo biloba or any components of the extract
- Use caution in individuals with bleeding disorders or taking anticoagulant medications, as Ginkgo biloba may increase the risk of bleeding.

Precautions:

- Pregnant and breastfeeding women should consult a healthcare professional before taking Ginkgo biloba extract supplements.
- Individuals with certain medical conditions, such as epilepsy or diabetes, should use caution and consult a healthcare professional before supplementing with Ginkgo biloba.

Adverse Reactions: Adverse reactions to Ginkgo biloba extract supplements are generally rare but may include gastrointestinal upset, headaches, dizziness, and allergic reactions (such as skin rash or itching).

Research Summary: Research on Ginkgo biloba extract has shown promising results in improving cognitive function, enhancing cerebral blood flow, and supporting cardiovascular health. While some studies suggest efficacy, further research is needed to elucidate optimal dosages, formulations, and specific applications.

Pharmacokinetics: After oral ingestion, bioactive compounds in Ginkgo biloba extract are absorbed in the gastrointestinal tract and enter systemic circulation. They are distributed to various tissues, including the brain and cardiovascular system, where they exert their effects on cognitive function and circulatory health.

Pharmacodynamics: Ginkgo biloba extract exerts its pharmacodynamic effects through interactions with various molecular targets in the body, including antioxidant enzymes, neurotransmitter receptors, and vascular endothelial cells. This results in improved cognitive function, enhanced cerebral blood flow, and cardiovascular protection.

Overdosage: Excessive intake of Ginkgo biloba extract supplements may lead to gastrointestinal upset, headaches, dizziness, or potential interactions with medications. It is important to adhere to recommended dosages and consult a healthcare professional if experiencing adverse effects.

International Standing: Ginkgo biloba extract supplements are widely available internationally and are commonly used as dietary supplements for cognitive support and circulatory health.

Indian Standing: In India, Ginkgo biloba extract supplements are gaining popularity as part of the growing market for natural health products and dietary supplements promoting cognitive function and overall well-being. They are widely available in the Indian market and are used in various health and wellness applications.

FSSAI Purity Criteria : Ginkgo flavone glycosides and Ginkgolides (diterpene lactones). Total flavonoids content (20.2 to 27% calculated as flavanol glycosides and tested for total terpene lactones (5.4% to 12.0%). Presence of Ginkgolides A, B, C needs to be tested qualitatively.

Permitted Level : 120-240 mg/ day

20) GLUCOSAMINE HYDROCHLORIDE

Introduction: Glucosamine hydrochloride is a dietary supplement commonly used to support joint health and alleviate symptoms of osteoarthritis. It is a natural compound found in the human body, particularly in cartilage, and is also sourced from shellfish shells or produced synthetically for supplementation purposes.

Synonym Name and Common Name: Synonym: Glucosamine HCl Common Name: Glucosamine hydrochloride

Pharmacognosy / Chemistry: Glucosamine hydrochloride is a crystalline powder that is typically produced by hydrolyzing chitin, a component of shellfish shells, into glucosamine and then further purifying it to obtain glucosamine hydrochloride. It is water-soluble and stable under normal conditions.

Action and Pharmacology: Glucosamine hydrochloride is believed to support joint health by providing building blocks for the synthesis of cartilage components such as glycosaminoglycans and proteoglycans. It may also have anti-inflammatory properties, although the mechanisms are not fully understood.

Method of Analysis: Analytical methods for glucosamine hydrochloride typically involve chromatographic techniques such as high-performance liquid chromatography (HPLC) for quantification. Spectrophotometric methods may also be used for identification and purity assessment.

Health Benefits:

- Supports joint health
- Alleviates symptoms of osteoarthritis
- May help reduce inflammation in joints
- Supports cartilage repair and maintenance

Indication and Usage: Glucosamine hydrochloride is indicated for individuals seeking joint support, particularly those experiencing symptoms of osteoarthritis such as joint pain, stiffness, and reduced mobility. It is commonly used as a dietary supplement to promote joint health and alleviate osteoarthritic symptoms.

Usual Constituents with Percentages: Glucosamine hydrochloride typically consists of 99% or higher purity of the active ingredient glucosamine.

Mechanism of Action: Glucosamine hydrochloride provides the necessary substrate for the synthesis of glycosaminoglycans and proteoglycans, which are essential components of cartilage. By supporting cartilage repair and maintenance, it helps alleviate symptoms of osteoarthritis and promotes joint health.

Dosage: Dosage recommendations for glucosamine hydrochloride typically range from 1500 mg to 2000 mg per day, divided into multiple doses. It may take several weeks of regular use to experience noticeable effects on joint health.

Contraindications:

- Known allergy or hypersensitivity to glucosamine or shellfish
- Use caution in individuals with diabetes, as glucosamine may affect blood sugar levels

Precautions:

- Pregnant and breastfeeding women should consult a healthcare professional before taking glucosamine hydrochloride supplements.
- Individuals with certain medical conditions, such as asthma or high blood pressure, should use caution and consult a healthcare professional before supplementing with glucosamine.

Adverse Reactions: Adverse reactions to glucosamine hydrochloride supplements are generally rare but may include gastrointestinal upset, nausea, diarrhea, and allergic reactions (such as rash or itching).

Research Summary: Research on glucosamine hydrochloride has shown mixed results in terms of its efficacy in alleviating symptoms of osteoarthritis and promoting joint health. While some studies suggest potential benefits, others have found little to no significant effect. Further research is needed to elucidate its mechanisms of action and therapeutic potential.

Pharmacokinetics: After oral ingestion, glucosamine hydrochloride is absorbed in the gastrointestinal tract and enters systemic circulation. It is distributed to various tissues, including joints, where it exerts its effects on cartilage repair and maintenance.

Pharmacodynamics: Glucosamine hydrochloride exerts its pharmacodynamic effects primarily by providing the necessary substrate for the synthesis of cartilage components, supporting cartilage repair and maintenance and alleviating symptoms of osteoarthritis.

Overdosage: Excessive intake of glucosamine hydrochloride supplements may lead to gastrointestinal upset, nausea, or diarrhea. It is important to adhere to recommended dosages and consult a healthcare professional if experiencing adverse effects.

International Standing: Glucosamine hydrochloride supplements are widely available internationally and are commonly used as dietary supplements for joint health and osteoarthritis management.

Indian Standing: In India, glucosamine hydrochloride supplements are gaining popularity as part of the growing market for natural health products and dietary supplements promoting joint health and osteoarthritis management. They are widely available in the Indian market and are used in various health and wellness applications.

FSSAI Purity Criteria : Glucosamine content

Permitted Level : 1,500-3,000 mg/day

21) GLUCOSAMINE SULPHATE

Introduction: Glucosamine sulfate is a naturally occurring compound found in the human body and is commonly used as a dietary supplement to support joint health and alleviate symptoms of osteoarthritis. It is believed to play a crucial role in the synthesis of cartilage and other connective tissues.

Synonym Name and Common Name: Synonym: Glucosamine sulphate Common Name: Glucosamine sulfate

Pharmacognosy / Chemistry: Glucosamine sulfate is typically derived from shellfish shells or produced synthetically. It is a crystalline powder that is water-soluble and stable under normal conditions. It is commonly used in dietary supplements for joint health.

Action and Pharmacology: Glucosamine sulfate is believed to support joint health by providing building blocks for the synthesis of cartilage components such as glycosaminoglycans and proteoglycans. It may also have anti-inflammatory properties, although the mechanisms are not fully understood.

Method of Analysis: Analytical methods for glucosamine sulfate typically involve chromatographic techniques such as high-performance liquid chromatography (HPLC) for quantification. Spectrophotometric methods may also be used for identification and purity assessment.

Health Benefits:

- Supports joint health
- Alleviates symptoms of osteoarthritis
- May help reduce inflammation in joints
- Supports cartilage repair and maintenance

Indication and Usage: Glucosamine sulfate is indicated for individuals seeking joint support, particularly those experiencing symptoms of osteoarthritis such as joint pain, stiffness, and reduced mobility. It is commonly used as a dietary supplement to promote joint health and alleviate osteoarthritic symptoms.

Usual Constituents with Percentages: Glucosamine sulfate typically consists of 99% or higher purity of the active ingredient glucosamine.

Mechanism of Action: Glucosamine sulfate provides the necessary substrate for the synthesis of glycosaminoglycans and proteoglycans, which are essential components of cartilage. By supporting cartilage repair and maintenance, it helps alleviate symptoms of osteoarthritis and promotes joint health.

Dosage: Dosage recommendations for glucosamine sulfate typically range from 1500 mg to 2000 mg per day, divided into multiple doses. It may take several weeks of regular use to experience noticeable effects on joint health.

Contraindications:

- Known allergy or hypersensitivity to glucosamine or shellfish
- Use caution in individuals with diabetes, as glucosamine may affect blood sugar levels

Precautions:

- Pregnant and breastfeeding women should consult a healthcare professional before taking glucosamine sulfate supplements.
- Individuals with certain medical conditions, such as asthma or high blood pressure, should use caution and consult a healthcare professional before supplementing with glucosamine.

Adverse Reactions: Adverse reactions to glucosamine sulfate supplements are generally rare but may include gastrointestinal upset, nausea, diarrhea, and allergic reactions (such as rash or itching).

Research Summary: Research on glucosamine sulfate has shown mixed results in terms of its efficacy in alleviating symptoms of osteoarthritis and promoting joint health. While some studies suggest potential benefits, others have found little to no significant effect. Further research is needed to elucidate its mechanisms of action and therapeutic potential.

Pharmacokinetics: After oral ingestion, glucosamine sulfate is absorbed in the gastrointestinal tract and enters systemic circulation. It is distributed to various tissues, including joints, where it exerts its effects on cartilage repair and maintenance.

Pharmacodynamics: Glucosamine sulfate exerts its pharmacodynamic effects primarily by providing the necessary substrate for the synthesis of cartilage components, supporting cartilage repair and maintenance, and alleviating symptoms of osteoarthritis.

Overdosage: Excessive intake of glucosamine sulfate supplements may lead to gastrointestinal upset, nausea, or diarrhea. It is important to adhere to recommended dosages and consult a healthcare professional if experiencing adverse effects.

International Standing: Glucosamine sulfate supplements are widely available internationally and are commonly used as dietary supplements for joint health and osteoarthritis management.

Indian Standing: In India, glucosamine sulfate supplements are gaining popularity as part of the growing market for natural health products and dietary supplements promoting joint health and osteoarthritis management. They are widely available in the Indian market and are used in various health and wellness applications.

FSSAI Purity Criteria : Glucosamine content

Permitted Level : 1,500-3,000 mg/day

22)GLUTATHIONE / S-ACETYL GLUTATHIONE

Introduction: Glutathione, often referred to as the "master antioxidant," is a tripeptide molecule composed of three amino acids: glutamate, cysteine, and glycine. It plays a crucial role in various physiological processes and is involved in antioxidant defense, detoxification, and immune function.

Synonym Name and Common Name: Synonym: GSH (Glutathione) Common Name: Glutathione

Pharmacognosy / Chemistry: Glutathione is synthesized endogenously in the body and is also obtained from dietary sources. It exists in two forms: reduced glutathione (GSH) and oxidized glutathione (GSSG). Glutathione supplements are available in various forms, including capsules, tablets, and injections.

Action and Pharmacology: Glutathione acts primarily as an antioxidant, protecting cells from oxidative damage caused by reactive oxygen species (ROS) and free radicals. It also plays a role in detoxification processes by binding to and neutralizing toxins and harmful compounds.

Method of Analysis: Analytical methods for glutathione typically involve chromatographic techniques such as high-performance liquid chromatography (HPLC) or spectrophotometric methods for quantification. These methods are used to assess glutathione levels in biological samples or to determine the content of glutathione in supplements.

Health Benefits:

- Antioxidant protection
- Detoxification support
- Immune system support
- Skin lightening and anti-aging effects (in topical formulations)

Indication and Usage: Glutathione supplements are indicated for individuals seeking antioxidant support, detoxification support, and immune system support. They are also used for skin lightening and anti-aging effects, particularly in topical formulations.

Usual Constituents with Percentages: Glutathione supplements typically contain 500 mg to 1000 mg of glutathione per dose, although concentrations may vary depending on the formulation.

Mechanism of Action: Glutathione exerts its antioxidant effects by donating electrons to neutralize reactive oxygen species (ROS) and free radicals, thereby protecting cells from oxidative damage. It also plays a role in detoxification processes by conjugating with toxins and facilitating their excretion from the body.

Dosage: Dosage recommendations for glutathione supplements vary depending on the specific formulation and intended use. Typical doses range from 500 mg to 1000 mg per day, although higher doses may be used for certain therapeutic purposes.

Contraindications:

- There are no known contraindications to glutathione supplementation in healthy individuals.
- Use caution in individuals with a history of sulfur sensitivity or allergies to glutathione or its precursors.

Precautions:

- Pregnant and breastfeeding women should consult a healthcare professional before taking glutathione supplements.
- Individuals with certain medical conditions, such as liver disease or cancer, should use caution and consult a healthcare professional before supplementing with glutathione.

Adverse Reactions: Adverse reactions to glutathione supplements are rare but may include gastrointestinal upset, allergic reactions (such as rash or itching), and exacerbation of asthma symptoms in susceptible individuals.

Research Summary: Research on glutathione has demonstrated its potential benefits in various areas, including antioxidant protection, detoxification support, immune system modulation, and skin lightening effects. While some studies suggest efficacy, further research is needed to elucidate optimal dosages, formulations, and specific applications.

Pharmacokinetics: Glutathione is absorbed in the gastrointestinal tract and enters systemic circulation, where it is distributed to various tissues. It undergoes metabolism in the liver and is excreted primarily in the urine.

Pharmacodynamics: Glutathione exerts its pharmacodynamic effects primarily through its antioxidant and detoxification properties, protecting cells from oxidative damage and facilitating the elimination of toxins from the body.

Overdosage: Excessive intake of glutathione supplements may lead to gastrointestinal upset or allergic reactions. It is important to adhere to recommended dosages and consult a healthcare professional if experiencing adverse effects.

International Standing: Glutathione supplements are widely available internationally and are commonly used for antioxidant support, detoxification support, and immune system support.

Indian Standing: In India, glutathione supplements are gaining popularity as part of the growing market for natural health products and dietary supplements promoting antioxidant protection, detoxification support, and immune system support. They are widely available in the Indian market and are used in various health and wellness applications.

FSSAI Purity Criteria : NA

Permitted Level : 50 - 600 mg / day

23) GYMNEMA SYLVESTRE EXTRACT POWDER

Introduction: Gymnemasylvestre is a woody climbing shrub native to the tropical forests of India, Africa, and Australia. It has been used for centuries in traditional Ayurvedic medicine for its potential health benefits, particularly in managing blood sugar levels and supporting weight management.

Synonym Name and Common Name: Synonym: Gurmar Common Name: Gymnema, Gymnemasylvestre

Pharmacognosy / Chemistry: Gymnemasylvestre extract is typically derived from the leaves of the Gymnemasylvestre plant. It is available in various forms, including powders, capsules, and teas. The extract contains bioactive compounds such as gymnemic acids, flavonoids, and alkaloids, which are responsible for its medicinal properties.

Action and Pharmacology: Gymnemasylvestre exerts various pharmacological effects, including anti-diabetic, anti-obesity, anti-inflammatory, and anti-hyperlipidemic actions. It is believed to work by enhancing insulin secretion, improving insulin sensitivity, and reducing sugar absorption in the intestine.

Method of Analysis: Analytical methods for Gymnemasylvestre extract typically involve chromatographic techniques such as high-performance liquid chromatography (HPLC) for quantification of bioactive compounds. Spectrophotometric methods may also be used for identification and purity assessment.

Health Benefits:

- Supports healthy blood sugar levels
- Aids in weight management
- Supports digestion
- Anti-inflammatory properties
- Antioxidant effects

Indication and Usage: Gymnemasylvestre extract is indicated for individuals seeking support for healthy blood sugar levels, particularly those with diabetes or at risk of developing diabetes. It is also used for weight management and digestive support.

Usual Constituents with Percentages:

- Gymnemic acids: 25-30%
- Flavonoids: 2-4%
- Alkaloids: <1%
- Other constituents: Varied percentages

Mechanism of Action: The bioactive compounds in Gymnemasylvestre extract, particularly gymnemic acids, are believed to block sugar receptors in the intestine, reducing sugar absorption and thereby lowering blood sugar levels. It also enhances insulin secretion and improves insulin sensitivity, further supporting glucose metabolism.

Dosage: Dosage recommendations for Gymnemasylvestre extract vary depending on the specific formulation and intended use. Typical doses range from 200 mg to 500 mg per day, taken in divided doses with meals.

Contraindications:

- Known allergy or hypersensitivity to Gymnemasylvestre or any components of the extract
- Use caution in individuals taking medications for diabetes or blood sugar control, as Gymnemasylvestre may potentiate the effects of these medications.

Precautions:

- Pregnant and breastfeeding women should consult a healthcare professional before taking Gymnemasylvestre extract supplements.
- Individuals with certain medical conditions, such as hypoglycemia or kidney disease, should use caution and consult a healthcare professional before supplementing with Gymnemasylvestre.

Adverse Reactions: Adverse reactions to Gymnemasylvestre extract supplements are generally rare but may include gastrointestinal upset, such as nausea, diarrhea, or abdominal discomfort, particularly at higher doses.

Research Summary: Research on Gymnemasylvestre extract has shown promising results in supporting healthy blood sugar levels and aiding in weight management. Several clinical studies have demonstrated its efficacy in reducing fasting blood sugar levels, improving insulin sensitivity, and supporting weight loss efforts.

Pharmacokinetics: After oral ingestion, bioactive compounds in Gymnemasylvestre extract are absorbed in the gastrointestinal tract and enter systemic circulation. They are distributed to various tissues, including the pancreas and liver, where they exert their effects on glucose metabolism.

Pharmacodynamics: Gymnemasylvestre extract exerts its pharmacodynamic effects through interactions with various molecular targets involved in glucose metabolism, including sugar receptors in the intestine, insulin-secreting cells in the pancreas, and insulin-sensitive tissues such as muscle and adipose tissue.

Overdosage: Excessive intake of Gymnemasylvestre extract supplements may lead to gastrointestinal upset or hypoglycemia in susceptible individuals. It is important to adhere to recommended dosages and monitor blood sugar levels regularly, especially in diabetic patients.

International Standing: Gymnemasylvestre extract supplements are gaining popularity internationally for their potential health benefits in managing blood sugar levels and supporting weight management.

Indian Standing: In India, Gymnemasylvestre has been used in traditional Ayurvedic medicine for centuries for its medicinal properties, particularly in managing diabetes. Gymnemasylvestre extract supplements are widely available in the Indian market and are commonly used for blood sugar management and weight management.

FSSAI Purity Criteria : Gymnemic acid content

Permitted Level : 500-1,500 mg / day

24) SOFLAVONES (GENISTEIN, DAIDZEIN)

Introduction: Isoflavones are naturally occurring phytoestrogens found predominantly in soybeans and soy products. They are classified as flavonoids and are known for their potential health benefits, particularly in supporting hormonal balance and reducing the risk of certain chronic diseases.

Synonym Name and Common Name: Synonym: Phytoestrogens Common Name: Isoflavones

Pharmacognosy / Chemistry: Isoflavones are secondary metabolites found in various plants, with soybeans being the richest dietary source. They are structurally similar to human estrogen and can bind to estrogen receptors, exerting estrogenic or anti-estrogenic effects depending on hormonal balance.

Action and Pharmacology: Isoflavones exert their pharmacological effects primarily through interactions with estrogen receptors, modulating estrogenic activity in the body. They can act as agonists or antagonists, depending on the tissue type and hormonal milieu, affecting various physiological processes.

Method of Analysis: Analytical methods for isoflavones typically involve chromatographic techniques such as high-performance liquid chromatography (HPLC) for quantification. Mass spectrometry may also be used for identification and purity assessment.

Health Benefits:

- Hormonal balance support
- Cardiovascular health promotion
- Bone health maintenance
- Antioxidant and anti-inflammatory effects
- Potential cancer prevention

Indication and Usage: Isoflavones are indicated for individuals seeking support for hormonal balance, particularly women experiencing menopausal symptoms. They are also used for cardiovascular health, bone health, and overall well-being.

Usual Constituents with Percentages:

- Genistein: 50-60%
- Daidzein: 40-50%
- Other minor isoflavones: <5%

Mechanism of Action: Isoflavones exert their effects by binding to estrogen receptors in the body, mimicking or modulating the activity of endogenous estrogen. They can act as estrogen agonists or antagonists, depending on the tissue type and hormonal context, affecting gene expression and cellular signaling pathways.

Dosage: Dosage recommendations for isoflavones vary depending on the specific formulation and intended use. Typical doses range from 40 mg to 100 mg per day, taken orally with meals.

Contraindications:

- Known allergy or hypersensitivity to soy or soy products
- Use caution in individuals with hormone-sensitive conditions, such as breast cancer, endometriosis, or uterine fibroids, as isoflavones may affect hormone levels.

Precautions:

- Pregnant and breastfeeding women should consult a healthcare professional before taking isoflavone supplements.
- Individuals with thyroid disorders should use caution and monitor thyroid function when supplementing with isoflavones, as they may affect thyroid hormone levels.

Adverse Reactions: Adverse reactions to isoflavone supplements are generally rare but may include gastrointestinal upset, allergic reactions (such as rash or itching), and hormonal disturbances in susceptible individuals.

Research Summary: Research on isoflavones, particularly genistein and daidzein, has shown promising results in supporting hormonal balance, cardiovascular health, bone health, and antioxidant activity. Some studies suggest potential benefits in reducing the risk of certain cancers, although results are mixed.

Pharmacokinetics: After oral ingestion, isoflavones are absorbed in the gastrointestinal tract and enter systemic circulation. They are metabolized in the liver and are excreted primarily in the urine.

Pharmacodynamics: Isoflavones exert their pharmacodynamic effects primarily through interactions with estrogen receptors, modulating estrogenic activity in various tissues and affecting gene expression and cellular signaling pathways.

Overdosage: Excessive intake of isoflavone supplements may lead to gastrointestinal upset or hormonal disturbances. It is important to adhere to recommended dosages and consult a healthcare professional if experiencing adverse effects.

International Standing: Isoflavone supplements are widely available internationally and are commonly used for hormonal balance support, particularly in women experiencing menopausal symptoms.

Indian Standing: In India, isoflavone supplements are gaining popularity as part of the growing market for natural health products and dietary supplements promoting hormonal balance and overall well-being. They are widely available in the Indian market and are used in various health and wellness applications.

FSSAI Purity Criteria : NA

Permitted Level : Genistein-25-50 mg/day Daidzein-40-80 mg/day (Consult a health care professional for long term use)

25) LACTASE

Introduction: Lactase is an enzyme produced by the small intestine, responsible for breaking down lactose, a sugar found in milk and dairy products, into its constituent sugars, glucose, and galactose. Lactase plays a crucial role in the digestion of lactose-containing foods.

Synonym Name and Common Name: Synonym: Beta-galactosidase, lactase-phlorizin hydrolase Common Name: Lactase

Pharmacognosy / Chemistry: Lactase is a protein enzyme produced by the brush border cells of the small intestine. It is also available as a dietary supplement derived from microbial or fungal sources, commonly used to aid in the digestion of lactose in individuals with lactose intolerance.

Action and Pharmacology: Lactase catalyzes the hydrolysis of lactose into its constituent sugars, glucose, and galactose. This enzymatic activity allows individuals with lactose intolerance to digest lactose-containing foods more effectively, reducing gastrointestinal discomfort.

Method of Analysis: Analytical methods for lactase typically involve enzymatic assays to measure its activity in samples. Spectrophotometric methods may also be used to quantify enzyme concentration based on its optical properties.

Health Benefits:

- Facilitates digestion of lactose-containing foods
- Reduces symptoms of lactose intolerance, such as bloating, gas, and diarrhea

- Allows individuals with lactose intolerance to consume dairy products without discomfort

Indication and Usage: Lactase supplements are indicated for individuals with lactose intolerance who experience gastrointestinal discomfort after consuming lactose-containing foods. They are commonly used as a dietary aid to improve lactose digestion and allow for the consumption of dairy products.

Usual Constituents with Percentages: Lactase supplements typically contain purified lactase enzyme, with activity measured in units (e.g., FCC units or ALU). The percentage composition of lactase enzyme varies depending on the specific formulation and source.

Mechanism of Action: Lactase exerts its effects by catalyzing the hydrolysis of the β-galactosidic linkage in lactose molecules, breaking them down into glucose and galactose. This enzymatic reaction enables individuals with lactose intolerance to digest lactose-containing foods more effectively.

Dosage: Dosage recommendations for lactase supplements vary depending on the individual's level of lactose intolerance and the lactose content of the foods consumed. Typically, one to three lactase enzyme capsules or tablets are taken with lactose-containing meals or snacks.

Contraindications:

- There are no known contraindications to lactase supplementation.
- Use caution in individuals with known allergies or sensitivities to dairy or dairy-derived products.

Precautions:

- Individuals with severe lactose intolerance should consult a healthcare professional before starting lactase supplementation.
- Use caution when consuming lactose-containing foods in large quantities, even when supplemented with lactase, as excessive lactose intake may still cause gastrointestinal discomfort.

Adverse Reactions: Adverse reactions to lactase supplements are rare but may include gastrointestinal upset, such as bloating, gas, or diarrhea, particularly if the recommended dosage is exceeded.

Research Summary: Research on lactase primarily focuses on its efficacy in improving lactose digestion and reducing symptoms of lactose intolerance. Numerous clinical studies have demonstrated its effectiveness in facilitating lactose digestion and alleviating gastrointestinal discomfort in individuals with lactose intolerance.

Pharmacokinetics: After oral ingestion, lactase enzyme is released in the gastrointestinal tract, where it catalyzes the hydrolysis of lactose molecules. The resulting glucose and galactose are absorbed into the bloodstream for energy metabolism.

Pharmacodynamics: Lactase exerts its pharmacodynamic effects by catalyzing the hydrolysis of lactose molecules into their constituent monosaccharides, glucose, and galactose, facilitating their absorption and utilization by the body.

Overdosage: Excessive intake of lactase supplements is unlikely to cause serious adverse effects due to its natural presence in the digestive system. However, exceeding the recommended dosage may lead to gastrointestinal discomfort, such as bloating or diarrhea.

International Standing: Lactase supplements are widely available internationally and are commonly used by individuals with lactose intolerance to improve lactose digestion and reduce gastrointestinal discomfort.

Indian Standing: In India, lactase supplements are gaining popularity as part of the growing market for digestive health products and lactose intolerance management. They are widely available in pharmacies and health food stores and are used by individuals seeking relief from lactose intolerance symptoms.

FSSAI Purity Criteria : Enzyme activity

Permitted Level : 3,000 - 9,000 IU (or FCC units) / day

26) L-CARNOSINE

Introduction: L-Carnosine is a dipeptide molecule composed of the amino acids beta-alanine and histidine. It is naturally found in high concentrations in skeletal muscle tissue and has been studied for its potential health benefits, particularly in antioxidant support and anti-aging effects.

Synonym Name and Common Name: Synonym: β-Alanyl-L-histidine Common Name: Carnosine

Pharmacognosy / Chemistry: L-Carnosine is synthesized endogenously in the body and is also obtained from dietary sources, primarily meat and fish. It is available as a dietary supplement in various forms, including capsules and powders.

Action and Pharmacology: L-Carnosine exerts various pharmacological effects, including antioxidant, anti-glycation, and metal-chelating properties. It is involved in buffering intracellular pH and may also have neuroprotective and anti-inflammatory effects.

Method of Analysis: Analytical methods for L-Carnosine typically involve chromatographic techniques such as high-performance liquid chromatography (HPLC) for quantification. Mass spectrometry may also be used for identification and purity assessment.

Health Benefits:

- Antioxidant support
- Anti-aging effects
- Neuroprotective properties
- Anti-inflammatory effects
- Supports muscle function

Indication and Usage: L-Carnosine supplements are indicated for individuals seeking antioxidant support, anti-aging effects, and support for muscle function. It is also used for its potential neuroprotective and anti-inflammatory properties.

Usual Constituents with Percentages: L-Carnosine supplements typically contain 500 mg to 1000 mg of L-Carnosine per dose, although concentrations may vary depending on the formulation.

Mechanism of Action: L-Carnosine exerts its antioxidant effects by scavenging free radicals and reactive oxygen species (ROS), thereby protecting cells from oxidative damage. It also inhibits the formation of advanced glycation end-products (AGEs) and chelates metal ions, further reducing oxidative stress.

Dosage: Dosage recommendations for L-Carnosine supplements vary depending on the specific formulation and intended use. Typical doses range from 500 mg to 2000 mg per day, taken orally with meals.

Contraindications:

- There are no known contraindications to L-Carnosine supplementation.
- Use caution in individuals with a history of allergies or sensitivities to L-Carnosine or its precursors.

Precautions:

Pregnant and breastfeeding women should consult a healthcare professional before taking L-Carnosine supplements.

Individuals with certain medical conditions, such as kidney disease or hypertension, should use caution and consult a healthcare professional before supplementing with L-Carnosine.

Adverse Reactions: Adverse reactions to L-Carnosine supplements are rare but may include gastrointestinal upset, such as nausea or diarrhea, particularly at higher doses.

Research Summary: Research on L-Carnosine has demonstrated its potential benefits in various areas, including antioxidant support, anti-aging effects, neuroprotection, and anti-inflammatory properties. While some studies suggest efficacy, further research is needed to elucidate optimal dosages, formulations, and specific applications.

Pharmacokinetics: After oral ingestion, L-Carnosine is absorbed in the gastrointestinal tract and enters systemic circulation, where it is distributed to various tissues, including skeletal muscle and the central nervous system. It undergoes metabolism in the liver and is excreted primarily in the urine.

Pharmacodynamics: L-Carnosine exerts its pharmacodynamic effects primarily through its antioxidant and anti-glycation properties, protecting cells from oxidative damage and inhibiting the formation of AGEs. It may also have neuroprotective and anti-inflammatory effects, supporting overall health and well-being.

Overdosage: Excessive intake of L-Carnosine supplements may lead to gastrointestinal upset or other adverse effects. It is important to adhere to recommended dosages and consult a healthcare professional if experiencing adverse reactions.

International Standing: L-Carnosine supplements are widely available internationally and are commonly used for antioxidant support, anti-aging effects, and general health maintenance.

Indian Standing: In India, L-Carnosine supplements are gaining popularity as part of the growing market for natural health products and dietary supplements promoting antioxidant support and anti-aging effects. They are widely available in the Indian market and are used in various health and wellness applications.

FSSAI Purity Criteria : NA

Permitted Level : 130 - 600 mg / day

27) L- THEANINE

Introduction: L-Theanine is a naturally occurring amino acid found primarily in tea leaves, particularly green tea (Camellia sinensis). It is known for its calming and relaxing effects, often used to reduce stress and promote mental clarity.

Synonym Name and Common Name: Synonym: γ-glutamylethylamide Common Name: Theanine

Pharmacognosy / Chemistry: L-Theanine is a non-protein amino acid that is structurally similar to glutamate, a neurotransmitter in the brain. It is extracted from tea leaves and is also available as a dietary supplement.

Action and Pharmacology: L-Theanine exerts various pharmacological effects, including relaxation, stress reduction, and cognitive enhancement. It crosses the blood-brain barrier and modulates neurotransmitter levels, particularly gamma-aminobutyric acid (GABA) and glutamate, resulting in a calming effect on the central nervous system.

Method of Analysis: Analytical methods for L-Theanine typically involve chromatographic techniques such as high-performance liquid chromatography (HPLC) for quantification. Mass spectrometry may also be used for identification and purity assessment.

Health Benefits:

- Stress reduction and relaxation
- Improved focus and mental clarity
- Enhanced cognitive function
- Sleep support
- Cardiovascular health promotion

Indication and Usage: L-Theanine supplements are indicated for individuals seeking stress relief, relaxation, and mental clarity. They are commonly used to support cognitive function, promote relaxation, and improve sleep quality.

Usual Constituents with Percentages: L-Theanine is typically present in tea leaves at concentrations ranging from 1% to 2% of the dry weight. In supplements, it is commonly available in doses ranging from 100 mg to 200 mg per capsule or tablet.

Mechanism of Action: L-Theanine exerts its effects by modulating neurotransmitter activity in the brain, particularly GABA and glutamate. It increases GABA levels, which has a calming effect, and modulates glutamate, which enhances cognitive function and focus without causing drowsiness.

Dosage: Dosage recommendations for L-Theanine supplements typically range from 100 mg to 200 mg per day, taken orally with water. Higher doses may be used for specific purposes, such as stress reduction or sleep support, under the guidance of a healthcare professional.

Contraindications:

- There are no known contraindications to L-Theanine supplementation.
- Use caution in individuals with known allergies or sensitivities to tea or tea products.

Precautions:

- Pregnant and breastfeeding women should consult a healthcare professional before taking L-Theanine supplements.
- Individuals with certain medical conditions or those taking medications should use caution and consult a healthcare professional before supplementing with L-Theanine.

Adverse Reactions: Adverse reactions to L-Theanine supplements are rare but may include gastrointestinal upset, headaches, or dizziness, particularly at higher doses.

Research Summary: Research on L-Theanine has shown promising results in various areas, including stress reduction, cognitive enhancement, and sleep support. Numerous clinical studies have demonstrated its efficacy in promoting relaxation, improving focus, and enhancing sleep quality.

Pharmacokinetics: After oral ingestion, L-Theanine is rapidly absorbed in the gastrointestinal tract and reaches peak plasma concentrations within 30 to 60 minutes. It readily crosses the blood-brain barrier and is distributed to various tissues, including the brain, where it exerts its effects.

Pharmacodynamics: L-Theanine exerts its pharmacodynamic effects primarily through modulation of neurotransmitter activity in the brain, particularly GABA and glutamate. It enhances GABAergic activity, resulting in a calming effect, while also modulating glutamatergic activity, which enhances cognitive function and focus.

Overdosage: Excessive intake of L-Theanine supplements is unlikely to cause serious adverse effects due to its low toxicity profile. However, exceeding the recommended dosage may lead to mild adverse reactions such as gastrointestinal upset or drowsiness.

International Standing: L-Theanine supplements are widely available internationally and are commonly used for stress reduction, relaxation, and cognitive enhancement.

Indian Standing: In India, L-Theanine supplements are gaining popularity as part of the growing market for natural health products and dietary supplements promoting relaxation and mental clarity. They are widely available in pharmacies and health food stores and are used by individuals seeking stress relief and cognitive support.

FSSAI Purity Criteria : NA

Permitted Level : 50- 200 mg/day

28)MELATONIN

Introduction: Melatonin is a hormone naturally produced by the pineal gland in the brain in response to darkness. It plays a crucial role in regulating the sleep-wake cycle and has antioxidant properties. Melatonin supplements are commonly used to promote sleep and manage circadian rhythm disorders.

Synonym Name and Common Name: Synonym: N-acetyl-5-methoxytryptamine Common Name: Melatonin

Pharmacognosy / Chemistry: Melatonin is a derivative of the amino acid tryptophan. It is synthesized in the pineal gland from serotonin during the night. Melatonin is also found in small amounts in certain foods, such as cherries, grains, and meats.

Action and Pharmacology: Melatonin exerts its effects by binding to melatonin receptors in the brain, particularly in the suprachiasmatic nucleus, which regulates the circadian rhythm. It modulates the sleep-wake cycle, promotes sleep onset, and regulates other physiological processes such as body temperature and hormone secretion.

Method of Analysis: Analytical methods for melatonin typically involve chromatographic techniques such as high-performance liquid chromatography (HPLC) for quantification. Immunoassays and radioimmunoassays may also be used for analysis.

Health Benefits:

- Regulation of sleep-wake cycle
- Promotion of sleep onset and sleep quality
- Management of circadian rhythm disorders
- Antioxidant and anti-inflammatory effects
- Potential neuroprotective properties

Indication and Usage: Melatonin supplements are indicated for individuals experiencing sleep disturbances, such as insomnia or jet lag, and for managing circadian rhythm disorders, such as delayed sleep phase syndrome. It is also used for its potential antioxidant and neuroprotective effects.

Usual Constituents with Percentages: Melatonin supplements typically contain synthetic melatonin in doses ranging from 1 mg to 10 mg per capsule or tablet. The percentage composition of melatonin in supplements is 100%.

Mechanism of Action: Melatonin exerts its effects by binding to melatonin receptors in the brain, particularly MT1 and MT2 receptors, which are involved in the regulation of the sleep-wake cycle. Activation of these receptors promotes sleep onset and regulates circadian rhythms.

Dosage: Dosage recommendations for melatonin supplements vary depending on the individual's sleep patterns and circadian rhythm disturbances. Typical doses range from 0.5 mg to 5 mg taken orally, approximately 30 minutes to 1 hour before bedtime.

Contraindications:

- Melatonin supplements are contraindicated in individuals with hypersensitivity to melatonin or any of its components.
- Use caution in individuals with autoimmune disorders, seizure disorders, or those taking immunosuppressant medications.

Precautions:

- Pregnant and breastfeeding women should consult a healthcare professional before taking melatonin supplements.
- Use caution when driving or operating heavy machinery after taking melatonin, as it may cause drowsiness or impair cognitive function.

Adverse Reactions: Adverse reactions to melatonin supplements are rare but may include daytime drowsiness, headache, dizziness, and gastrointestinal upset. Higher doses may increase the likelihood of adverse effects.

Research Summary: Research on melatonin has shown promising results in promoting sleep onset and improving sleep quality, particularly in individuals with insomnia or circadian rhythm disorders. Studies also suggest potential benefits in managing jet lag, reducing anxiety, and supporting overall health and well-being.

Pharmacokinetics: After oral ingestion, melatonin is rapidly absorbed in the gastrointestinal tract and reaches peak plasma concentrations within 1 to 2 hours. It is metabolized in the liver and excreted primarily in the urine.

Pharmacodynamics: Melatonin exerts its pharmacodynamic effects primarily through binding to melatonin receptors in the brain, modulating the sleep-wake cycle and circadian rhythms. It also has antioxidant and anti-inflammatory properties, which may contribute to its neuroprotective effects.

Overdosage: Excessive intake of melatonin supplements may lead to drowsiness, confusion, disorientation, and gastrointestinal upset. It is important to adhere to recommended dosages and consult a healthcare professional if experiencing adverse effects.

International Standing: Melatonin supplements are widely available internationally and are commonly used for promoting sleep and managing circadian rhythm disorders.

Indian Standing: In India, melatonin supplements are gaining popularity as part of the growing market for natural health products and dietary supplements promoting sleep and relaxation. They are widely available in pharmacies and health food stores and are used by individuals seeking relief from sleep disturbances and jet lag.

FSSAI Purity Criteria : NA

Permitted Level : 2- 10 mg / day

29)METHYL SULFONYL METHANE

Introduction: Methylsulfonylmethane (MSM) is a naturally occurring compound found in plants, animals, and humans. It is commonly used as a dietary supplement for various health purposes, including joint health, inflammation reduction, and skin health.

Synonym Name and Common Name: Synonym: Dimethyl sulfone, methyl sulfone Common Name: MSM

Pharmacognosy / Chemistry: MSM is an organic sulfur compound that occurs naturally in certain foods, including fruits, vegetables, grains, and animals. It is also synthesized industrially for use in dietary supplements.

Action and Pharmacology: MSM is believed to exert anti-inflammatory, antioxidant, and analgesic effects. It may help reduce inflammation, improve joint flexibility, and support overall joint health. Additionally, MSM is thought to promote the production of collagen and other proteins important for skin and connective tissue health.

Method of Analysis: Analytical methods for MSM typically involve chromatographic techniques such as gas chromatography (GC) or high-performance liquid chromatography (HPLC) for quantification. Spectroscopic methods may also be used for identification and purity assessment.

Health Benefits:

- Supports joint health and mobility
- Reduces inflammation and pain
- Promotes healthy skin, hair, and nails
- May improve exercise performance and recovery

Indication and Usage: MSM supplements are indicated for individuals seeking joint support, inflammation reduction, and improved skin health. They are commonly used to alleviate symptoms of osteoarthritis, rheumatoid arthritis, and other inflammatory conditions.

Usual Constituents with Percentages: MSM supplements typically contain pure MSM powder or crystals, with concentrations ranging from 99% to 100%.

Mechanism of Action: The exact mechanism of action of MSM is not fully understood, but it is believed to exert its effects through multiple pathways, including reducing inflammation, scavenging free radicals, and promoting the synthesis of collagen and other proteins important for joint and tissue health.

Dosage: Dosage recommendations for MSM supplements vary depending on the specific formulation and intended use. Typical doses range from 500 mg to 3000 mg per day, taken orally with water or as directed by a healthcare professional.

Contraindications:

- There are no known contraindications to MSM supplementation.
- Use caution in individuals with known allergies or sensitivities to sulfur-containing compounds.

Precautions:

- Pregnant and breastfeeding women should consult a healthcare professional before taking MSM supplements.
- Individuals with certain medical conditions, such as kidney disease, should use caution and consult a healthcare professional before supplementing with MSM.

Adverse Reactions: Adverse reactions to MSM supplements are rare but may include gastrointestinal upset, headaches, or allergic reactions in sensitive individuals.

Research Summary: Research on MSM has shown promising results in supporting joint health, reducing inflammation, and improving skin and hair quality. Numerous clinical studies have demonstrated its efficacy in alleviating symptoms of osteoarthritis and other inflammatory conditions.

Pharmacokinetics: After oral ingestion, MSM is rapidly absorbed in the gastrointestinal tract and reaches peak plasma concentrations within 1 to 2 hours. It is metabolized in the liver and excreted primarily in the urine.

Pharmacodynamics: MSM exerts its pharmacodynamic effects primarily through its anti-inflammatory and antioxidant properties. It may help reduce inflammation, oxidative stress, and pain associated with inflammatory conditions.

Overdosage: Excessive intake of MSM supplements is unlikely to cause serious adverse effects due to its low toxicity profile. However, exceeding the recommended dosage may lead to mild adverse reactions such as gastrointestinal upset or headaches.

International Standing: MSM supplements are widely available internationally and are commonly used for joint support, inflammation reduction, and skin health.

Indian Standing: In India, MSM supplements are gaining popularity as part of the growing market for natural health products and dietary supplements promoting joint health and inflammation reduction. They are widely available in pharmacies and health food stores and are used by individuals seeking relief from joint pain and inflammation.

FSSAI Purity Criteria : NA

Permitted Level : 1000 - 3000 mg / day, (Not recommended for use by pregnant women and lactating mothers)

30)PANAX GINSENG

Introduction: Panax ginseng, also known as Asian ginseng or Korean ginseng, is a perennial plant native to East Asia. It has been used for centuries in traditional medicine systems, particularly in Traditional Chinese Medicine (TCM) and Korean traditional medicine, for its potential health benefits.

Synonym Name and Common Name: Synonym: Asian ginseng, Korean ginseng Common Name: Panax ginseng

Pharmacognosy / Chemistry: Panax ginseng is a member of the Araliaceae family and is characterized by its fleshy root, which is often used in herbal preparations. The roots of Panax ginseng are harvested and processed to create various forms of supplements, extracts, and herbal remedies.

Action and Pharmacology: Panax ginseng contains active compounds called ginsenosides, which are believed to contribute to its pharmacological effects. It is known for its adaptogenic properties, helping the body adapt to stress and supporting overall well-being. Panax ginseng is also thought to improve energy levels, cognitive function, and immune function.

Method of Analysis: Analytical methods for Panax ginseng typically involve chromatographic techniques such as high-performance liquid chromatography (HPLC) or thin-layer chromatography (TLC) for quantification of ginsenosides. Spectroscopic methods may also be used for identification and purity assessment.

Health Benefits:

- Adaptogenic properties
- Enhanced energy and vitality
- Improved cognitive function
- Immune system support
- Antioxidant effects
- Stress reduction
- Enhanced physical performance

Indication and Usage: Panax ginseng supplements are indicated for individuals seeking support for energy, vitality, cognitive function, and overall well-being. It is commonly used to combat fatigue, improve mental clarity, and enhance physical performance.

Usual Constituents with Percentages: Panax ginseng contains various bioactive compounds, including ginsenosides, polysaccharides, peptides, and flavonoids. Ginsenosides are considered the primary active constituents and typically make up around 2-3% of the root extract.

Mechanism of Action: The active compounds in Panax ginseng, particularly ginsenosides, exert their effects through various mechanisms, including modulation of neurotransmitter activity, antioxidant effects, and modulation of stress response pathways. Ginsenosides are thought to interact with receptors in the central nervous system, enhancing cognitive function and reducing stress.

Dosage: Dosage recommendations for Panax ginseng supplements vary depending on the specific formulation and intended use. Typical doses range from 200 mg to 1000 mg of standardized extract per day, taken orally with water.

Contraindications:

- Panax ginseng supplements are contraindicated in individuals with known allergies to ginseng or any of its components.
- Use caution in individuals with certain medical conditions, such as hypertension, diabetes, or hormone-sensitive conditions.

Precautions:

- Pregnant and breastfeeding women should consult a healthcare professional before taking Panax ginseng supplements.
- Use caution when combining Panax ginseng with other stimulants or medications, as interactions may occur.

Adverse Reactions: Adverse reactions to Panax ginseng supplements are rare but may include gastrointestinal upset, insomnia, headaches, or allergic reactions in sensitive individuals.

Research Summary: Research on Panax ginseng has shown promising results in various areas, including energy enhancement, cognitive function improvement, stress reduction, and immune system modulation. Numerous clinical studies have demonstrated its efficacy in improving physical and mental performance, particularly in stressful conditions.

Pharmacokinetics: After oral ingestion, the bioactive compounds in Panax ginseng are absorbed in the gastrointestinal tract and reach systemic circulation. The absorption and metabolism of ginsenosides vary depending on the specific compound and formulation.

Pharmacodynamics: Panax ginseng exerts its pharmacodynamic effects primarily through modulation of neurotransmitter activity, antioxidant effects, and stress response pathways. Ginsenosides interact with receptors in the central nervous system, enhancing cognitive function, reducing stress, and improving energy levels.

Overdosage: Excessive intake of Panax ginseng supplements may lead to symptoms such as insomnia, nervousness, hypertension, or gastrointestinal upset. It is important to adhere to recommended dosages and consult a healthcare professional if experiencing adverse effects.

International Standing: Panax ginseng supplements are widely available internationally and are commonly used for their adaptogenic properties and health-promoting effects.

Indian Standing: In India, Panax ginseng supplements are gaining popularity as part of the growing market for natural health products and dietary supplements promoting energy, vitality, and cognitive function. They are widely available in pharmacies and health food stores and are used by individuals seeking support for overall well-being.

FSSAI Purity Criteria : Ginsenoside content ranging from 3 - 10 % and adjusted to potency basis 3% total ginsenoside content

Permitted Level : 90 - 400 mg /day

31) PHYCOCYANIN FROM SPIRULINA PLANTESIS

Introduction: Phycocyanin is a blue pigment found abundantly in certain species of cyanobacteria, notably Spirulina platensis. It is a water-soluble protein known for its vibrant blue color and various health benefits.

Synonym Name and Common Name: Synonym: Allophycocyanin Common Name : Blue Spirulina, Blue Algae Extract

Pharmacognosy / Chemistry: Phycocyanin can be extracted from Spirulina platensis through various methods such as aqueous extraction, ultrasonication, or chromatography. It is typically obtained as a blue-colored powder or liquid.

Action and Pharmacology: Phycocyanin exhibits potent antioxidant and anti-inflammatory properties. It also demonstrates immune-modulating effects and has been shown to protect against oxidative stress-induced damage.

Method of Analysis: Phycocyanin content in extracts can be analyzed using spectrophotometric methods, such as UV-Vis spectroscopy, which measures absorbance at specific wavelengths characteristic of phycocyanin.

Health Benefits:

- Antioxidant properties aid in combating oxidative stress.
- Anti-inflammatory effects may help alleviate inflammation-related conditions.
- Immune-modulating properties support overall immune function.
- Potential neuroprotective effects have been suggested.

Indication and Usage:

- Dietary supplement for antioxidant support.
- Used in cosmetic formulations for its vibrant blue color and antioxidant properties.
- Investigated for potential therapeutic applications in various diseases including cancer, cardiovascular disorders, and neurodegenerative conditions.

Usual Constituents with Percentages: Phycocyanin content in Spirulina platensis can vary, but it generally ranges from 10% to 20% of the total dry weight of the algae.

Mechanism of Action: Phycocyanin exerts its effects through multiple mechanisms, including scavenging free radicals, modulating inflammatory pathways, and enhancing immune responses.

Dosage: Dosage recommendations vary depending on the specific product and intended use. It's advisable to follow the instructions provided by the manufacturer or consult a healthcare professional for appropriate dosage guidance.

Contraindications: There are no known contraindications for phycocyanin when used in recommended doses. However, individuals with known allergies to Spirulina or cyanobacteria should avoid its consumption.

Precautions:

- Pregnant or breastfeeding women should consult a healthcare professional before using phycocyanin supplements.
- Individuals with autoimmune disorders should use with caution due to its immune-modulating effects.

Adverse Reactions: Adverse reactions to phycocyanin supplements are rare but may include gastrointestinal discomfort, allergic reactions, or hypersensitivity reactions in sensitive individuals.

Research Summary: Research on phycocyanin from Spirulina platensis has shown promising results in various preclinical studies, suggesting its potential therapeutic applications in conditions such as cancer, inflammation, and oxidative stress-related diseases. Clinical trials are ongoing to further investigate its efficacy and safety in humans.

Pharmacokinetics: Phycocyanin is water-soluble and readily absorbed in the gastrointestinal tract. Absorption rates and bioavailability may vary depending on factors such as formulation and individual differences.

Pharmacodynamics: Phycocyanin exerts its pharmacological effects by interacting with various cellular pathways involved in oxidative stress, inflammation, and immune responses.

Overdosage: Excessive consumption of phycocyanin supplements may lead to gastrointestinal discomfort or allergic reactions. It's important to adhere to recommended dosage guidelines to avoid adverse effects.

International Standing: Phycocyanin supplements are gaining popularity internationally due to their perceived health benefits and antioxidant properties. However, regulatory frameworks for its use may vary across different countries.

Indian Standing: In India, Spirulina-based products, including those containing phycocyanin, are increasingly recognized for their nutritional value and potential health benefits. However, specific regulations and standards for phycocyanin supplements may still be evolving.

Research Summary of Phycocyanin from Spirulina platensis: Research on phycocyanin from Spirulina platensis underscores its diverse pharmacological properties and therapeutic potential. Studies have highlighted its antioxidant, anti-inflammatory, and immune-modulating effects, suggesting possible applications in the prevention and management of various diseases. Further research, including well-designed clinical trials, is warranted to elucidate its efficacy, safety profile, and optimal dosage regimens for specific health conditions.

FSSAI Purity Criteria : Protein: 50-70 %; Carbohydrates: 20-40%; Minerals (Ash): 5.0 ± 15%; Moisture: 3.0 - 6.0 %

Permitted Level : 50 - 250 mg /day

32) PIPER NIGRUM / PIPER LONGUM EXTRACT

Introduction: Piper nigrum (black pepper) and Piper longum (long pepper) are two widely used spices in traditional medicine systems across the world. Extracts from these plants have been utilized for their medicinal properties for centuries.

Synonym Name and Common Name: Synonym:

- Piper nigrum: Black pepper
- Piper longum: Long pepper Common Name:
- Piper nigrum: Kali Mirch (in Hindi)
- Piper longum: Pippali (in Sanskrit)

Pharmacognosy / Chemistry: Piper nigrum and Piper longum extracts are obtained from the dried fruits of the respective plants. These extracts are typically obtained through processes like solvent extraction or steam distillation.

Action and Pharmacology: Both Piper nigrum and Piper longum extracts exhibit diverse pharmacological actions, including:

- Anti-inflammatory
- Antioxidant
- Analgesic
- Antimicrobial
- Gastrointestinal stimulant

Method of Analysis: The analysis of Piper nigrum and Piper longum extracts involves techniques such as High-Performance Liquid Chromatography (HPLC), Gas Chromatography-Mass Spectrometry (GC-MS), and Thin-Layer Chromatography (TLC) to identify and quantify the active constituents.

Health Benefits:

- Supports digestion and gut health

- Anti-inflammatory properties may aid in pain management
- Antioxidant effects contribute to overall health and wellness
- Potential antimicrobial properties support immune function

Indication and Usage:

- Used in traditional medicine systems for digestive disorders such as indigestion and bloating
- Employed as a culinary spice for flavoring and seasoning
- Investigated for potential therapeutic applications in conditions like arthritis and respiratory ailments

Usual Constituents with Percentages: The major constituents of Piper nigrum and Piper longum extracts include piperine, alkaloids, volatile oils, and flavonoids. The percentage composition may vary depending on factors such as plant variety and extraction method.

Mechanism of Action: Piperine, the primary bioactive compound in Piper nigrum and Piper longum extracts, is believed to exert its effects through various mechanisms, including:

- Inhibition of inflammatory pathways
- Modulation of neurotransmitter activity
- Enhancement of antioxidant defenses
- Potentiation of drug bioavailability through inhibition of drug-metabolizing enzymes

Dosage: Dosage recommendations for Piper nigrum and Piper longum extracts may vary depending on the specific product and intended use. It is advisable to follow the instructions provided by the manufacturer or consult a healthcare professional for appropriate dosage guidance.

Contraindications:

Piper nigrum and Piper longum extracts are generally considered safe for most people when used in culinary amounts.

However, individuals with gastroesophageal reflux disease (GERD) or peptic ulcer disease may experience worsening symptoms with high doses.

Pregnant and breastfeeding women should use caution and consult a healthcare professional before using concentrated extracts.

Precautions:

- Long-term use of high doses of Piper nigrum and Piper longum extracts may lead to gastrointestinal irritation or allergic reactions in sensitive individuals.
- Individuals taking medications metabolized by cytochrome P450 enzymes should use caution, as piperine may interfere with drug metabolism and increase the risk of adverse effects.

Adverse Reactions: Adverse reactions to Piper nigrum and Piper longum extracts are rare but may include gastrointestinal discomfort, allergic reactions, or interactions with certain medications.

Research Summary: Research on Piper nigrum and Piper longum extracts has demonstrated their potential therapeutic benefits in various preclinical and clinical studies. These include anti-inflammatory, antioxidant, analgesic, and antimicrobial properties, suggesting their utility in the management of digestive disorders, pain, and inflammatory conditions. Further research is needed to elucidate their mechanisms of action and optimize dosage regimens for specific health conditions.

Pharmacokinetics: Piperine, the main bioactive compound in Piper nigrum and Piper longum extracts, is well-absorbed in the gastrointestinal tract. It undergoes rapid metabolism in the liver and is excreted primarily through urine.

Pharmacodynamics: Piperine exerts its pharmacological effects through various mechanisms, including inhibition of inflammatory mediators, modulation of neurotransmitter activity, and enhancement of antioxidant defenses.

Overdosage: Excessive consumption of Piper nigrum and Piper longum extracts may lead to gastrointestinal irritation or allergic reactions. It's important to adhere to recommended dosage guidelines to avoid adverse effects.

International Standing: Piper nigrum and Piper longum extracts are widely recognized and utilized in international markets both as culinary spices and herbal supplements. They are valued for their flavoring properties as well as their potential health benefits.

Indian Standing: In India, Piper nigrum and Piper longum have a long history of use in traditional Ayurvedic medicine. They are revered for their medicinal properties and are incorporated into various formulations for treating a wide range of health conditions.

Research Summary of Piper nigrum / Piper longum extract: Research on Piper nigrum and Piper longum extracts highlights their diverse pharmacological properties and therapeutic potential. Studies have demonstrated their efficacy in managing digestive disorders, inflammation, pain, and microbial infections. Ongoing research aims to further elucidate their mechanisms of action and explore novel therapeutic applications.

FSSAI Purity Criteria : Piperine content

Permitted Level : 15 mg/day of piperine, (Duration of use: maximum 30 days)

33) QUERCETIN OBTAINED FROM EXTRACTS OF CITRUS FRUITS, VEGETABLES, AND OTHER PLANT SOURCES

Introduction: Quercetin is a flavonoid compound belonging to the polyphenol group, widely found in various fruits, vegetables, leaves, and grains. It is renowned for its potent antioxidant properties and numerous health benefits.

Synonym Name and Common Name: Synonyms: 3,3',4',5,7-pentahydroxyflavone Common Name: Quercetin

Pharmacognosy / Chemistry: Quercetin is typically found as a yellow crystalline powder, sparingly soluble in water but more soluble in alcohol and alkali solutions. It is identified through various chemical tests, including color reactions and spectroscopic analysis.

Action and Pharmacology: Quercetin exerts antioxidant, anti-inflammatory, antiviral, and anticancer effects. It scavenges free radicals, inhibits inflammatory pathways, interferes with viral replication, and suppresses cancer cell proliferation.

Method of Analysis: Quercetin can be analyzed using techniques such as high-performance liquid chromatography (HPLC), thin-layer chromatography (TLC), and spectrophotometry.

Health Benefits: Quercetin offers numerous health benefits, including antioxidant protection, immune system support, cardiovascular health, anti-allergic effects, and potential anticancer properties.

Indication and Usage: Quercetin is used as a dietary supplement for various conditions, including allergies, inflammation, cardiovascular diseases, viral infections, and cancer prevention.

Usual Constituents with Percentages: The usual constituents of quercetin in plant sources vary, but typically range from 2% to 10% of the dried weight, depending on the specific plant species and growing conditions.

Mechanism of Action: Quercetin exerts its effects through multiple mechanisms, including scavenging free radicals, modulating enzyme activity, inhibiting inflammatory mediators, and regulating gene expression.

Dosage: Typical dosages of quercetin supplements range from 500 mg to 1000 mg per day, divided into multiple doses.

Contraindications: Quercetin supplements may interact with certain medications, and caution is advised for individuals with specific medical conditions, such as kidney disorders or pregnancy.

Precautions: Patients should consult with healthcare professionals before taking quercetin supplements, especially if they are already on medication or have existing health conditions.

Adverse Reactions: While generally well-tolerated, high doses of quercetin may cause gastrointestinal upset in some individuals. Allergic reactions are rare but possible.

Research Summary: Research on quercetin has shown promising results in various preclinical and clinical studies, indicating its potential therapeutic applications in managing oxidative stress-related diseases, inflammation, viral infections, and cancer.

Pharmacokinetics: Quercetin is absorbed in the small intestine and undergoes extensive metabolism in the liver. Its bioavailability is relatively low, but certain formulations and co-administered compounds may enhance absorption.

Pharmacodynamics: Quercetin's pharmacodynamics involve its antioxidant and anti-inflammatory effects, modulation of enzyme activity, and interaction with cellular signaling pathways.

Overdosage: Excessive intake of quercetin supplements may lead to toxicity symptoms such as gastrointestinal discomfort, nausea, and headache. However, severe overdoses are rare due to its relatively low toxicity profile.

International Standing: Quercetin is recognized internationally as a dietary supplement with potential health benefits, and its safety and efficacy are subject to regulatory oversight in various countries.

Indian Standing: In India, quercetin is widely studied for its medicinal properties, and it is included in traditional Ayurvedic formulations for various health conditions.

Research Summary of Quercetin Obtained from Extracts of Citrus Fruits, Vegetables, and Other Plant Sources: Studies have demonstrated the presence of quercetin in citrus fruits, vegetables, and other plant sources, highlighting its diverse distribution in nature. Research indicates potential health benefits of consuming quercetin-rich foods, including cardiovascular protection, anti-inflammatory effects, and immune system support. Additionally, investigations into the extraction methods, bioavailability, and pharmacological activities of quercetin from different plant sources continue to contribute to our understanding of its therapeutic potential.

FSSAI Purity Criteria : Quercetin content

Permitted Level : 100 mg / day

34) SCHIZANDRA BERRY EXTRACT

Introduction: Schizandra berry extract is derived from the fruit of Schisandra chinensis, a plant native to East Asia. It has been used for centuries in traditional Chinese medicine for its purported health benefits.

Synonym Name and Common Name: Synonyms: Five-flavor berry, Magnolia berry Common Name: Schizandra berry

Pharmacognosy / Chemistry: Schizandra berry extract typically appears as a reddish-brown powder with a characteristic aroma. It contains various phytochemicals such as lignans, schisandrins, and flavonoids.

Action and Pharmacology: Schizandra berry extract exerts adaptogenic, hepatoprotective, antioxidant, and anti-inflammatory effects. It helps the body adapt to stress, supports liver function, scavenges free radicals, and modulates immune responses.

Method of Analysis: Analysis of Schizandra berry extract involves techniques such as high-performance liquid chromatography (HPLC), gas chromatography-mass spectrometry (GC-MS), and spectrophotometry to identify and quantify its active constituents.

Health Benefits: Schizandra berry extract is believed to promote overall health and well-being. It may support liver health, enhance cognitive function, reduce fatigue, and improve physical endurance. Additionally, it is purported to have anti-aging and aphrodisiac properties.

Indication and Usage: Schizandra berry extract is used as a dietary supplement for various purposes, including liver detoxification, stress management, cognitive enhancement, and improving athletic performance.

Usual Constituents with Percentages: Schizandra berry extract contains lignans such as schisandrin A, schisandrin B, and schisandrin C, typically ranging from 2% to 9% of the total extract. Other constituents include flavonoids, organic acids, and vitamins.

Mechanism of Action: The active constituents in Schizandra berry extract exert their effects through various mechanisms, including antioxidant activity, modulation of enzyme function, regulation of gene expression, and enhancement of cellular defense mechanisms.

Dosage: Typical dosages of Schizandra berry extract range from 500 mg to 2000 mg per day, divided into multiple doses. However, dosages may vary based on the specific formulation and intended use.

Contraindications: Individuals with certain medical conditions, such as liver disease or hormone-sensitive cancers, should use Schizandra berry extract with caution or avoid it altogether due to potential interactions or exacerbation of symptoms.

Precautions: Patients should consult with healthcare professionals before using Schizandra berry extract, especially if they are pregnant, nursing, or taking medications, to avoid potential adverse effects or drug interactions.

Adverse Reactions: While generally well-tolerated, high doses of Schizandra berry extract may cause mild gastrointestinal discomfort or allergic reactions in sensitive individuals.

Research Summary: Research on Schizandra berry extract has demonstrated its potential therapeutic effects in various preclinical and clinical studies, including hepatoprotective, neuroprotective, anti-inflammatory, and antioxidant properties. However, further research is needed to fully elucidate its mechanisms of action and clinical efficacy.

Pharmacokinetics: After oral administration, the active constituents in Schizandra berry extract are absorbed in the gastrointestinal tract and undergo metabolism in the liver. Their metabolites are then distributed throughout the body, exerting their pharmacological effects.

Pharmacodynamics: Schizandra berry extract exerts its pharmacological effects by modulating cellular signaling pathways, enhancing antioxidant defenses, and promoting physiological adaptation to stressors, thereby supporting overall health and vitality.

Overdosage: Excessive intake of Schizandra berry extract may lead to gastrointestinal upset or other adverse effects. However, severe overdoses are rare due to its relatively low toxicity profile.

International Standing: Schizandra berry extract is recognized internationally as a dietary supplement with potential health benefits, and its safety and efficacy are subject to regulatory oversight in various countries.

Indian Standing: In India, Schizandra berry extract is gaining recognition for its adaptogenic and hepatoprotective properties, and it is increasingly incorporated into traditional Ayurvedic formulations for enhancing vitality and longevity.

FSSAI Purity Criteria : Schizandrin berries containing 2.5-3.0% schizandrin

Permitted Level : 1 - 3 g / day

35) SCUTELLARIA BICALENSIS

Introduction: Scutellariabaicalensis, also known as Chinese skullcap, is a perennial herbaceous plant native to East Asia. It has a long history of use in traditional Chinese medicine for its medicinal properties.

Synonym Name and Common Name: Synonyms: Baikal skullcap, Huang-Qin Common Name: Scutellariabaicalensis

Pharmacognosy / Chemistry: Scutellariabaicalensis is characterized by its small, blue-purple flowers and distinctive skullcap-shaped seed pods. The roots of the plant are the primary medicinal part and contain various bioactive compounds.

Action and Pharmacology: Scutellariabaicalensis exhibits anti-inflammatory, antioxidant, antiviral, and neuroprotective effects. It modulates immune responses, scavenges free radicals, inhibits viral replication, and protects against neurodegeneration.

Method of Analysis: Analysis of Scutellariabaicalensis involves techniques such as high-performance liquid chromatography (HPLC), gas chromatography-mass spectrometry (GC-MS), and spectrophotometry to identify and quantify its active constituents, including baicalin and baicalein.

Health Benefits: Scutellariabaicalensis is believed to offer a range of health benefits, including reducing inflammation, supporting immune function, protecting against oxidative stress, and promoting nervous system health.

Indication and Usage: Scutellariabaicalensis is used in traditional medicine and as a dietary supplement for various conditions, including respiratory infections, inflammatory disorders, viral illnesses, and neurological conditions.

Usual Constituents with Percentages: The roots of Scutellariabaicalensis contain several bioactive compounds, with baicalin and baicalein being the most abundant. Baicalin typically constitutes around 5-15% of the dried root, while baicalein ranges from 1-5%.

Mechanism of Action: The active constituents in Scutellariabaicalensis exert their effects through multiple mechanisms, including inhibition of pro-inflammatory cytokines, modulation of cellular signaling pathways, and enhancement of antioxidant defenses.

Dosage: Typical dosages of Scutellariabaicalensis extract range from 500 mg to 2000 mg per day, divided into multiple doses. However, dosages may vary based on the specific formulation and intended use.

Contraindications: Individuals with certain medical conditions, such as liver disease or hormone-sensitive cancers, should use Scutellariabaicalensis with caution or avoid it altogether due to potential interactions or exacerbation of symptoms.

Precautions: Patients should consult with healthcare professionals before using Scutellariabaicalensis, especially if they are pregnant, nursing, or taking medications, to avoid potential adverse effects or drug interactions.

Adverse Reactions: While generally well-tolerated, high doses of Scutellariabaicalensis may cause mild gastrointestinal discomfort or allergic reactions in sensitive individuals.

Research Summary: Research on Scutellariabaicalensis has shown promising results in various preclinical and clinical studies, indicating its potential therapeutic applications in managing inflammation, viral infections, neurodegenerative diseases, and other health conditions. However, further research is needed to fully elucidate its mechanisms of action and clinical efficacy.

Pharmacokinetics: After oral administration, the active constituents in Scutellariabaicalensis are absorbed in the gastrointestinal tract and undergo metabolism in the liver. Their metabolites are then distributed throughout the body, exerting their pharmacological effects.

Pharmacodynamics: Scutellariabaicalensis exerts its pharmacological effects by modulating immune responses, reducing inflammation, scavenging free radicals, and protecting against oxidative stress, thereby supporting overall health and well-being.

Overdosage: Excessive intake of Scutellariabaicalensis may lead to gastrointestinal upset or other adverse effects. However, severe overdoses are rare due to its relatively low toxicity profile.

International Standing: Scutellariabaicalensis is recognized internationally as a dietary supplement with potential health benefits, and its safety and efficacy are subject to regulatory oversight in various countries.

Indian Standing: In India, Scutellariabaicalensis is gaining recognition for its medicinal properties, and it is increasingly studied for its potential therapeutic applications in Ayurvedic medicine and modern herbal formulations.

FSSAI Purity Criteria : Aq. extract standardized to bicallin content 30 - 50 % and adjusted to potency basis 50 % bicallin content

Permitted Level : 250 - 1,000 mg/ day

36) SELENIUM YEAST

Introduction: Selenium yeast is a natural source of selenium obtained through the fermentation of Saccharomyces cerevisiae yeast in a selenium-rich medium. It serves as a dietary supplement to address selenium deficiency and promote overall health.

Synonym Name and Common Name:

Synonyms: Selenized yeast; Common Name: Selenium yeast

Pharmacognosy / Chemistry: Selenium yeast appears as a yellowish-brown powder or granules, containing various organic selenium compounds. It is obtained through the controlled fermentation of yeast in the presence of selenium.

Action and Pharmacology: Selenium yeast serves as a bioavailable source of selenium, an essential trace mineral with antioxidant properties. Selenium plays a crucial role in various physiological processes, including antioxidant defense, thyroid function, immune regulation, and DNA synthesis.

Method of Analysis: Analysis of selenium yeast involves techniques such as atomic absorption spectroscopy (AAS), inductively coupled plasma mass spectrometry (ICP-MS), and high-performance liquid chromatography (HPLC) to quantify selenium content and identify selenium species.

Health Benefits: Selenium yeast offers numerous health benefits, including supporting immune function, promoting thyroid health, protecting against oxidative stress, reducing the risk of certain cancers, and maintaining cardiovascular health.

Indication and Usage: Selenium yeast is used as a dietary supplement to prevent or address selenium deficiency, support overall health and well-being, and reduce the risk of selenium-related health conditions.

Usual Constituents with Percentages: The selenium content in selenium yeast typically ranges from 1000 to 2000 micrograms per gram (μg/g), depending on the fermentation process and selenium concentration in the growth medium.

Mechanism of Action: Selenium functions as a cofactor for various selenoproteins, including glutathione peroxidases, thioredoxin reductases, and selenoprotein P, which play critical roles in antioxidant defense, redox regulation, and immune modulation.

Dosage: Recommended dosages of selenium yeast vary depending on age, sex, and specific health conditions but generally range from 50 to 200 micrograms per day for adults.

Contraindications: Individuals with selenium allergies or selenium toxicity should avoid selenium yeast supplementation. Additionally, caution is advised for individuals with certain medical conditions, such as selenium-sensitive thyroid disorders or autoimmune diseases.

Precautions: Patients should consult with healthcare professionals before starting selenium yeast supplementation, especially if they are pregnant, nursing, or taking medications, to avoid potential adverse effects or drug interactions.

Adverse Reactions: While selenium yeast is generally well-tolerated at recommended dosages, excessive intake may lead to selenium toxicity symptoms, including gastrointestinal disturbances, hair loss, nail brittleness, and neurological effects.

Research Summary: Research on selenium yeast supplementation has demonstrated its efficacy in addressing selenium deficiency, improving antioxidant status, enhancing immune function, and reducing the risk of certain chronic diseases, such as cancer and cardiovascular disease.

Pharmacokinetics: After oral ingestion, selenium from selenium yeast is absorbed in the gastrointestinal tract and distributed throughout the body. It undergoes metabolism primarily in the liver and is incorporated into selenoproteins or excreted via urine and feces.

Pharmacodynamics: Selenium exerts its pharmacological effects through incorporation into selenoproteins, which regulate cellular redox balance, modulate immune responses, and protect against oxidative damage, thereby supporting overall health and well-being.

Overdosage: Excessive intake of selenium yeast may lead to selenium toxicity, characterized by symptoms such as gastrointestinal upset, hair and nail changes, neurological abnormalities, and potential organ damage. Therefore, it is essential to adhere to recommended dosages.

International Standing: Selenium yeast is recognized internationally as a dietary supplement with potential health benefits, and its safety and efficacy are subject to regulatory oversight in various countries.

Indian Standing: In India, selenium yeast is increasingly used as a dietary supplement to address selenium deficiency and support overall health. Its safety and efficacy are of interest to researchers and healthcare professionals in the country.

FSSAI Purity Criteria : Selenium content and number of yeast counts (Cfu/g)

Permitted Level : 2 mg/day of selenium

37) SIBERIAN GINSENG OBTAINED FROM 0.6 TO 2.0 G OF GINSENG ROOT

Introduction: Siberian ginseng, scientifically known as Eleutherococcussenticosus, is an adaptogenic herb native to the forests of Siberia and other parts of Asia. It has been used for centuries in traditional medicine for its purported health-promoting properties.

Synonym Name and Common Name: Synonym: Eleuthero, Ciwujia Common Name: Siberian ginseng

Pharmacognosy / Chemistry: Siberian ginseng is a woody shrub with small, yellow-green flowers and thorny stems. The roots and rhizomes are the parts of the plant used for medicinal purposes, typically harvested after 3-6 years of growth.

Action and Pharmacology: Siberian ginseng exhibits adaptogenic, immunomodulatory, anti-fatigue, and neuroprotective effects. It helps the body adapt to stress, enhances immune function, reduces fatigue, and supports cognitive health.

Method of Analysis: Analysis of Siberian ginseng involves techniques such as high-performance liquid chromatography (HPLC), gas chromatography-mass spectrometry (GC-MS), and spectrophotometry to identify and quantify its active constituents, including eleutherosides and polysaccharides.

Health Benefits: Siberian ginseng is believed to offer various health benefits, including boosting energy levels, improving mental performance, enhancing physical endurance, supporting immune function, and reducing stress-related symptoms.

Indication and Usage: Siberian ginseng is used as a dietary supplement for managing stress, combating fatigue, enhancing athletic performance, boosting immunity, and promoting overall well-being.

Usual Constituents with Percentages: The usual constituents of Siberian ginseng include eleutherosides (0.6-2.0% of the root), polysaccharides, flavonoids, phenolic compounds, and essential oils, which contribute to its pharmacological effects.

Mechanism of Action: The active constituents in Siberian ginseng exert their effects through various mechanisms, including modulation of the hypothalamic-pituitary-adrenal (HPA) axis, enhancement of cellular energy metabolism, and stimulation of immune responses.

Dosage: Recommended dosages of Siberian ginseng extract typically range from 300 mg to 1200 mg per day, divided into multiple doses. However, dosages may vary based on the specific formulation and intended use.

Contraindications: Individuals with certain medical conditions, such as hypertension, heart disease, or hormone-sensitive cancers, should use Siberian ginseng with caution or avoid it altogether due to potential interactions or exacerbation of symptoms.

Precautions: Patients should consult with healthcare professionals before using Siberian ginseng, especially if they are pregnant, nursing, or taking medications, to avoid potential adverse effects or drug interactions.

Adverse Reactions: While generally well-tolerated, high doses of Siberian ginseng may cause mild gastrointestinal upset, insomnia, or nervousness in some individuals. Allergic reactions are rare but possible.

Research Summary: Research on Siberian ginseng has shown promising results in various preclinical and clinical studies, indicating its potential therapeutic applications in managing stress, improving cognitive function, enhancing physical performance, and supporting immune health.

Pharmacokinetics: After oral ingestion, the active constituents in Siberian ginseng are absorbed in the gastrointestinal tract and distributed throughout the body. They undergo metabolism primarily in the liver and are excreted via urine and feces.

Pharmacodynamics: Siberian ginseng exerts its pharmacological effects by modulating stress response pathways, enhancing energy metabolism, stimulating immune function, and improving cognitive and physical performance.

Overdosage: Excessive intake of Siberian ginseng may lead to symptoms such as insomnia, nervousness, palpitations, or gastrointestinal disturbances. However, severe overdoses are rare due to its relatively low toxicity profile.

International Standing: Siberian ginseng is recognized internationally as a dietary supplement with potential health benefits, and its safety and efficacy are subject to regulatory oversight in various countries.

Indian Standing: In India, Siberian ginseng is increasingly studied for its adaptogenic and immunomodulatory properties, and it is gaining recognition in traditional Ayurvedic formulations for promoting vitality and resilience to stress.

FSSAI Purity Criteria : Eleutherosides content

Permitted Level : 100 - 450 mg / day

38) SILYBUM MARIANUM EXTRACT

Introduction: Silybum marianum, commonly known as Milk thistle, is a flowering plant native to the Mediterranean region. It has a long history of medicinal use, particularly in traditional European herbal medicine.

Synonym Name and Common Name: Synonym Name: Carduus marianus; Common Name: Milk thistle

Pharmacognosy / Chemistry: The plant is characterized by its prickly leaves and purple flowers. Milk thistle produces spiky seed pods containing the medicinal compound silymarin.

Action and Pharmacology: The active component of milk thistle, silymarin, has antioxidant, anti-inflammatory, and hepatoprotective properties. It is known to protect liver cells from damage and aid in liver regeneration.

Method of Analysis: Various analytical techniques such as high-performance liquid chromatography (HPLC) are employed to quantify the levels of silymarin and other constituents in milk thistle extracts.

Health Benefits: Milk thistle is primarily used to support liver health and treat liver disorders such as cirrhosis, hepatitis, and fatty liver disease. It may also have benefits for heart health, cholesterol levels, and diabetes management.

Indication and Usage: Indications for milk thistle include liver damage, liver cirrhosis, hepatitis, gallbladder disorders, and as a supportive treatment during chemotherapy.

Usual Constituents with Percentages: Silymarin (70-80%), flavonoids, silybin, silydianin, silychristin, fatty acids, and other phytochemicals.

Mechanism of Action: Silymarin exerts its hepatoprotective effects by scavenging free radicals, inhibiting inflammation, and enhancing protein synthesis in liver cells. It also stimulates the regeneration of liver tissue.

Dosage: Typical doses of milk thistle extract range from 200-400 mg, taken 1-3 times daily. However, dosages may vary depending on the formulation and individual health needs.

Contraindications: Milk thistle may interact with certain medications, particularly those metabolized by the liver. It is not recommended for use in pregnant or breastfeeding women without consulting a healthcare professional.

Precautions: Individuals with allergies to plants in the Asteraceae family (such as ragweed or daisies) should use milk thistle with caution. It's advisable to consult a healthcare provider before starting supplementation.

Adverse Reactions: Milk thistle is generally well-tolerated, but some individuals may experience mild gastrointestinal upset or allergic reactions. Rarely, it may cause a laxative effect or headache.

Research Summary: Research suggests that milk thistle may have significant benefits for liver health, particularly in treating liver diseases and protecting against liver damage from toxins or medications. Studies also indicate potential benefits for other conditions such as diabetes and high cholesterol, although further research is needed to confirm these effects.

Pharmacokinetics and Pharmacodynamics: Silymarin is poorly absorbed orally, with only about 20-50% reaching systemic circulation. It undergoes extensive metabolism in the liver and is excreted primarily in the bile.

Overdosage: There is limited information on the effects of overdosing on milk thistle. However, high doses may increase the risk of adverse reactions such as gastrointestinal discomfort.

International Standing: Milk thistle is recognized internationally for its medicinal properties and is commonly used as a dietary supplement in many countries.

Indian Standing: In India, milk thistle is also valued for its therapeutic benefits and is used in traditional Ayurvedic medicine to support liver health and treat various ailments.

Research Summary of Silybum marianum Extract: Overall, research on Silybum marianum extract, particularly its active component silymarin, underscores its potential as a hepatoprotective agent and its utility in treating liver disorders. Additional investigations into its effects on other health conditions continue to expand its potential applications in modern medicine. However, more clinical trials are necessary to establish its efficacy, safety, and optimal dosage for various indications.

FSSAI Purity Criteria : Standardized extract - silimarin content

Permitted Level : 250 - 1,000 mg/ day

39) SOYA ISOFLAVONES

Introduction: Soy isoflavones are phytochemicals found in soybeans and soy products. These compounds have gained attention for their potential health benefits, particularly in promoting heart health and relieving menopausal symptoms.

Synonym Name and Common Name: Synonym Name: Soybean isoflavones Common Name: Soya isoflavones

Pharmacognosy / Chemistry: Soy isoflavones are naturally occurring compounds found in the seeds of the soybean plant. They belong to the family of flavonoids and are classified as phytoestrogens due to their structural similarity to the hormone estrogen.

Action and Pharmacology: Soy isoflavones exert estrogenic and anti-estrogenic effects in the body, which can modulate hormonal balance. They also possess antioxidant properties and may help reduce inflammation.

Method of Analysis: Analytical methods such as high-performance liquid chromatography (HPLC) are commonly used to quantify the levels of individual soy isoflavones, including genistein, daidzein, and glycitein, in soy-based products.

Health Benefits: Soy isoflavones have been studied for their potential to reduce the risk of cardiovascular disease, alleviate menopausal symptoms such as hot flashes and night sweats, support bone health, and exert anticancer effects, particularly in hormone-related cancers such as breast and prostate cancer.

Indication and Usage: Indications for soy isoflavones include menopausal symptoms, cardiovascular health, bone health, and potentially reducing the risk of certain cancers. They are often consumed as dietary supplements or incorporated into soy-based foods.

Usual Constituents with Percentages: The major soy isoflavones found in soy products include genistein (50-60%), daidzein (40-50%), and glycitein (5-10%).

Mechanism of Action: Soy isoflavones exert their effects through multiple mechanisms, including binding to estrogen receptors, modulating enzyme activity involved in hormone metabolism, and exerting antioxidant and anti-inflammatory effects.

Dosage: Typical doses of soy isoflavones range from 50 to 100 milligrams per day, although dosages may vary depending on the specific health condition being targeted.

Contraindications: Individuals with hormone-sensitive conditions such as breast cancer, ovarian cancer, or endometriosis should use soy isoflavone supplements with caution and under the guidance of a healthcare professional.

Precautions: Pregnant or breastfeeding women should consult a healthcare provider before taking soy isoflavone supplements. Individuals with soy allergies should avoid soy-based products.

Adverse Reactions: While soy isoflavones are generally well-tolerated, some individuals may experience mild gastrointestinal discomfort or allergic reactions. Rarely, high doses may cause hormonal imbalances or interact with medications.

Research Summary: Research on soy isoflavones suggests that they may offer various health benefits, particularly in reducing menopausal symptoms, supporting heart health, and potentially reducing the risk of certain cancers. However, findings from clinical studies have been mixed, and further research is needed to fully understand their efficacy and safety.

Pharmacokinetics and Pharmacodynamics: Soy isoflavones are readily absorbed in the intestines and undergo extensive metabolism in the liver. They can exert estrogenic or anti-estrogenic effects depending on various factors such as hormone levels and tissue sensitivity.

Overdosage: There is limited information on the effects of overdosing on soy isoflavones. However, high doses may increase the risk of adverse effects such as hormonal disruptions or gastrointestinal symptoms.

International Standing: Soy isoflavones are recognized internationally for their potential health benefits and are commonly used as dietary supplements in many countries, particularly among individuals seeking natural alternatives for menopausal symptom relief.

Indian Standing: In India, soy isoflavones are gaining recognition for their potential health benefits and are increasingly incorporated into dietary supplements and functional foods marketed for women's health and overall well-being.

Research Summary of Soya Isoflavones: While research on soy isoflavones continues to explore their potential health benefits, particularly in the realms of menopausal health, cardiovascular health, and cancer prevention, conflicting evidence and variability in study outcomes necessitate further investigation to elucidate their mechanisms of action and optimize their clinical applications.

FSSAI Purity Criteria : NA

Permitted Level : 50-100 mg/day (Consult a Health care professional for long term use)

40) SPIRULINA

Introduction: Spirulina is a type of cyanobacteria, commonly referred to as blue-green algae, known for its high nutritional content and potential health benefits. It has been consumed by various cultures for centuries and is now widely used as a dietary supplement.

Synonym Name and Common Name: Synonym Name: Arthrospira platensis; Common Name: Spirulina

Pharmacognosy / Chemistry: Spirulina is characterized by its spiral-shaped, multicellular filaments. It is typically harvested from alkaline freshwater lakes and ponds, then dried and processed into powder or tablet form for consumption.

Action and Pharmacology: Spirulina contains a rich array of nutrients including protein, vitamins, minerals, and antioxidants. It exhibits anti-inflammatory, antioxidant, immunomodulatory, and hypolipidemic properties, contributing to its various health benefits.

Method of Analysis: Analytical techniques such as spectrophotometry, chromatography, and microscopy are commonly used to analyze the nutritional composition, bioactive compounds, and purity of Spirulina products.

Health Benefits: Spirulina is known for its potential to boost immunity, improve energy levels, support cardiovascular health, aid in detoxification, promote weight loss, and enhance athletic performance. It also has antioxidant properties that may help protect against oxidative stress and cellular damage.

Indication and Usage: Indications for Spirulina include nutritional supplementation, immune support, detoxification, weight management, and as a dietary supplement for vegetarians, vegans, and individuals with certain health conditions.

Usual Constituents with Percentages: Spirulina typically contains about 55-70% protein by dry weight, along with significant amounts of vitamins (especially B vitamins), minerals (such as iron and calcium), essential fatty acids, and antioxidants like phycocyanin.

Mechanism of Action: The bioactive compounds in Spirulina exert their effects through various mechanisms, including antioxidant activity, modulation of immune function, regulation of lipid metabolism, and anti-inflammatory actions.

Dosage: Recommended dosages of Spirulina vary depending on individual health goals and specific formulations. Typical doses range from 1 to 8 grams per day, divided into several smaller doses.

Contraindications: Individuals with phenylketonuria (PKU) should avoid Spirulina due to its high phenylalanine content. Additionally, those with autoimmune diseases, allergies to seafood, or hypersensitivities to Spirulina should use caution or avoid its consumption.

Precautions: It is advisable to purchase Spirulina supplements from reputable sources to ensure quality and safety. Pregnant or breastfeeding women, as well as individuals with underlying health conditions, should consult a healthcare professional before using Spirulina supplements.

Adverse Reactions: While Spirulina is generally well-tolerated, some individuals may experience mild gastrointestinal symptoms such as nausea, diarrhea, or stomach cramps. Allergic reactions, although rare, can occur in sensitive individuals.

Research Summary: Research on Spirulina has demonstrated its potential health benefits in various areas, including immune support, antioxidant protection, cardiovascular health, weight management, and exercise performance. While many studies show promising results, further research is needed to elucidate its mechanisms of action and optimize its clinical applications.

Pharmacokinetics and Pharmacodynamics: After ingestion, the nutrients and bioactive compounds in Spirulina are absorbed in the gastrointestinal tract and distributed throughout the body. Spirulina's effects on metabolism, immune function, and oxidative stress are mediated by its rich nutritional profile and bioactive constituents.

Overdosage: There is limited information on the effects of overdosing on Spirulina. However, excessive consumption may lead to gastrointestinal discomfort or allergic reactions in sensitive individuals.

International Standing: Spirulina is recognized internationally as a valuable dietary supplement and functional food, with widespread consumption and availability in many countries due to its nutritional benefits and potential health-promoting effects.

Indian Standing: In India, Spirulina is gaining popularity as a nutritional supplement and superfood. It is cultivated and marketed by various organizations to address malnutrition, support public health initiatives, and promote sustainable agriculture.

Research Summary of Spirulina: While Spirulina has been extensively studied for its nutritional composition and potential health benefits, ongoing research aims to further elucidate its therapeutic properties, optimize dosage regimens, and explore its applications in various health conditions, including immune disorders, metabolic syndrome, neurodegenerative diseases, and cancer.

FSSAI Purity Criteria : (Protein (min.) - 55%, carbohydrates (max.)-30%, fats (lipid) ± not more than 10%, minerals (ash)-5-10%, moisture- 3-6% (also fatty acid profile to be mentioned on the package)

Permitted Level : 500 - 3,000 mg / day

41) UNDENATURED TYPE II COLLAGEN

Introduction: Undenatured type II collagen is a form of collagen derived from chicken cartilage. It is known for its potential health benefits, particularly in supporting joint health and relieving symptoms of arthritis.

Synonym Name and Common Name: Synonym Name: UC-II Common Name: Undenatured Collagen Type II

Pharmacognosy / Chemistry: Undenatured type II collagen is a protein extracted from the cartilage of chicken sternum. It undergoes minimal processing to preserve its native structure and bioactivity.

Action and Pharmacology: Undenatured type II collagen works by modulating the immune response in the joints. It helps regulate the production of inflammatory cytokines, thereby reducing joint inflammation and supporting cartilage repair.

Method of Analysis: Analytical methods such as enzyme-linked immunosorbent assay (ELISA) and high-performance liquid chromatography (HPLC) are commonly used to analyze the concentration and purity of undenatured type II collagen in supplements.

Health Benefits: Undenatured type II collagen is primarily used to support joint health and alleviate symptoms of arthritis, including pain, stiffness, and reduced mobility. It may also have benefits for skin health and wound healing.

Indication and Usage: Indications for undenatured type II collagen include osteoarthritis, rheumatoid arthritis, joint pain, and inflammation. It is typically consumed as a dietary supplement in capsule or powder form.

Usual Constituents with Percentages: Undenatured type II collagen is composed mainly of collagen proteins, with type II collagen being the predominant form. The exact percentage of collagen content may vary depending on the source and processing method.

Mechanism of Action: Undenatured type II collagen works by interacting with immune cells in the gut-associated lymphoid tissue (GALT), which helps induce oral tolerance to type II collagen. This process reduces the immune system's overreaction to collagen in the joints, thereby reducing inflammation and preserving joint health.

Dosage: Typical dosages of undenatured type II collagen range from 20 to 40 milligrams per day, although dosages may vary depending on the specific product and individual health needs.

Contraindications: Undenatured type II collagen is generally considered safe for most individuals. However, individuals with allergies to chicken or collagen should avoid its consumption. Pregnant or breastfeeding women should consult a healthcare professional before using collagen supplements.

Precautions: It is important to ensure that undenatured type II collagen supplements are sourced from reputable manufacturers to ensure quality and purity. Individuals with underlying health conditions should consult a healthcare provider before starting supplementation.

Adverse Reactions: While undenatured type II collagen is generally well-tolerated, some individuals may experience mild gastrointestinal symptoms such as bloating, gas, or diarrhea. Allergic reactions are rare but possible in individuals with sensitivities to chicken or collagen.

Research Summary: Research on undenatured type II collagen suggests that it may offer significant benefits for joint health, particularly in reducing inflammation and alleviating symptoms of arthritis. Clinical studies have demonstrated its efficacy in improving joint function, reducing pain, and slowing the progression of joint degeneration.

Pharmacokinetics and Pharmacodynamics: After oral ingestion, undenatured type II collagen is broken down into smaller peptides in the gastrointestinal tract and absorbed into the bloodstream. These peptides then interact with immune cells in the gut-associated lymphoid tissue (GALT), leading to the induction of oral tolerance and modulation of the immune response in the joints.

Overdosage: There is limited information on the effects of overdosing on undenatured type II collagen. However, excessive consumption may increase the risk of gastrointestinal discomfort or allergic reactions in sensitive individuals.

International Standing: Undenatured type II collagen supplements are recognized internationally for their potential health benefits, particularly in supporting joint health and relieving symptoms of arthritis.

Indian Standing: In India, undenatured type II collagen supplements are gaining popularity as a natural remedy for joint pain and arthritis. They are available through various channels, including pharmacies, health food stores, and online retailers.

Research Summary of Undenatured Type II Collagen: Overall, research on undenatured type II collagen supports its efficacy in promoting joint health and alleviating symptoms of arthritis. Clinical studies have demonstrated its ability to reduce inflammation, improve joint function, and enhance the quality of life for individuals with osteoarthritis and rheumatoid arthritis. Further research is ongoing to explore its mechanisms of action and potential applications in other health conditions.

FSSAI Purity Criteria : NA

Permitted Level : 40 mg/day

42) VACCINIUM MYRSTILLUS EXTRACT

Introduction: Vaccinium myrtillus extract is derived from the bilberry plant, a species closely related to blueberries. It has been used for centuries in traditional medicine for its potential health benefits.

Synonym Name and Common Name: Synonym Name: Bilberry extract Common Name: Bilberry

Pharmacognosy / Chemistry: Vaccinium myrtillus extract is obtained from the fruit of the bilberry plant, which is a small, dark-blue berry similar in appearance to blueberries. The extract is typically standardized to contain specific bioactive compounds such as anthocyanins.

Action and Pharmacology: Bilberry extract is rich in anthocyanins, flavonoids, and other antioxidants. It exhibits anti-inflammatory, antioxidant, and vasoprotective properties, which contribute to its various health benefits.

Method of Analysis: Analytical methods such as high-performance liquid chromatography (HPLC) and spectrophotometry are commonly used to quantify the levels of active compounds, particularly anthocyanins, in bilberry extract.

Health Benefits: Bilberry extract is known for its potential to improve vision and eye health, enhance circulation, support cardiovascular health, reduce inflammation, and protect against oxidative damage.

Indication and Usage: Indications for bilberry extract include eye conditions such as macular degeneration, cataracts, and diabetic retinopathy, as well as circulatory disorders, varicose veins, and general antioxidant support.

Usual Constituents with Percentages: Bilberry extract typically contains around 25-36% anthocyanins, along with other flavonoids, phenolic acids, and tannins.

Mechanism of Action: The bioactive compounds in bilberry extract, particularly anthocyanins, exert their effects by scavenging free radicals, reducing inflammation, improving microcirculation, and enhancing antioxidant enzyme activity.

Dosage: Typical dosages of bilberry extract range from 80 to 160 milligrams per day, standardized to contain 25% anthocyanins. However, dosages may vary depending on the specific health condition being targeted.

Contraindications: Bilberry extract is generally considered safe for most individuals. However, individuals with allergies to berries or other plant compounds should use caution. Pregnant or breastfeeding women should consult a healthcare professional before using bilberry extract.

Precautions: It is advisable to purchase bilberry extract from reputable sources to ensure quality and purity. Individuals with underlying health conditions or those taking medications should consult a healthcare provider before starting supplementation.

Adverse Reactions: While bilberry extract is generally well-tolerated, some individuals may experience mild gastrointestinal symptoms such as nausea or upset stomach. Allergic reactions are rare but possible in individuals with sensitivities to berries.

Research Summary: Research on bilberry extract suggests that it may offer various health benefits, particularly in supporting eye health, improving circulation, and providing antioxidant protection. Clinical studies have demonstrated its efficacy in reducing symptoms of eye conditions such as macular degeneration and diabetic retinopathy.

Pharmacokinetics and Pharmacodynamics: After oral ingestion, the bioactive compounds in bilberry extract are absorbed in the gastrointestinal tract and distributed throughout the body. They exert their effects through antioxidant, anti-inflammatory, and vasoprotective mechanisms.

Overdosage: There is limited information on the effects of overdosing on bilberry extract. However, excessive consumption may increase the risk of adverse reactions such as gastrointestinal upset or allergic symptoms.

International Standing: Bilberry extract is recognized internationally for its potential health benefits and is commonly used as a dietary supplement in many countries, particularly in Europe and North America.

Indian Standing: In India, bilberry extract is gaining recognition for its therapeutic properties and is increasingly used in traditional and complementary medicine practices.

Research Summary of Vaccinium myrtillus Extract: Overall, research on bilberry extract supports its potential benefits for vision and eye health, cardiovascular health, and antioxidant protection. Clinical studies have shown promising results in various health conditions, although further research is needed to fully elucidate its mechanisms of action and optimize its clinical applications.

FSSAI Purity Criteria : Anthocyanin content

Permitted Level : 50 - 600 mg / day

43) ZEAXANTHIN

Introduction: Zeaxanthin is a naturally occurring carotenoid pigment found in various fruits and vegetables. It belongs to the xanthophyll family of compounds and is known for its potential health benefits, particularly in supporting eye health.

Synonym Name and Common Name: Synonym Name: β-cryptoxanthin Common Name: Zeaxanthin

Pharmacognosy / Chemistry: Zeaxanthin is a yellow-orange pigment found in plants, algae, and some microorganisms. It is commonly present in foods such as corn, peppers, spinach, and egg yolks.

Action and Pharmacology: Zeaxanthin acts as a powerful antioxidant, protecting cells from oxidative damage caused by free radicals. It also plays a role in filtering harmful blue light and protecting the eyes from age-related macular degeneration (AMD) and other eye conditions.

Method of Analysis: Analytical methods such as high-performance liquid chromatography (HPLC) and spectrophotometry are commonly used to analyze and quantify the levels of zeaxanthin in food products and dietary supplements.

Health Benefits: Zeaxanthin is primarily known for its potential benefits in supporting eye health, particularly in reducing the risk of age-related macular degeneration (AMD), cataracts, and other eye disorders. It may also have antioxidant and anti-inflammatory properties that contribute to overall health and well-being.

Indication and Usage: Indications for zeaxanthin supplementation include age-related macular degeneration (AMD), cataracts, diabetic retinopathy, and general eye health support. It is commonly consumed as a dietary supplement in combination with other carotenoids such as lutein.

Usual Constituents with Percentages: Zeaxanthin is typically found in foods and supplements alongside other carotenoids such as lutein. The exact percentage of zeaxanthin content may vary depending on the source and processing method.

Mechanism of Action: Zeaxanthin acts as an antioxidant by neutralizing free radicals and reducing oxidative stress in the eyes. It also absorbs harmful blue light, protecting the retina from damage and preserving visual acuity.

Dosage: Typical dosages of zeaxanthin range from 2 to 10 milligrams per day, although dosages may vary depending on the specific health condition being targeted and individual health needs.

Contraindications: Zeaxanthin is generally considered safe for most individuals when consumed in recommended amounts from dietary sources or supplements. However, individuals with allergies to carotenoids or other plant compounds should use caution.

Precautions: It is advisable to consult a healthcare professional before starting zeaxanthin supplementation, particularly for individuals with underlying health conditions or those taking medications. Pregnant or breastfeeding women should also seek medical advice.

Adverse Reactions: Zeaxanthin is generally well-tolerated, and adverse reactions are rare. However, some individuals may experience mild gastrointestinal symptoms such as nausea or diarrhea.

Research Summary: Research on zeaxanthin suggests that it may offer significant benefits for eye health, particularly in reducing the risk of age-related macular degeneration (AMD) and other eye conditions. Clinical studies have demonstrated its efficacy in improving visual function and slowing the progression of AMD.

Pharmacokinetics and Pharmacodynamics: After ingestion, zeaxanthin is absorbed in the gastrointestinal tract and transported to various tissues, including the eyes, where it accumulates in the macula. Its antioxidant and light-filtering properties help protect the retina from oxidative damage and blue light-induced stress.

Overdosage: There is limited information on the effects of overdosing on zeaxanthin. However, excessive consumption may increase the risk of adverse effects such as gastrointestinal discomfort or allergic reactions in sensitive individuals.

International Standing: Zeaxanthin is recognized internationally for its potential health benefits, particularly in supporting eye health and preventing age-related macular degeneration (AMD). It is commonly used as a dietary supplement in many countries.

Indian Standing: In India, zeaxanthin is gaining recognition for its therapeutic properties and is increasingly used in dietary supplements marketed for eye health and overall well-being.

Research Summary of Zeaxanthin: Overall, research on zeaxanthin supports its potential benefits for eye health, particularly in reducing the risk of age-related macular degeneration (AMD) and other eye disorders. Clinical studies have shown promising results, although further research is needed to fully elucidate its mechanisms of action and optimize its clinical applications.

FSSAI Purity Criteria : NA

Permitted Level : 4 mg/day

44) CAMELLIA SINENSIS, BLACK /GREEN TEA EXTRACT, STANDARDIZED POWDER

Introduction: Camellia sinensis, commonly known as tea plant, is famous worldwide for its leaves used to produce various types of tea. Black and green tea extracts derived from Camellia sinensis have gained popularity for their potential health benefits.

Synonym Name and Common Name: Synonym Name: Tea extract; Common Name: Black tea extract, Green tea extract

Pharmacognosy / Chemistry: Camellia sinensis extracts are derived from the leaves of the tea plant. Black tea extract is obtained from leaves that have been fermented and oxidized, while green tea extract is derived from unfermented leaves. Both extracts contain bioactive compounds with potential health benefits.

Action and Pharmacology: Black and green tea extracts contain polyphenols, particularly catechins and theaflavins, which exhibit antioxidant, anti-inflammatory, and cardioprotective properties. These compounds help scavenge free radicals, reduce inflammation, and support cardiovascular health.

Method of Analysis: Analytical methods such as high-performance liquid chromatography (HPLC) and spectrophotometry are commonly used to analyze and quantify the levels of polyphenols and other bioactive compounds in black and green tea extracts.

Health Benefits: Black and green tea extracts are associated with various health benefits, including antioxidant protection, cardiovascular health support, weight management, improved cognitive function, and potential cancer prevention.

Indication and Usage: Indications for black and green tea extracts include promoting heart health, boosting metabolism, supporting weight loss, enhancing cognitive function, and providing antioxidant support. They are commonly consumed as dietary supplements or added to food and beverage products.

Usual Constituents with Percentages: Black tea extract typically contains around 20-30% polyphenols, while green tea extract may contain higher percentages of polyphenols, ranging from 30-40%. The specific composition may vary depending on factors such as processing methods and growing conditions.

Mechanism of Action: The polyphenols in black and green tea extracts exert their effects through antioxidant activity, anti-inflammatory mechanisms, and modulation of various signaling pathways involved in cardiovascular health, metabolism, and cognitive function.

Dosage: Typical dosages of black and green tea extracts vary depending on the specific product and desired health outcomes. However, standardized extracts are often dosed in the range of 200-500 milligrams per day.

Contraindications: Individuals with caffeine sensitivity or cardiovascular conditions should use caution when consuming black tea extract, as it contains caffeine. Green tea extract may interact with certain medications or exacerbate liver conditions in high doses.

Precautions: It is advisable to consult a healthcare professional before starting black or green tea extract supplementation, particularly for individuals with underlying health conditions or those taking medications. Pregnant or breastfeeding women should also seek medical advice.

Adverse Reactions: While black and green tea extracts are generally well-tolerated, some individuals may experience side effects such as gastrointestinal discomfort, insomnia, or jitteriness due to their caffeine content. Allergic reactions are rare but possible in sensitive individuals.

Research Summary: Research on black and green tea extracts suggests that they may offer various health benefits, particularly in supporting cardiovascular health, metabolism, cognitive function, and antioxidant protection. Clinical studies have demonstrated their efficacy in improving markers of health and reducing the risk of chronic diseases.

Pharmacokinetics and Pharmacodynamics: After oral ingestion, the bioactive compounds in black and green tea extracts are absorbed in the gastrointestinal tract and distributed throughout the body. They exert their effects through antioxidant mechanisms, modulation of enzyme activity, and interaction with various cellular pathways.

Overdosage: Consuming excessive amounts of black or green tea extract, particularly in concentrated forms, may lead to adverse effects such as insomnia, nervousness, gastrointestinal upset, or increased heart rate due to their caffeine content.

International Standing: Black and green tea extracts are recognized internationally for their potential health benefits and are commonly consumed as dietary supplements or incorporated into food and beverage products.

Indian Standing: In India, black and green tea extracts are gaining popularity for their therapeutic properties and are increasingly used in dietary supplements and functional foods marketed for health and wellness.

Research Summary of Camellia sinensis Black/Green Tea Extract, Standardized Powder: Overall, research on black and green tea extracts supports their potential benefits for cardiovascular health, metabolism, cognitive function, and antioxidant protection. Clinical studies have shown promising results, although further research is needed to fully elucidate their mechanisms of action and optimize their clinical applications.

FSSAI Purity Criteria : NA

Permitted Level : 0.5 g - 2 g/day

45) CAMELLIA SINENSIS-TEA CATECHINS

Introduction: Camellia sinensis, commonly known as tea plant, is widely cultivated for its leaves, which are used to produce various types of tea. Tea catechins are bioactive compounds found in tea leaves, particularly in green tea, and are associated with numerous health benefits.

Synonym Name and Common Name: Synonym Name: Tea polyphenols Common Name: Tea catechins

Pharmacognosy / Chemistry: Tea catechins are polyphenolic compounds found predominantly in the leaves of the Camellia sinensis plant. They belong to the flavonoid family and are abundant in green tea, although smaller amounts can also be found in black and oolong teas.

Action and Pharmacology: Tea catechins exhibit antioxidant, anti-inflammatory, and antimicrobial properties. They also have potential anticancer effects, support cardiovascular health, improve metabolic function, and enhance cognitive function.

Method of Analysis: Analytical methods such as high-performance liquid chromatography (HPLC) and spectrophotometry are commonly used to analyze and quantify the levels of tea catechins in tea leaves, extracts, and dietary supplements.

Health Benefits: Tea catechins are associated with various health benefits, including antioxidant protection, cardiovascular health support, weight management, improved cognitive function, cancer prevention, and antimicrobial activity.

Indication and Usage: Indications for tea catechin supplementation include promoting heart health, supporting weight loss, enhancing cognitive function, reducing the risk of cancer, and providing antioxidant support. They are commonly consumed as dietary supplements or incorporated into food and beverage products.

Usual Constituents with Percentages: Tea catechins include compounds such as epicatechin (EC), epicatechin gallate (ECG), epigallocatechin (EGC), and epigallocatechin gallate (EGCG). EGCG is the most abundant and biologically active catechin, typically comprising around 50-80% of the total catechin content in green tea extracts.

Mechanism of Action: The antioxidant and anti-inflammatory properties of tea catechins help protect cells from oxidative stress and inflammation. They also modulate various signaling pathways involved in metabolism, cardiovascular function, cognitive health, and cancer development.

Dosage: Typical dosages of tea catechin supplements vary depending on the specific product and desired health outcomes. However, standardized extracts are often dosed in the range of 200-500 milligrams per day.

Contraindications: Individuals with caffeine sensitivity or cardiovascular conditions should use caution when consuming tea catechin supplements, as they may contain caffeine. Pregnant or breastfeeding women should also seek medical advice before use.

Precautions: It is advisable to consult a healthcare professional before starting tea catechin supplementation, particularly for individuals with underlying health conditions or those taking medications. Excessive consumption of tea catechins may lead to adverse effects such as gastrointestinal discomfort or caffeine-related side effects.

Adverse Reactions: While tea catechin supplements are generally well-tolerated, some individuals may experience mild side effects such as gastrointestinal upset, insomnia, nervousness, or increased heart rate due to their caffeine content.

Research Summary: Research on tea catechins suggests that they may offer various health benefits, particularly in supporting cardiovascular health, metabolism, cognitive function, cancer prevention, and antioxidant protection. Clinical studies have demonstrated their efficacy in improving markers of health and reducing the risk of chronic diseases.

Pharmacokinetics and Pharmacodynamics: After oral ingestion, tea catechins are absorbed in the gastrointestinal tract and distributed throughout the body. They exert their effects through antioxidant mechanisms, modulation of enzyme activity, and interaction with various cellular pathways involved in health and disease.

Overdosage: Consuming excessive amounts of tea catechins, particularly in concentrated forms, may lead to adverse effects such as gastrointestinal discomfort, insomnia, nervousness, or caffeine-related side effects.

International Standing: Tea catechins are recognized internationally for their potential health benefits and are commonly consumed as dietary supplements or incorporated into food and beverage products.

Indian Standing: In India, tea catechin supplements are gaining recognition for their therapeutic properties and are increasingly used in dietary supplements and functional foods marketed for health and wellness.

Research Summary of Camellia sinensis-Tea Catechins: Overall, research on tea catechins supports their potential benefits for cardiovascular health, metabolism, cognitive function, cancer prevention, and antioxidant protection. Clinical studies have shown promising results, although further research is needed to fully elucidate their mechanisms of action and optimize their clinical applications.

FSSAI Purity Criteria : NA

Permitted Level : 0.7 g/day

Part B

Enzymes

1) ALPHA AMYLASE

Introduction: Alpha-amylase is an enzyme primarily involved in the breakdown of starch and glycogen into simpler sugars such as maltose and glucose. It plays a crucial role in the digestion of carbohydrates in the human body.

Synonym Name and Common Name: Synonym Name: 1,4-alpha-D-glucan glucanohydrolase Common Name: Alpha-amylase

Pharmacognosy/Chemistry: Alpha-amylase is a glycoside hydrolase enzyme that hydrolyzes alpha-1,4 glycosidic bonds in polysaccharides like starch and glycogen. It is produced by various organisms, including humans, animals, plants, and microorganisms. Commercially, it is often derived from microbial or fungal sources.

Action and Pharmacology: Alpha-amylase catalyzes the hydrolysis of starch molecules into smaller polysaccharides, dextrins, and ultimately into maltose and glucose. It initiates the digestion of dietary carbohydrates in the mouth and continues its action in the small intestine, where pancreatic alpha-amylase further breaks down starch into simple sugars for absorption.

Method of Analysis: The activity of alpha-amylase can be measured using various methods, including spectrophotometric assays, iodine-based assays, and enzyme activity assays based on the hydrolysis of starch. These methods determine the rate of starch breakdown by monitoring the release of reducing sugars or changes in starch viscosity.

Health Benefits: Alpha-amylase plays a crucial role in carbohydrate digestion, facilitating the breakdown of dietary starch into absorbable sugars. Adequate activity of alpha-amylase is essential for proper nutrient absorption and energy metabolism. However, excessive or insufficient alpha-amylase activity may contribute to metabolic disorders such as diabetes and obesity.

Indication and Usage: Alpha-amylase is used in various industries, including food and beverage, textile, pharmaceutical, and detergent industries. In food processing, it is employed to convert starch into sugars for sweetening or fermentation processes. In pharmaceuticals, it may be used in digestive enzyme supplements to aid carbohydrate digestion.

Usual Constituents with Percentages: Alpha-amylase is typically produced as a purified enzyme preparation with high specific activity. The exact constituents and percentages may vary depending on the source and manufacturing process. In commercial formulations, alpha-amylase is often standardized to ensure consistent enzyme activity.

Mechanism of Action: Alpha-amylase acts on the alpha-1,4 glycosidic bonds present in starch molecules, breaking them down into shorter oligosaccharides and ultimately into maltose and glucose. This process involves the hydrolysis of the glycosidic bonds through the addition of water molecules, resulting in the cleavage of the polysaccharide chain.

Dosage: The dosage of alpha-amylase depends on its intended use and formulation. In food processing, the amount of enzyme added is based on factors such as the substrate concentration, desired reaction rate, and processing conditions. In pharmaceutical formulations or enzyme supplements, dosages are determined based on the specific activity of the enzyme and the recommended therapeutic or functional effect.

Contraindications: Alpha-amylase supplements are generally safe when used as directed. However, individuals with known allergies to fungal proteins or those with sensitivity to enzyme preparations should avoid products containing alpha-amylase. In rare cases, excessive enzyme activity may lead to gastrointestinal discomfort or allergic reactions.

Precautions: Individuals with pre-existing medical conditions, such as pancreatic disorders or diabetes, should consult with a healthcare professional before using alpha-amylase supplements. Pregnant or breastfeeding women should also seek medical advice before supplementation.

Adverse Reactions: Adverse reactions to alpha-amylase supplements are rare but may include gastrointestinal symptoms such as bloating, gas, abdominal discomfort, or diarrhea, particularly in individuals with sensitive digestive systems. Allergic reactions to enzyme preparations are possible in sensitive individuals and may manifest as skin rash, itching, or respiratory symptoms.

Research Standing: Alpha-amylase is a well-studied enzyme with extensive research supporting its role in carbohydrate digestion and its applications in various industries. Research continues to explore novel sources, purification methods, and applications of alpha-amylase in food processing, biotechnology, and medicine.

Pharmacokinetics and Pharmacodynamics: Alpha-amylase is an enzyme that acts extracellularly in the digestive system, primarily in the mouth and small intestine. It is secreted by the salivary glands and pancreas and functions to hydrolyze starch into simpler sugars. Alpha-amylase activity is influenced by factors such as pH, temperature, substrate concentration, and the presence of inhibitors or activators.

Overdosage: Overconsumption of alpha-amylase supplements beyond recommended dosages may lead to excessive breakdown of starch and subsequent spikes in blood sugar levels. Individuals with conditions such as diabetes should monitor their blood glucose levels closely when using alpha-amylase supplements to avoid hyperglycemia.

2) ALPHA-GALACTOSIDASE

Introduction: Alpha-galactosidase is an enzyme that catalyzes the hydrolysis of alpha-galactosidic bonds in carbohydrates, particularly in complex sugars such as raffinose and stachyose. It is commonly used as a dietary supplement to aid in the digestion of certain foods, particularly those containing oligosaccharides that can cause gas and bloating.

Synonym Name and Common Name: Synonym Name: α-GAL Common Name: Alpha-galactosidase

Pharmacognosy/Chemistry: Alpha-galactosidase is a glycoside hydrolase enzyme that belongs to the family of exoglycosidases. It is produced by various organisms, including humans, plants, and microorganisms. Commercially, it is often derived from microbial sources such as Aspergillus niger.

Action and Pharmacology: Alpha-galactosidase acts by breaking down complex carbohydrates, specifically alpha-galactosides found in certain foods like beans, legumes, and cruciferous vegetables. By hydrolyzing these sugars into simpler forms, it helps alleviate symptoms of gas, bloating, and discomfort associated with their digestion.

Method of Analysis: The activity of alpha-galactosidase can be measured using various enzymatic assays that monitor the hydrolysis of specific substrates such as p-nitrophenyl-alpha-D-galactopyranoside (pNPG). These assays typically involve spectrophotometric or fluorometric detection methods.

Health Benefits: The primary health benefit of alpha-galactosidase is its ability to reduce gastrointestinal discomfort associated with the consumption of certain foods rich in alpha-galactosides. By aiding in the digestion of these complex carbohydrates, it helps alleviate symptoms such as gas, bloating, and abdominal discomfort.

Indication and Usage: Alpha-galactosidase supplements are commonly used to improve digestive health, particularly in individuals who experience gas and bloating after consuming certain foods. They are often taken before meals containing high amounts of alpha-galactosides to prevent or reduce digestive discomfort.

Usual Constituents with Percentages: Alpha-galactosidase supplements typically contain purified enzyme preparations with standardized activity levels. The exact constituents and percentages may vary depending on the formulation and manufacturer.

Mechanism of Action: Alpha-galactosidase catalyzes the hydrolysis of alpha-galactosidic bonds in oligosaccharides such as raffinose and stachyose. This enzymatic reaction results in the breakdown of these complex carbohydrates into simpler sugars that can be readily absorbed and metabolized by the body, reducing the risk of fermentation and gas production in the gut.

Dosage: The dosage of alpha-galactosidase supplements varies depending on the individual's needs and the specific formulation. It is typically recommended to take one or two capsules before meals containing high amounts of alpha-galactosides, such as beans or cruciferous vegetables.

Contraindications: Alpha-galactosidase supplements are generally considered safe for most individuals when taken as directed. However, individuals with known allergies or hypersensitivity to the enzyme or any of its components should avoid its use.

Precautions: It is advisable to consult a healthcare professional before starting alpha-galactosidase supplementation, especially for individuals with underlying medical conditions or those taking medications. Pregnant and breastfeeding women should also seek medical advice before use.

Adverse Reactions: Adverse reactions to alpha-galactosidase supplements are rare but may include mild gastrointestinal symptoms such as nausea, diarrhea, or abdominal cramps. Allergic reactions are possible in sensitive individuals and may manifest as skin rash, itching, or swelling.

Research Standing: Alpha-galactosidase has been extensively studied for its role in improving digestive health and reducing symptoms of gastrointestinal discomfort. Research continues to explore its efficacy, safety, and potential applications in various clinical conditions related to carbohydrate malabsorption and gut health.

Pharmacokinetics and Pharmacodynamics: Alpha-galactosidase is orally administered and acts locally within the gastrointestinal tract. It is not absorbed systemically and exerts its enzymatic activity within the lumen of the small intestine, where it catalyzes the hydrolysis of alpha-galactosides.

Overdosage: Overconsumption of alpha-galactosidase supplements beyond recommended dosages is unlikely to cause serious adverse effects due to its localized action in the gut. However, excessive intake may lead to gastrointestinal upset or diarrhea in some individuals.

3) AMYLASE

Introduction: Amylase is a digestive enzyme that plays a crucial role in the breakdown of complex carbohydrates into simpler sugars, such as starches into maltose and glucose. It is produced in various organs, including the pancreas and salivary glands, and is essential for the digestion and absorption of dietary carbohydrates.

Synonym Name and Common Name: Synonym Name: α-Amylase, pancreatic amylase Common Name: Amylase

Pharmacognosy/Chemistry: Amylase is a type of enzyme classified as a glycoside hydrolase, specifically an endoamylase, which cleaves alpha-1,4-glycosidic linkages in polysaccharides like starch and glycogen. It exists in multiple forms, including alpha-amylase, beta-amylase, and gamma-amylase, each with different substrate specificities and optimal pH ranges.

Action and Pharmacology: Amylase catalyzes the hydrolysis of starch and glycogen molecules, breaking down their complex structures into shorter oligosaccharides and ultimately into glucose and maltose. This enzymatic activity is essential for the digestion and absorption of carbohydrates in the small intestine.

Method of Analysis: The activity of amylase can be measured using various enzymatic assays that monitor the hydrolysis of starch or related substrates. These assays often involve colorimetric or spectrophotometric detection methods to quantify the rate of substrate degradation.

Health Benefits: The primary health benefit of amylase is its role in facilitating the digestion of carbohydrates, ensuring the efficient utilization of dietary starches and glycogen for energy production and metabolic processes.

Indication and Usage: Amylase supplements are not typically used therapeutically but may be prescribed in cases of pancreatic insufficiency or other conditions associated with impaired carbohydrate digestion. In clinical settings, amylase levels in blood or urine may be monitored to diagnose pancreatic disorders or assess digestive function.

Usual Constituents with Percentages: Amylase supplements contain purified enzyme preparations derived from microbial or animal sources, often with standardized activity levels measured in international units (IU) or enzymatic activity units.

Mechanism of Action: Amylase catalyzes the hydrolysis of alpha-1,4-glycosidic bonds in starch and glycogen molecules, cleaving them into shorter polysaccharides, maltose, and glucose. This enzymatic breakdown enhances the accessibility of carbohydrates for further digestion by other enzymes and facilitates their absorption in the small intestine.

Dosage: The dosage of amylase supplements varies depending on the specific indication and formulation. It is typically administered orally in the form of tablets, capsules, or solutions, often in conjunction with other digestive enzymes.

Contraindications: Amylase supplements are generally considered safe for most individuals when taken as directed. However, individuals with known allergies or hypersensitivity to amylase or any of its components should avoid its use.

Precautions: It is advisable to consult a healthcare professional before starting amylase supplementation, especially for individuals with underlying medical conditions or those taking medications. Pregnant and breastfeeding women should also seek medical advice before use.

Adverse Reactions: Adverse reactions to amylase supplements are rare but may include mild gastrointestinal symptoms such as nausea, diarrhea, or abdominal discomfort. Allergic reactions are possible in sensitive individuals and may manifest as skin rash, itching, or swelling.

Research Standing: Amylase is a well-studied enzyme with extensive research conducted on its biochemical properties, physiological functions, and clinical applications. Ongoing research aims to further elucidate its role in carbohydrate metabolism and its potential therapeutic uses in various medical conditions.

Pharmacokinetics and Pharmacodynamics: Amylase is orally administered and acts within the gastrointestinal tract to catalyze the hydrolysis of dietary carbohydrates. It is not absorbed systemically but exerts its enzymatic activity locally in the lumen of the small intestine, where it facilitates carbohydrate digestion.

Overdosage: Overconsumption of amylase supplements beyond recommended dosages is unlikely to cause serious adverse effects due to its localized action in the gut. However, excessive intake may lead to gastrointestinal upset or diarrhea in some individuals.

International Standing: Amylase is recognized as an essential digestive enzyme worldwide and is commonly used in various industries, including food processing, brewing, and pharmaceuticals.

Indian Standing: Amylase supplements are available in the Indian market and are used in clinical practice as needed for digestive support and diagnostic purposes. Research on amylase and its applications is also conducted in Indian academic and medical institutions.

4) AMYLOGLUCOSIDASE

Introduction: Amyloglucosidase, also known as glucoamylase or glucan 1,4-alpha-glucosidase, is an enzyme that catalyzes the hydrolysis of starch and related polysaccharides into glucose molecules. It plays a crucial role in various industrial processes, including food and beverage production, as well as in clinical applications for carbohydrate digestion and analysis.

Synonym Name and Common Name: Synonym Name: Glucoamylase, Glucan 1,4-alpha-glucosidase Common Name: Amyloglucosidase

Pharmacognosy/Chemistry: Amyloglucosidase is a type of glycoside hydrolase enzyme that specifically cleaves alpha-1,4-glycosidic bonds in starch molecules, releasing glucose units. It is produced by various microorganisms, including fungi and bacteria, and is commonly used in industrial processes and research applications.

Action and Pharmacology: Amyloglucosidase acts on starch molecules, breaking down the polysaccharide chains into glucose units through successive hydrolysis of alpha-1,4-glycosidic linkages. This enzymatic activity is essential for the conversion of complex carbohydrates into simpler sugars for energy production and metabolic processes.

Method of Analysis: The activity of amyloglucosidase can be measured using enzymatic assays that monitor the hydrolysis of starch or related substrates, coupled with detection methods such as colorimetry or spectrophotometry. These assays provide quantitative data on enzyme activity and are widely used in research and industrial settings.

Health Benefits: Amyloglucosidase supplementation is not typically used for health benefits but may be beneficial in cases of carbohydrate malabsorption or as a digestive aid for individuals with impaired starch digestion.

Indication and Usage: Amyloglucosidase is used in various industrial processes, including brewing, starch processing, and food production, to facilitate the conversion of starch into glucose and other fermentable sugars. It is also employed in clinical laboratories for carbohydrate analysis and in research applications for enzymatic studies.

Usual Constituents with Percentages: Amyloglucosidase supplements contain purified enzyme preparations derived from microbial sources, often with standardized activity levels measured in enzyme units (e.g., SKB or AGU).

Mechanism of Action: Amyloglucosidase catalyzes the hydrolysis of alpha-1,4-glycosidic bonds in starch molecules, liberating glucose units from the polysaccharide chains. This enzymatic breakdown enhances the availability of glucose for energy metabolism and other cellular processes.

Dosage: The dosage of amyloglucosidase supplements varies depending on the specific application and desired enzymatic activity. It is typically administered in appropriate concentrations for industrial processes or analytical assays.

Contraindications: Amyloglucosidase supplements are generally safe for consumption and do not have specific contraindications. However, individuals with known allergies or hypersensitivity to fungal proteins may experience adverse reactions and should avoid its use.

Precautions: It is advisable to handle amyloglucosidase preparations with care to prevent contamination and maintain enzymatic activity. Standard laboratory safety protocols should be followed when working with this enzyme.

Adverse Reactions: Adverse reactions to amyloglucosidase supplements are rare but may include gastrointestinal symptoms such as bloating, gas, or diarrhea, particularly in individuals with carbohydrate malabsorption or sensitivity.

Research Standing: Amyloglucosidase is a well-studied enzyme with extensive research conducted on its biochemical properties, industrial applications, and potential therapeutic uses. Ongoing research continues to explore its role in carbohydrate metabolism and its applications in various fields.

Pharmacokinetics and Pharmacodynamics : Amyloglucosidase is orally administered and acts within the gastrointestinal tract to catalyze the hydrolysis of starch molecules into glucose. It is not absorbed systemically but exerts its enzymatic activity locally in the intestinal lumen.

Overdosage: Overconsumption of amyloglucosidase supplements is unlikely to cause systemic toxicity due to its localized action in the gut. However, excessive intake may lead to gastrointestinal discomfort or disturbances in carbohydrate metabolism.

International Standing: Amyloglucosidase is recognized internationally as a key enzyme in various industrial processes, including food and beverage production, biofuel manufacturing, and pharmaceutical applications.

Indian Standing: Amyloglucosidase supplements are available in the Indian market and are used in industrial processes and research applications. Research on amyloglucosidase and its enzymatic properties is also conducted in Indian academic and industrial settings.

5)CELLULASE

Introduction: Cellulase is an enzyme that catalyzes the hydrolysis of cellulose, breaking it down into smaller polysaccharides and eventually glucose. It plays a crucial role in various industrial processes and has potential applications in biofuel production, textile manufacturing, and food processing.

Synonym Name and Common Name: Synonym Name: Cellulolytic enzymes Common Name: Cellulase

Pharmacognosy/Chemistry: Cellulase enzymes are produced by various microorganisms, including bacteria and fungi, as well as some plants and animals. They belong to the class of glycoside hydrolase enzymes and consist of multiple subunits with distinct catalytic activities.

Action and Pharmacology: Cellulase catalyzes the hydrolysis of cellulose, breaking the beta-1,4-glycosidic bonds between glucose units in the cellulose polymer. This enzymatic action results in the release of glucose and other oligosaccharides, which can be further metabolized or utilized in various processes.

Method of Analysis: The activity of cellulase can be measured using enzymatic assays that monitor the hydrolysis of cellulose or cellulose analogs, coupled with detection methods such as colorimetry or spectrophotometry. These assays provide quantitative data on enzyme activity and are widely used in research and industrial settings.

Health Benefits: Cellulase supplementation is not typically used for health benefits but may have indirect effects on digestion and nutrient absorption by breaking down dietary cellulose in the gastrointestinal tract.

Indication and Usage: Cellulase is used in various industrial processes, including biofuel production, paper and pulp industry, textile manufacturing, and food processing, to degrade cellulose-containing materials and facilitate the release of sugars and other components.

Usual Constituents with Percentages: Cellulase supplements contain purified enzyme preparations derived from microbial or fungal sources, often with standardized activity levels measured in enzyme units (e.g., FPU or CU).

Mechanism of Action: Cellulase enzymes possess specific domains that bind to cellulose molecules, allowing them to cleave the beta-1,4-glycosidic bonds between glucose units. This enzymatic hydrolysis results in the depolymerization of cellulose into smaller fragments and ultimately glucose.

Dosage: The dosage of cellulase supplements varies depending on the specific application and desired enzymatic activity. It is typically administered in appropriate concentrations for industrial processes or analytical assays.

Contraindications: Cellulase supplements are generally safe for consumption and do not have specific contraindications. However, individuals with known allergies or hypersensitivity to fungal proteins may experience adverse reactions and should avoid its use.

Precautions: It is advisable to handle cellulase preparations with care to prevent contamination and maintain enzymatic activity. Standard laboratory safety protocols should be followed when working with this enzyme.

Adverse Reactions: Adverse reactions to cellulase supplements are rare but may include gastrointestinal symptoms such as bloating, gas, or diarrhea, particularly in individuals with cellulose intolerance or sensitivity.

Research Standing: Cellulase is a well-studied enzyme with extensive research conducted on its biochemical properties, industrial applications, and potential therapeutic uses. Ongoing research continues to explore its role in cellulose degradation, biofuel production, and environmental remediation.

Pharmacokinetics and Pharmacodynamics: Cellulase is orally administered and acts within the gastrointestinal tract to catalyze the hydrolysis of cellulose. It is not absorbed systemically but exerts its enzymatic activity locally in the intestinal lumen or within industrial processes.

Overdosage: Overconsumption of cellulase supplements is unlikely to cause systemic toxicity due to its localized action in the gut or industrial processes. However, excessive intake may lead to gastrointestinal discomfort or disturbances in cellulose metabolism.

International Standing: Cellulase enzymes are recognized internationally as essential catalysts in various industrial processes and research applications. They are widely used in biotechnology, bioenergy, and environmental sectors across the globe.

Indian Standing: Cellulase supplements and research on cellulase enzymes are prevalent in the Indian market and scientific community. India has significant expertise in the production and application of cellulase enzymes for diverse industrial and research purposes.

6) DIASTASE

Introduction: Diastase is an enzyme complex primarily composed of α-amylase and glucoamylase, which catalyzes the hydrolysis of starch into simpler sugars like maltose and glucose. It is widely used in various industries, including food and beverage, pharmaceuticals, and textiles.

Synonym Name and Common Name: Synonym Name: Amylase Common Name: Diastase

Pharmacognosy/Chemistry: Diastase is derived from various sources, including plants, animals, and microorganisms. It consists mainly of α-amylase and glucoamylase enzymes, which belong to the class of glycoside hydrolases. These enzymes act synergistically to break down starch molecules into smaller sugar units.

Action and Pharmacology: Diastase catalyzes the hydrolysis of starch molecules by breaking the α-1,4-glycosidic bonds between glucose units. This enzymatic action results in the production of maltose, maltotriose, and glucose, which can be further metabolized or utilized in various metabolic processes.

Method of Analysis: The activity of diastase can be measured using enzymatic assays that monitor the hydrolysis of starch substrates, coupled with detection methods such as colorimetry or spectrophotometry. These assays provide quantitative data on enzyme activity and are widely used in research and industrial settings.

Health Benefits: Diastase supplementation is not typically used for health benefits, but it may aid in digestion and improve the availability of glucose from starchy foods.

Indication and Usage: Diastase is used in various industrial processes, including brewing, baking, sugar production, and pharmaceutical formulations, to convert starch into fermentable sugars or as a digestive aid in enzyme supplements.

Usual Constituents with Percentages: Diastase preparations typically contain a mixture of α-amylase and glucoamylase enzymes derived from microbial or fungal sources. The activity of these enzymes is measured in enzyme units (e.g., SKB, DU) to indicate their potency.

Mechanism of Action: α-Amylase enzymes in diastase initially hydrolyze the α-1,4-glycosidic bonds in starch molecules, producing maltose, maltotriose, and dextrins. Glucoamylase further breaks down these oligosaccharides into glucose units through the hydrolysis of α-1,4 and α-1,6-glycosidic bonds.

Dosage: The dosage of diastase supplements varies depending on the specific application and desired enzymatic activity. It is typically administered in appropriate concentrations for industrial processes or digestive aid supplements.

Contraindications: Diastase supplements are generally safe for consumption and do not have specific contraindications. However, individuals with known allergies or hypersensitivity to fungal proteins may experience adverse reactions and should avoid its use.

Precautions: It is advisable to handle diastase preparations with care to prevent contamination and maintain enzymatic activity. Standard laboratory safety protocols should be followed when working with this enzyme.

Adverse Reactions: Adverse reactions to diastase supplements are rare but may include gastrointestinal symptoms such as bloating, gas, or diarrhea, particularly in individuals with starch intolerance or sensitivity.

Research Standing: Diastase is a well-studied enzyme complex with extensive research conducted on its biochemical properties, industrial applications, and potential therapeutic uses. Ongoing research continues to explore its role in starch hydrolysis, enzyme kinetics, and biotechnological applications.

Pharmacokinetics and Pharmacodynamics: Diastase is orally administered and acts within the gastrointestinal tract to catalyze the hydrolysis of starch. It is not absorbed systemically but exerts its enzymatic activity locally in the intestinal lumen or within industrial processes.

Overdosage: Overconsumption of diastase supplements is unlikely to cause systemic toxicity due to its localized action in the gut or industrial processes. However, excessive intake may lead to gastrointestinal discomfort or disturbances in starch metabolism.

International Standing: Diastase enzymes are recognized internationally as essential catalysts in various industrial processes, particularly in the food and beverage industry. They are widely used for starch hydrolysis and sugar production worldwide.

Indian Standing: Diastase supplements and research on diastase enzymes are prevalent in the Indian market and scientific community. India has significant expertise in the production and application of diastase enzymes for diverse industrial and research purposes.

7) GLUCOAMYLASE

Introduction: Glucoamylase is an enzyme that belongs to the class of glycoside hydrolases, specifically the family of amylases. It plays a crucial role in catalyzing the hydrolysis of starch and related carbohydrates into glucose molecules. Glucoamylase is widely utilized in various industries, including food and beverage, brewing, and biofuel production.

Synonym Name and Common Name: Synonym Name: Amyloglucosidase Common Name: Glucoamylase

Pharmacognosy/Chemistry: Glucoamylase is derived from various sources, including fungi, bacteria, and yeasts. It is a glycoprotein enzyme composed of amino acids arranged in a specific sequence, forming the active site responsible for substrate binding and catalysis. Glucoamylase is often produced through fermentation processes using microbial strains engineered for high enzyme yields.

Action and Pharmacology: Glucoamylase catalyzes the hydrolysis of α-1,4 and α-1,6-glycosidic bonds present in starch molecules, amylopectin, and related polysaccharides. This enzymatic action releases glucose units from the non-reducing ends of the polysaccharide chains, resulting in the production of maltose and free glucose.

Method of Analysis: The activity of glucoamylase can be quantitatively determined using enzymatic assays that monitor the hydrolysis of starch or maltose substrates coupled with colorimetric or spectrophotometric detection methods. These assays provide valuable information on enzyme activity and kinetics.

Health Benefits: Glucoamylase supplementation is not typically used for direct health benefits but may indirectly support digestive processes by facilitating the breakdown of complex carbohydrates into absorbable glucose units.

Indication and Usage: Glucoamylase is widely used in various industrial applications, including starch processing, brewing, baking, and biofuel production. It is employed to convert starch substrates into fermentable sugars, enhance sugar yields, and improve product quality.

Usual Constituents with Percentages: Glucoamylase preparations typically contain the enzyme as the active ingredient, often in purified form or as a concentrated enzyme extract. The percentage composition of glucoamylase in commercial preparations varies depending on the specific enzyme activity required for a particular application.

Mechanism of Action: Glucoamylase hydrolyzes the α-1,4 and α-1,6-glycosidic bonds present in starch molecules and related polysaccharides. It cleaves these bonds from the non-reducing ends of the polysaccharide chains, releasing glucose units as the primary end product of hydrolysis.

Dosage: The dosage of glucoamylase depends on the specific application and desired enzymatic activity. It is typically used in appropriate concentrations for industrial processes, enzymatic assays, or as a component of enzyme supplements.

Contraindications: Glucoamylase supplements are generally safe for consumption and do not have specific contraindications. However, individuals with known allergies or hypersensitivity to fungal proteins may experience adverse reactions and should avoid its use.

Precautions: It is advisable to handle glucoamylase preparations with care to prevent contamination and maintain enzymatic activity. Standard laboratory safety protocols should be followed when working with this enzyme.

Adverse Reactions: Adverse reactions to glucoamylase supplements are rare but may include gastrointestinal symptoms such as bloating, gas, or diarrhea, particularly in individuals with starch intolerance or sensitivity.

Research Standing: Glucoamylase is a well-studied enzyme with extensive research conducted on its biochemical properties, industrial applications, and potential therapeutic uses. Ongoing research continues to explore its role in starch hydrolysis, enzyme engineering, and biotechnological applications.

Pharmacokinetics and Pharmacodynamics: Glucoamylase is orally administered and acts within the gastrointestinal tract to catalyze the hydrolysis of starch. It is not absorbed systemically but exerts its enzymatic activity locally in the intestinal lumen or within industrial processes.

Overdosage: Overconsumption of glucoamylase supplements is unlikely to cause systemic toxicity due to its localized action in the gut or industrial processes. However, excessive intake may lead to gastrointestinal discomfort or disturbances in carbohydrate metabolism.

International Standing: Glucoamylase enzymes are recognized internationally as essential catalysts in various industrial processes, particularly in the food and beverage industry. They are widely used for starch hydrolysis, sugar production, and biofuel fermentation worldwide.

Indian Standing: Glucoamylase supplements and research on glucoamylase enzymes are prevalent in the Indian market and scientific community. India has significant expertise in the production and application of glucoamylase enzymes for diverse industrial and research purposes.

8) HEMICELLULASE

Introduction: Hemicellulase is an enzyme that plays a crucial role in the breakdown of hemicellulose, a complex carbohydrate found in plant cell walls. It belongs to the class of carbohydrase enzymes and is widely used in various industrial and biomedical applications due to its ability to hydrolyze hemicellulose into simpler sugars.

Synonym Name and Common Name: Synonym: Xylanase Common Name: Hemicellulase

Pharmacognosy/Chemistry: Hemicellulase is a glycoside hydrolase enzyme that specifically targets the bonds within hemicellulose molecules. It is produced by various microorganisms, including bacteria and fungi, and can be extracted from their cultures for commercial use. The enzyme is a proteinaceous substance with a specific tertiary structure critical for its catalytic activity.

Action and Pharmacology: Hemicellulase acts by breaking down the glycosidic bonds present in hemicellulose molecules, thereby releasing simple sugars like xylose, glucose, and mannose. This enzymatic action facilitates the conversion of complex plant materials into fermentable sugars, which can be utilized in industries such as biofuel production, food processing, and animal feed.

Method of Analysis: The activity of hemicellulase can be determined using various analytical methods, including spectrophotometry, chromatography, and enzymatic assays. These methods assess the enzyme's ability to hydrolyze hemicellulose substrates and measure the rate of sugar release.

Health Benefits: Hemicellulase supplementation may offer several health benefits, including improved digestion of dietary fiber, enhanced nutrient absorption, and relief from digestive discomforts like bloating and gas. Additionally, hemicellulase enzymes may help individuals with dietary restrictions, such as those following a high-fiber or plant-based diet.

Indication and Usage: Hemicellulase supplements are commonly used to support digestive health and optimize the breakdown of dietary fibers from plant sources. They are often included in digestive enzyme formulations or taken as standalone supplements to aid in the digestion of high-fiber meals.

Usual Constituents with Percentages: The usual constituents of hemicellulase supplements typically include the enzyme hemicellulase itself, often derived from microbial sources such as Aspergillus niger or Trichoderma reesei. The percentages of hemicellulase enzyme in commercial formulations can vary depending on the product and manufacturer.

Mechanism of Action: Hemicellulase functions by catalyzing the hydrolysis of the glycosidic bonds in hemicellulose molecules, leading to the breakdown of complex polysaccharides into simpler sugars. This enzymatic process enhances the accessibility of nutrients encapsulated within plant cell walls, promoting their absorption and utilization by the body.

Dosage: The recommended dosage of hemicellulase supplements can vary depending on factors such as the individual's dietary habits, digestive health, and specific needs. It is advisable to follow the dosage instructions provided by the manufacturer or consult a healthcare professional for personalized recommendations.

Contraindications: Individuals with known allergies or sensitivities to microbial enzymes or any components of hemicellulase supplements should avoid their use. Additionally, individuals with certain medical conditions or those taking medications should consult a healthcare provider before starting hemicellulase supplementation.

Precautions: It is important to use hemicellulase supplements as directed and avoid exceeding the recommended dosage. Pregnant or nursing women, as well as children, should consult a healthcare professional before using hemicellulase supplements. Additionally, individuals with digestive disorders or gastrointestinal issues should seek medical advice before supplementation.

Adverse Reactions: Although rare, potential adverse reactions to hemicellulase supplements may include gastrointestinal discomfort, such as bloating, gas, or diarrhea. Individuals experiencing persistent or severe adverse effects should discontinue use and consult a healthcare provider.

Research Standing: Research on the efficacy and safety of hemicellulase supplementation is ongoing, with studies exploring its potential benefits for digestive health, nutrient absorption, and dietary management. While some research supports the use of hemicellulase enzymes for improving digestion and gastrointestinal function, further clinical trials are needed to establish its effectiveness conclusively.

Pharmacokinetics and Pharmacodynamics: The pharmacokinetics and pharmacodynamics of hemicellulase enzymes involve their interaction with dietary hemicellulose substrates in the gastrointestinal tract. Following oral ingestion, hemicellulase enzymes exert their catalytic activity within the digestive system, facilitating the hydrolysis of hemicellulose molecules into absorbable sugars.

Overdosage: Overdosage of hemicellulase supplements may lead to excessive enzymatic activity in the gastrointestinal tract, potentially causing digestive discomfort, diarrhea, or nutrient malabsorption. It is essential to adhere to recommended dosages and usage guidelines to minimize the risk of adverse effects.

International Standing: Hemicellulase supplements are available internationally and are commonly used in various industries, including food processing, biofuel production, and animal feed. Regulatory standards and guidelines for hemicellulase products may vary across different countries and regions.

Indian Standing: In India, hemicellulase supplements are gaining popularity as digestive aids and dietary supplements. They are available in various forms, including capsules, tablets, and powders, and are marketed for their digestive health benefits.

Research Summary: Research on hemicellulase enzymes encompasses a wide range of applications, from industrial processes to biomedical uses. Studies have investigated their role in enhancing the efficiency of biofuel production, improving the digestibility of animal feed, and optimizing the extraction of valuable compounds from plant materials. Additionally, research continues to explore the potential therapeutic benefits of hemicellulase supplementation for digestive disorders, metabolic health, and overall well-being.

9) INVERTASE

Introduction: Invertase is an enzyme essential for the hydrolysis of sucrose into its constituent monosaccharides, glucose, and fructose. This enzymatic process is pivotal in various biological and industrial processes, including carbohydrate metabolism in living organisms and the production of sweeteners and confectionery.

Synonym Name and Common Name: Synonym: β-fructofuranosidase Common Name: Invertase

Pharmacognosy/Chemistry: Invertase belongs to the class of glycoside hydrolase enzymes and is widely distributed in nature, found in microorganisms, plants, and animals. It is a proteinaceous substance with a specific tertiary structure crucial for its catalytic activity. Commercially, invertase is often derived from yeast sources such as Saccharomyces cerevisiae.

Action and Pharmacology: Invertase catalyzes the hydrolysis of sucrose, a disaccharide composed of glucose and fructose, into its monosaccharide components. This enzymatic action increases the availability of glucose and fructose for absorption and utilization in various metabolic pathways. Invertase is essential for carbohydrate digestion and energy metabolism in living organisms.

Method of Analysis: The activity of invertase can be determined using various analytical methods, including spectrophotometry, chromatography, and enzymatic assays. These methods assess the enzyme's ability to hydrolyze sucrose substrates and measure the rate of glucose and fructose release.

Health Benefits: Invertase supplementation may offer several health benefits, including improved digestion of sucrose-containing foods, enhanced nutrient absorption, and regulation of blood sugar levels. Additionally, invertase enzymes may be used to alleviate digestive discomfort associated with sucrose intolerance or malabsorption.

Indication and Usage: Invertase supplements are commonly used to support digestive health and optimize the breakdown of sucrose in the diet. They are often included in digestive enzyme formulations or taken as standalone supplements to aid in the digestion of sucrose-rich foods and beverages.

Usual Constituents with Percentages: The usual constituents of invertase supplements typically include the enzyme invertase itself, derived from microbial sources such as yeast. The percentages of invertase enzyme in commercial formulations can vary depending on the product and manufacturer.

Mechanism of Action: Invertase functions by catalyzing the hydrolysis of the glycosidic bond in sucrose molecules, resulting in the cleavage of the disaccharide into its constituent monosaccharides, glucose, and fructose. This enzymatic process increases the availability of simple sugars for absorption and utilization by the body.

Dosage: The recommended dosage of invertase supplements can vary depending on factors such as the individual's dietary habits, digestive health, and specific needs. It is advisable to follow the dosage instructions provided by the manufacturer or consult a healthcare professional for personalized recommendations.

Contraindications: Individuals with known allergies or sensitivities to yeast-derived products or any components of invertase supplements should avoid their use. Additionally, individuals with certain medical conditions or those taking medications should consult a healthcare provider before starting invertase supplementation.

Precautions: It is important to use invertase supplements as directed and avoid exceeding the recommended dosage. Pregnant or nursing women, as well as children, should consult a healthcare professional before using invertase supplements. Additionally, individuals with digestive disorders or gastrointestinal issues should seek medical advice before supplementation.

Adverse Reactions: Although rare, potential adverse reactions to invertase supplements may include gastrointestinal discomfort, such as bloating, gas, or diarrhea. Individuals experiencing persistent or severe adverse effects should discontinue use and consult a healthcare provider.

Research Standing: Research on the efficacy and safety of invertase supplementation is ongoing, with studies exploring its potential benefits for digestive health, nutrient absorption, and carbohydrate metabolism. While some research supports the use of invertase enzymes for improving sucrose digestion and gastrointestinal function, further clinical trials are needed to establish its effectiveness conclusively.

Pharmacokinetics and Pharmacodynamics: The pharmacokinetics and pharmacodynamics of invertase enzymes involve their interaction with dietary sucrose substrates in the gastrointestinal tract. Following oral ingestion, invertase enzymes exert their catalytic activity within the digestive system, facilitating the hydrolysis of sucrose molecules into absorbable glucose and fructose.

Overdosage: Overdosage of invertase supplements may lead to excessive enzymatic activity in the gastrointestinal tract, potentially causing digestive discomfort, diarrhea, or nutrient malabsorption. It is essential to adhere to recommended dosages and usage guidelines to minimize the risk of adverse effects.

International Standing: Invertase supplements are available internationally and are commonly used in various industries, including food processing, beverage production, and pharmaceuticals. Regulatory standards and guidelines for invertase products may vary across different countries and regions.

Indian Standing: In India, invertase supplements are utilized in food processing and confectionery industries for their ability to hydrolyze sucrose and produce invert sugar. They are also available as digestive enzyme supplements for individuals seeking support for sucrose digestion and gastrointestinal health.

Research Summary: Research on invertase enzymes spans various fields, including food science, biotechnology, and medicine. Studies have investigated their role in improving sucrose digestion, enhancing the shelf life of food products, and optimizing industrial processes for sugar production. Additionally, research continues to explore the potential therapeutic benefits of invertase supplementation for individuals with digestive disorders, metabolic conditions, and carbohydrate intolerance.

10) LACTOPEROXIDASE

Introduction: Lactoperoxidase is an enzyme found in various mammalian secretions, including milk, saliva, and tears. It plays a crucial role in innate immunity and antimicrobial defense by catalyzing the oxidation of thiocyanate ions in the presence of hydrogen peroxide, resulting in the generation of antimicrobial compounds.

Synonym Name and Common Name: Synonym: Salivary peroxidase Common Name: Lactoperoxidase

Pharmacognosy/Chemistry: Lactoperoxidase is a heme-containing glycoprotein enzyme belonging to the peroxidase family. It is structurally similar to other mammalian peroxidases and contains a prosthetic heme group essential for its catalytic activity. Lactoperoxidase is primarily isolated from milk sources, particularly bovine milk.

Action and Pharmacology: Lactoperoxidase acts as a natural antimicrobial agent by catalyzing the oxidation of thiocyanate ions in the presence of hydrogen peroxide, generating hypothiocyanite, a potent antimicrobial compound. This enzymatic process inhibits the growth of bacteria, fungi, and other microorganisms, contributing to the preservation of milk and other biological fluids.

Method of Analysis: The activity of lactoperoxidase can be determined using various analytical methods, including spectrophotometry, enzymatic assays, and immunoassays. These methods assess the enzyme's ability to catalyze the oxidation of substrates and measure the production of antimicrobial compounds.

Health Benefits: Lactoperoxidase supplementation may offer several health benefits, including enhanced antimicrobial protection, improved oral health, and support for immune function. Additionally, lactoperoxidase enzymes may be used in various industrial and biomedical applications, including food preservation and wound care.

Indication and Usage: Lactoperoxidase supplements are commonly used to support oral and dental health, enhance immune function, and provide natural antimicrobial protection. They may be included in oral care products such as mouthwashes and toothpaste or taken as dietary supplements to promote overall well-being.

Usual Constituents with Percentages: The usual constituents of lactoperoxidase supplements typically include the enzyme lactoperoxidase itself, derived from milk or other mammalian sources. The percentages of lactoperoxidase enzyme in commercial formulations can vary depending on the product and manufacturer.

Mechanism of Action: Lactoperoxidase functions by catalyzing the oxidation of thiocyanate ions in the presence of hydrogen peroxide, leading to the production of hypothiocyanite, a reactive antimicrobial compound. This enzymatic process inhibits the growth and proliferation of microorganisms, thereby contributing to innate immunity and antimicrobial defense.

Dosage: The recommended dosage of lactoperoxidase supplements can vary depending on factors such as the individual's health status, age, and specific needs. It is advisable to follow the dosage instructions provided by the manufacturer or consult a healthcare professional for personalized recommendations.

Contraindications: Individuals with known allergies or sensitivities to milk proteins or any components of lactoperoxidase supplements should avoid their use. Additionally, individuals with certain medical conditions or those taking medications should consult a healthcare provider before starting lactoperoxidase supplementation.

Precautions: It is important to use lactoperoxidase supplements as directed and avoid exceeding the recommended dosage. Pregnant or nursing women, as well as children, should consult a healthcare professional before using lactoperoxidase supplements. Additionally, individuals with compromised immune function or chronic health conditions should seek medical advice before supplementation.

Adverse Reactions: Although rare, potential adverse reactions to lactoperoxidase supplements may include allergic reactions, gastrointestinal discomfort, or skin irritation. Individuals experiencing persistent or severe adverse effects should discontinue use and consult a healthcare provider.

Research Standing: Research on the efficacy and safety of lactoperoxidase supplementation is ongoing, with studies investigating its potential benefits for oral health, immune function, and antimicrobial defense. While some research supports the use of lactoperoxidase enzymes for promoting oral hygiene and inhibiting microbial growth, further clinical trials are needed to establish its effectiveness conclusively.

Pharmacokinetics and Pharmacodynamics: The pharmacokinetics and pharmacodynamics of lactoperoxidase enzymes involve their interaction with substrates and cofactors in biological fluids and tissues. Following oral ingestion or topical application, lactoperoxidase enzymes exert their antimicrobial activity locally, contributing to innate immunity and antimicrobial defense mechanisms.

Overdosage: Overdosage of lactoperoxidase supplements is unlikely due to their natural occurrence in biological fluids and tissues. However, excessive supplementation may lead to imbalances in microbial flora or allergic reactions in sensitive individuals. It is essential to adhere to recommended dosages and usage guidelines to minimize the risk of adverse effects.

International Standing: Lactoperoxidase supplements are available internationally and are commonly used in various industries, including food processing, oral care, and pharmaceuticals. Regulatory standards and guidelines for lactoperoxidase products may vary across different countries and regions.

Indian Standing: In India, lactoperoxidase enzymes are utilized in food processing and preservation, particularly in the dairy industry. They are also included in oral care products and dietary supplements for their antimicrobial properties and potential health benefits.

Research Summary: Research on lactoperoxidase enzymes encompasses a wide range of applications, including food preservation, oral care, and biomedical uses. Studies have investigated their role in inhibiting microbial growth, promoting oral hygiene, and enhancing immune function. Additionally, research continues to explore the potential therapeutic benefits of lactoperoxidase supplementation for individuals with oral infections, immune disorders, and microbial imbalances.

11) LIPASE

Introduction: Lipase is an enzyme that plays a crucial role in the digestion and metabolism of dietary fats. It catalyzes the hydrolysis of triglycerides into fatty acids and glycerol, facilitating their absorption and utilization by the body. Lipase enzymes are produced in various organs, including the pancreas, liver, and stomach, and are essential for lipid digestion and nutrient absorption.

Synonym Name and Common Name: Synonym: Triacylglycerol lipase Common Name: Lipase

Pharmacognosy/Chemistry: Lipase is a type of hydrolase enzyme belonging to the class of esterases. It is a proteinaceous substance with a specific tertiary structure critical for its catalytic activity. Lipase enzymes are produced by various organisms, including humans, animals, plants, and microorganisms, and play diverse roles in lipid metabolism and cellular function.

Action and Pharmacology: Lipase catalyzes the hydrolysis of triglycerides, the primary constituents of dietary fats, into fatty acids and glycerol. This enzymatic process occurs in the gastrointestinal tract and is essential for the digestion and absorption of dietary lipids. Lipase enzymes also play a role in various metabolic pathways, including lipid metabolism and energy production.

Method of Analysis: The activity of lipase can be determined using various analytical methods, including spectrophotometry, chromatography, and enzymatic assays. These methods assess the enzyme's ability to hydrolyze triglyceride substrates and measure the rate of fatty acid release.

Health Benefits: Lipase supplementation may offer several health benefits, including improved digestion of dietary fats, enhanced nutrient absorption, and support for gastrointestinal health. Additionally, lipase enzymes may be used in various industrial and biomedical applications, including food processing, pharmaceuticals, and biotechnology.

Indication and Usage: Lipase supplements are commonly used to support digestive health and optimize the breakdown of dietary fats. They may be included in digestive enzyme formulations or taken as standalone supplements to aid in the digestion of high-fat meals and alleviate symptoms of fat malabsorption.

Usual Constituents with Percentages: The usual constituents of lipase supplements typically include the enzyme lipase itself, derived from microbial or animal sources. The percentages of lipase enzyme in commercial formulations can vary depending on the product and manufacturer.

Mechanism of Action: Lipase functions by catalyzing the hydrolysis of ester bonds in triglyceride molecules, leading to the cleavage of fatty acids from the glycerol backbone. This enzymatic process increases the solubility of dietary fats and enhances their absorption across the intestinal mucosa, facilitating their utilization by the body.

Dosage: The recommended dosage of lipase supplements can vary depending on factors such as the individual's dietary habits, digestive health, and specific needs. It is advisable to follow the dosage instructions provided by the manufacturer or consult a healthcare professional for personalized recommendations.

Contraindications: Individuals with known allergies or sensitivities to microbial or animal-derived enzymes or any components of lipase supplements should avoid their use. Additionally, individuals with certain medical conditions or those taking medications should consult a healthcare provider before starting lipase supplementation.

Precautions: It is important to use lipase supplements as directed and avoid exceeding the recommended dosage. Pregnant or nursing women, as well as children, should consult a healthcare professional before using lipase supplements. Additionally, individuals with digestive disorders or gastrointestinal issues should seek medical advice before supplementation.

Adverse Reactions: Although rare, potential adverse reactions to lipase supplements may include gastrointestinal discomfort, such as bloating, gas, or diarrhea. Individuals experiencing persistent or severe adverse effects should discontinue use and consult a healthcare provider.

Research Standing: Research on the efficacy and safety of lipase supplementation is ongoing, with studies exploring its potential benefits for digestive health, nutrient absorption, and fat metabolism. While some research supports the use of lipase enzymes for improving fat digestion and gastrointestinal function, further clinical trials are needed to establish its effectiveness conclusively.

Pharmacokinetics and Pharmacodynamics: The pharmacokinetics and pharmacodynamics of lipase enzymes involve their interaction with dietary fats and lipids in the gastrointestinal tract. Following oral ingestion, lipase enzymes exert their catalytic activity within the digestive system, facilitating the hydrolysis of triglyceride molecules into absorbable fatty acids and glycerol.

Overdosage: Overdosage of lipase supplements may lead to excessive enzymatic activity in the gastrointestinal tract, potentially causing digestive discomfort or diarrhea. It is essential to adhere to recommended dosages and usage guidelines to minimize the risk of adverse effects.

International Standing: Lipase supplements are available internationally and are commonly used in various industries, including food processing, pharmaceuticals, and healthcare. Regulatory standards and guidelines for lipase products may vary across different countries and regions.

Indian Standing: In India, lipase enzymes are utilized in food processing, pharmaceuticals, and healthcare for their role in lipid digestion and metabolism. They are also included in digestive enzyme formulations and dietary supplements for individuals seeking support for fat digestion and gastrointestinal health.

Research Summary: Research on lipase enzymes spans various fields, including food science, nutrition, and medicine. Studies have investigated their role in improving fat digestion, enhancing nutrient absorption, and supporting gastrointestinal function. Additionally, research continues to explore the potential therapeutic benefits of lipase supplementation for individuals with digestive disorders, metabolic conditions, and fat malabsorption syndromes.

12) MALTASE

Introduction: Maltase is an enzyme essential for the hydrolysis of maltose, a disaccharide composed of two glucose molecules. It plays a crucial role in carbohydrate digestion and metabolism, breaking down maltose into its constituent glucose units for absorption and utilization by the body.

Synonym Name and Common Name: Synonym: α-glucosidase Common Name: Maltase

Pharmacognosy/Chemistry: Maltase is a glycoside hydrolase enzyme that specifically targets the α-1,4-glycosidic bond in maltose molecules. It is produced by various organisms, including humans, animals, plants, and microorganisms, and is involved in carbohydrate metabolism and energy production.

Action and Pharmacology: Maltase catalyzes the hydrolysis of maltose, releasing glucose molecules as a result. This enzymatic process occurs in the small intestine, where maltase enzymes are secreted by the intestinal mucosa and brush border cells. The liberated glucose is then absorbed across the intestinal lining and utilized by the body for energy.

Method of Analysis: The activity of maltase can be determined using various analytical methods, including spectrophotometry, chromatography, and enzymatic assays. These methods assess the enzyme's ability to hydrolyze maltose substrates and measure the rate of glucose release.

Health Benefits: Maltase supplementation may offer several health benefits, including improved digestion of maltose-containing foods, enhanced nutrient absorption, and support for carbohydrate metabolism. Additionally, maltase enzymes may be used in various industrial and biomedical applications, including food processing, pharmaceuticals, and biotechnology.

Indication and Usage: Maltase supplements are commonly used to support digestive health and optimize the breakdown of maltose in the diet. They may be included in digestive enzyme formulations or taken as standalone supplements to aid in the digestion of maltose-rich foods and alleviate symptoms of carbohydrate intolerance.

Usual Constituents with Percentages: The usual constituents of maltase supplements typically include the enzyme maltase itself, derived from microbial or plant sources. The percentages of maltase enzyme in commercial formulations can vary depending on the product and manufacturer.

Mechanism of Action: Maltase functions by catalyzing the hydrolysis of the α-1,4-glycosidic bond in maltose molecules, leading to the release of glucose units. This enzymatic process increases the availability of glucose for absorption across the intestinal lining, facilitating its utilization by the body for energy production and metabolic processes.

Dosage: The recommended dosage of maltase supplements can vary depending on factors such as the individual's dietary habits, digestive health, and specific needs. It is advisable to follow the dosage instructions provided by the manufacturer or consult a healthcare professional for personalized recommendations.

Contraindications: Individuals with known allergies or sensitivities to microbial or plant-derived enzymes or any components of maltase supplements should avoid their use. Additionally, individuals with certain medical conditions or those taking medications should consult a healthcare provider before starting maltase supplementation.

Precautions: It is important to use maltase supplements as directed and avoid exceeding the recommended dosage. Pregnant or nursing women, as well as children, should consult a healthcare professional before using maltase supplements. Additionally, individuals with digestive disorders or gastrointestinal issues should seek medical advice before supplementation.

Adverse Reactions: Although rare, potential adverse reactions to maltase supplements may include gastrointestinal discomfort, such as bloating, gas, or diarrhea. Individuals experiencing persistent or severe adverse effects should discontinue use and consult a healthcare provider.

Research Standing: Research on the efficacy and safety of maltase supplementation is ongoing, with studies exploring its potential benefits for digestive health, nutrient absorption, and carbohydrate metabolism. While some research supports the use of maltase enzymes for improving maltose digestion and gastrointestinal function, further clinical trials are needed to establish its effectiveness conclusively.

Pharmacokinetics and Pharmacodynamics: The pharmacokinetics and pharmacodynamics of maltase enzymes involve their interaction with maltose substrates in the gastrointestinal tract. Following oral ingestion, maltase enzymes exert their catalytic activity within the digestive system, facilitating the hydrolysis of maltose molecules into absorbable glucose units.

Overdosage: Overdosage of maltase supplements is unlikely due to their natural occurrence in the body and food sources. However, excessive supplementation may lead to imbalances in carbohydrate metabolism or gastrointestinal discomfort. It is essential to adhere to recommended dosages and usage guidelines to minimize the risk of adverse effects.

International Standing: Maltase supplements are available internationally and are commonly used in various industries, including food processing, pharmaceuticals, and healthcare. Regulatory standards and guidelines for maltase products may vary across different countries and regions.

Indian Standing: In India, maltase enzymes are utilized in food processing, pharmaceuticals, and healthcare for their role in carbohydrate digestion and metabolism. They are also included in digestive enzyme formulations and dietary supplements for individuals seeking support for maltose digestion and gastrointestinal health.

Research Summary: Research on maltase enzymes encompasses a wide range of applications, including food science, nutrition, and medicine. Studies have investigated their role in improving maltose digestion, enhancing nutrient absorption, and supporting gastrointestinal function. Additionally, research continues to explore the potential therapeutic benefits of maltase supplementation for individuals with digestive disorders, metabolic conditions, and carbohydrate intolerance.

13) NATTOKINASE ENZYME

Introduction: Nattokinase is a potent fibrinolytic enzyme derived from the traditional Japanese food natto, which is made from fermented soybeans. It has gained attention for its potential health benefits, particularly in supporting cardiovascular health and promoting blood circulation.

Synonym Name and Common Name: Synonym: Subtilisin NAT Common Name: Nattokinase

Pharmacognosy/Chemistry: Nattokinase is a serine protease enzyme belonging to the subtilisin family. It is produced by the bacterium Bacillus subtilis during the fermentation process of soybeans to produce natto. Nattokinase is a proteinaceous substance with a specific tertiary structure essential for its enzymatic activity.

Action and Pharmacology: Nattokinase exhibits potent fibrinolytic activity, meaning it has the ability to dissolve fibrin, a protein involved in blood clot formation. By breaking down fibrin, nattokinase promotes blood flow and helps maintain healthy circulation. Additionally, nattokinase may have antithrombotic and anti-inflammatory effects, further contributing to its cardiovascular benefits.

Method of Analysis: The activity of nattokinase can be determined using various analytical methods, including chromogenic assays, fibrin plate assays, and enzyme-linked immunosorbent assays (ELISA). These methods assess the enzyme's ability to degrade fibrin substrates and measure its fibrinolytic activity.

Health Benefits: Nattokinase supplementation may offer several health benefits, including improved cardiovascular health, enhanced blood circulation, and support for overall vascular function. Additionally, nattokinase has been studied for its potential role in reducing blood viscosity, lowering blood pressure, and preventing thrombotic events.

Indication and Usage: Nattokinase supplements are commonly used to support cardiovascular health and promote blood flow. They may be recommended for individuals at risk of cardiovascular disease, thrombotic events, or those seeking to maintain healthy blood circulation. Nattokinase is often included in heart health formulations or taken as a standalone supplement.

Usual Constituents with Percentages: The usual constituents of nattokinase supplements primarily include the enzyme nattokinase itself, derived from fermentation of Bacillus subtilis cultures. The percentages of nattokinase enzyme in commercial formulations can vary depending on the product and manufacturer.

Mechanism of Action: Nattokinase functions by breaking down fibrin, a key component of blood clots, through its potent fibrinolytic activity. This enzymatic process dissolves existing blood clots and prevents their formation, leading to improved blood flow and reduced risk of thrombotic events.

Dosage: The recommended dosage of nattokinase supplements can vary depending on factors such as the individual's health status, cardiovascular risk factors, and specific needs. It is advisable to follow the dosage instructions provided by the manufacturer or consult a healthcare professional for personalized recommendations.

Contraindications: Individuals with known bleeding disorders, those taking anticoagulant or antiplatelet medications, or undergoing surgery should avoid nattokinase supplementation without consulting a healthcare professional.

Additionally, individuals with hypersensitivity to soy or any components of nattokinase supplements should avoid their use.

Precautions: It is important to use nattokinase supplements cautiously, especially in individuals with bleeding disorders or those taking anticoagulant medications. Pregnant or nursing women, as well as individuals with certain medical conditions, should consult a healthcare professional before using nattokinase supplements.

Adverse Reactions: Although rare, potential adverse reactions to nattokinase supplements may include gastrointestinal discomfort, allergic reactions, or increased risk of bleeding in susceptible individuals. Individuals experiencing persistent or severe adverse effects should discontinue use and seek medical attention.

Research Standing: Research on the efficacy and safety of nattokinase supplementation is ongoing, with studies investigating its potential benefits for cardiovascular health, blood circulation, and thrombosis prevention. While some research supports the use of nattokinase for improving fibrinolysis and reducing cardiovascular risk, further clinical trials are needed to establish its effectiveness conclusively.

Pharmacokinetics and Pharmacodynamics: The pharmacokinetics and pharmacodynamics of nattokinase involve its absorption, distribution, metabolism, and elimination within the body. Following oral ingestion, nattokinase is absorbed from the gastrointestinal tract and exerts its fibrinolytic activity in the bloodstream, promoting the breakdown of fibrin and improving blood flow.

Overdosage: Overdosage of nattokinase supplements may increase the risk of bleeding or hemorrhagic events, particularly in individuals with bleeding disorders or those taking anticoagulant medications. It is essential to adhere to recommended dosages and usage guidelines to minimize the risk of adverse effects.

International Standing: Nattokinase supplements are available internationally and are commonly used in various countries, particularly in Asia and North America, for their cardiovascular benefits. Regulatory standards and guidelines for nattokinase products may vary across different regions.

Indian Standing: In India, nattokinase supplements are gaining popularity for their potential cardiovascular benefits and blood clot prevention. They are available through online retailers and specialty health stores, and their usage is increasing among individuals seeking natural alternatives for heart health support.

Research Summary: Research on nattokinase encompasses a broad range of studies, including in vitro, animal, and clinical trials. Studies have investigated its fibrinolytic activity, cardiovascular effects, and potential therapeutic applications for conditions such as thrombosis, hypertension, and atherosclerosis. While some research supports the cardiovascular benefits of nattokinase supplementation, further clinical evidence is needed to validate its efficacy and safety for widespread use.

14) PANCREATIN

Introduction: Pancreatin is a mixture of digestive enzymes derived from the pancreas of animals, usually pigs or cows. It contains several enzymes, including amylase, lipase, and protease, which play essential roles in the digestion and absorption of carbohydrates, fats, and proteins.

Synonym Name and Common Name: Synonym: Pancreatic enzyme Common Name: Pancreatin

Pharmacognosy/Chemistry: Pancreatin is a complex mixture of enzymes produced by the exocrine cells of the pancreas. It contains primarily amylase, lipase, and protease enzymes, along with other minor enzymes and cofactors. Pancreatin is available in both powdered and tablet forms for medicinal and dietary supplement use.

Action and Pharmacology: Pancreatin enzymes facilitate the breakdown of complex nutrients, including carbohydrates, fats, and proteins, into smaller molecules that can be absorbed by the intestines. This enzymatic action is essential for proper digestion and nutrient absorption, ensuring the body receives essential nutrients for energy and cellular function.

Method of Analysis: The activity of pancreatin enzymes can be determined using various analytical methods, including enzymatic assays, chromatography, and spectrophotometry. These methods assess the enzyme's ability to hydrolyze specific substrates and measure the rate of digestion under controlled conditions.

Health Benefits: Pancreatin supplementation may offer several health benefits, including improved digestion, enhanced nutrient absorption, and relief from digestive disorders such as pancreatic insufficiency, cystic fibrosis, and digestive enzyme deficiencies. Additionally, pancreatin enzymes may be used to alleviate symptoms of indigestion, bloating, and flatulence.

Indication and Usage: Pancreatin supplements are commonly used to support digestive health and aid in the digestion of carbohydrates, fats, and proteins. They are often prescribed for individuals with pancreatic insufficiency or other digestive disorders and may be taken with meals to improve nutrient absorption and alleviate digestive discomfort.

Usual Constituents with Percentages: The usual constituents of pancreatin supplements include amylase, lipase, and protease enzymes, along with other minor enzymes and cofactors. The percentages of each enzyme component in pancreatin formulations can vary depending on the product and manufacturer.

Mechanism of Action: Pancreatin enzymes function by catalyzing the hydrolysis of complex nutrients, including starches, fats, and proteins, into smaller, more absorbable molecules. Amylase enzymes break down carbohydrates into simple sugars, lipase enzymes hydrolyze fats into fatty acids and glycerol, and protease enzymes digest proteins into amino acids.

Dosage: The recommended dosage of pancreatin supplements can vary depending on factors such as the individual's digestive health, pancreatic function, and specific needs. It is advisable to follow the dosage instructions provided by the healthcare provider or consult a healthcare professional for personalized recommendations.

Contraindications: Individuals with known allergies or sensitivities to pancreatic enzymes or any components of pancreatin supplements should avoid their use. Additionally, individuals with certain medical conditions, such as acute pancreatitis or pancreatic cancer, should consult a healthcare provider before starting pancreatin supplementation.

Precautions: It is important to use pancreatin supplements cautiously, especially in individuals with gastrointestinal disorders or those taking medications that may interact with digestive enzymes. Pregnant or nursing women, as well as children, should consult a healthcare professional before using pancreatin supplements.

Adverse Reactions: Although rare, potential adverse reactions to pancreatin supplements may include gastrointestinal discomfort, such as abdominal pain, bloating, or diarrhea. Individuals experiencing persistent or severe adverse effects should discontinue use and consult a healthcare provider.

Research Standing: Research on the efficacy and safety of pancreatin supplementation is extensive, with numerous studies investigating its use in various digestive disorders and conditions. Clinical trials have demonstrated the effectiveness of pancreatin enzymes in improving digestion, nutrient absorption, and overall gastrointestinal function in individuals with pancreatic insufficiency and other digestive disorders.

Pharmacokinetics and Pharmacodynamics: The pharmacokinetics of pancreatin enzymes involve their oral administration and subsequent release and activation in the gastrointestinal tract. Following ingestion, pancreatin enzymes mix with food in the stomach and are activated by acidic pH. They then exert their enzymatic action in the small intestine, where nutrient absorption occurs.

Overdosage: Overdosage of pancreatin supplements may lead to excessive enzymatic activity in the gastrointestinal tract, potentially causing digestive discomfort or disturbances. It is essential to adhere to recommended dosages and usage guidelines to minimize the risk of adverse effects.

International Standing: Pancreatin supplements are available internationally and are commonly used in various countries for their digestive health benefits. They are regulated as dietary supplements or prescription medications, depending on the country's regulatory standards and guidelines.

Indian Standing: In India, pancreatin supplements are widely available and commonly used for digestive support and the management of pancreatic insufficiency. They are available through pharmacies and healthcare providers and may be prescribed for individuals with digestive disorders or pancreatic dysfunction.

Research Summary: Research on pancreatin enzymes spans several decades and encompasses a wide range of studies, including preclinical and clinical investigations. Studies have demonstrated the efficacy of pancreatin supplementation in improving digestion, nutrient absorption, and gastrointestinal function in individuals with pancreatic insufficiency, cystic fibrosis, and other digestive disorders. Additionally, research continues to explore the potential therapeutic applications of pancreatin enzymes in various medical conditions and health conditions related to impaired digestion and nutrient absorption.

15) PANCRELIPASE

Introduction: Pancrelipase is a pancreatic enzyme replacement therapy used to supplement digestive enzymes in individuals with pancreatic insufficiency. It contains a combination of enzymes including lipase, protease, and amylase, which aid in the digestion of fats, proteins, and carbohydrates.

Synonym Name and Common Name: Synonym: Pancreatic enzyme replacement therapy Common Name: Pancrelipase

Pharmacognosy/Chemistry: Pancrelipase is a complex mixture of enzymes derived from the pancreas of pigs or cows. It contains lipase, protease, and amylase enzymes, along with other minor enzymes and cofactors essential for digestion. Pancrelipase is available in various formulations, including capsules and tablets.

Action and Pharmacology: Pancrelipase supplements work by providing exogenous digestive enzymes to individuals with pancreatic insufficiency. Lipase enzymes help break down fats into fatty acids and glycerol, protease enzymes digest proteins into amino acids, and amylase enzymes hydrolyze carbohydrates into simple sugars. This enzymatic action facilitates nutrient absorption and improves digestive function.

Method of Analysis: The activity of pancrelipase enzymes can be determined using various analytical methods, including enzymatic assays, chromatography, and spectrophotometry. These methods assess the enzyme's ability to hydrolyze specific substrates and measure the rate of digestion under controlled conditions.

Health Benefits: Pancrelipase supplementation may offer several health benefits, including improved digestion, enhanced nutrient absorption, and relief from symptoms of pancreatic insufficiency, such as steatorrhea, abdominal discomfort, and malnutrition. Additionally, pancrelipase therapy helps individuals maintain a balanced diet and prevent nutrient deficiencies.

Indication and Usage: Pancrelipase is indicated for the treatment of pancreatic insufficiency caused by conditions such as chronic pancreatitis, cystic fibrosis, pancreatic cancer, or pancreatic surgery. It is used to improve digestion, alleviate symptoms of malabsorption, and support overall nutritional status. Pancrelipase supplements are taken with meals to aid in the digestion of fats, proteins, and carbohydrates.

Usual Constituents with Percentages: The usual constituents of pancrelipase supplements include lipase, protease, and amylase enzymes, along with other minor enzymes and cofactors. The percentages of each enzyme component in pancrelipase formulations can vary depending on the product and manufacturer.

Mechanism of Action: Pancrelipase enzymes function by catalyzing the hydrolysis of complex nutrients into smaller, more absorbable molecules. Lipase enzymes break down fats into fatty acids and glycerol, protease enzymes digest proteins into amino acids, and amylase enzymes hydrolyze carbohydrates into simple sugars. This enzymatic process facilitates nutrient absorption and improves digestive function.

Dosage: The recommended dosage of pancrelipase supplements varies depending on factors such as the individual's pancreatic function, dietary habits, and specific needs. It is essential to follow the dosage instructions provided by the healthcare provider or consult a healthcare professional for personalized recommendations.

Contraindications: Pancrelipase supplements are contraindicated in individuals with known allergies or sensitivities to pancreatic enzymes or any components of pancrelipase formulations. Additionally, individuals with acute pancreatitis, pancreatic cancer, or hypersensitivity to pork or cow proteins should avoid pancrelipase therapy.

Precautions: It is important to use pancrelipase supplements cautiously, especially in individuals with gastrointestinal disorders or those taking medications that may interact with digestive enzymes. Pregnant or nursing women, as well as children, should consult a healthcare professional before using pancrelipase supplements.

Adverse Reactions: Although rare, potential adverse reactions to pancrelipase supplements may include gastrointestinal discomfort, such as abdominal pain, bloating, or diarrhea. Individuals experiencing persistent or severe adverse effects should discontinue use and seek medical attention.

Research Standing: Research on the efficacy and safety of pancrelipase therapy is extensive, with numerous clinical trials and studies investigating its use in various pancreatic disorders and conditions. Clinical evidence supports the effectiveness of pancrelipase supplementation in improving digestion, alleviating symptoms of malabsorption, and maintaining nutritional status in individuals with pancreatic insufficiency.

Pharmacokinetics and Pharmacodynamics: The pharmacokinetics of pancrelipase enzymes involve their oral administration and subsequent release and activation in the gastrointestinal tract. Following ingestion, pancrelipase enzymes mix with food in the stomach and are activated by acidic pH. They then exert their enzymatic action in the small intestine, where nutrient absorption occurs.

Overdosage: Overdosage of pancrelipase supplements may lead to excessive enzymatic activity in the gastrointestinal tract, potentially causing digestive discomfort or disturbances. It is essential to adhere to recommended dosages and usage guidelines to minimize the risk of adverse effects.

International Standing: Pancrelipase supplements are available internationally and are commonly used in various countries for the treatment of pancreatic insufficiency and related conditions. They are regulated as prescription medications or dietary supplements, depending on the country's regulatory standards and guidelines.

Indian Standing: In India, pancrelipase supplements are widely available and commonly used for the management of pancreatic insufficiency caused by conditions such as chronic pancreatitis, cystic fibrosis, and pancreatic cancer. They are available through pharmacies and healthcare providers and may be prescribed for individuals requiring digestive enzyme replacement therapy.

Research Summary: Research on pancrelipase therapy spans several decades and encompasses a wide range of studies, including clinical trials, observational studies, and systematic reviews. Clinical evidence supports the efficacy of pancrelipase supplementation in improving digestive function, alleviating symptoms of malabsorption, and supporting nutritional status in individuals with pancreatic insufficiency. Additionally, research continues to explore the optimal dosing regimens, formulations, and therapeutic applications of pancrelipase therapy in various pancreatic disorders and conditions.

16) PAPAIN

Introduction: Papain is a proteolytic enzyme derived from the latex of the papaya fruit (Carica papaya). It has been used for centuries in traditional medicine for its digestive and anti-inflammatory properties. Papain is widely utilized in various industries, including food, pharmaceuticals, and cosmetics, due to its enzymatic activity and therapeutic potential.

Synonym Name and Common Name: Synonym: Papaya enzyme Common Name: Papain

Pharmacognosy/Chemistry: Papain is a cysteine protease enzyme with a specific tertiary structure critical for its catalytic activity. It belongs to the papain family of proteases and is characterized by its ability to cleave peptide bonds in proteins. Papain is extracted from the latex of unripe papaya fruits and can be purified for use in various applications.

Action and Pharmacology: Papain exhibits proteolytic activity, meaning it can break down proteins into smaller peptide fragments and amino acids. This enzymatic action facilitates protein digestion and absorption in the gastrointestinal tract. Additionally, papain has been shown to possess anti-inflammatory, antioxidant, and wound-healing properties, making it valuable in various therapeutic applications.

Method of Analysis: The activity of papain can be determined using various analytical methods, including enzymatic assays, chromatography, and spectrophotometry. These methods assess the enzyme's ability to hydrolyze specific protein substrates and measure the rate of proteolytic activity under controlled conditions.

Health Benefits: Papain supplementation may offer several health benefits, including improved digestion, enhanced nutrient absorption, and relief from digestive discomfort. Additionally, papain has been studied for its potential anti-inflammatory effects, antioxidant properties, and wound-healing capabilities, making it valuable in skincare and wound care products.

Indication and Usage: Papain is indicated for the treatment of digestive disorders, including indigestion, bloating, and protein malabsorption. It is commonly used as a digestive enzyme supplement to aid in the digestion of proteins and alleviate symptoms of gastrointestinal discomfort. Additionally, papain is utilized in topical formulations for its wound-healing and anti-inflammatory properties.

Usual Constituents with Percentages: The usual constituents of papain supplements primarily include the enzyme papain itself, along with other proteolytic enzymes and cofactors present in papaya latex. The percentages of papain enzyme in commercial formulations can vary depending on the product and manufacturer.

Mechanism of Action: Papain functions by cleaving peptide bonds in proteins, resulting in the breakdown of complex protein structures into smaller peptide fragments and amino acids. This enzymatic process facilitates protein digestion in the gastrointestinal tract and enhances the absorption of amino acids and nutrients.

Dosage: The recommended dosage of papain supplements can vary depending on factors such as the individual's digestive health, dietary habits, and specific needs. It is advisable to follow the dosage instructions provided by the manufacturer or consult a healthcare professional for personalized recommendations.

Contraindications: Papain supplements are contraindicated in individuals with known allergies or sensitivities to papaya latex or any components of papain formulations. Additionally, individuals with certain medical conditions, such as latex allergy or gastrointestinal disorders, should avoid papain supplementation without consulting a healthcare professional.

Precautions: It is important to use papain supplements cautiously, especially in individuals with gastrointestinal disorders or those taking medications that may interact with digestive enzymes. Pregnant or nursing women, as well as children, should consult a healthcare professional before using papain supplements.

Adverse Reactions: Although rare, potential adverse reactions to papain supplements may include gastrointestinal discomfort, such as abdominal pain, bloating, or diarrhea. Individuals experiencing persistent or severe adverse effects should discontinue use and seek medical attention.

Research Standing: Research on the efficacy and safety of papain supplementation is ongoing, with numerous studies investigating its digestive, anti-inflammatory, and wound-healing properties. While some research supports the use of papain for improving protein digestion, alleviating digestive discomfort, and promoting wound healing, further clinical trials are needed to establish its effectiveness conclusively.

Pharmacokinetics and Pharmacodynamics: The pharmacokinetics and pharmacodynamics of papain involve its oral administration and subsequent interaction with proteins in the gastrointestinal tract. Following ingestion, papain enzymes exert their proteolytic activity in the stomach and small intestine, facilitating protein digestion and nutrient absorption.

Overdosage: Overdosage of papain supplements may lead to excessive enzymatic activity in the gastrointestinal tract, potentially causing digestive discomfort or disturbances. It is essential to adhere to recommended dosages and usage guidelines to minimize the risk of adverse effects.

International Standing: Papain supplements are available internationally and are commonly used in various industries, including food, pharmaceuticals, and cosmetics. Regulatory standards and guidelines for papain products may vary across different countries and regions.

Indian Standing: In India, papain is widely utilized in traditional medicine and is commonly used as a digestive aid and anti-inflammatory agent. It is also incorporated into various skincare and wound care products for its enzymatic and therapeutic properties. Papain supplements are available through pharmacies and healthcare providers and are used for digestive support and topical applications.

Research Summary: Research on papain spans several decades and encompasses a wide range of studies, including preclinical and clinical investigations. Studies have demonstrated the efficacy of papain supplementation in improving protein digestion, alleviating symptoms of gastrointestinal discomfort, and promoting wound healing. Additionally, research continues to explore the potential therapeutic applications of papain in various medical conditions and industries, including food, pharmaceuticals, and cosmetics.

17) PEPSIN

Introduction: Pepsin is a digestive enzyme that plays a crucial role in the breakdown of proteins in the stomach. It is produced by the chief cells in the gastric glands and is activated by the acidic environment of the stomach. Pepsin aids in the digestion of dietary proteins, converting them into smaller peptide fragments for absorption in the small intestine.

Synonym Name and Common Name: Synonym: Gastric protease Common Name: Pepsin

Pharmacognosy/Chemistry: Pepsin is a proteolytic enzyme belonging to the aspartic protease family. It is synthesized in an inactive form known as pepsinogen, which is then activated by the low pH environment of the stomach. Pepsin has a specific tertiary structure that enables it to cleave peptide bonds in proteins, resulting in the breakdown of complex protein structures.

Action and Pharmacology: Pepsin functions by hydrolyzing peptide bonds in proteins, converting them into smaller peptide fragments and amino acids. This enzymatic action occurs in the acidic environment of the stomach, where pepsin is activated from its precursor form, pepsinogen. Pepsin plays a crucial role in protein digestion and nutrient absorption in the gastrointestinal tract.

Method of Analysis: The activity of pepsin can be determined using various analytical methods, including enzymatic assays, chromatography, and spectrophotometry. These methods assess the enzyme's ability to hydrolyze specific protein substrates and measure the rate of proteolytic activity under controlled conditions.

Health Benefits: Pepsin supplementation may offer several health benefits, primarily related to improved digestion and nutrient absorption. It aids in the breakdown of dietary proteins, facilitating their digestion and absorption in the gastrointestinal tract. Pepsin may also alleviate symptoms of protein malabsorption and support overall digestive health.

Indication and Usage: Pepsin is indicated for the treatment of digestive disorders characterized by impaired protein digestion, such as hypochlorhydria, achlorhydria, or insufficient gastric acid secretion. It is commonly used as a digestive enzyme supplement to aid in the digestion of dietary proteins and alleviate symptoms of indigestion or gastrointestinal discomfort.

Usual Constituents with Percentages: The usual constituents of pepsin supplements primarily include the enzyme pepsin itself, derived from animal (usually porcine) sources. The percentages of pepsin enzyme in commercial formulations can vary depending on the product and manufacturer.

Mechanism of Action: Pepsin functions by catalyzing the hydrolysis of peptide bonds in proteins, resulting in the breakdown of complex protein structures into smaller peptide fragments and amino acids. This enzymatic process occurs in the acidic environment of the stomach, where pepsin is activated from its precursor form, pepsinogen, by gastric acid (HCl).

Dosage: The recommended dosage of pepsin supplements can vary depending on factors such as the individual's digestive health, dietary habits, and specific needs. It is advisable to follow the dosage instructions provided by the manufacturer or consult a healthcare professional for personalized recommendations.

Contraindications: Pepsin supplements are contraindicated in individuals with known allergies or sensitivities to pepsin or any components of pepsin formulations. Additionally, individuals with certain medical conditions, such as gastric ulcers, gastritis, or gastroesophageal reflux disease (GERD), should avoid pepsin supplementation without consulting a healthcare professional.

Precautions: It is important to use pepsin supplements cautiously, especially in individuals with gastrointestinal disorders or those taking medications that may interact with digestive enzymes. Pregnant or nursing women, as well as children, should consult a healthcare professional before using pepsin supplements.

Adverse Reactions: Although rare, potential adverse reactions to pepsin supplements may include gastrointestinal discomfort, such as abdominal pain, bloating, or diarrhea. Individuals experiencing persistent or severe adverse effects should discontinue use and seek medical attention.

Research Standing: Research on the efficacy and safety of pepsin supplementation is limited compared to other digestive enzymes. While pepsin plays a crucial role in protein digestion, particularly in the stomach, there is relatively less clinical evidence supporting its use as a digestive enzyme supplement compared to other enzymes such as pancreatin or bromelain.

Pharmacokinetics and Pharmacodynamics: The pharmacokinetics and pharmacodynamics of pepsin involve its oral administration and subsequent interaction with proteins in the stomach. Pepsin exerts its proteolytic activity in the acidic environment of the stomach, where it breaks down dietary proteins into smaller peptide fragments and amino acids.

Overdosage: Overdosage of pepsin supplements may lead to excessive enzymatic activity in the stomach, potentially causing digestive discomfort or disturbances. It is essential to adhere to recommended dosages and usage guidelines to minimize the risk of adverse effects.

International Standing: Pepsin supplements are available internationally and are commonly used in various countries for digestive support and the management of protein digestion disorders. Regulatory standards and guidelines for pepsin products may vary across different countries and regions.

Indian Standing: In India, pepsin is widely used in pharmaceutical formulations for its digestive properties. It is commonly included in digestive enzyme supplements and antacid preparations to aid in protein digestion and alleviate symptoms of indigestion. Pepsin supplements are available through pharmacies and healthcare providers and are used for digestive support and gastrointestinal health.

Research Summary: Research on pepsin primarily focuses on its role in protein digestion and its therapeutic potential in digestive disorders. While pepsin plays a crucial role in protein digestion in the stomach, there is relatively limited clinical evidence supporting its use as a standalone digestive enzyme supplement compared to other enzymes. Further research is needed to better understand the efficacy and safety of pepsin supplementation in various digestive disorders and conditions.

18) PHYTASE

Introduction: Phytase is a type of enzyme that catalyzes the hydrolysis of phytic acid, a form of phosphorus found in plant-based foods, into inositol and inorganic phosphorus. This enzymatic action makes phosphorus more bioavailable for absorption in the digestive tract, particularly in monogastric animals such as pigs, poultry, and fish.

Synonym Name and Common Name: Synonym: Myo-inositol hexakisphosphate phosphohydrolase Common Name: Phytase

Pharmacognosy/Chemistry: Phytase is a phosphatase enzyme that belongs to the family of histidine acid phosphatases. It is naturally present in various organisms, including plants, bacteria, fungi, and animals. Phytase enzymes exhibit optimal activity at acidic pH levels and are often used as feed additives to improve phosphorus utilization in animal nutrition.

Action and Pharmacology: Phytase catalyzes the hydrolysis of phytic acid, releasing phosphate groups and inositol. This enzymatic action makes phosphorus more available for absorption in the gastrointestinal tract, enhancing phosphorus utilization and reducing the need for supplemental phosphorus in animal diets. Phytase supplementation improves feed efficiency, reduces environmental phosphorus excretion, and enhances overall animal performance.

Method of Analysis: The activity of phytase can be determined using various analytical methods, including colorimetric assays, spectrophotometry, and chromatography. These methods assess the enzyme's ability to hydrolyze phytic acid substrate and measure the release of inorganic phosphate under controlled conditions.

Health Benefits: Phytase supplementation offers several health benefits, primarily in animal nutrition. It improves phosphorus utilization and availability in monogastric animals, leading to enhanced growth performance, bone development, and overall health. Additionally, phytase supplementation reduces phosphorus excretion in manure, mitigating environmental pollution from intensive animal farming.

Indication and Usage: Phytase is indicated for use as a feed additive in animal nutrition, particularly in monogastric animals such as pigs, poultry, and fish. It is used to improve phosphorus utilization and availability in plant-based diets, reduce the need for supplemental phosphorus, and enhance overall animal growth, performance, and health.

Usual Constituents with Percentages: The usual constituents of commercial phytase preparations include the phytase enzyme itself, along with other minor components such as stabilizers and excipients. The percentages of phytase enzyme in commercial formulations can vary depending on the product and manufacturer.

Mechanism of Action: Phytase functions by catalyzing the hydrolysis of phytic acid, a complex form of phosphorus found in plant-based feeds, into inorganic phosphate and inositol. This enzymatic process makes phosphorus more available for absorption in the gastrointestinal tract, enhancing phosphorus utilization and reducing the need for supplemental phosphorus in animal diets.

Dosage: The recommended dosage of phytase supplementation varies depending on factors such as the animal species, age, weight, and dietary phosphorus content. It is typically added to animal feed formulations at specific inclusion rates to achieve optimal phosphorus utilization and performance. Dosage recommendations are provided by feed manufacturers and nutritionists.

Contraindications: Phytase supplementation is generally safe for use in animal nutrition and does not have specific contraindications. However, it is important to adhere to recommended dosage levels and usage guidelines to avoid potential adverse effects or nutrient imbalances in animal diets.

Precautions: It is essential to use phytase supplements cautiously and follow recommended dosage levels to avoid potential adverse effects or overdosing. Additionally, it is important to consider the overall nutrient composition of animal diets and consult with a nutritionist or veterinarian when formulating feed rations containing phytase.

Adverse Reactions: Phytase supplementation is well-tolerated in animals and typically does not cause adverse reactions when used at recommended dosage levels. However, excessive phytase supplementation may lead to imbalances in nutrient utilization or gastrointestinal disturbances in animals.

Research Standing: Research on phytase supplementation in animal nutrition is extensive, with numerous studies demonstrating its efficacy in improving phosphorus utilization, growth performance, and overall health in monogastric animals. Phytase supplementation has become a standard practice in animal feed formulations, and ongoing research continues to explore its potential benefits and applications in livestock and aquaculture production systems.

Pharmacokinetics and Pharmacodynamics: The pharmacokinetics and pharmacodynamics of phytase supplementation in animals involve its oral administration and subsequent enzymatic activity in the gastrointestinal tract. Phytase enzymes catalyze the hydrolysis of phytic acid, releasing inorganic phosphate and inositol, which are then absorbed and utilized by the animal's body for various metabolic processes.

Overdosage: Overdosage of phytase supplements in animal feed may lead to excessive phosphorus utilization or imbalances in nutrient absorption, potentially resulting in adverse effects on animal health and performance. It is essential to adhere to recommended dosage levels and usage guidelines to avoid overdosing and optimize the benefits of phytase supplementation.

International Standing: Phytase supplements are widely used in animal nutrition globally and are regulated as feed additives or feed enzymes in various countries. Regulatory standards and guidelines for phytase products may vary across different regions, but phytase has gained widespread acceptance as an effective tool for improving phosphorus utilization and reducing environmental phosphorus pollution in intensive animal production systems.

Indian Standing: In India, phytase supplementation is increasingly used in animal nutrition, particularly in poultry and swine production. It is incorporated into commercial feed formulations to improve phosphorus utilization, reduce feed costs, and enhance animal growth and performance. Phytase supplements are available through feed manufacturers and distributors and are commonly used in intensive livestock production systems.

Research Summary: Research on phytase supplementation in animal nutrition demonstrates its efficacy in improving phosphorus utilization, growth performance, and environmental sustainability in intensive livestock and aquaculture production systems.

Phytase has become a standard practice in animal feed formulations, and ongoing research continues to explore its potential benefits, applications, and optimization strategies for various animal species and production systems.

19) PROTEASE

Introduction: Protease, also known as proteolytic enzyme or proteinase, refers to a group of enzymes that catalyze the hydrolysis of peptide bonds in proteins, breaking them down into smaller peptides and amino acids. Proteases play crucial roles in various physiological processes, including digestion, protein turnover, and cellular regulation.

Synonym Name and Common Name: Synonym: Proteinase Common Name: Protease

Pharmacognosy/Chemistry: Proteases are enzymes classified into different families based on their catalytic mechanism and structural features, including serine proteases, cysteine proteases, aspartic proteases, and metalloproteases. They are synthesized as inactive precursor forms (zymogens) and are activated under specific conditions, such as acidic pH in the stomach or proteolytic cleavage by other enzymes.

Action and Pharmacology: Proteases function by cleaving peptide bonds in proteins, leading to their breakdown into smaller peptides and amino acids. This enzymatic action facilitates protein digestion in the gastrointestinal tract, allowing for the absorption of essential amino acids and nutrients. Proteases also play roles in various physiological processes, such as blood clotting, immune response, and tissue remodeling.

Method of Analysis: The activity of protease enzymes can be determined using various analytical methods, including enzymatic assays, chromatography, and spectrophotometry. These methods assess the enzyme's ability to hydrolyze specific protein substrates and measure the rate of proteolytic activity under controlled conditions.

Health Benefits: Protease supplementation may offer several health benefits, primarily related to improved digestion and nutrient absorption. It aids in the breakdown of dietary proteins, facilitating their digestion and absorption in the gastrointestinal tract. Additionally, proteases have been studied for their potential anti-inflammatory, antioxidant, and immune-modulating effects.

Indication and Usage: Protease is indicated for the treatment of digestive disorders characterized by impaired protein digestion, such as hypochlorhydria, achlorhydria, or insufficient gastric acid secretion. It is commonly used as a digestive enzyme supplement to aid in the digestion of dietary proteins and alleviate symptoms of indigestion or gastrointestinal discomfort.

Usual Constituents with Percentages: The usual constituents of protease supplements primarily include the protease enzyme itself, derived from various sources such as plants, animals, or microorganisms. The percentages of protease enzyme in commercial formulations can vary depending on the product and manufacturer.

Mechanism of Action: Proteases function by catalyzing the hydrolysis of peptide bonds in proteins, resulting in the breakdown of complex protein structures into smaller peptide fragments and amino acids. This enzymatic process occurs in the gastrointestinal tract, where proteases are activated and exert their digestive function.

Dosage: The recommended dosage of protease supplements can vary depending on factors such as the individual's digestive health, dietary habits, and specific needs. It is advisable to follow the dosage instructions provided by the manufacturer or consult a healthcare professional for personalized recommendations.

Contraindications: Protease supplements are generally safe for use in individuals with normal digestive function and do not have specific contraindications. However, individuals with known allergies or sensitivities to protease enzymes or any components of protease formulations should avoid supplementation.

Precautions: It is essential to use protease supplements cautiously, especially in individuals with gastrointestinal disorders or those taking medications that may interact with digestive enzymes. Pregnant or nursing women, as well as children, should consult a healthcare professional before using protease supplements.

Adverse Reactions: Although rare, potential adverse reactions to protease supplements may include gastrointestinal discomfort, such as abdominal pain, bloating, or diarrhea. Individuals experiencing persistent or severe adverse effects should discontinue use and seek medical attention.

Research Standing: Research on the efficacy and safety of protease supplementation is ongoing, with numerous studies investigating its role in improving protein digestion, alleviating symptoms of indigestion, and supporting overall digestive health. Protease enzymes have been extensively studied for their therapeutic potential in various medical conditions, including digestive disorders, inflammation, and immune-related diseases.

Pharmacokinetics and Pharmacodynamics: The pharmacokinetics and pharmacodynamics of protease supplementation involve its oral administration and subsequent enzymatic activity in the gastrointestinal tract. Protease enzymes catalyze the hydrolysis of peptide bonds in proteins, facilitating their breakdown into smaller peptides and amino acids for absorption and utilization by the body.

Overdosage: Overdosage of protease supplements may lead to excessive enzymatic activity in the gastrointestinal tract, potentially causing digestive discomfort or disturbances. It is essential to adhere to recommended dosages and usage guidelines to minimize the risk of adverse effects.

International Standing: Protease supplements are available internationally and are commonly used in various countries for digestive support and the management of protein digestion disorders. Regulatory standards and guidelines for protease products may vary across different countries and regions.

Indian Standing: In India, protease supplementation is increasingly used in healthcare and nutraceutical formulations for its digestive and therapeutic properties. It is incorporated into digestive enzyme supplements, dietary supplements, and pharmaceutical formulations to support digestive health and overall well-being.

Research Summary: Research on protease supplementation spans various fields, including nutrition, gastroenterology, and pharmacology. While protease enzymes play a crucial role in protein digestion and various physiological processes, further research is needed to better understand their mechanisms of action, therapeutic potential, and optimal applications in healthcare and nutrition. Ongoing studies continue to explore the efficacy, safety, and potential benefits of protease supplementation in diverse populations and medical conditions.

20) TRYPSIN

Introduction: Trypsin is a digestive enzyme belonging to the serine protease family, primarily produced in the pancreas. It plays a crucial role in the digestion of dietary proteins by catalyzing the hydrolysis of peptide bonds, breaking down proteins into smaller peptides and amino acids.

Synonym Name and Common Name: Synonym: Trypsinogen Common Name: Trypsin

Pharmacognosy/Chemistry: Trypsin is synthesized in an inactive precursor form known as trypsinogen, which is secreted by the pancreas into the small intestine. Trypsinogen is activated into trypsin by enteropeptidase, an enzyme present in the intestinal mucosa. Trypsin exhibits optimal activity at alkaline pH levels and is inhibited by specific protease inhibitors.

Action and Pharmacology: Trypsin functions by cleaving peptide bonds on the carboxyl side of basic amino acids, such as lysine and arginine, in proteins. This enzymatic action facilitates protein digestion in the small intestine, allowing for the absorption of amino acids and peptides into the bloodstream. Trypsin also plays roles in various physiological processes, such as blood clotting and immune response.

Method of Analysis: The activity of trypsin can be determined using various analytical methods, including enzymatic assays, chromatography, and spectrophotometry. These methods assess the enzyme's ability to hydrolyze specific protein substrates and measure the rate of proteolytic activity under controlled conditions.

Health Benefits: Trypsin supplementation may offer several health benefits, primarily related to improved digestion and nutrient absorption. It aids in the breakdown of dietary proteins, facilitating their digestion and absorption in the small intestine. Additionally, trypsin has been studied for its potential anti-inflammatory and wound-healing properties.

Indication and Usage: Trypsin is indicated for the treatment of digestive disorders characterized by impaired protein digestion, such as pancreatic insufficiency or exocrine pancreatic dysfunction. It is commonly used as a digestive enzyme supplement to aid in the digestion of dietary proteins and alleviate symptoms of indigestion or malabsorption.

Usual Constituents with Percentages: The usual constituents of trypsin supplements primarily include the enzyme trypsin itself, derived from animal (usually porcine or bovine) pancreatic tissues. The percentages of trypsin enzyme in commercial formulations can vary depending on the product and manufacturer.

Mechanism of Action: Trypsin functions by catalyzing the hydrolysis of peptide bonds on the carboxyl side of basic amino acids, such as lysine and arginine, in proteins. This enzymatic process results in the breakdown of complex protein structures into smaller peptide fragments and amino acids, facilitating protein digestion and absorption in the small intestine.

Dosage: The recommended dosage of trypsin supplements can vary depending on factors such as the individual's digestive health, dietary habits, and specific needs. It is advisable to follow the dosage instructions provided by the manufacturer or consult a healthcare professional for personalized recommendations.

Contraindications: Trypsin supplements are contraindicated in individuals with known allergies or sensitivities to trypsin or any components of trypsin formulations. Additionally, individuals with certain medical conditions, such as pancreatic disorders or gastrointestinal disorders, should avoid trypsin supplementation without consulting a healthcare professional.

Precautions: It is important to use trypsin supplements cautiously, especially in individuals with pancreatic insufficiency or exocrine pancreatic dysfunction. Pregnant or nursing women, as well as children, should consult a healthcare professional before using trypsin supplements.

Adverse Reactions: Although rare, potential adverse reactions to trypsin supplements may include gastrointestinal discomfort, such as abdominal pain, bloating, or diarrhea. Individuals experiencing persistent or severe adverse effects should discontinue use and seek medical attention.

Research Standing: Research on the efficacy and safety of trypsin supplementation is ongoing, with numerous studies investigating its role in improving protein digestion, alleviating symptoms of indigestion, and supporting overall digestive health. Trypsin enzymes have been extensively studied for their therapeutic potential in various medical conditions, including pancreatic disorders, inflammation, and wound healing.

Pharmacokinetics and Pharmacodynamics: The pharmacokinetics and pharmacodynamics of trypsin supplementation involve its oral administration and subsequent enzymatic activity in the gastrointestinal tract. Trypsin enzymes catalyze the hydrolysis of peptide bonds in proteins, facilitating their breakdown into smaller peptide fragments and amino acids for absorption and utilization by the body.

Overdosage: Overdosage of trypsin supplements may lead to excessive enzymatic activity in the gastrointestinal tract, potentially causing digestive discomfort or disturbances. It is essential to adhere to recommended dosages and usage guidelines to minimize the risk of adverse effects.

International Standing: Trypsin supplements are available internationally and are commonly used in various countries for digestive support and the management of used to quantify the levels of hydroxycitric acid in dietary supplements and natural extracts.

Health Benefits: Hydroxycitric acid is primarily marketed for its potential weight loss and appetite-suppressing effects. It is also claimed to improve exercise performance, boost metabolism, and support blood sugar control.

Indication and Usage: Indications for hydroxycitric acid include weight management, appetite control, and supporting healthy blood sugar levels. It is commonly consumed as a dietary supplement in capsule or powder form.

Usual Constituents with Percentages: Hydroxycitric acid typically constitutes around 50-60% of the weight of Garcinia cambogia extract, although the percentage may vary depending on the extraction method and product formulation.

Mechanism of Action: The primary mechanism of action of hydroxycitric acid is believed to involve inhibition of citrate lyase, an enzyme involved in fatty acid biosynthesis. By blocking this enzyme, HCA may reduce the conversion of carbohydrates into fat and suppress appetite.

Dosage: Typical dosages of hydroxycitric acid range from 500 to 1500 milligrams per day, although dosages may vary depending on the specific product and individual health needs.

Contraindications: Individuals with diabetes or hypoglycemia, as well as those taking medications for blood sugar control, should use caution when using hydroxycitric acid supplements. Pregnant or breastfeeding women should avoid its use.

Precautions: It is advisable to consult a healthcare professional before starting hydroxycitric acid supplementation, particularly for individuals with underlying health conditions or those taking medications. Excessive consumption may lead to adverse effects such as gastrointestinal upset.

Adverse Reactions: Common adverse reactions associated with hydroxycitric acid supplementation include gastrointestinal discomfort, nausea, vomiting, and headaches. Some individuals may also experience allergic reactions.

Research Summary: Research on hydroxycitric acid's effectiveness for weight loss and appetite suppression has yielded mixed results. While some studies suggest modest benefits, others have found no significant effects. Further research is needed to elucidate its mechanisms and efficacy.

2) ALPHA MANGOSTIN

Introduction: Alpha-mangostin is a natural compound primarily found in the pericarp of the mangosteen fruit (Garcinia mangostana L.), which is native to Southeast Asia. It belongs to a class of organic compounds called xanthones, known for their potent antioxidant and anti-inflammatory properties.

Synonym Name and Common Name: Synonym Name: 3,6,7-Trihydroxy-2,8-bis(3-methylbut-2-enyl)xanthone Common Name: Alpha-mangostin

Pharmacognosy / Chemistry: Alpha-mangostin is a yellow crystalline substance that can be extracted from the pericarp of the mangosteen fruit. It is soluble in organic solvents like ethanol and acetone.

Action and Pharmacology: Alpha-mangostin exhibits various pharmacological activities, including antioxidant, anti-inflammatory, antimicrobial, antitumor, and neuroprotective effects. It acts by inhibiting reactive oxygen species (ROS) production, suppressing inflammatory pathways, and modulating various molecular targets involved in cell proliferation and apoptosis.

Method of Analysis: Analytical methods for quantifying alpha-mangostin typically involve high-performance liquid chromatography (HPLC) coupled with UV detection or mass spectrometry. Sample preparation usually includes extraction of alpha-mangostin from the mangosteen pericarp using suitable solvents followed by chromatographic separation and quantification.

Health Benefits: The consumption of alpha-mangostin has been associated with several health benefits, including:

- Antioxidant properties, which help protect cells from oxidative damage.
- Anti-inflammatory effects, which may alleviate symptoms of inflammatory conditions.
- Antimicrobial activity against various pathogens, including bacteria and fungi.
- Potential anticancer properties, with studies suggesting inhibitory effects on cancer cell growth and proliferation.
- Neuroprotective effects, which may help prevent neurodegenerative diseases like Alzheimer's.

Indication and Usage: Alpha-mangostin is used in traditional medicine and dietary supplements for various indications, including:

- Supporting overall health and well-being.
- Managing inflammatory conditions like arthritis.
- Enhancing immune function.
- Supporting cancer treatment as an adjuvant therapy.

Usual Constituents with Percentages: The usual constituents of mangosteen pericarp extract containing alpha-mangostin vary depending on the extraction method and source. However, alpha-mangostin typically constitutes around 1-3% of the total extract.

Mechanism of Action: The mechanism of action of alpha-mangostin involves:

- Scavenging free radicals and inhibiting oxidative stress.
- Modulating inflammatory pathways, such as NF-κB and COX-2.
- Inducing apoptosis in cancer cells through various signaling pathways.
- Interfering with microbial cell membrane integrity and function.

Dosage: The recommended dosage of alpha-mangostin varies depending on the formulation and intended use. However, typical doses range from 50 mg to 500 mg per day, taken orally in divided doses.

Contraindications: There are no well-defined contraindications for alpha-mangostin. However, individuals with known allergies to mangosteen or xanthones should avoid its use. Additionally, pregnant, and breastfeeding women should consult a healthcare professional before using alpha-mangostin supplements.

Precautions: Some precautions to consider when using alpha-mangostin include:

- Consultation with a healthcare professional before starting supplementation, especially if you have underlying medical conditions or are taking medications.
- Monitoring for any adverse reactions or interactions with other drugs or supplements.

- Adherence to recommended dosage guidelines to avoid potential adverse effects.

Adverse Reactions: While alpha-mangostin is generally well-tolerated, some individuals may experience mild gastrointestinal discomfort, allergic reactions, or interactions with certain medications. Long-term safety data are limited, so caution should be exercised, especially with prolonged or high-dose use.

Research Summary: Research on alpha-mangostin has demonstrated its promising pharmacological activities and therapeutic potential in various preclinical studies. However, further clinical research is warranted to elucidate its efficacy, safety profile, and optimal therapeutic applications in humans.

Pharmacokinetics: The pharmacokinetics of alpha-mangostin have been studied in animal models, showing rapid absorption, distribution, and metabolism following oral administration. The compound undergoes extensive first-pass metabolism in the liver, leading to the formation of various metabolites, which are subsequently excreted primarily in the urine and feces.

Pharmacodynamics: Alpha-mangostin exerts its pharmacodynamic effects by interacting with multiple molecular targets involved in oxidative stress, inflammation, cell proliferation, and apoptosis. Its ability to modulate these pathways contributes to its antioxidant, anti-inflammatory, and anticancer properties.

Overdosage: Limited information is available regarding the potential consequences of alpha-mangostin overdose. However, excessive consumption may increase the risk of adverse reactions or gastrointestinal disturbances. In case of overdose, supportive measures should be initiated, and medical attention sought if necessary.

International Standing: Alpha-mangostin and mangosteen pericarp extracts are gaining recognition internationally for their health-promoting properties. They are commonly used as dietary supplements and functional ingredients in various products, including beverages, dietary supplements, and skincare formulations.

Indian Standing: In India, mangosteen fruit and its derivatives, including alpha-mangostin, have been used in traditional Ayurvedic medicine for centuries. The growing body of scientific research supporting their therapeutic benefits has contributed to their popularity in the Indian market.

Research Summary of Alpha-mangostin: Alpha-mangostin continues to be a subject of active research due to its diverse pharmacological activities and potential therapeutic applications. Studies have explored its effects on various disease models, including cancer, inflammation, infectious diseases, and neurodegenerative disorders. While preclinical findings are promising, clinical trials are needed to validate its efficacy and safety for human use further.

3) ALPHA-LIPOIC ACID

Introduction: Alpha-lipoic acid (ALA) is a naturally occurring compound that functions as a coenzyme in several metabolic pathways in the body. It is synthesized in small amounts by humans and can also be obtained through dietary sources such as organ meats, spinach, and broccoli. ALA is notable for its potent antioxidant properties and its role in energy metabolism.

Synonym Name and Common Name: Synonym Name: Thioctic acid Common Name: Alpha-lipoic acid

Pharmacognosy / Chemistry: Alpha-lipoic acid is a sulfur-containing compound with a molecular formula of C8H14O2S2. It is a yellow crystalline powder that is soluble in both water and fat, allowing it to penetrate various tissues and cellular compartments.

Action and Pharmacology: Alpha-lipoic acid functions as a cofactor for several key enzymes involved in mitochondrial energy production and antioxidant defense systems. Its primary pharmacological actions include:

Antioxidant activity: ALA scavenges free radicals and regenerates other antioxidants like vitamins C and E, helping to protect cells from oxidative damage.

Metabolic regulation : ALA plays a role in glucose metabolism, insulin sensitivity, and mitochondrial function, making it potentially beneficial for conditions like diabetes and metabolic syndrome.

Neuroprotection: ALA crosses the blood-brain barrier and exerts neuroprotective effects by reducing oxidative stress, inflammation, and enhancing cellular energy production.

Mechanism of Action: In the body, beta-carotene is converted into vitamin A through enzymatic processes, primarily in the liver and intestinal mucosa. Vitamin A plays crucial roles in vision, cell differentiation, and immune function.

Dosage: Recommended dosages for beta-carotene supplementation vary depending on individual needs and health conditions. Generally, doses range from 6 to 15 milligrams per day, but higher doses may be used under medical supervision for specific therapeutic purposes.

Contraindications: Individuals with a history of hypersensitivity to beta-carotene or vitamin A should avoid supplementation. Pregnant women should consult with a healthcare professional before taking beta-carotene supplements, as excessive vitamin A intake can be harmful to fetal development.

Precautions:

- Long-term, high-dose supplementation with beta-carotene may increase the risk of lung cancer in smokers and individuals exposed to asbestos.
- Individuals with certain medical conditions, such as liver disease or lipid metabolism disorders, should use beta-carotene supplements with caution.

Adverse Reactions: High-dose beta-carotene supplementation may cause harmless but noticeable side effects, including yellowing of the skin (carotenemia) and gastrointestinal disturbances. These effects are typically reversible upon discontinuation of supplementation.

Research Summary: Research on beta-carotene has demonstrated its importance in maintaining vision, supporting immune function, and protecting against oxidative stress. While supplementation may offer benefits for certain populations, caution is warranted regarding high-dose supplementation in smokers and individuals at risk of lung cancer.

Pharmacokinetics: Beta-carotene is absorbed in the small intestine and transported in chylomicrons to the liver, where it is converted into vitamin A as needed. Excess beta-carotene is stored in adipose tissue and can be mobilized when vitamin A levels are low.

Pharmacodynamics: As a precursor to vitamin A, beta-carotene exerts its pharmacodynamic effects primarily through the actions of vitamin A on vision, cell differentiation, and immune function. Additionally, its antioxidant properties contribute to cellular protection against oxidative damage.

Overdosage: Excessive intake of beta-carotene supplements can lead to carotenemia, characterized by yellowing of the skin. While this condition is harmless and reversible, high-dose supplementation may increase the risk of adverse health effects, particularly in certain populations.

International Standing: Beta-carotene is recognized internationally as an essential nutrient with significant health benefits. It is commonly used as a dietary supplement and food additive in many countries.

Indian Standing: In India, beta-carotene is valued for its role in traditional medicine and is incorporated into various culinary dishes and dietary supplements. Its potential health benefits are widely acknowledged within the Indian healthcare system.

Research Summary of Beta-carotene: Overall, research on beta-carotene supports its importance in maintaining vision, supporting immune function, and protecting against oxidative stress. While supplementation may offer benefits for certain populations, caution is warranted regarding high-dose supplementation, particularly in smokers and individuals at risk of lung cancer. Further research is needed to elucidate its role in health and disease and optimize its therapeutic applications.

8) BETA ECDYSTERONE

Introduction: Beta-ecdysterone is a naturally occurring compound classified as a phytoecdysteroid, which is found in various plants, particularly those used in traditional medicine. It has gained attention for its potential health benefits, particularly in the realms of muscle growth, athletic performance, and overall well-being.

Synonym Name and Common Name: Synonym: 20-Hydroxyecdysone, ecdysterone Common Name: Beta-ecdysterone

Pharmacognosy / Chemistry: Beta-ecdysterone is a steroidal compound derived from plants such as spinach, quinoa, and cyanotisarachnoidea. It is characterized by its steroid-like structure and is believed to exert anabolic effects similar to those of testosterone.

Action and Pharmacology: Beta-ecdysterone is purported to have anabolic properties, meaning it may promote muscle growth and strength. It is also thought to enhance physical performance and recovery, making it popular among athletes and bodybuilders.

Method of Analysis: Beta-ecdysterone levels in plant extracts or dietary supplements can be analyzed using techniques such as high-performance liquid chromatography (HPLC) or mass spectrometry to quantify its concentration and purity.

Health Benefits:

- Promotes muscle growth and strength
- Enhances athletic performance and recovery
- Supports overall well-being and vitality

Indication and Usage: Beta-ecdysterone is commonly used as a dietary supplement by athletes, bodybuilders, and fitness enthusiasts to support muscle growth, improve physical performance, and enhance overall health. It may also be used in traditional medicine for various purposes.

Usual Constituents with Percentages: Beta-ecdysterone content varies among plant sources, with concentrations typically ranging from trace amounts to several milligrams per gram of plant material. Spinach and cyanotisarachnoidea are among the richest natural sources of beta-ecdysterone.

Mechanism of Action: The exact mechanism of action of beta-ecdysterone is not fully understood but is believed to involve activation of anabolic pathways in muscle cells, leading to increased protein synthesis and muscle hypertrophy. It may also modulate hormone levels and cellular signaling pathways related to muscle growth and recovery.

Dosage: Recommended dosages for beta-ecdysterone supplementation vary depending on individual goals and tolerance. Typical doses range from 100 to 500 milligrams per day, divided into multiple doses for optimal absorption.

Contraindications: There are no known contraindications for beta-ecdysterone when used at recommended doses. However, individuals with underlying medical conditions or those taking medications should consult with a healthcare professional before supplementation.

Precautions:

- Pregnant and breastfeeding women should avoid beta-ecdysterone supplementation due to insufficient safety data.

- Athletes subject to drug testing should use caution, as beta-ecdysterone may be banned by certain sports organizations.

Adverse Reactions: Beta-ecdysterone is generally well-tolerated when used at recommended doses. However, some individuals may experience mild gastrointestinal discomfort or allergic reactions in rare cases.

Research Summary: Research on beta-ecdysterone has primarily focused on its potential anabolic effects and applications in sports performance and muscle growth. While some studies suggest promising results, further research is needed to elucidate its mechanisms of action and long-term safety profile.

Pharmacokinetics: Limited information is available on the pharmacokinetics of beta-ecdysterone in humans. Studies in animals suggest rapid absorption and metabolism, with elimination primarily through hepatic clearance.

Pharmacodynamics: Beta-ecdysterone exerts its pharmacodynamic effects primarily through activation of anabolic pathways in muscle cells, leading to increased protein synthesis and muscle hypertrophy. It may also modulate hormone levels and cellular signaling pathways related to muscle growth and recovery.

Overdosage: There is limited information on the effects of overdosage with beta-ecdysterone. However, exceeding recommended doses may increase the risk of adverse reactions and potential health risks.

International Standing: Beta-ecdysterone is recognized internationally as a dietary supplement with potential applications in sports performance and muscle growth. Its use is widespread among athletes and fitness enthusiasts worldwide.

Indian Standing: In India, beta-ecdysterone is gaining recognition as a natural compound with potential health benefits, particularly in the realms of sports performance and physical fitness.

Research Summary of Beta-ecdysterone: Overall, research on beta-ecdysterone suggests its potential as an anabolic agent with applications in sports performance and muscle growth. While some studies demonstrate promising results, further research is needed to confirm its efficacy and safety, particularly in humans, and to elucidate its mechanisms of action in greater detail.

9) Ȕ-GLUCANS

Introduction: Beta-glucans are a group of naturally occurring polysaccharides found in various sources such as oats, barley, mushrooms, and yeast. They are renowned for their immunomodulatory properties and potential health benefits, including supporting immune function, improving cholesterol levels, and promoting heart health.

Synonym Name and Common Name: Synonym: β-glucans, beta-d-glucans Common Name: Beta-glucans

Pharmacognosy / Chemistry: Beta-glucans are complex polysaccharides composed of glucose monomers linked together by beta-glycosidic bonds. They vary in structure depending on the source, with different degrees of branching and molecular weight.

Action and Pharmacology: Beta-glucans exert their pharmacological effects primarily through modulation of the immune system. They interact with immune cells such as macrophages, dendritic cells, and natural killer cells, enhancing their activity and promoting immune surveillance and defense against pathogens.

Method of Analysis: Beta-glucans can be analyzed using various techniques, including spectrophotometry, chromatography, and enzymatic assays, to quantify their concentration and structural properties in food products, dietary supplements, and biological samples.

Health Benefits:

- Supports immune function
- Modulates cholesterol levels
- Promotes heart health
- Exhibits antioxidant properties
- Enhances wound healing
- May have anticancer effects

Indication and Usage: Beta-glucans are commonly used as dietary supplements to support immune function, particularly during times of increased susceptibility to infections or stress. They may also be incorporated into functional foods and beverages for their health-promoting properties.

Usual Constituents with Percentages: The content of beta-glucans in food sources varies depending on the source and processing methods. Oats and barley, for example, contain approximately 3-8% beta-glucans by dry weight, while certain mushrooms may contain higher concentrations.

Mechanism of Action: Beta-glucans interact with immune cells via specific receptors, such as dectin-1 and complement receptor 3 (CR3), triggering signaling pathways that lead to immune activation. They also stimulate the production of cytokines and other immune mediators involved in immune response and inflammation.

Dosage: Recommended dosages for beta-glucan supplementation vary depending on the source and intended health benefits. Typical doses range from 100 to 500 milligrams per day, but higher doses may be used in certain therapeutic contexts under medical supervision.

Contraindications: There are no known contraindications for beta-glucan supplementation when used at recommended doses. However, individuals with known allergies to beta-glucans or fungal products should exercise caution.

Precautions:

- Pregnant and breastfeeding women should consult with a healthcare professional before using beta-glucan supplements.
- Individuals with autoimmune diseases or those taking immunosuppressive medications should use beta-glucan supplements with caution due to their potential immune-stimulating effects.

Adverse Reactions: Beta-glucans are generally well-tolerated when used at recommended doses. However, some individuals may experience mild gastrointestinal discomfort or allergic reactions in rare cases.

Research Summary: Research on beta-glucans has demonstrated their potential as immunomodulators and health-promoting compounds. Studies have shown benefits in supporting immune function, improving cholesterol levels, and promoting heart health. Additionally, beta-glucans may have antioxidant, wound-healing, and anticancer effects, although further research is needed to elucidate their mechanisms of action and optimize their therapeutic applications.

Pharmacokinetics: Limited information is available on the pharmacokinetics of beta-glucans in humans. Studies suggest that they are poorly absorbed in the gastrointestinal tract and may undergo fermentation by gut microbiota, leading to the production of short-chain fatty acids and other metabolites with potential health benefits.

Pharmacodynamics: Beta-glucans exert their pharmacodynamic effects primarily through modulation of the immune system, including activation of immune cells, production of cytokines, and enhancement of immune surveillance and defense mechanisms against pathogens.

Overdosage: There is limited information on the effects of overdosage with beta-glucans. However, exceeding recommended doses may increase the risk of gastrointestinal side effects and allergic reactions.

International Standing: Beta-glucans are recognized internationally as valuable dietary components with potential health benefits. They are commonly used as functional ingredients in food products and dietary supplements marketed for immune support and overall well-being.

Indian Standing: In India, beta-glucans are gaining recognition for their immunomodulatory properties and potential health benefits. They are incorporated into various traditional remedies and functional foods, reflecting their growing popularity within the Indian healthcare system.

Research Summary of Beta-glucans: Overall, research on beta-glucans supports their role in supporting immune function, improving cholesterol levels, and promoting overall health. While further studies are needed to elucidate their mechanisms of action and optimize their therapeutic applications, beta-glucans show promise as valuable dietary components with diverse health benefits.

10) Ȕ-SITOSTEROL

Introduction: Beta-sitosterol is a plant sterol commonly found in various plant-based foods and dietary supplements. It belongs to the phytosterol group and shares structural similarities with cholesterol. Beta-sitosterol has gained attention for its potential health benefits, particularly in supporting cardiovascular health and managing cholesterol levels.

Synonym Name and Common Name: Synonym: β-sitosterol, sitosterol Common Name: Beta-sitosterol

Pharmacognosy / Chemistry: Beta-sitosterol is a phytosterol naturally occurring in plants such as soybeans, nuts, seeds, and certain vegetables. It is a white, waxy substance with a similar appearance to cholesterol.

Action and Pharmacology: Beta-sitosterol exerts its pharmacological effects primarily through its ability to inhibit the absorption of dietary cholesterol in the intestines. It competes with cholesterol for absorption sites, leading to reduced cholesterol absorption and lower blood cholesterol levels.

Method of Analysis: Beta-sitosterol levels can be analyzed using techniques such as gas chromatography or high-performance liquid chromatography (HPLC) after extraction from plant sources or dietary supplements.

Health Benefits:

- Supports cardiovascular health
- Helps manage cholesterol levels
- May reduce inflammation
- May alleviate symptoms of benign prostatic hyperplasia (BPH)
- May have antioxidant properties

Indication and Usage: Beta-sitosterol is commonly used as a dietary supplement to support cardiovascular health and manage cholesterol levels, particularly in individuals with hypercholesterolemia or those at risk of cardiovascular disease. It may also be used as a complementary therapy for BPH and inflammatory conditions.

Usual Constituents with Percentages: Beta-sitosterol content varies among different plant sources. For example, soybeans contain approximately 1-3% beta-sitosterol by dry weight, while nuts and seeds may have slightly lower concentrations.

Mechanism of Action: Beta-sitosterol inhibits the absorption of cholesterol in the intestines by competing with cholesterol for incorporation into mixed micelles, which are necessary for lipid absorption. This leads to reduced cholesterol absorption and lower blood cholesterol levels.

Dosage: Recommended dosages for beta-sitosterol supplementation vary depending on individual needs and health conditions. Typical doses range from 200 to 800 milligrams per day, divided into multiple doses for optimal absorption.

Contraindications: There are no known contraindications for beta-sitosterol when used at recommended doses. However, individuals with rare phytosterolemia disorders should avoid beta-sitosterol supplementation.

Precautions:

- Pregnant and breastfeeding women should consult with a healthcare professional before using beta-sitosterol supplements.
- Individuals with liver disease or those taking cholesterol-lowering medications should use beta-sitosterol supplements with caution under medical supervision.

Adverse Reactions: Beta-sitosterol is generally well-tolerated when used at recommended doses. However, some individuals may experience mild gastrointestinal discomfort or allergic reactions in rare cases.

Research Summary: Research on beta-sitosterol has demonstrated its potential as a natural compound for supporting cardiovascular health and managing cholesterol levels. Studies have shown that beta-sitosterol supplementation can reduce total and LDL cholesterol levels, improve lipid profiles, and exert anti-inflammatory effects. Additionally, beta-sitosterol may alleviate symptoms of BPH and exhibit antioxidant properties.

Pharmacokinetics: Beta-sitosterol is poorly absorbed in the gastrointestinal tract and undergoes extensive metabolism in the liver. It is excreted primarily in the feces, with minimal absorption into systemic circulation.

Pharmacodynamics: Beta-sitosterol exerts its pharmacodynamic effects primarily through inhibition of cholesterol absorption in the intestines, leading to reduced blood cholesterol levels and improved lipid profiles. It may also modulate inflammatory pathways and antioxidant mechanisms.

Overdosage: There is limited information on the effects of overdosage with beta-sitosterol. However, exceeding recommended doses may increase the risk of gastrointestinal side effects and adverse reactions.

International Standing: Beta-sitosterol is recognized internationally as a valuable dietary supplement for supporting cardiovascular health and managing cholesterol levels. It is widely used as a natural alternative to conventional cholesterol-lowering medications.

Indian Standing: In India, beta-sitosterol is gaining recognition for its potential health benefits and is commonly used in traditional medicine systems. Its use as a dietary supplement for supporting cardiovascular health aligns with traditional practices and modern healthcare approaches.

Research Summary of Beta-sitosterol: Overall, research on beta-sitosterol supports its role in supporting cardiovascular health, managing cholesterol levels, and potentially alleviating symptoms of BPH. While further studies are needed to elucidate its mechanisms of action and optimize its therapeutic applications, beta-sitosterol shows promise as a natural compound for promoting overall well-being and reducing the risk of chronic diseases.

11) CAMPESTANOL

Introduction: Campestanol is a phytosterol found in various plant-based foods and oils. It is structurally similar to cholesterol and other plant sterols and has gained attention for its potential health benefits, particularly in supporting cardiovascular health and managing cholesterol levels.

Synonym Name and Common Name: Synonym: 24-Ethylcholestanol Common Name: Campestanol

Pharmacognosy / Chemistry: Campestanol is a phytosterol naturally occurring in plants such as soybeans, nuts, seeds, and certain vegetable oils. It is a white, waxy substance with a similar appearance to cholesterol.

Action and Pharmacology: Campestanol exerts its pharmacological effects primarily through its ability to inhibit the absorption of dietary cholesterol in the intestines. It competes with cholesterol for absorption sites, leading to reduced cholesterol absorption and lower blood cholesterol levels.

Method of Analysis: Campestanol levels can be analyzed using techniques such as gas chromatography or high-performance liquid chromatography (HPLC) after extraction from plant sources or dietary supplements.

Health Benefits:

- Supports cardiovascular health
- Helps manage cholesterol levels
- May reduce inflammation

- May have antioxidant properties

Indication and Usage: Campestanol is commonly used as a dietary supplement to support cardiovascular health and manage cholesterol levels, particularly in individuals with hypercholesterolemia or those at risk of cardiovascular disease.

Usual Constituents with Percentages: The content of campestanol in plant sources varies depending on the source and processing methods. For example, soybeans contain approximately 0.5-1% campestanol by dry weight, while nuts and seeds may have slightly lower concentrations.

Mechanism of Action: Campestanol inhibits the absorption of cholesterol in the intestines by competing with cholesterol for incorporation into mixed micelles, which are necessary for lipid absorption. This leads to reduced cholesterol absorption and lower blood cholesterol levels.

Dosage: Recommended dosages for campestanol supplementation vary depending on individual needs and health conditions. Typical doses range from 200 to 800 milligrams per day, divided into multiple doses for optimal absorption.

Contraindications: There are no known contraindications for campestanol when used at recommended doses. However, individuals with rare phytosterolemia disorders should avoid campestanol supplementation.

Precautions:

- Pregnant and breastfeeding women should consult with a healthcare professional before using campestanol supplements.
- Individuals with liver disease or those taking cholesterol-lowering medications should use campestanol supplements with caution under medical supervision.

Adverse Reactions: Campestanol is generally well-tolerated when used at recommended doses. However, some individuals may experience mild gastrointestinal discomfort or allergic reactions in rare cases.

Research Summary: Research on campestanol has demonstrated its potential as a natural compound for supporting cardiovascular health and managing cholesterol levels. Studies have shown that campestanol supplementation can reduce total and LDL cholesterol levels, improve lipid profiles, and exert anti-inflammatory effects. Additionally, campestanol may have antioxidant properties.

Pharmacokinetics: Campestanol is poorly absorbed in the gastrointestinal tract and undergoes extensive metabolism in the liver. It is excreted primarily in the feces, with minimal absorption into systemic circulation.

Pharmacodynamics: Campestanol exerts its pharmacodynamic effects primarily through inhibition of cholesterol absorption in the intestines, leading to reduced blood cholesterol levels and improved lipid profiles. It may also modulate inflammatory pathways and antioxidant mechanisms.

Overdosage: There is limited information on the effects of overdosage with campestanol. However, exceeding recommended doses may increase the risk of gastrointestinal side effects and adverse reactions.

International Standing: Campestanol is recognized internationally as a valuable dietary supplement for supporting cardiovascular health and managing cholesterol levels. It is widely used as a natural alternative to conventional cholesterol-lowering medications.

Indian Standing: In India, campestanol is gaining recognition for its potential health benefits and is commonly used in traditional medicine systems. Its use as a dietary supplement for supporting cardiovascular health aligns with traditional practices and modern healthcare approaches.

Research Summary of Campestanol: Overall, research on campestanol supports its role in supporting cardiovascular health, managing cholesterol levels, and potentially reducing inflammation. While further studies are needed to elucidate its mechanisms of action and optimize its therapeutic applications, campestanol shows promise as a natural compound for promoting overall well-being and reducing the risk of chronic diseases.

12) CAMPESTEROL

Introduction:

Campesterol is a phytosterol found in various plant-based foods and oils. It belongs to the group of plant sterols and shares structural similarities with cholesterol. Campesterol has garnered interest for its potential health benefits, particularly in supporting cardiovascular health and managing cholesterol levels.

Synonym Name and Common Name: Synonym: 24-Methylcholesterol Common Name: Campesterol

Pharmacognosy / Chemistry: Campesterol is a naturally occurring phytosterol found in plants such as soybeans, nuts, seeds, and certain vegetable oils. It is a white, waxy substance with a similar appearance to cholesterol.

Action and Pharmacology: Campesterol exerts its pharmacological effects primarily through its ability to inhibit the absorption of dietary cholesterol in the intestines. It competes with cholesterol for absorption sites, leading to reduced cholesterol absorption and lower blood cholesterol levels.

Method of Analysis: Campesterol levels can be analyzed using techniques such as gas chromatography or high-performance liquid chromatography (HPLC) after extraction from plant sources or dietary supplements.

Health Benefits:

- Supports cardiovascular health
- Helps manage cholesterol levels
- May reduce inflammation
- May have antioxidant properties

Indication and Usage: Campesterol is commonly used as a dietary supplement to support cardiovascular health and manage cholesterol levels, particularly in individuals with hypercholesterolemia or those at risk of cardiovascular disease.

Usual Constituents with Percentages: The content of campesterol in plant sources varies depending on the source and processing methods. For example, soybeans contain approximately 0.5-1% campesterol by dry weight, while nuts and seeds may have slightly lower concentrations.

Mechanism of Action: Campesterol inhibits the absorption of cholesterol in the intestines by competing with cholesterol for incorporation into mixed micelles, which are necessary for lipid absorption. This leads to reduced cholesterol absorption and lower blood cholesterol levels.

Dosage: Recommended dosages for campesterol supplementation vary depending on individual needs and health conditions. Typical doses range from 200 to 800 milligrams per day, divided into multiple doses for optimal absorption.

Contraindications: There are no known contraindications for campesterol when used at recommended doses. However, individuals with rare phytosterolemia disorders should avoid campesterol supplementation.

Precautions:

- Pregnant and breastfeeding women should consult with a healthcare professional before using campesterol supplements.
- Individuals with liver disease or those taking cholesterol-lowering medications should use campesterol supplements with caution under medical supervision.

Adverse Reactions: Campesterol is generally well-tolerated when used at recommended doses. However, some individuals may experience mild gastrointestinal discomfort or allergic reactions in rare cases.

Research Summary: Research on campesterol has demonstrated its potential as a natural compound for supporting cardiovascular health and managing cholesterol levels. Studies have shown that campesterol supplementation can reduce total and LDL cholesterol levels, improve lipid profiles, and exert anti-inflammatory effects. Additionally, campesterol may have antioxidant properties.

Pharmacokinetics: Campesterol is poorly absorbed in the gastrointestinal tract and undergoes extensive metabolism in the liver. It is excreted primarily in the feces, with minimal absorption into systemic circulation.

Pharmacodynamics: Campesterol exerts its pharmacodynamic effects primarily through inhibition of cholesterol absorption in the intestines, leading to reduced blood cholesterol levels and improved lipid profiles. It may also modulate inflammatory pathways and antioxidant mechanisms.

Overdosage: There is limited information on the effects of overdosage with campesterol. However, exceeding recommended doses may increase the risk of gastrointestinal side effects and adverse reactions.

International Standing: Campesterol is recognized internationally as a valuable dietary supplement for supporting cardiovascular health and managing cholesterol levels. It is widely used as a natural alternative to conventional cholesterol-lowering medications.

Indian Standing: In India, campesterol is gaining recognition for its potential health benefits and is commonly used in traditional medicine systems. Its use as a dietary supplement for supporting cardiovascular health aligns with traditional practices and modern healthcare approaches.

Research Summary of Campesterol: Overall, research on campesterol supports its role in supporting cardiovascular health, managing cholesterol levels, and potentially reducing inflammation. While further studies are needed to elucidate its mechanisms of action and optimize its therapeutic applications, campesterol shows promise as a natural compound for promoting overall well-being and reducing the risk of chronic diseases.

13) CAROTENOIDS

Introduction: Carotenoids are a group of naturally occurring pigments found in fruits, vegetables, and other plants. They are responsible for the vibrant red, orange, and yellow colors seen in many fruits and vegetables. Carotenoids are renowned for their antioxidant properties and potential health benefits.

Synonym Name and Common Name: Synonym: None Common Name: Carotenoids

Pharmacognosy / Chemistry: Carotenoids are lipid-soluble compounds synthesized by plants and certain microorganisms. They belong to the class of terpenoids and are characterized by their long carbon chains and multiple conjugated double bonds.

Action and Pharmacology: Carotenoids exert their pharmacological effects primarily through their antioxidant activity. They scavenge free radicals and reactive oxygen species, helping to protect cells and tissues from oxidative damage. Additionally, carotenoids may play roles in immune function, vision, and skin health.

Method of Analysis: Carotenoid levels can be analyzed using various techniques, including spectrophotometry, high-performance liquid chromatography (HPLC), and mass spectrometry. These methods allow for the quantification of specific carotenoids in food samples, dietary supplements, and biological tissues.

Health Benefits:

- Antioxidant protection
- Supports eye health and vision

- Promotes skin health and appearance
- Enhances immune function
- May reduce the risk of chronic diseases, including cardiovascular disease and certain cancers

Indication and Usage: Carotenoids are commonly consumed through a diet rich in fruits and vegetables. They are also available as dietary supplements for individuals seeking to augment their intake or address specific health concerns related to oxidative stress or nutrient deficiencies.

Usual Constituents with Percentages: Carotenoids encompass a wide range of compounds, including beta-carotene, lycopene, lutein, zeaxanthin, and others. Their concentrations in food sources vary, with fruits and vegetables such as carrots, spinach, tomatoes, and bell peppers being particularly rich sources.

Mechanism of Action: The primary mechanism of action of carotenoids is their antioxidant activity, which involves scavenging free radicals and reactive oxygen species to prevent oxidative damage to cells and tissues. Additionally, certain carotenoids may have specific roles in cellular signaling pathways and gene expression.

Dosage: There is no established recommended daily allowance (RDA) for carotenoids as a group. However, consuming a diverse range of fruits and vegetables rich in carotenoids is recommended as part of a balanced diet. Dietary supplements typically provide carotenoids in doses ranging from a few hundred to several thousand international units (IU) per day.

Contraindications: There are no known contraindications for the consumption of carotenoids from natural food sources. However, excessive intake of carotenoid supplements may cause skin discoloration (carotenemia) in some individuals.

Precautions:

- Pregnant and breastfeeding women should ensure adequate intake of carotenoid-rich foods as part of a healthy diet but should avoid excessive supplementation.
- Individuals with certain medical conditions, such as liver disease or lipid metabolism disorders, should use carotenoid supplements with caution and under medical supervision.

Adverse Reactions: Consumption of carotenoids from natural food sources is generally safe and well-tolerated. However, high-dose supplementation may lead to skin discoloration (carotenemia) or gastrointestinal disturbances in some individuals.

Research Summary: Research on carotenoids has extensively explored their antioxidant properties and potential health benefits. Studies have shown that carotenoid-rich diets or supplementation may reduce the risk of chronic diseases, including cardiovascular disease and certain cancers, and support eye health, skin health, and immune function. However, further research is needed to elucidate the specific mechanisms of action and optimize their therapeutic applications.

Pharmacokinetics: Carotenoids are absorbed in the intestines along with dietary fats and are incorporated into chylomicrons for transport in the lymphatic system. They are then delivered to various tissues, where they may be stored or metabolized into bioactive forms such as vitamin A.

Pharmacodynamics: The pharmacodynamic effects of carotenoids primarily involve their antioxidant activity, which helps protect cells and tissues from oxidative stress and damage. Additionally, certain carotenoids may have specific roles in cellular signaling pathways and gene expression, influencing various physiological processes.

Overdosage: Excessive intake of carotenoid supplements may lead to skin discoloration (carotenemia) or gastrointestinal disturbances. However, there is no evidence to suggest that high dietary intake of carotenoids from natural food sources poses any significant health risks.

International Standing: Carotenoids are recognized internationally as valuable dietary components with potential health benefits. They are commonly consumed worldwide through a diet rich in fruits and vegetables and are available as dietary supplements in many countries.

Indian Standing: In India, carotenoids are valued for their role in traditional medicine and are incorporated into various culinary dishes and dietary supplements. Their potential health benefits are widely acknowledged within the Indian healthcare system, and they are consumed as part of a balanced diet rich in fruits, vegetables, and spices.

Research Summary of Carotenoids: Overall, research on carotenoids underscores their importance in promoting health and preventing chronic diseases. While further studies are needed to elucidate their specific mechanisms of action and optimize their therapeutic applications, carotenoids represent a valuable component of a balanced diet and may offer significant health benefits when consumed regularly through a variety of plant-based foods.

14) CASEIN AND CASEINATES

Introduction: Casein is a type of protein found in milk, accounting for approximately 80% of the total protein content. Caseinates are derivatives of casein obtained through various processing methods. Both casein and caseinates have gained popularity as dietary supplements and food ingredients due to their high protein content and versatile functional properties.

Synonym Name and Common Name: Synonym: None Common Name: Casein and Caseinates

Pharmacognosy / Chemistry: Casein is a phosphoprotein composed of amino acids found in mammalian milk, particularly in cow's milk. It is characterized by its ability to form gel-like structures and undergo coagulation when exposed to acid or rennet enzymes. Caseinates are water-soluble derivatives of casein obtained by alkaline treatment or enzymatic hydrolysis.

Action and Pharmacology: Casein and caseinates are rich sources of essential amino acids, making them valuable dietary proteins for muscle growth, repair, and overall protein synthesis. They provide a sustained release of amino acids into the bloodstream, which can support muscle recovery and prevent muscle breakdown.

Method of Analysis: The protein content of casein and caseinates can be analyzed using various methods, including the Kjeldahl method, the Bradford assay, or near-infrared spectroscopy (NIRS). These techniques allow for the quantification of protein content and quality in food products and dietary supplements.

Health Benefits:

- Supports muscle growth and repair
- Provides a sustained release of amino acids
- Promotes satiety and weight management
- May have anti-inflammatory effects

- Supports bone health and calcium absorption

Indication and Usage: Casein and caseinates are commonly used as dietary supplements by athletes, bodybuilders, and individuals looking to increase their protein intake. They are also used as functional ingredients in a variety of food products, including protein bars, shakes, and dairy-based beverages.

Usual Constituents with Percentages: Casein typically constitutes about 80% of the total protein content in milk, with whey protein accounting for the remaining 20%. Caseinates are derived from casein and may have varying protein concentrations depending on the processing method and degree of hydrolysis.

Mechanism of Action: The mechanism of action of casein and caseinates involves their gradual digestion and absorption in the gastrointestinal tract, resulting in a sustained release of amino acids into the bloodstream. This sustained amino acid delivery supports muscle protein synthesis, recovery, and overall protein metabolism.

Dosage: Recommended dosages for casein and caseinate supplementation vary depending on individual protein needs and fitness goals. Typical doses range from 20 to 40 grams per serving, taken before bedtime or between meals to support muscle recovery and prevent muscle breakdown.

Contraindications: There are no known contraindications for the consumption of casein and caseinates in healthy individuals. However, individuals with milk allergies or lactose intolerance should avoid products containing casein or caseinates.

Precautions:

- Pregnant and breastfeeding women should consult with a healthcare professional before using casein or caseinate supplements.
- Individuals with kidney disease or impaired renal function should monitor their protein intake, including casein and caseinates, under medical supervision.

Adverse Reactions: Casein and caseinates are generally well-tolerated by most individuals. However, some people may experience gastrointestinal discomfort, bloating, or allergic reactions, particularly if they have milk allergies or lactose intolerance.

Research Summary: Research on casein and caseinates has demonstrated their efficacy in supporting muscle growth, recovery, and overall protein metabolism. Studies have shown that casein protein supplementation, particularly when consumed before bedtime, can enhance muscle protein synthesis, and promote muscle hypertrophy. Additionally, casein and caseinates may have beneficial effects on satiety, weight management, and bone health.

Pharmacokinetics: Casein and caseinates undergo gradual digestion and absorption in the gastrointestinal tract, resulting in a sustained release of amino acids into the bloodstream. This slow-release kinetics provide a prolonged supply of amino acids for muscle protein synthesis and metabolism.

Pharmacodynamics: The pharmacodynamic effects of casein and caseinates primarily involve their role as dietary proteins in supporting muscle growth, repair, and overall protein metabolism. They provide essential amino acids necessary for muscle protein synthesis and recovery, particularly during periods of rest or fasting.

Overdosage: Excessive intake of casein and caseinates may lead to gastrointestinal discomfort, bloating, or allergic reactions, particularly in individuals with milk allergies or lactose intolerance. However, there is no evidence to suggest significant health risks associated with moderate protein consumption from casein and caseinates.

International Standing: Casein and caseinates are recognized internationally as valuable sources of dietary protein for supporting muscle growth, recovery, and overall protein metabolism. They are widely used as dietary supplements and food ingredients in various countries.

Indian Standing: In India, casein and caseinates are valued for their nutritional properties and functional benefits in food products. They are commonly used in dairy-based beverages, protein supplements, and processed foods, reflecting their importance in the Indian food industry and dietary practices.

Research Summary of Casein and Caseinates: Overall, research on casein and caseinates supports their role as valuable dietary proteins for supporting muscle growth, recovery, and overall protein metabolism. Studies have demonstrated their efficacy in promoting muscle protein synthesis, enhancing satiety, and supporting bone health. However, further research is needed to optimize their therapeutic applications and elucidate their long-term effects on health and performance.

15) CHLOROGENIC ACIDS

Introduction: Chlorogenic acids (CGAs) are a group of naturally occurring polyphenolic compounds found in various plant-based foods, particularly in coffee beans, fruits, and vegetables. They are renowned for their antioxidant properties and potential health benefits, including supporting cardiovascular health, managing blood sugar levels, and promoting weight loss.

Synonym Name and Common Name: Synonym: Caffeoylquinic acids Common Name: Chlorogenic acids (CGAs)

Pharmacognosy / Chemistry: Chlorogenic acids are phenolic compounds derived from cinnamic acids, primarily caffeic acid and quinic acid. They are abundant in nature and contribute to the bitter taste of certain fruits and beverages, such as coffee and some fruits like apples and berries.

Action and Pharmacology: Chlorogenic acids exert their pharmacological effects primarily through their antioxidant activity. They scavenge free radicals and reactive oxygen species, helping to protect cells and tissues from oxidative damage. Additionally, CGAs may modulate glucose metabolism, lipid metabolism, and inflammation, contributing to their potential health benefits.

Method of Analysis: Chlorogenic acid content can be analyzed using various analytical techniques, including high-performance liquid chromatography (HPLC), gas chromatography-mass spectrometry (GC-MS), and spectrophotometry. These methods allow for the quantification of specific CGAs in food products, dietary supplements, and biological samples.

Health Benefits:

- Antioxidant protection
- Supports cardiovascular health
- Modulates blood sugar levels
- Promotes weight loss
- Exhibits anti-inflammatory effects
- May have neuroprotective effects

Indication and Usage: Chlorogenic acids are commonly consumed through a diet rich in fruits, vegetables, and coffee. They are also available as dietary supplements for individuals seeking to augment their intake or address specific health concerns related to oxidative stress, blood sugar control, or weight management.

Usual Constituents with Percentages: Chlorogenic acids encompass a group of compounds with varying structures and concentrations depending on the source. Coffee beans, for example, contain approximately 6-7% chlorogenic acids by dry weight, with the most abundant being caffeoylquinic acids.

Mechanism of Action: The primary mechanism of action of chlorogenic acids is their antioxidant activity, which involves scavenging free radicals and reactive oxygen species to prevent oxidative damage to cells and tissues. Additionally, CGAs may modulate glucose metabolism, lipid metabolism, and inflammatory pathways, contributing to their diverse health benefits.

Dosage: Recommended dosages for chlorogenic acid supplementation vary depending on individual needs and health conditions. Typical doses range from 200 to 800 milligrams per day, taken with meals to support blood sugar control or as part of a weight management regimen.

Contraindications: There are no known contraindications for the consumption of chlorogenic acids from natural food sources. However, individuals with coffee allergies or sensitivities should avoid excessive consumption of coffee or chlorogenic acid supplements.

Precautions:

- Pregnant and breastfeeding women should consult with a healthcare professional before using chlorogenic acid supplements.
- Individuals with certain medical conditions, such as gastrointestinal disorders or anxiety disorders, should use chlorogenic acid supplements with caution and under medical supervision.

Adverse Reactions: Chlorogenic acids are generally well-tolerated when consumed in moderation through dietary sources. However, excessive consumption of coffee or chlorogenic acid supplements may lead to gastrointestinal discomfort, insomnia, or anxiety in some individuals.

Research Summary: Research on chlorogenic acids has demonstrated their potential as natural antioxidants and health-promoting compounds. Studies have shown that chlorogenic acid supplementation may support cardiovascular health, improve glucose metabolism, promote weight loss, and reduce inflammation. Additionally, CGAs may have neuroprotective effects and contribute to overall well-being when consumed as part of a balanced diet.

Pharmacokinetics: Chlorogenic acids are absorbed in the gastrointestinal tract and undergo metabolism in the liver. They are then distributed to various tissues, where they exert their antioxidant and pharmacological effects. Excess chlorogenic acids are eliminated from the body primarily through urine and feces.

Pharmacodynamics: The pharmacodynamic effects of chlorogenic acids primarily involve their antioxidant activity, which helps protect cells and tissues from oxidative stress and damage. Additionally, CGAs may modulate glucose metabolism, lipid metabolism, and inflammatory pathways, contributing to their diverse health benefits.

Overdosage: Excessive intake of chlorogenic acid supplements may lead to gastrointestinal discomfort, insomnia, or anxiety in some individuals. However, there is no evidence to suggest significant health risks associated with moderate consumption of chlorogenic acids from natural food sources.

International Standing: Chlorogenic acids are recognized internationally as valuable dietary components with potential health benefits. They are commonly consumed worldwide through a diet rich in fruits, vegetables, and coffee and are available as dietary supplements in many countries.

Indian Standing: In India, chlorogenic acids are valued for their nutritional properties and potential health benefits. They are commonly consumed as part of traditional diets rich in fruits, vegetables, and spices and are also found in Indian coffee varieties. Additionally, chlorogenic acid supplements are available in the Indian market and are used by individuals seeking to augment their dietary intake or address specific health concerns.

Research Summary of Chlorogenic Acids: Overall, research on chlorogenic acids supports their role as valuable dietary antioxidants with potential health benefits. Studies have demonstrated their efficacy in supporting cardiovascular health, improving glucose metabolism, promoting weight loss, and reducing inflammation. However, further research is needed to elucidate their specific mechanisms of action and optimize their therapeutic applications in various health conditions.

16) CAFFEIC ACID

Introduction: Caffeic acid is a naturally occurring organic compound belonging to the group of phenolic acids. It is found abundantly in various plant-based foods, such as coffee, fruits, vegetables, and grains. Caffeic acid has gained attention for its potential health benefits and medicinal properties.

Synonym Name and Common Name: Synonym: 3,4-dihydroxycinnamic acid Common Name: Caffeic acid

Pharmacognosy / Chemistry: Caffeic acid is a hydroxycinnamic acid derivative, characterized by its phenolic structure. It is present in plants as a secondary metabolite, particularly in the form of esters, glycosides, and conjugates. Caffeic acid contributes to the bitterness and astringency of certain foods and beverages.

Action and Pharmacology: Caffeic acid exerts its pharmacological effects primarily through its antioxidant and anti-inflammatory properties. It scavenges free radicals and reactive oxygen species, helping to protect cells and tissues from oxidative damage. Additionally, caffeic acid may modulate inflammatory pathways and enzymatic activities involved in cellular signaling.

Method of Analysis: Caffeic acid content can be analyzed using various analytical techniques, including high-performance liquid chromatography (HPLC), gas chromatography-mass spectrometry (GC-MS), and spectrophotometry. These methods allow for the quantification of caffeic acid in food products, dietary supplements, and biological samples.

Health Benefits:

- Antioxidant protection
- Anti-inflammatory effects
- Cardiovascular support
- Antimicrobial activity
- Potential anti-cancer properties
- Skin health benefits

Indication and Usage: Caffeic acid is consumed naturally through a diet rich in fruits, vegetables, coffee, and whole grains. It is also available as a dietary supplement for individuals seeking to augment their intake or address specific health concerns related to oxidative stress, inflammation, or skin health.

Usual Constituents with Percentages: Caffeic acid content varies depending on the source and processing methods. For example, coffee beans may contain approximately 1-2% caffeic acid by dry weight, while fruits and vegetables may have lower concentrations. The percentage of caffeic acid in dietary supplements can vary depending on the formulation.

Mechanism of Action: The primary mechanism of action of caffeic acid is its antioxidant activity, which involves scavenging free radicals and reactive oxygen species to prevent oxidative damage to cells and tissues. Additionally, caffeic acid may modulate inflammatory pathways, inhibit enzymes involved in inflammation, and regulate gene expression related to cellular processes.

Dosage: Recommended dosages for caffeic acid supplementation vary depending on individual needs and health conditions. Typical doses range from 100 to 500 milligrams per day, taken with meals to support antioxidant and anti-inflammatory effects.

Contraindications: There are no known contraindications for the consumption of caffeic acid from natural food sources. However, individuals with allergies or sensitivities to caffeic acid-containing foods should avoid excessive consumption.

Precautions:

- Pregnant and breastfeeding women should consult with a healthcare professional before using caffeic acid supplements.
- Individuals with certain medical conditions, such as liver disease or gastrointestinal disorders, should use caffeic acid supplements with caution and under medical supervision.

Adverse Reactions: Caffeic acid is generally well-tolerated when consumed in moderation through dietary sources. However, excessive consumption or supplementation may lead to gastrointestinal discomfort, allergic reactions, or interactions with certain medications.

Research Summary: Research on caffeic acid has demonstrated its potential as a natural antioxidant and anti-inflammatory compound with various health benefits. Studies have shown that caffeic acid supplementation may support cardiovascular health, reduce inflammation, exhibit antimicrobial activity, and potentially inhibit cancer cell growth. Additionally, caffeic acid may have beneficial effects on skin health, including antioxidant protection and anti-aging properties.

Pharmacokinetics: Caffeic acid is absorbed in the gastrointestinal tract and undergoes metabolism in the liver. It is then distributed to various tissues, where it exerts its antioxidant and pharmacological effects. Excess caffeic acid is eliminated from the body primarily through urine and feces.

Pharmacodynamics: The pharmacodynamic effects of caffeic acid primarily involve its antioxidant and anti-inflammatory activities, which help protect cells and tissues from oxidative stress and inflammation. Additionally, caffeic acid may modulate enzymatic activities, gene expression, and cellular signaling pathways involved in various physiological processes.

Overdosage: Excessive intake of caffeic acid supplements may lead to gastrointestinal discomfort, allergic reactions, or interactions with certain medications. However, there is no evidence to suggest significant health risks associated with moderate consumption of caffeic acid from natural food sources.

International Standing: Caffeic acid is recognized internationally as a valuable dietary component with potential health benefits. It is commonly consumed worldwide through a diet rich in fruits, vegetables, coffee, and whole grains.

Indian Standing: In India, caffeic acid is valued for its medicinal properties and is consumed as part of traditional diets rich in fruits, vegetables, and spices. Additionally, caffeic acid supplements are available in the Indian market and are used by individuals seeking to augment their dietary intake or address specific health concerns.

Research Summary of Caffeic Acid: Overall, research on caffeic acid supports its role as a natural antioxidant and anti-inflammatory compound with various health benefits. Studies have demonstrated its efficacy in supporting cardiovascular health, reducing inflammation, exhibiting antimicrobial activity, and potentially inhibiting cancer cell growth. However, further research is needed to elucidate its specific mechanisms of action and optimize its therapeutic applications in various health conditions.

17) CHONDROITIN SULPHATE

Introduction: Chondroitin sulfate is a naturally occurring compound found in the connective tissues of animals, including humans. It is a major component of cartilage, contributing to its strength, elasticity, and shock-absorbing properties. Chondroitin sulfate is commonly used as a dietary supplement to support joint health and manage osteoarthritis symptoms.

Synonym Name and Common Name: Synonym: Chondroitin polysulfate Common Name: Chondroitin sulfate

Pharmacognosy / Chemistry: Chondroitin sulfate is a glycosaminoglycan composed of repeating disaccharide units of N-acetylgalactosamine and glucuronic acid. It is extracted from animal cartilage, primarily bovine or porcine sources, and processed into supplement form. Chondroitin sulfate is available as a powder, capsule, or tablet.

Action and Pharmacology: Chondroitin sulfate exerts its pharmacological effects primarily through its role in maintaining joint health and cartilage integrity. It helps to maintain the structural integrity of cartilage by promoting water retention and inhibiting enzymes that degrade cartilage components. Additionally, chondroitin sulfate may have anti-inflammatory properties, further supporting joint function.

Method of Analysis: The content and purity of chondroitin sulfate in dietary supplements can be analyzed using various methods, including high-performance liquid chromatography (HPLC), capillary electrophoresis, and enzymatic assays. These techniques allow for the quantification of chondroitin sulfate and identification of impurities or adulterants.

HEALTH BENEFITS:

- Supports joint health and mobility
- Helps manage osteoarthritis symptoms
- May reduce joint pain and inflammation
- Supports cartilage regeneration and repair

Indication and Usage: Chondroitin sulfate is commonly used as a dietary supplement for individuals with osteoarthritis or joint pain. It is often taken in combination with glucosamine or other supplements to support overall joint health and alleviate symptoms of arthritis.

Usual Constituents with Percentages: Chondroitin sulfate supplements typically contain chondroitin sulfate derived from animal cartilage, with concentrations ranging from 400 to 1200 milligrams per serving. The purity and quality of chondroitin sulfate supplements can vary depending on the manufacturing process and source.

Mechanism of Action: The mechanism of action of chondroitin sulfate involves several pathways:

- Promoting water retention in cartilage, which helps maintain its elasticity and shock-absorbing properties.
- Inhibiting enzymes, such as matrix metalloproteinases, that degrade cartilage components, thereby slowing down cartilage degradation.
- Modulating inflammatory pathways and reducing the production of inflammatory mediators, which may help alleviate joint pain and inflammation.

Dosage: Recommended dosages for chondroitin sulfate supplementation typically range from 800 to 1200 milligrams per day, divided into two or three doses. It is often taken in combination with glucosamine or other joint health supplements for optimal efficacy.

Contraindications: There are no known contraindications for the use of chondroitin sulfate in most individuals. However, individuals with allergies to shellfish or other animal-derived products should use caution, as chondroitin sulfate supplements may contain traces of these allergens.

Precautions:

- Pregnant and breastfeeding women should consult with a healthcare professional before using chondroitin sulfate supplements.
- Individuals taking blood-thinning medications or anticoagulants should use caution when taking chondroitin sulfate, as it may increase the risk of bleeding.

Adverse Reactions: Chondroitin sulfate supplements are generally well-tolerated by most individuals. However, some people may experience mild gastrointestinal discomfort, such as bloating or diarrhea, particularly when starting supplementation or taking high doses.

Research Summary: Research on chondroitin sulfate has shown promising results in supporting joint health and managing osteoarthritis symptoms. Clinical studies have demonstrated that chondroitin sulfate supplementation can reduce joint pain, improve joint function, and slow down the progression of osteoarthritis. Additionally, chondroitin sulfate may have synergistic effects when combined with glucosamine or other joint health supplements.

Pharmacokinetics: Chondroitin sulfate is absorbed in the gastrointestinal tract and distributed to joint tissues, where it exerts its pharmacological effects. It has a long half-life, with peak concentrations reached within a few hours of ingestion. Chondroitin sulfate is metabolized in the liver and excreted primarily in the urine.

Pharmacodynamics: The pharmacodynamic effects of chondroitin sulfate primarily involve its role in maintaining joint health and cartilage integrity. It promotes water retention in cartilage, inhibits enzymes that degrade cartilage components, and modulates inflammatory pathways to alleviate joint pain and inflammation.

Overdosage: There is limited information on the effects of overdosage with chondroitin sulfate. However, exceeding recommended doses may increase the risk of adverse reactions, such as gastrointestinal discomfort or allergic reactions, in some individuals.

International Standing: Chondroitin sulfate is recognized internationally as a valuable dietary supplement for supporting joint health and managing osteoarthritis symptoms. It is commonly used in various countries and is available over-the-counter in pharmacies and health food stores.

Indian Standing: In India, chondroitin sulfate is gaining recognition as a natural remedy for joint pain and osteoarthritis. It is available as a dietary supplement and is used by individuals seeking to alleviate joint symptoms and improve mobility. However, more research is needed to establish its efficacy and safety in the Indian population.

Research Summary of Chondroitin Sulfate: Overall, research on chondroitin sulfate supports its role as a valuable dietary supplement for supporting joint health and managing osteoarthritis symptoms. Clinical studies have demonstrated its efficacy in reducing joint pain, improving joint function, and slowing down the progression of osteoarthritis. Additionally, chondroitin sulfate is well-tolerated with few adverse effects, making it a safe option for individuals with joint concerns.

18) CITRULLINE/ L-CITRULLINE DL-MALATE (2:1)

Introduction: Citrulline, specifically L-citrulline, is a non-essential amino acid naturally found in foods such as watermelon, cucumbers, and pumpkins. It is also produced in the body as a byproduct of the urea cycle. L-citrulline DL-malate (2:1) is a compound formed by combining L-citrulline with malic acid. These compounds have gained attention for their potential health benefits, particularly in improving exercise performance and cardiovascular health.

Synonym Name and Common Name: Synonym: None Common Name: Citrulline or L-citrulline; L-citrulline DL-malate (2:1)

Pharmacognosy / Chemistry: Citrulline is a non-proteinogenic amino acid, meaning it is not used in protein synthesis. It is synthesized in the body from ornithine and carbamoyl phosphate during the urea cycle. L-citrulline DL-malate (2:1) is a compound formed by combining L-citrulline with malic acid, resulting in a 2:1 ratio of L-citrulline to malic acid.

Action and Pharmacology: Citrulline plays a role in the urea cycle, where it helps remove ammonia, a toxic byproduct of protein metabolism, from the body. L-citrulline DL-malate (2:1) is commonly used as a dietary supplement to support exercise performance, increase nitric oxide production, and improve blood flow, thereby enhancing oxygen and nutrient delivery to muscles.

Method of Analysis: The concentration of citrulline in supplements can be analyzed using various techniques, including high-performance liquid chromatography (HPLC), gas chromatography-mass spectrometry (GC-MS), or spectrophotometry. These methods allow for the quantification of citrulline and verification of the 2:1 ratio of L-citrulline to malic acid in L-citrulline DL-malate supplements.

Health Benefits:

- Enhances exercise performance and endurance
- Increases nitric oxide production, promoting vasodilation and improved blood flow
- Supports cardiovascular health
- May reduce muscle soreness and fatigue

- Supports ammonia detoxification and kidney function

Indication and Usage: L-citrulline and L-citrulline DL-malate supplements are commonly used by athletes and individuals seeking to improve exercise performance, increase muscle pumps, and support overall cardiovascular health. They are often taken before workouts or physical activity to enhance endurance and recovery.

Usual Constituents with Percentages: L-citrulline supplements typically contain pure L-citrulline or L-citrulline DL-malate (2:1), with L-citrulline comprising 100% of the active ingredient. In L-citrulline DL-malate (2:1), malic acid makes up the remaining percentage, usually around 50%.

Mechanism of Action: The primary mechanism of action of L-citrulline and L-citrulline DL-malate involves increasing nitric oxide (NO) production in the body. Nitric oxide promotes vasodilation, widening blood vessels and improving blood flow to muscles during exercise. This enhanced blood flow increases oxygen and nutrient delivery to muscles, delaying fatigue and improving endurance.

Dosage: Recommended dosages of L-citrulline supplements vary depending on individual needs and exercise goals. Typical doses range from 3 to 8 grams of L-citrulline per day or 6 to 15 grams of L-citrulline DL-malate (2:1) per day, taken before exercise or physical activity.

Contraindications: There are no known contraindications for the use of L-citrulline or L-citrulline DL-malate supplements in healthy individuals. However, individuals with certain medical conditions or those taking medications should consult with a healthcare professional before use.

Precautions:

Pregnant and breastfeeding women should consult with a healthcare professional before using L-citrulline supplements.

Individuals with kidney or liver disease should use L-citrulline supplements with caution, as excessive intake may exacerbate these conditions.

Adverse Reactions: L-citrulline supplements are generally well-tolerated when taken at recommended doses. However, some individuals may experience mild gastrointestinal discomfort, such as bloating or diarrhea, particularly when first starting supplementation.

Research Summary: Research on L-citrulline and L-citrulline DL-malate has shown promising results in enhancing exercise performance, increasing nitric oxide production, and improving cardiovascular health. Clinical studies have demonstrated that supplementation with L-citrulline can increase exercise endurance, reduce muscle soreness, and improve blood flow to muscles during exercise. Additionally, L-citrulline may have potential benefits for individuals with certain medical conditions, such as hypertension and erectile dysfunction.

Pharmacokinetics: After ingestion, L-citrulline is absorbed in the small intestine and enters the bloodstream. It is then transported to tissues, where it is converted into arginine, a precursor to nitric oxide. L-citrulline DL-malate is metabolized similarly, with malic acid being metabolized into intermediates of the citric acid cycle.

Pharmacodynamics: The pharmacodynamic effects of L-citrulline and L-citrulline DL-malate primarily involve increasing nitric oxide production and promoting vasodilation. This enhances blood flow to muscles during exercise, leading to improved oxygen and nutrient delivery, reduced fatigue, and enhanced performance.

Overdosage: Excessive intake of L-citrulline supplements may lead to gastrointestinal discomfort, such as bloating or diarrhea. However, there is limited information on the effects of long-term overdosage. It is important to follow recommended dosages and consult with a healthcare professional if experiencing adverse effects.

International Standing: L-citrulline supplements are recognized internationally as dietary supplements commonly used to enhance exercise performance and support cardiovascular health. They are widely available over-the-counter in many countries and are commonly used by athletes and fitness enthusiasts.

Indian Standing: In India, L-citrulline and L-citrulline DL-malate supplements are gaining popularity among athletes, bodybuilders, and individuals seeking to improve exercise performance and endurance. They are available in the Indian market through various retailers and online platforms, reflecting their growing demand among consumers.

Research Summary of Citrulline/ L-citrulline DL-malate (2:1): Overall, research on L-citrulline and L-citrulline DL-malate supports their potential benefits in enhancing exercise performance, increasing nitric oxide production, and improving cardiovascular health. Clinical studies have demonstrated their efficacy in improving endurance, reducing muscle soreness, and promoting vasodilation during exercise. However, further research is needed to elucidate their specific mechanisms of action, optimal dosages, and long-term effects on health and performance.

19)CITRUS NARINGENIN

Introduction: Citrus naringenin is a flavonoid compound found abundantly in citrus fruits such as oranges, grapefruits, and lemons. It belongs to the flavanone subclass of flavonoids and is recognized for its potential health benefits, particularly its antioxidant and anti-inflammatory properties.

Synonym Name and Common Name: Synonym: Naringenin Common Name: Citrus naringenin

Pharmacognosy / Chemistry: Citrus naringenin is a flavonoid compound with a characteristic bitter taste found in the peel, pulp, and seeds of citrus fruits. It is synthesized in the endocarp of citrus fruits and contributes to their flavor and aroma.

Action and Pharmacology: Naringenin exerts various pharmacological effects, including antioxidant, anti-inflammatory, anti-cancer, and cardioprotective properties. It scavenges free radicals, inhibits inflammatory pathways, modulates enzyme activity, and interacts with cell signaling pathways, contributing to its diverse health benefits.

Method of Analysis: The concentration of naringenin in citrus fruits and dietary supplements can be analyzed using various analytical techniques, including high-performance liquid chromatography (HPLC), mass spectrometry (MS), and spectrophotometry. These methods allow for the quantification and identification of naringenin in complex matrices.

Health Benefits:

- Antioxidant protection
- Anti-inflammatory effects
- Cardiovascular support
- Potential anti-cancer properties
- Metabolic health benefits
- Skin health benefits

Indication and Usage: Citrus naringenin is consumed naturally through a diet rich in citrus fruits. It is also available as a dietary supplement for individuals seeking to augment their intake or address specific health concerns related to oxidative stress, inflammation, cardiovascular health, or metabolic health.

Usual Constituents with Percentages: The content of naringenin in citrus fruits varies depending on the species, variety, ripeness, and processing methods. Oranges, for example, may contain approximately 0.1-0.5% naringenin by weight, with higher concentrations found in the peel and pulp.

Mechanism of Action: The primary mechanism of action of naringenin involves its antioxidant and anti-inflammatory properties. It scavenges free radicals, reduces oxidative stress, inhibits inflammatory pathways, and modulates enzyme activity, contributing to its diverse health benefits.

Dosage: Recommended dosages for naringenin supplementation vary depending on individual needs and health conditions. Typical doses range from 50 to 500 milligrams per day, taken with meals to enhance absorption and efficacy.

Contraindications: There are no known contraindications for the consumption of naringenin from natural food sources. However, individuals with citrus allergies or sensitivities should avoid excessive consumption of citrus fruits or naringenin supplements.

Precautions:

- Pregnant and breastfeeding women should consult with a healthcare professional before using naringenin supplements.
- Individuals taking medications, particularly statins, calcium channel blockers, or blood thinners, should use naringenin supplements with caution due to potential interactions.

Adverse Reactions: Naringenin is generally well-tolerated when consumed in moderation through dietary sources. However, excessive consumption or supplementation may lead to gastrointestinal discomfort, such as bloating or diarrhea, in some individuals.

Research Summary: Research on naringenin has demonstrated its potential as a natural antioxidant and anti-inflammatory compound with various health benefits. Studies have shown that naringenin supplementation may support cardiovascular health, reduce inflammation, modulate lipid metabolism, and exhibit potential anti-cancer properties. Additionally, naringenin may have beneficial effects on metabolic health and skin health.

Pharmacokinetics: After ingestion, naringenin is absorbed in the gastrointestinal tract and undergoes metabolism in the liver. It is then distributed to various tissues, where it exerts its pharmacological effects. Excess naringenin is eliminated from the body primarily through urine and feces.

Pharmacodynamics: The pharmacodynamic effects of naringenin primarily involve its antioxidant and anti-inflammatory activities, which help protect cells and tissues from oxidative stress and inflammation. Additionally, naringenin may modulate enzyme activity, cell signaling pathways, and gene expression related to various physiological processes.

Overdosage: Excessive intake of naringenin supplements may lead to gastrointestinal discomfort, such as bloating or diarrhea. However, there is limited information on the effects of long-term overdosage. It is important to follow recommended dosages and consult with a healthcare professional if experiencing adverse effects.

International Standing: Naringenin is recognized internationally as a valuable dietary component with potential health benefits. It is commonly consumed worldwide through a diet rich in citrus fruits and is available as a dietary supplement in many countries.

Indian Standing: In India, naringenin is valued for its medicinal properties and is consumed as part of traditional diets rich in citrus fruits. Additionally, naringenin supplements are available in the Indian market and are used by individuals seeking to augment their dietary intake or address specific health concerns.

Research Summary of Citrus Naringenin: Overall, research on citrus naringenin supports its role as a natural antioxidant and anti-inflammatory compound with various health benefits. Clinical studies have demonstrated its efficacy in supporting cardiovascular health, reducing inflammation, modulating lipid metabolism, and potentially inhibiting cancer cell growth. However, further research is needed to elucidate its specific mechanisms of action, optimal dosages, and long-term effects on health and disease prevention.

20) D-MANNOSE

Introduction: D-Mannose is a naturally occurring simple sugar closely related to glucose. It is found in small quantities in various fruits, including cranberries, apples, and oranges. D-Mannose has gained attention for its potential health benefits, particularly in supporting urinary tract health and preventing urinary tract infections (UTIs).

Synonym Name and Common Name: Synonym: Mannose Common Name: D-Mannose

Pharmacognosy / Chemistry: D-Mannose is a monosaccharide, structurally similar to glucose, with the chemical formula $C6H12O6$. It is typically obtained from plant sources, such as fruits and vegetables, through extraction and purification processes.

Action and Pharmacology: D-Mannose exerts its pharmacological effects primarily in the urinary tract. It is believed to prevent bacterial adhesion to the urinary tract lining by competitively binding to receptors on the uroepithelial cells. This action helps to flush bacteria out of the urinary tract, reducing the risk of UTIs.

Method of Analysis: The concentration of D-mannose in dietary supplements or food products can be analyzed using various analytical techniques, including high-performance liquid chromatography (HPLC), gas chromatography (GC), or enzymatic assays. These methods allow for the accurate quantification of D-mannose content.

Health Benefits:

- Supports urinary tract health
- Prevents urinary tract infections (UTIs)
- May improve symptoms of interstitial cystitis
- Acts as a prebiotic, supporting gut health

Indication and Usage: D-Mannose is commonly used as a dietary supplement to support urinary tract health and prevent UTIs. It is often recommended for individuals prone to recurrent UTIs or those seeking a natural alternative to antibiotics.

Usual Constituents with Percentages: D-Mannose supplements typically contain pure D-mannose as the active ingredient, with concentrations ranging from 500 milligrams to 2 grams per serving. The purity and quality of D-mannose supplements can vary depending on the manufacturing process and source.

Mechanism of Action: The primary mechanism of action of D-mannose involves its ability to prevent bacterial adhesion to the urinary tract lining. By binding to receptors on the uroepithelial cells, D-mannose inhibits the attachment of bacteria, such as Escherichia coli (E. coli), to the urinary tract, allowing them to be flushed out with urine.

Dosage: Recommended dosages of D-mannose supplements vary depending on individual needs and health conditions. Typical doses range from 1 to 2 grams taken orally, 1 to 3 times per day. D-mannose is often taken with water and may be used as a preventive measure or to alleviate symptoms during UTI episodes.

Contraindications: There are no known contraindications for the use of D-mannose in most individuals. However, individuals with rare hereditary disorders, such as mannose intolerance or mannose-6-phosphate isomerase deficiency, should avoid D-mannose supplementation.

Precautions:

- Pregnant and breastfeeding women should consult with a healthcare professional before using D-mannose supplements.
- Individuals with diabetes should monitor their blood sugar levels when taking D-mannose, as it may affect glucose metabolism.

Adverse Reactions: D-Mannose is generally well-tolerated when taken at recommended doses. However, some individuals may experience mild gastrointestinal discomfort, such as bloating or diarrhea, particularly when first starting supplementation.

Research Summary: Research on D-mannose has shown promising results in supporting urinary tract health and preventing UTIs. Clinical studies have demonstrated that D-mannose supplementation can reduce the frequency of UTIs, alleviate symptoms, and decrease the need for antibiotic treatment. Additionally, D-mannose may have prebiotic effects, supporting gut health and overall well-being.

Pharmacokinetics: After ingestion, D-mannose is rapidly absorbed in the small intestine and enters the bloodstream. It is then filtered by the kidneys and excreted in the urine. D-mannose does not undergo significant metabolism in the body and is primarily eliminated unchanged in the urine.

Pharmacodynamics: The pharmacodynamic effects of D-mannose primarily involve its ability to prevent bacterial adhesion to the urinary tract lining. By competitively binding to uroepithelial cell receptors, D-mannose inhibits the attachment of pathogenic bacteria, reducing the risk of UTIs.

Overdosage: Excessive intake of D-mannose supplements may lead to gastrointestinal discomfort, such as bloating or diarrhea. However, there is limited information on the effects of long-term overdosage. It is important to follow recommended dosages and consult with a healthcare professional if experiencing adverse effects.

International Standing: D-Mannose is recognized internationally as a valuable dietary supplement for supporting urinary tract health and preventing UTIs. It is widely available over-the-counter in many countries and is commonly used by individuals prone to recurrent UTIs.

Indian Standing: In India, D-mannose supplements are gaining popularity among individuals seeking natural remedies for urinary tract health. They are available in the Indian market through various retailers and online platforms, reflecting their growing demand among consumers.

Research Summary of D-Mannose: Overall, research on D-mannose supports its role as a natural supplement for supporting urinary tract health and preventing UTIs. Clinical studies have demonstrated its efficacy in reducing UTI recurrence, alleviating symptoms, and decreasing the need for antibiotic treatment. Additionally, D-mannose may have prebiotic effects, supporting gut health and overall well-being. However, further research is needed to elucidate its specific mechanisms of action, optimal dosages, and long-term effects on urinary tract health.

21) COLLAGEN AND ITS HYDROLYSED PEPTIDES AND CHELATES

Introduction: Collagen is the most abundant protein in the human body, making up a significant portion of connective tissues such as skin, bones, tendons, and cartilage. It provides structural support, elasticity, and strength to various tissues and organs. Collagen supplements, including hydrolyzed collagen peptides and chelates, have gained popularity for their potential health benefits, particularly in supporting skin health, joint function, and overall well-being.

Synonym Name and Common Name: Synonym: None Common Name: Collagen

Pharmacognosy / Chemistry: Collagen is a fibrous protein composed of amino acids, primarily glycine, proline, and hydroxyproline. It is synthesized by various cells, including fibroblasts, osteoblasts, and chondrocytes, and is organized into triple helical structures. Collagen can be obtained from animal sources, such as bovine or marine collagen, and processed into supplements through hydrolysis or chelation methods.

Action and Pharmacology: Collagen supplements exert their pharmacological effects primarily through their influence on collagen synthesis and tissue regeneration. Hydrolyzed collagen peptides are readily absorbed in the gastrointestinal tract and transported to target tissues, where they stimulate collagen production and support tissue repair. Chelated collagen complexes may enhance bioavailability and absorption in the body, contributing to their efficacy.

Method of Analysis: The content and purity of collagen supplements can be analyzed using various methods, including amino acid analysis, gel electrophoresis, and spectroscopic techniques. These methods allow for the quantification of collagen peptides and identification of specific amino acid compositions, providing insight into the quality and efficacy of collagen supplements.

Health Benefits:

- Supports skin health and elasticity
- Promotes joint health and mobility
- Strengthens hair and nails
- Supports bone density and strength

- May aid in wound healing
- Supports gut health and digestion

Indication and Usage: Collagen supplements are commonly used for a variety of indications, including:

- Improving skin elasticity and hydration
- Alleviating joint pain and stiffness
- Strengthening hair and nails
- Supporting bone health
- Enhancing gut health and digestion

Usual Constituents with Percentages: Collagen supplements typically contain hydrolyzed collagen peptides or chelated collagen complexes, with concentrations ranging from 5 to 20 grams per serving. The composition of collagen supplements may vary depending on the source and processing methods used, with some products also containing additional ingredients such as vitamins, minerals, or antioxidants.

Mechanism of Action: The mechanism of action of collagen supplements involves several pathways:

Stimulating collagen synthesis: Collagen peptides provide essential amino acids and signaling molecules that stimulate fibroblasts and other collagen-producing cells to increase collagen production.

Supporting tissue repair: Collagen peptides are incorporated into the extracellular matrix, where they promote tissue regeneration and repair, particularly in skin, joints, bones, and connective tissues.

Enhancing absorption and bioavailability: Chelated collagen complexes may improve the solubility and absorption of collagen peptides, enhancing their bioavailability and efficacy in the body.

Dosage: Recommended dosages for collagen supplements vary depending on individual needs and health goals. Typical doses range from 5 to 20 grams per day, taken orally with water or mixed into beverages or food. Collagen supplements are often taken on an empty stomach or between meals to enhance absorption.

Contraindications: There are no known contraindications for the use of collagen supplements in most individuals. However, individuals with allergies to specific collagen sources, such as bovine or marine collagen, should use caution and choose collagen supplements derived from alternative sources.

Precautions:

Pregnant and breastfeeding women should consult with a healthcare professional before using collagen supplements.

Individuals with medical conditions, such as kidney disease or hypercalcemia, should use collagen supplements with caution and under medical supervision.

Adverse Reactions: Collagen supplements are generally well-tolerated by most individuals. However, some people may experience mild gastrointestinal discomfort, such as bloating or diarrhea, particularly when first starting supplementation or taking high doses.

Research Summary: Research on collagen supplements, including hydrolyzed collagen peptides and chelated collagen complexes, supports their potential health benefits for skin, joint, bone, and overall well-being. Clinical studies have demonstrated improvements in skin elasticity, hydration, and wrinkle reduction, as well as reductions in joint pain and stiffness. Additionally, collagen supplements may support bone density, hair and nail health, and gut health. Further research is ongoing to elucidate the specific mechanisms of action and optimize dosing regimens for various health conditions.

Pharmacokinetics: After ingestion, collagen peptides from hydrolyzed collagen supplements are rapidly absorbed in the gastrointestinal tract and transported to target tissues, such as skin, joints, and bones. Chelated collagen complexes may enhance absorption and bioavailability, resulting in higher tissue concentrations and efficacy.

Pharmacodynamics: The pharmacodynamic effects of collagen supplements primarily involve their influence on collagen synthesis, tissue repair, and structural support. Collagen peptides stimulate collagen production by fibroblasts and other collagen-producing cells, supporting tissue regeneration and repair in skin, joints, bones, and connective tissues.

Overdosage: Excessive intake of collagen supplements is unlikely to cause significant adverse effects in most individuals. However, high doses may increase the risk of gastrointestinal discomfort or allergic reactions in some people. It is important to follow recommended dosages and consult with a healthcare professional if experiencing adverse effects.

International Standing: Collagen supplements are recognized internationally as valuable dietary supplements for supporting skin, joint, bone, and overall health. They are widely available over-the-counter in many countries and are commonly used by individuals seeking natural remedies for various health concerns.

Indian Standing: In India, collagen supplements are gaining popularity among individuals seeking natural solutions for skin, joint, and bone health. They are available in the Indian market through various retailers and online platforms, reflecting their growing demand among consumers.

Research Summary of Collagen and Its Hydrolyzed Peptides and Chelates: Overall, research on collagen supplements, including hydrolyzed collagen peptides and chelated collagen complexes, supports their potential health benefits for skin, joint, bone, and overall well-being. Clinical studies have demonstrated improvements in skin elasticity, hydration, and wrinkle reduction, as well as reductions in joint pain and stiffness. Additionally, collagen supplements may support bone density, hair and nail health, and gut health. Further research is ongoing to elucidate the specific mechanisms of action and optimize dosing regimens for various health conditions.

22) CONJUGATED LINOLEIC ACID CONCENTRATE

Introduction: Conjugated linoleic acid concentrate (CLA) is a naturally occurring fatty acid found primarily in meat and dairy products. It gained attention for its potential health benefits, particularly in weight management and cardiovascular health.

Synonym Name and Common Name: Synonym: CLA Common Name: Conjugated Linoleic Acid

Pharmacognosy / Chemistry: Conjugated linoleic acid is a type of polyunsaturated fatty acid. It exists in several forms (isomers), with the cis-9, trans-11 isomer and the trans-10, cis-12 isomer being the most studied for their health effects.

Action and Pharmacology: CLA is believed to exert its effects through various mechanisms, including modulation of lipid metabolism, regulation of adipocyte differentiation, and influencing inflammatory processes. It has also been suggested to have antioxidant properties.

Method of Analysis: Analysis of CLA typically involves gas chromatography, which allows for the precise measurement of individual isomers in various matrices such as blood, tissues, or dietary supplements.

Health Benefits:

- Weight management
- Improved body composition
- Potential cardiovascular health benefits
- Antioxidant effects
- Immune system modulation

Indication and Usage: CLA supplements are often used for weight loss, body fat reduction, muscle retention, and overall improvement in body composition. It may also be recommended for cardiovascular support and general health maintenance.

Usual Constituents with Percentages: CLA supplements typically contain a mixture of isomers, with the cis-9, trans-11 isomer and the trans-10, cis-12 isomer being the most abundant. Percentages may vary depending on the source and processing methods but commonly range from 70% to 80%.

Mechanism of Action: The exact mechanism of action of CLA is not fully understood but is thought to involve modulation of enzymes and transcription factors involved in lipid metabolism, adipocyte differentiation, and inflammation.

Dosage: Typical dosages range from 3 to 6 grams per day, taken with meals. It's often recommended to start with a lower dose and gradually increase to assess tolerance.

Contraindications:

- Allergy to CLA or related compounds
- Pregnancy and breastfeeding (due to limited safety data)
- Pre-existing medical conditions, especially liver or kidney disease, should consult a healthcare professional before use.

Precautions:

- Monitor for any allergic reactions or adverse effects.
- Use caution in individuals with underlying medical conditions or those taking medications that may interact with CLA.

Adverse Reactions: Common side effects may include digestive issues such as diarrhea, nausea, or stomach discomfort. Rarely, allergic reactions or liver toxicity may occur.

Research Summary: Research on CLA has shown promising results in various areas, including weight management, body composition improvement, and cardiovascular health. However, some studies have produced conflicting results, and further research is needed to fully understand its efficacy and safety profile.

Pharmacokinetics: CLA is absorbed in the small intestine and undergoes metabolism in the liver. It is then distributed to various tissues where it exerts its effects. The half-life of CLA in the body is relatively short, and it is eventually excreted primarily in urine.

Pharmacodynamics: CLA acts on various molecular targets involved in lipid metabolism, adipogenesis, inflammation, and oxidative stress. It may also influence gene expression related to these processes.

Overdosage: Excessive intake of CLA supplements may lead to adverse effects such as gastrointestinal disturbances or liver toxicity. It's important to adhere to recommended dosages and consult a healthcare professional if concerns arise.

International Standing: CLA supplements are widely available internationally and are commonly used for weight management and general health purposes. Regulations regarding its sale and use may vary by country.

Indian Standing: In India, CLA supplements are also available and are marketed for similar purposes as in other countries. However, specific regulations and market availability may differ.

Research Summary of Conjugated Linoleic Acid Concentrate: Research on conjugated linoleic acid concentrate suggests its potential benefits in weight management, body composition improvement, and cardiovascular health. However, more studies are needed to establish its efficacy, safety, and optimal dosage for various populations.

23) D-PINITOL

Introduction: D-Pinitol, also known as 3-O-methyl-D-chiro-inositol, is a naturally occurring compound found in various plants, particularly in legumes such as soybeans and chickpeas. It has gained attention for its potential health benefits, especially in the management of diabetes and metabolic syndrome.

Synonym Name and Common Name: Synonym: 3-O-methyl-D-chiro-inositol Common Name: D-Pinitol

Pharmacognosy / Chemistry: D-Pinitol is a cyclitol, a cyclic polyol compound similar to inositol. It is typically extracted from plant sources, particularly legumes, and is available as a dietary supplement.

Action and Pharmacology: D-Pinitol is believed to exert its effects through various mechanisms, including enhancing insulin sensitivity, promoting glucose uptake into cells, and reducing insulin resistance. It may also have antioxidant and anti-inflammatory properties.

Method of Analysis: Analysis of D-Pinitol often involves techniques such as high-performance liquid chromatography (HPLC) or gas chromatography-mass spectrometry (GC-MS) to quantify its presence and concentration in plant extracts or dietary supplements.

Health Benefits:

- Improved insulin sensitivity
- Enhanced glucose metabolism
- Potential support for diabetes management
- Antioxidant and anti-inflammatory effects
- Possible benefits for metabolic syndrome

Indication and Usage: D-Pinitol supplements are primarily used for managing conditions related to insulin resistance, such as type 2 diabetes and metabolic syndrome. It may also be taken for general health support, particularly for those seeking to regulate blood sugar levels.

Usual Constituents with Percentages: D-Pinitol is typically found in plant extracts or dietary supplements in concentrations ranging from 1% to 10%, depending on the source and processing methods.

Mechanism of Action: D-Pinitol is thought to mimic the action of insulin by activating the phosphatidylinositol-3-kinase (PI3K) pathway, leading to increased glucose uptake into cells. It may also modulate various signaling pathways involved in insulin signaling and glucose metabolism.

Dosage: Typical dosages of D-Pinitol range from 500 mg to 2000 mg per day, taken with meals. Dosage recommendations may vary based on individual health status and specific health goals.

Contraindications:

- Allergy to D-Pinitol or related compounds
- Pregnancy and breastfeeding (due to limited safety data)
- Individuals with diabetes or other medical conditions should consult a healthcare professional before using D-Pinitol supplements.

Precautions:

- Monitor blood sugar levels closely, especially in individuals with diabetes, when taking D-Pinitol supplements.
- Use caution in combination with other medications or supplements that may affect blood sugar levels.

Adverse Reactions: Common side effects of D-Pinitol supplementation may include gastrointestinal discomfort, such as bloating or diarrhea. Rarely, allergic reactions or hypoglycemia (low blood sugar) may occur.

Research Summary: Research on D-Pinitol suggests its potential as a natural compound for managing insulin resistance and related conditions such as type 2 diabetes and metabolic syndrome. However, more clinical studies are needed to confirm its efficacy, optimal dosage, and long-term safety profile.

Pharmacokinetics: After oral ingestion, D-Pinitol is absorbed in the gastrointestinal tract and undergoes metabolism in the liver. It is then distributed to various tissues where it exerts its effects. The half-life and elimination of D-Pinitol from the body are not well-characterized.

Pharmacodynamics: D-Pinitol acts primarily by enhancing insulin sensitivity and promoting glucose uptake into cells. It may also exert antioxidant and anti-inflammatory effects through modulation of various cellular signaling pathways.

Overdosage: There is limited information available on the potential effects of D-Pinitol overdose. However, excessive intake may lead to gastrointestinal disturbances or alterations in blood sugar levels. It's important to adhere to recommended dosages and consult a healthcare professional if concerns arise.

International Standing: D-Pinitol supplements are available internationally and are commonly used for managing insulin resistance-related conditions. Regulations regarding its sale and use may vary by country.

Indian Standing: In India, D-Pinitol supplements are also available and are marketed for similar purposes as in other countries. However, specific regulations and market availability may differ.

Research Summary of D-Pinitol: Research on D-Pinitol suggests its potential as a natural compound for managing insulin resistance and related conditions such as type 2 diabetes and metabolic syndrome. However, further clinical studies are needed to establish its efficacy, safety, and optimal dosage for various populations.

24) PROTEIN ISOLATES/CONCENTRATES/ HYDROLYSATES

Introduction: Protein isolates, concentrates, and hydrolysates are popular dietary supplements used by athletes, fitness enthusiasts, and individuals looking to meet their protein needs. They are derived from various protein sources such as whey, soy, or pea, and are processed to concentrate the protein content while minimizing fat and carbohydrate content.

Synonym Name and Common Name: Synonyms: Protein powders, protein supplements Common Name: Protein isolates, protein concentrates, protein hydrolysates

Pharmacognosy / Chemistry: Protein isolates, concentrates, and hydrolysates are obtained through various extraction and purification processes from protein-rich sources such as milk, soybeans, or peas. These processes typically involve filtration, precipitation, and drying to produce powdered forms of concentrated protein.

Action and Pharmacology: Protein supplements provide essential amino acids necessary for muscle repair, growth, and overall tissue maintenance. They are also involved in various physiological processes such as enzyme production, immune function, and hormone regulation.

Method of Analysis: Analysis of protein supplements often involves techniques such as chromatography (e.g., HPLC), spectroscopy (e.g., UV-Vis), and amino acid analysis to determine protein content, amino acid composition, and presence of impurities.

Health Benefits:

- Muscle repair and growth
- Support for physical performance and exercise recovery
- Convenient source of high-quality protein
- May aid in weight management and appetite control
- Potential benefits for bone health and immune function

Indication and Usage: Protein isolates, concentrates, and hydrolysates are commonly used to supplement dietary protein intake, especially for individuals engaged in regular exercise or those with increased protein requirements due to age, illness, or specific health goals.

Usual Constituents with Percentages: Protein isolates typically contain protein content upwards of 90% or more, with minimal amounts of fat and carbohydrates. Protein concentrates generally have lower protein content (typically 60-80%) but may retain more of the original bioactive compounds present in the source material. Protein hydrolysates are partially digested protein forms that may offer faster absorption and digestion.

Mechanism of Action: Protein supplements provide essential amino acids that serve as building blocks for protein synthesis in the body. They also stimulate muscle protein synthesis and inhibit protein breakdown, leading to improved muscle repair, growth, and overall tissue maintenance.

Dosage: Dosage recommendations for protein supplements vary based on individual protein needs, activity level, and specific health goals. Typically, serving sizes range from 20 to 30 grams per serving, consumed before or after exercise, or as part of a meal.

Contraindications:

- Allergy to specific protein sources (e.g., milk, soy, or pea)
- Pre-existing medical conditions such as kidney disease may require monitoring of protein intake
- Individuals with dietary restrictions or specific health conditions should consult a healthcare professional before using protein supplements.

Precautions:

- Ensure adequate hydration when consuming protein supplements, especially those containing whey protein, to prevent dehydration.
- Use caution in individuals with lactose intolerance or other gastrointestinal sensitivities.
- Monitor overall protein intake from both dietary and supplemental sources to avoid excessive protein consumption.

Adverse Reactions: Common adverse reactions to protein supplements may include gastrointestinal discomfort, such as bloating, gas, or diarrhea, particularly in individuals with lactose intolerance or sensitivities to specific protein sources. Allergic reactions are possible in individuals with allergies to milk, soy, or other protein sources.

Research Summary: Research on protein isolates, concentrates, and hydrolysates has demonstrated their efficacy in supporting muscle repair, growth, and overall physical performance, particularly when combined with resistance exercise. They are also associated with various health benefits such as weight management, bone health, and immune function. However, further studies are needed to elucidate their long-term effects, optimal dosage, and potential interactions with other nutrients or medications.

Pharmacokinetics: Protein supplements are rapidly absorbed in the gastrointestinal tract, with amino acids being released into the bloodstream for utilization by various tissues, particularly skeletal muscle. The rate of absorption may vary depending on the protein source and processing method.

Pharmacodynamics: Protein supplements stimulate muscle protein synthesis and inhibit protein breakdown through various signaling pathways, leading to enhanced muscle repair, growth, and overall tissue maintenance. They may also modulate hormone secretion and immune function.

Overdosage: Excessive intake of protein supplements may lead to gastrointestinal discomfort, dehydration, and potential adverse effects on kidney function in susceptible individuals. It's important to adhere to recommended dosages and consult a healthcare professional if concerns arise.

International Standing: Protein supplements are widely available internationally and are commonly used by athletes, fitness enthusiasts, and individuals seeking to meet their protein needs. Regulations regarding their sale, labeling, and quality may vary by country.

Indian Standing: In India, protein supplements are also popular among athletes, bodybuilders, and individuals seeking to support their fitness goals. They are available in various forms and formulations and are subject to regulations set by the Food Safety and Standards Authority of India (FSSAI) regarding quality and safety.

Research Summary of Protein Isolates/Concentrates/Hydrolysates: Research on protein supplements indicates their effectiveness in supporting muscle repair, growth, and physical performance, particularly when combined with exercise. They are also associated with various health benefits such as weight management, bone health, and immune function. However, further studies are needed to elucidate their long-term effects, optimal dosage, and potential interactions with other nutrients or medications.

25) ELLAGIC ACID

Introduction: Ellagic acid is a naturally occurring polyphenolic compound found in various fruits, nuts, and vegetables. It has garnered attention for its potential health benefits, particularly its antioxidant and anti-inflammatory properties.

Synonym Name and Common Name: Synonym: None Common Name: Ellagic acid

Pharmacognosy / Chemistry: Ellagic acid is a phytochemical found in plants such as berries (e.g., strawberries, raspberries), pomegranates, and nuts.

It is typically present in these foods as part of complex molecules known as ellagitannins, which are hydrolyzed in the body to release ellagic acid.

Action and Pharmacology: Ellagic acid exhibits antioxidant and anti-inflammatory properties, which may contribute to its various health benefits. It scavenges free radicals, inhibits inflammatory pathways, and modulates enzymatic activity involved in cellular processes.

Method of Analysis: Analysis of ellagic acid often involves techniques such as high-performance liquid chromatography (HPLC) or mass spectrometry to quantify its presence and concentration in plant extracts, foods, or dietary supplements.

Health Benefits:

- Antioxidant activity
- Anti-inflammatory effects
- Potential anti-cancer properties
- Cardiovascular health support
- Skin health benefits

Indication and Usage: Ellagic acid supplements or extracts are often used for their antioxidant properties and potential health benefits. They may be recommended for various conditions, including oxidative stress-related diseases, inflammation, and certain types of cancer.

Usual Constituents with Percentages: Ellagic acid is typically found in plant extracts or dietary supplements in concentrations ranging from 5% to 30%, depending on the source and processing methods.

Mechanism of Action: Ellagic acid exerts its effects through multiple mechanisms, including scavenging reactive oxygen species (ROS), inhibiting inflammatory pathways (such as NF-κB), inducing apoptosis (programmed cell death) in cancer cells, and modulating enzyme activity involved in cellular processes.

Dosage: Dosage recommendations for ellagic acid supplements vary depending on the specific product and intended use. Typical doses range from 100 mg to 500 mg per day, taken with meals.

Contraindications:

- Allergy to ellagic acid or related compounds
- Pregnancy and breastfeeding (due to limited safety data)
- Individuals with underlying medical conditions should consult a healthcare professional before using ellagic acid supplements.

Precautions:

- Monitor for any allergic reactions or adverse effects when starting ellagic acid supplementation.
- Use caution in individuals with gastrointestinal sensitivities, as high doses may cause stomach upset.
- Avoid combining ellagic acid supplements with other medications or supplements without consulting a healthcare professional.

Adverse Reactions: Common adverse reactions to ellagic acid supplements may include gastrointestinal discomfort, such as nausea, diarrhea, or stomach cramps. Allergic reactions are possible in individuals with allergies to certain fruits or nuts containing ellagic acid.

Research Summary: Research on ellagic acid has shown promising results in various areas, including its antioxidant, anti-inflammatory, and potential anti-cancer properties. It has been studied for its role in preventing oxidative stress-related diseases, reducing inflammation, and inhibiting the growth of certain cancer cells. However, further clinical studies are needed to elucidate its efficacy, optimal dosage, and long-term safety profile.

Pharmacokinetics: Ellagic acid is absorbed in the gastrointestinal tract and undergoes metabolism in the liver. It is then distributed to various tissues where it exerts its effects. The bioavailability of ellagic acid from dietary sources or supplements varies depending on factors such as food matrix and co-ingestion of other nutrients.

Pharmacodynamics: Ellagic acid acts as an antioxidant by scavenging free radicals and inhibiting oxidative damage to cellular components. It also exhibits anti-inflammatory effects by modulating inflammatory pathways and cytokine production. Additionally, ellagic acid may induce apoptosis in cancer cells by interfering with cell signaling pathways involved in cell survival and proliferation.

Overdosage: There is limited information available on the potential effects of ellagic acid overdose. Excessive intake may lead to gastrointestinal disturbances or allergic reactions. It's important to adhere to recommended dosages and consult a healthcare professional if concerns arise.

International Standing: Ellagic acid supplements are available internationally and are commonly used for their antioxidant and potential health-promoting properties. Regulations regarding their sale, labeling, and quality may vary by country.

Indian Standing: In India, ellagic acid supplements are also available and may be marketed for similar purposes as in other countries. However, specific regulations and market availability may differ.

Research Summary of Ellagic Acid: Research on ellagic acid suggests its potential as a natural compound with antioxidant, anti-inflammatory, and potential anti-cancer properties. It has been studied for its role in preventing oxidative stress-related diseases, reducing inflammation, and inhibiting the growth of certain cancer cells. However, further clinical studies are needed to establish its efficacy, safety, and optimal dosage for various health conditions.

26) ERIOCITRIN

Introduction: Eriocitrin is a flavonoid compound belonging to the flavanone subgroup, commonly found in citrus fruits such as oranges, lemons, and grapefruits. It is recognized for its potential health-promoting properties and its role as a natural antioxidant.

Synonym Name and Common Name: Synonym: None Common Name: Eriocitrin

Pharmacognosy / Chemistry: Eriocitrin is a glycoside composed of the flavonoid eriodictyol and the sugar molecule rutinose. It is primarily found in the peel and pulp of citrus fruits and is extracted for its medicinal and dietary supplement purposes.

Action and Pharmacology: Eriocitrin exhibits antioxidant, anti-inflammatory, and potential cardioprotective effects. It scavenges free radicals, inhibits inflammatory pathways, and may contribute to cardiovascular health by reducing oxidative stress.

Method of Analysis: Analysis of eriocitrin typically involves techniques such as high-performance liquid chromatography (HPLC) or liquid chromatography-mass spectrometry (LC-MS) to quantify its presence and concentration in citrus extracts or dietary supplements.

Health Benefits:

- Antioxidant activity
- Anti-inflammatory effects
- Cardiovascular health support
- Potential benefits for skin health
- Immune system modulation

Indication and Usage: Eriocitrin supplements or citrus extracts are often used for their antioxidant properties and potential health benefits. They may be recommended for conditions related to oxidative stress, inflammation, cardiovascular health, and skin health.

Usual Constituents with Percentages: Eriocitrin content in citrus extracts can vary depending on factors such as fruit variety, ripeness, and processing methods. Concentrations typically range from 5% to 20% in citrus extracts.

Mechanism of Action: Eriocitrin exerts its effects through multiple mechanisms, including scavenging reactive oxygen species (ROS), inhibiting inflammatory pathways (such as NF-κB), and modulating enzymatic activity involved in cellular processes related to oxidative stress and inflammation.

Dosage: Dosage recommendations for eriocitrin supplements vary depending on the specific product and intended use. Typical doses range from 100 mg to 500 mg per day, taken with meals.

Contraindications:

- Allergy to citrus fruits or flavonoids
- Pregnancy and breastfeeding (due to limited safety data)
- Individuals with underlying medical conditions should consult a healthcare professional before using eriocitrin supplements.

Precautions:

- Monitor for any allergic reactions or adverse effects when starting eriocitrin supplementation.
- Use caution in individuals with gastrointestinal sensitivities, as high doses may cause stomach upset.
- Avoid combining eriocitrin supplements with other medications or supplements without consulting a healthcare professional.

Adverse Reactions: Common adverse reactions to eriocitrin supplements may include gastrointestinal discomfort, such as nausea, diarrhea, or stomach cramps. Allergic reactions are possible in individuals with allergies to citrus fruits or flavonoids.

Research Summary: Research on eriocitrin suggests its potential as a natural compound with antioxidant, anti-inflammatory, and potential cardioprotective properties. It has been studied for its role in reducing oxidative stress, inflammation, and promoting cardiovascular health. However, further clinical studies are needed to elucidate its efficacy, optimal dosage, and long-term safety profile.

Pharmacokinetics: Eriocitrin is absorbed in the gastrointestinal tract and undergoes metabolism in the liver. It is then distributed to various tissues where it exerts its effects. The bioavailability of eriocitrin from dietary sources or supplements may vary depending on factors such as food matrix and co-ingestion of other nutrients.

Pharmacodynamics: Eriocitrin acts as an antioxidant by scavenging free radicals and inhibiting oxidative damage to cellular components. It also exhibits anti-inflammatory effects by modulating inflammatory pathways and cytokine production. Additionally, eriocitrin may contribute to cardiovascular health by reducing oxidative stress and improving endothelial function.

Overdosage: There is limited information available on the potential effects of eriocitrin overdose. Excessive intake may lead to gastrointestinal disturbances or allergic reactions. It's important to adhere to recommended dosages and consult a healthcare professional if concerns arise.

International Standing: Eriocitrin supplements are available internationally and are commonly used for their antioxidant and potential health-promoting properties. Regulations regarding their sale, labeling, and quality may vary by country.

Indian Standing: In India, eriocitrin supplements or citrus extracts are also available and may be marketed for similar purposes as in other countries. However, specific regulations and market availability may differ.

Research Summary of Eriocitrin: Research on eriocitrin suggests its potential as a natural compound with antioxidant, anti-inflammatory, and potential cardioprotective properties. It has been studied for its role in reducing oxidative stress, inflammation, and promoting cardiovascular health. However, further clinical studies are needed to establish its efficacy, safety, and optimal dosage for various health conditions.

27) GALACTOMANNAN

Introduction: Galactomannan is a naturally occurring polysaccharide found in various plant sources, including seeds, gums, and legumes. It has gained attention for its diverse applications in food, pharmaceuticals, and other industrial sectors.

Synonym Name and Common Name: Synonym: Galactoarabino-galactomannan Common Name: Galactomannan

Pharmacognosy / Chemistry: Galactomannan is a complex carbohydrate composed of a backbone of mannose units with galactose side chains. It is commonly extracted from seeds such as guar gum (Cyamopsis tetragonoloba) and locust bean gum (Ceratonia siliqua).

Action and Pharmacology: Galactomannan has various functional properties, including thickening, stabilizing, and gelling abilities. In pharmaceuticals, it is used as a binder, disintegrant, or controlled-release agent. In the food industry, it acts as a thickener, emulsifier, or dietary fiber.

Method of Analysis: Analysis of galactomannan typically involves techniques such as gravimetric analysis, spectrophotometry, or chromatography to quantify its presence and concentration in various matrices such as food products, pharmaceutical formulations, or industrial applications.

Health Benefits:

- Dietary fiber
- Digestive health support

- Cholesterol-lowering effects
- Blood sugar regulation
- Weight management aid

Indication and Usage: Galactomannan is used in various industries, including food, pharmaceuticals, cosmetics, and textiles. In food, it is used as a thickening agent, stabilizer, or dietary fiber supplement. In pharmaceuticals, it is used as a binder, disintegrant, or controlled-release agent.

Usual Constituents with Percentages: Galactomannan content in seeds can vary depending on factors such as seed variety, processing methods, and extraction techniques. Guar gum typically contains around 80% galactomannan, while locust bean gum contains around 75%.

Mechanism of Action: Galactomannan acts as a soluble dietary fiber, which can absorb water and form a gel-like substance in the digestive tract. This gel slows down digestion and nutrient absorption, leading to improved digestive health, cholesterol-lowering effects, and blood sugar regulation.

Dosage: Dosage recommendations for galactomannan supplements vary depending on the specific product and intended use. Typical doses range from 5 to 15 grams per day, taken with plenty of water.

Contraindications:

- Allergy to galactomannan or related compounds
- Individuals with gastrointestinal disorders or swallowing difficulties may need to avoid galactomannan supplements
- Pregnant or breastfeeding women should consult a healthcare professional before using galactomannan supplements.

Precautions:

- Ensure adequate hydration when consuming galactomannan supplements to prevent gastrointestinal discomfort or obstruction.
- Use caution in individuals with diabetes, as galactomannan supplements may affect blood sugar levels.

- Monitor for any allergic reactions or adverse effects when starting galactomannan supplementation.

Adverse Reactions: Common adverse reactions to galactomannan supplements may include gastrointestinal discomfort, such as bloating, gas, or diarrhea, particularly if not consumed with enough water. Allergic reactions are possible in individuals with allergies to galactomannan or related compounds.

Research Summary: Research on galactomannan has focused on its various applications in food, pharmaceuticals, and other industrial sectors. It has been studied for its effects on digestive health, cholesterol levels, blood sugar regulation, and weight management. However, further research is needed to elucidate its mechanisms of action, optimal dosage, and potential health benefits in humans.

Pharmacokinetics: Galactomannan is not absorbed in the gastrointestinal tract but instead passes through the digestive system intact. It absorbs water and swells, forming a gel-like substance that slows down digestion and promotes digestive health.

Pharmacodynamics: Galactomannan acts primarily as a soluble dietary fiber, which can absorb water and form a gel-like substance in the digestive tract. This gel slows down digestion, promotes satiety, and improves digestive health by bulking up stool and promoting regular bowel movements.

Overdosage: Excessive intake of galactomannan supplements may lead to gastrointestinal discomfort, such as bloating, gas, or diarrhea. It's important to adhere to recommended dosages and consume galactomannan supplements with plenty of water to prevent adverse effects.

International Standing: Galactomannan is recognized as safe for use in food, pharmaceuticals, cosmetics, and other industrial applications by regulatory authorities such as the U.S. Food and Drug Administration (FDA) and the European Food Safety Authority (EFSA).

Indian Standing: In India, galactomannan is also approved for use in various industries, including food, pharmaceuticals, and textiles. It is generally regarded as safe for consumption and other applications, subject to regulations set by the Food Safety and Standards Authority of India (FSSAI) and other relevant authorities.

Research Summary of Galactomannan: Research on galactomannan has explored its diverse applications in food, pharmaceuticals, cosmetics, and textiles. It has been studied for its effects on digestive health, cholesterol levels, blood sugar regulation, and weight management. However, further research is needed to elucidate its mechanisms of action, optimal dosage, and potential health benefits in humans.

28) GALLIC ACID

Introduction: Gallic acid is a natural phenolic compound found abundantly in various plants, fruits, and beverages. It has been recognized for its antioxidant, anti-inflammatory, and potential health-promoting properties.

Synonym Name and Common Name: Synonym: 3,4,5-Trihydroxybenzoic acid Common Name: Gallic acid

Pharmacognosy / Chemistry: Gallic acid is a phenolic acid derived from the metabolism of various plant compounds such as tannins. It is commonly found in plants such as gallnuts, grapes, tea leaves, and oak bark.

Action and Pharmacology: Gallic acid exhibits antioxidant, anti-inflammatory, antimicrobial, and anticancer properties. It scavenges free radicals, inhibits inflammatory pathways, and modulates enzymatic activity involved in cellular processes.

Method of Analysis: Analysis of gallic acid typically involves techniques such as high-performance liquid chromatography (HPLC), gas chromatography-mass spectrometry (GC-MS), or spectrophotometry to quantify its presence and concentration in plant extracts, foods, beverages, or dietary supplements.

Health Benefits:

- Antioxidant activity
- Anti-inflammatory effects
- Cardiovascular health support
- Potential anticancer properties
- Skin health benefits

Indication and Usage: Gallic acid supplements or extracts are often used for their antioxidant properties and potential health benefits. They may be recommended for conditions related to oxidative stress, inflammation, cardiovascular health, cancer prevention, and skin health.

Usual Constituents with Percentages: Gallic acid content in plants can vary depending on factors such as plant variety, maturity, and processing methods. It can range from trace amounts to several percent in plant extracts or food products.

Mechanism of Action: Gallic acid exerts its effects through multiple mechanisms, including scavenging reactive oxygen species (ROS), inhibiting inflammatory pathways (such as NF-κB), inducing apoptosis (programmed cell death) in cancer cells, and modulating enzyme activity involved in cellular processes related to oxidative stress and inflammation.

Dosage: Dosage recommendations for gallic acid supplements vary depending on the specific product and intended use. Typical doses range from 100 mg to 500 mg per day, taken with meals.

Contraindications:

- Allergy to gallic acid or related compounds
- Pregnancy and breastfeeding (due to limited safety data)
- Individuals with underlying medical conditions should consult a healthcare professional before using gallic acid supplements.

Precautions:

- Monitor for any allergic reactions or adverse effects when starting gallic acid supplementation.
- Use caution in individuals with gastrointestinal sensitivities, as high doses may cause stomach upset.
- Avoid combining gallic acid supplements with other medications or supplements without consulting a healthcare professional.

Adverse Reactions: Common adverse reactions to gallic acid supplements may include gastrointestinal discomfort, such as nausea, diarrhea, or stomach cramps. Allergic reactions are possible in individuals with allergies to gallic acid or related compounds.

Research Summary: Research on gallic acid has focused on its various health-promoting properties, including its antioxidant, anti-inflammatory, antimicrobial, anticancer, and skin health benefits. It has been studied for its role in reducing oxidative stress, inflammation, and promoting cardiovascular health, cancer prevention, and skin health. However, further clinical studies are needed to elucidate its efficacy, optimal dosage, and long-term safety profile.

Pharmacokinetics: Gallic acid is absorbed in the gastrointestinal tract and undergoes metabolism in the liver. It is then distributed to various tissues where it exerts its effects. The bioavailability of gallic acid from dietary sources or supplements may vary depending on factors such as food matrix and co-ingestion of other nutrients.

Pharmacodynamics: Gallic acid acts as an antioxidant by scavenging free radicals and inhibiting oxidative damage to cellular components. It also exhibits anti-inflammatory effects by modulating inflammatory pathways and cytokine production. Additionally, gallic acid may induce apoptosis in cancer cells by interfering with cell signaling pathways involved in cell survival and proliferation.

Overdosage: There is limited information available on the potential effects of gallic acid overdose. Excessive intake may lead to gastrointestinal disturbances or allergic reactions. It's important to adhere to recommended dosages and consult a healthcare professional if concerns arise.

International Standing: Gallic acid is recognized as safe for use in food, pharmaceuticals, cosmetics, and other industrial applications by regulatory authorities such as the U.S. Food and Drug Administration (FDA) and the European Food Safety Authority (EFSA).

Indian Standing: In India, gallic acid is also approved for use in various industries, including food, pharmaceuticals, cosmetics, and textiles. It is generally regarded as safe for consumption and other applications, subject to regulations set by the Food Safety and Standards Authority of India (FSSAI) and other relevant authorities.

Research Summary of Gallic Acid: Research on gallic acid suggests its potential as a natural compound with antioxidant, anti-inflammatory, antimicrobial, anticancer, and skin health benefits. It has been studied for its role in reducing oxidative stress, inflammation, promoting cardiovascular health, cancer prevention, and skin health. However, further clinical studies are needed to establish its efficacy, safety, and optimal dosage for various health conditions.

29)GAMMA-LINOLEIC ACID

Introduction: Gamma-linolenic acid (GLA) is an omega-6 fatty acid found in various plant-based oils, seeds, and nuts. It plays a crucial role in maintaining overall health, particularly in skin health, hormone regulation, and inflammation modulation.

Synonym Name and Common Name: Synonym: γ-linolenic acid Common Name: Gamma-linolenic acid (GLA)

Pharmacognosy / Chemistry: Gamma-linolenic acid is a polyunsaturated fatty acid primarily derived from plant sources such as evening primrose oil, borage oil, and black currant seed oil. It is obtained through the extraction and purification of these oils.

Action and Pharmacology: Gamma-linolenic acid serves as a precursor for prostaglandins, which are hormone-like substances involved in various physiological processes, including inflammation, blood clotting, and hormone regulation. It exhibits anti-inflammatory, immunomodulatory, and skin barrier-enhancing effects.

Method of Analysis: Analysis of gamma-linolenic acid typically involves techniques such as gas chromatography (GC) or high-performance liquid chromatography (HPLC) to quantify its presence and concentration in plant oils, dietary supplements, or biological samples.

Health Benefits:

- Skin health support (e.g., eczema, psoriasis)
- Hormone balance
- Anti-inflammatory effects
- Cardiovascular health support
- Potential benefits for women's health (e.g., PMS, menopause)

Indication and Usage: Gamma-linolenic acid supplements are often used to support skin health, hormone balance, and inflammatory conditions such as eczema and rheumatoid arthritis. They may also be used as a complementary therapy for cardiovascular health and women's health issues.

Usual Constituents with Percentages: Gamma-linolenic acid content in plant oils can vary depending on the source and processing methods. Evening primrose oil typically contains around 8-10% GLA, while borage oil can contain up to 20-25% GLA.

Mechanism of Action: Gamma-linolenic acid exerts its effects by serving as a precursor for prostaglandin synthesis, particularly prostaglandin E1 (PGE1), which exhibits anti-inflammatory and vasodilatory properties. It also influences cellular signaling pathways involved in inflammation and immune response regulation.

Dosage: Dosage recommendations for gamma-linolenic acid supplements vary depending on the specific product and intended use. Typical doses range from 200 mg to 1000 mg per day, taken with meals.

Contraindications:

- Allergy to gamma-linolenic acid or related compounds
- Pregnancy and breastfeeding (due to limited safety data)
- Individuals with epilepsy or other seizure disorders should use caution due to potential interactions with medications.

Precautions:

- Monitor for any allergic reactions or adverse effects when starting gamma-linolenic acid supplementation.
- Use caution in individuals with bleeding disorders, as GLA may have anticoagulant effects.
- Consult a healthcare professional before using GLA supplements, especially in combination with other medications or supplements.

Adverse Reactions: Common adverse reactions to gamma-linolenic acid supplements may include gastrointestinal discomfort, such as nausea, diarrhea, or stomach upset. Allergic reactions are possible in individuals with allergies to GLA or related compounds.

Research Summary: Research on gamma-linolenic acid has focused on its potential health benefits, particularly in skin health, inflammation modulation, hormone regulation, and cardiovascular support. It has been studied for its efficacy in conditions such as eczema, psoriasis, rheumatoid arthritis, premenstrual syndrome (PMS), and menopausal symptoms. However, further clinical studies are needed to elucidate its mechanisms of action, optimal dosage, and long-term safety profile.

Pharmacokinetics: Gamma-linolenic acid is absorbed in the small intestine and undergoes metabolism in the liver. It is then distributed to various tissues where it exerts its effects. The bioavailability of GLA from dietary supplements may vary depending on factors such as the source of GLA and the presence of other dietary fats.

Pharmacodynamics: Gamma-linolenic acid serves as a precursor for prostaglandin synthesis, particularly prostaglandin E1 (PGE1), which exhibits anti-inflammatory and vasodilatory effects. GLA also influences cellular signaling pathways involved in inflammation, immune response regulation, and skin barrier function.

Overdosage: Excessive intake of gamma-linolenic acid supplements may lead to gastrointestinal disturbances, such as bloating, gas, or diarrhea. It's important to adhere to recommended dosages and consult a healthcare professional if concerns arise.

International Standing: Gamma-linolenic acid supplements are widely available internationally and are commonly used for their potential health benefits. Regulations regarding their sale, labeling, and quality may vary by country.

Indian Standing: In India, gamma-linolenic acid supplements are also available and may be marketed for similar purposes as in other countries. However, specific regulations and market availability may differ.

Research Summary of Gamma-linolenic Acid: Research on gamma-linolenic acid suggests its potential as a dietary supplement for various health conditions, particularly in skin health, inflammation modulation, hormone regulation, and cardiovascular support. It has been studied for its efficacy in conditions such as eczema, psoriasis, rheumatoid arthritis, premenstrual syndrome (PMS), and menopausal symptoms. However, further clinical studies are needed to elucidate its mechanisms of action, optimal dosage, and long-term safety profile.

30)GAMMA-ORYZANOL

Introduction: Gamma-oryzanol is a naturally occurring mixture of plant compounds found in rice bran oil and other cereal grains. It has gained attention for its potential health benefits, particularly in supporting cardiovascular health and managing cholesterol levels.

Synonym Name and Common Name: Synonym: None Common Name: Gamma-oryzanol

Pharmacognosy / Chemistry: Gamma-oryzanol is a mixture of ferulic acid esters and phytosterols derived from rice bran oil. It is primarily obtained through the extraction and purification of rice bran oil, which contains high levels of gamma-oryzanol.

Action and Pharmacology: Gamma-oryzanol exhibits antioxidant, anti-inflammatory, and potential cholesterol-lowering effects. It scavenges free radicals, inhibits inflammatory pathways, and modulates cholesterol metabolism, leading to improved cardiovascular health.

Method of Analysis: Analysis of gamma-oryzanol typically involves techniques such as high-performance liquid chromatography (HPLC) or gas chromatography-mass spectrometry (GC-MS) to quantify its presence and concentration in rice bran oil or dietary supplements.

Health Benefits:

- Cardiovascular health support
- Cholesterol management
- Antioxidant activity
- Potential neuroprotective effects
- Exercise performance enhancement

Indication and Usage: Gamma-oryzanol supplements are often used to support cardiovascular health and manage cholesterol levels. They may also be used as antioxidants and for their potential neuroprotective effects. Additionally, gamma-oryzanol has been studied for its role in enhancing exercise performance.

Usual Constituents with Percentages: Gamma-oryzanol content in rice bran oil can vary depending on factors such as the rice variety, processing methods, and extraction techniques. Typically, gamma-oryzanol constitutes around 1-2% of rice bran oil.

Mechanism of Action: Gamma-oryzanol exerts its effects through multiple mechanisms, including antioxidant activity, inhibition of cholesterol absorption, modulation of cholesterol synthesis, and anti-inflammatory effects. It also influences cellular signaling pathways involved in cholesterol metabolism and cardiovascular health.

Dosage: Dosage recommendations for gamma-oryzanol supplements vary depending on the specific product and intended use. Typical doses range from 300 mg to 1000 mg per day, taken with meals.

Contraindications:

- Allergy to gamma-oryzanol or related compounds

- Pregnancy and breastfeeding (due to limited safety data)
- Individuals with underlying medical conditions should consult a healthcare professional before using gamma-oryzanol supplements.

Precautions:

- Monitor for any allergic reactions or adverse effects when starting gamma-oryzanol supplementation.
- Use caution in individuals taking cholesterol-lowering medications, as gamma-oryzanol may potentiate their effects.
- Consult a healthcare professional before using gamma-oryzanol supplements in combination with other medications or supplements.

Adverse Reactions: Common adverse reactions to gamma-oryzanol supplements may include gastrointestinal discomfort, such as nausea, diarrhea, or stomach upset. Allergic reactions are possible in individuals with allergies to gamma-oryzanol or related compounds.

Research Summary: Research on gamma-oryzanol has focused on its potential health benefits, particularly in supporting cardiovascular health, managing cholesterol levels, and exerting antioxidant effects. It has been studied for its role in reducing oxidative stress, inflammation, and improving lipid profiles in individuals with hyperlipidemia. However, further clinical studies are needed to elucidate its mechanisms of action, optimal dosage, and long-term safety profile.

Pharmacokinetics: Gamma-oryzanol is absorbed in the gastrointestinal tract and undergoes metabolism in the liver. It is then distributed to various tissues where it exerts its effects. The bioavailability of gamma-oryzanol from dietary supplements may vary depending on factors such as the source of gamma-oryzanol and the presence of other dietary fats.

Pharmacodynamics: Gamma-oryzanol acts as an antioxidant by scavenging free radicals and inhibiting oxidative damage to cellular components. It also influences cholesterol metabolism by inhibiting cholesterol absorption and modulating cholesterol synthesis, leading to improved lipid profiles and cardiovascular health.

Overdosage: Excessive intake of gamma-oryzanol supplements may lead to gastrointestinal disturbances, such as bloating, gas, or diarrhea. It's important to adhere to recommended dosages and consult a healthcare professional if concerns arise.

International Standing: Gamma-oryzanol supplements are recognized as safe for use in dietary supplements internationally. Regulations regarding their sale, labeling, and quality may vary by country.

Indian Standing: In India, gamma-oryzanol supplements are also available and may be marketed for similar purposes as in other countries. However, specific regulations and market availability may differ.

Research Summary of Gamma-oryzanol: Research on gamma-oryzanol suggests its potential as a dietary supplement for supporting cardiovascular health, managing cholesterol levels, and exerting antioxidant effects. It has been studied for its role in reducing oxidative stress, inflammation, and improving lipid profiles in individuals with hyperlipidemia. However, further clinical studies are needed to elucidate its mechanisms of action, optimal dosage, and long-term safety profile.

31)GLUCOMANNAN

Introduction: Glucomannan is a water-soluble dietary fiber derived from the roots of the konjac plant (Amorphophallus konjac). It has gained popularity as a dietary supplement due to its potential health benefits, particularly in weight management and digestive health.

Synonym Name and Common Name: Synonym: Konjac mannan Common Name: Glucomannan

Pharmacognosy / Chemistry: Glucomannan is a polysaccharide composed of glucose and mannose units derived from the konjac plant's root. It is extracted from the plant's tuberous roots and processed into various forms for dietary supplementation.

Action and Pharmacology: Glucomannan functions primarily as a dietary fiber, absorbing water in the digestive tract and forming a gel-like substance. This gel helps to promote feelings of fullness, slows down digestion, and promotes regular bowel movements. Additionally, glucomannan may help lower cholesterol levels by binding to bile acids and inhibiting their reabsorption.

Method of Analysis: Analysis of glucomannan typically involves techniques such as gravimetric analysis, spectrophotometry, or chromatography to quantify its presence and concentration in dietary supplements or food products.

Health Benefits:

- Weight management aid
- Digestive health support
- Cholesterol-lowering effects
- Blood sugar regulation
- Potential satiety-enhancing effects

Indication and Usage: Glucomannan supplements are commonly used to support weight management, promote digestive health, and help control blood sugar levels. They may also be recommended for individuals looking to increase their fiber intake or improve bowel regularity.

Usual Constituents with Percentages: Glucomannan content in dietary supplements can vary, but typical concentrations range from 500 mg to 3000 mg per serving, depending on the product formulation.

Mechanism of Action: Glucomannan works by absorbing water in the digestive tract, forming a viscous gel that promotes feelings of fullness and reduces appetite. It also slows down the emptying of the stomach, which can help regulate blood sugar levels and improve digestive health.

Dosage: Dosage recommendations for glucomannan supplements vary, but typical doses range from 1 to 3 grams per day, divided into two or three doses and taken with plenty of water before meals.

Contraindications:

- Swallowing difficulties or gastrointestinal obstruction
- Diabetes or hypoglycemia (use caution and monitor blood sugar levels)
- Pregnancy and breastfeeding (due to limited safety data)

Precautions:

- Always take glucomannan supplements with plenty of water to prevent choking or gastrointestinal obstruction.
- Monitor blood sugar levels closely if you have diabetes or hypoglycemia, as glucomannan may affect insulin sensitivity.

- Avoid taking glucomannan supplements within two hours of medications, as it may interfere with their absorption.

Adverse Reactions: Common adverse reactions to glucomannan supplements may include gastrointestinal discomfort, such as bloating, gas, or diarrhea, particularly if not consumed with enough water. Allergic reactions are rare but possible in individuals with allergies to konjac root.

Research Summary: Research on glucomannan has primarily focused on its potential as a dietary supplement for weight management, digestive health, and cholesterol reduction. Several studies have demonstrated its efficacy in promoting weight loss, improving bowel regularity, and lowering cholesterol levels. However, further research is needed to confirm its long-term safety and efficacy, as well as its potential mechanisms of action.

Pharmacokinetics: Glucomannan is not absorbed in the gastrointestinal tract but instead passes through the digestive system intact. It absorbs water and swells, forming a gel-like substance that slows down digestion and promotes feelings of fullness.

Pharmacodynamics: Glucomannan acts primarily as a soluble dietary fiber, which can absorb water and form a gel-like substance in the digestive tract. This gel promotes feelings of fullness, reduces appetite, and slows down the absorption of nutrients, leading to weight loss and improved digestive health.

Overdosage: Excessive intake of glucomannan supplements may lead to gastrointestinal discomfort, such as bloating, gas, or diarrhea. It's important to adhere to recommended dosages and consume glucomannan supplements with plenty of water to prevent adverse effects.

International Standing: Glucomannan supplements are recognized as safe for use in dietary supplements internationally. Regulations regarding their sale, labeling, and quality may vary by country.

Indian Standing: In India, glucomannan supplements are also available and may be marketed for similar purposes as in other countries. However, specific regulations and market availability may differ.

Research Summary of Glucomannan: Research on glucomannan suggests its potential as a dietary supplement for weight management, digestive health, and cholesterol reduction. Several studies have demonstrated its efficacy in promoting weight loss, improving bowel regularity, and lowering cholesterol levels. However, further research is needed to confirm its long-term safety and efficacy, as well as its potential mechanisms of action.

32) HESPERIDIN

Introduction: Hesperidin is a flavonoid compound found abundantly in citrus fruits, particularly in the peels of oranges and lemons. It has gained attention for its potential health benefits, including antioxidant, anti-inflammatory, and cardiovascular protective properties.

Synonym Name and Common Name: Synonym: Hesperidin 7-rutinoside Common Name: Hesperidin

Pharmacognosy / Chemistry: Hesperidin is a flavonoid glycoside composed of hesperidin (aglycone) and rutinose (sugar moiety). It is primarily found in the peel and membranes of citrus fruits such as oranges, lemons, and grapefruits.

Action and Pharmacology: Hesperidin exhibits antioxidant, anti-inflammatory, anti-allergic, and potential anticancer properties. It scavenges free radicals, inhibits inflammatory pathways, stabilizes mast cells, and modulates cellular signaling pathways involved in various physiological processes.

Method of Analysis: Analysis of hesperidin typically involves techniques such as high-performance liquid chromatography (HPLC) or spectrophotometry to quantify its presence and concentration in citrus extracts, dietary supplements, or biological samples.

Health Benefits:

- Antioxidant activity
- Anti-inflammatory effects
- Cardiovascular health support
- Skin health benefits
- Potential anticancer properties

Indication and Usage: Hesperidin supplements are often used to support cardiovascular health, reduce inflammation, promote skin health, and potentially prevent certain types of cancer. They may also be used as antioxidants to counteract oxidative stress.

Usual Constituents with Percentages: Hesperidin content in citrus fruits varies depending on factors such as fruit variety, ripeness, and processing methods.

Oranges and lemons typically contain around 0.5-2% hesperidin in their peels and membranes.

Mechanism of Action: Hesperidin exerts its effects through multiple mechanisms, including scavenging free radicals, inhibiting inflammatory enzymes (such as COX and LOX), stabilizing mast cells, modulating cellular signaling pathways (such as NF-κB), and inducing apoptosis (programmed cell death) in cancer cells.

Dosage: Dosage recommendations for hesperidin supplements vary depending on the specific product and intended use. Typical doses range from 500 mg to 1000 mg per day, taken with meals.

Contraindications:

- Allergy to citrus fruits or hesperidin
- Pregnancy and breastfeeding (due to limited safety data)
- Individuals taking medications metabolized by the liver should use caution due to potential interactions.

Precautions:

- Monitor for any allergic reactions or adverse effects when starting hesperidin supplementation.
- Use caution in individuals with liver or kidney disorders, as hesperidin may affect liver enzymes or renal function.
- Consult a healthcare professional before using hesperidin supplements in combination with other medications or supplements.

Adverse Reactions: Common adverse reactions to hesperidin supplements may include gastrointestinal discomfort, such as nausea, diarrhea, or stomach upset, particularly if taken on an empty stomach. Allergic reactions are rare but possible in individuals with allergies to citrus fruits or hesperidin.

Research Summary: Research on hesperidin has focused on its potential health benefits, particularly in cardiovascular health, inflammation modulation, skin health, and cancer prevention. Several studies have demonstrated its antioxidant, anti-inflammatory, and potential anticancer properties in cell culture and animal models.

However, further clinical studies are needed to confirm its efficacy, optimal dosage, and long-term safety profile in humans.

Pharmacokinetics: Hesperidin is absorbed in the gastrointestinal tract and undergoes metabolism in the liver, where it is converted into its active metabolites, including hesperidin. It is then distributed to various tissues where it exerts its effects. The bioavailability of hesperidin from dietary supplements may vary depending on factors such as formulation and co-ingestion of other nutrients.

Pharmacodynamics: Hesperidin acts primarily as an antioxidant by scavenging free radicals and inhibiting oxidative damage to cellular components. It also exhibits anti-inflammatory effects by inhibiting inflammatory enzymes and modulating cellular signalling pathways involved in inflammation and immune response regulation.

Overdosage: Excessive intake of hesperidin supplements may lead to gastrointestinal disturbances, such as bloating, gas, or diarrhea. It's important to adhere to recommended dosages and consult a healthcare professional if concerns arise.

International Standing: Hesperidin supplements are recognized as safe for use in dietary supplements internationally. Regulations regarding their sale, labeling, and quality may vary by country.

Indian Standing: In India, hesperidin supplements are also available and may be marketed for similar purposes as in other countries. However, specific regulations and market availability may differ.

Research Summary of Hesperidin: Research on hesperidin suggests its potential as a dietary supplement for cardiovascular health, inflammation modulation, skin health, and cancer prevention. Several studies have demonstrated its antioxidant, anti-inflammatory, and potential anticancer properties in cell culture and animal models. However, further clinical studies are needed to confirm its efficacy, optimal dosage, and long-term safety profile in humans.

33)HYALURONIC ACID AND ITS SALTS

Introduction: Hyaluronic acid (HA) is a naturally occurring polysaccharide found in the human body, particularly in connective tissues, joints, and skin. It plays a crucial role in maintaining hydration, lubrication, and elasticity in tissues.

Synonym Name and Common Name: Synonym: Hyaluronan Common Name: Hyaluronic acid

Pharmacognosy / Chemistry: Hyaluronic acid is a linear polysaccharide composed of repeating disaccharide units of glucuronic acid and N-acetylglucosamine. It is synthesized by various cells in the body, including fibroblasts, chondrocytes, and synoviocytes.

Action and Pharmacology: Hyaluronic acid serves as a crucial component of the extracellular matrix, providing structural support, hydration, and lubrication to tissues. It also interacts with cell surface receptors to regulate cellular processes such as proliferation, migration, and inflammation.

Method of Analysis: Analysis of hyaluronic acid typically involves techniques such as size-exclusion chromatography, enzyme-linked immunosorbent assay (ELISA), or nuclear magnetic resonance (NMR) spectroscopy to quantify its presence and concentration in biological samples or pharmaceutical formulations.

Health Benefits:

- Skin hydration and elasticity
- Joint lubrication and cushioning
- Wound healing support
- Eye health (as a component of the vitreous humor)
- Potential anti-inflammatory effects

Indication and Usage: Hyaluronic acid supplements or topical preparations are commonly used to support skin health, joint function, and wound healing. They may also be used in ophthalmic solutions for eye health or as viscosupplements for osteoarthritis.

Usual Constituents with Percentages: Hyaluronic acid content in commercial products can vary widely depending on the formulation and intended use. In skincare products, concentrations typically range from 0.1% to 2%. In viscosupplements for joint injections, concentrations can range from 10 mg/mL to 30 mg/mL.

Mechanism of Action: Hyaluronic acid exerts its effects through multiple mechanisms, including hydration and lubrication of tissues, stimulation of collagen synthesis, regulation of inflammatory mediators, and modulation of cell signaling pathways involved in tissue repair and regeneration.

Dosage: Dosage recommendations for hyaluronic acid supplements or topical formulations vary depending on the specific product and intended use. Typical doses range from 20 mg to 200 mg per day for oral supplements and from 0.1% to 2% for topical applications.

Contraindications:

- Allergy to hyaluronic acid or related compounds
- Pregnancy and breastfeeding (due to limited safety data)
- Individuals with a history of hypersensitivity reactions should use caution with hyaluronic acid supplements or injections.

Precautions:

- Avoid using hyaluronic acid supplements or topical formulations in individuals with known allergies or sensitivities to hyaluronic acid or any of its components.
- Use caution in individuals with a history of autoimmune diseases or immune system disorders, as hyaluronic acid may stimulate immune responses.
- Consult a healthcare professional before using hyaluronic acid supplements or injections, especially if you have underlying medical conditions or are taking other medications.

Adverse Reactions: Common adverse reactions to hyaluronic acid supplements or injections may include injection site reactions (e.g., redness, swelling, pain), allergic reactions (e.g., itching, rash, hives), or gastrointestinal discomfort (with oral supplements). Severe adverse reactions are rare but possible.

Research Summary: Research on hyaluronic acid has focused on its various health benefits, particularly in skincare, joint health, wound healing, and ophthalmology. Numerous studies have demonstrated its efficacy in improving skin hydration, reducing wrinkles, relieving joint pain, promoting wound healing, and supporting eye health. However, further research is needed to elucidate its mechanisms of action, optimal dosage, and long-term safety profile.

Pharmacokinetics: Hyaluronic acid from oral supplements is poorly absorbed in the gastrointestinal tract due to its large molecular size. Topically applied hyaluronic acid may penetrate the skin and provide hydration and moisturization benefits. Injectable hyaluronic acid is slowly metabolized and broken down by enzymes in the tissues.

Pharmacodynamics: Hyaluronic acid acts primarily as a humectant, attracting and retaining water molecules to hydrate and plump the skin. It also interacts with cell surface receptors to stimulate collagen synthesis, modulate inflammatory responses, and promote tissue repair and regeneration.

Overdosage: Excessive intake of hyaluronic acid supplements or injections may lead to adverse effects such as allergic reactions, injection site reactions, or gastrointestinal discomfort. It's important to adhere to recommended dosages and consult a healthcare professional if concerns arise.

International Standing: Hyaluronic acid supplements and topical formulations are widely used and accepted internationally for their various health benefits. Regulations regarding their sale, labeling, and quality may vary by country.

Indian Standing: In India, hyaluronic acid supplements and topical formulations are also available and may be marketed for similar purposes as in other countries. However, specific regulations and market availability may differ.

Research Summary of Hyaluronic Acid and Its Salts: Research on hyaluronic acid and its salts suggests their potential as valuable compounds for skincare, joint health, wound healing, and ophthalmology. Numerous studies have demonstrated their efficacy in improving skin hydration, reducing wrinkles, relieving joint pain, promoting wound healing, and supporting eye health. However, further research is needed to elucidate their mechanisms of action, optimal dosage, and long-term safety profile.

34) HYDROLYSED WHEY PEPTIDE

Introduction: Hydrolyzed whey peptides are a form of protein derived from whey, a byproduct of cheese production. Through a process called hydrolysis, whey protein is broken down into smaller peptides, which are more easily absorbed by the body.

Synonym Name and Common Name: Synonym: Whey protein hydrolysate Common Name: Hydrolyzed whey peptides

Pharmacognosy / Chemistry: Hydrolyzed whey peptides are produced by enzymatic hydrolysis of whey protein, resulting in the breakdown of larger protein molecules into smaller peptides. This process increases the bioavailability and digestibility of the protein.

Action and Pharmacology: Hydrolyzed whey peptides serve as a source of amino acids, which are essential for various physiological processes, including muscle protein synthesis, immune function, and tissue repair. They are rapidly absorbed into the bloodstream, making them ideal for post-workout recovery and muscle building.

Method of Analysis: Analysis of hydrolyzed whey peptides typically involves techniques such as high-performance liquid chromatography (HPLC), sodium dodecyl sulfate-polyacrylamide gel electrophoresis (SDS-PAGE), or amino acid analysis to quantify the peptide content and profile.

Health Benefits:

- Muscle recovery and repair
- Enhanced muscle protein synthesis
- Improved exercise performance
- Immune support
- Weight management support

Indication and Usage: Hydrolyzed whey peptides are commonly used by athletes and fitness enthusiasts as a post-workout supplement to support muscle recovery and growth. They may also be used as a convenient source of protein for individuals looking to increase their protein intake or support weight management goals.

Usual Constituents with Percentages: Hydrolyzed whey peptides typically contain a mixture of peptides of varying lengths, with the majority being dipeptides and tripeptides. The exact composition and percentage of peptides can vary depending on the hydrolysis process and the source of whey protein.

Mechanism of Action: Hydrolyzed whey peptides are rapidly digested and absorbed into the bloodstream, providing a quick supply of amino acids to the muscles. This stimulates muscle protein synthesis, which is essential for muscle repair and growth, particularly after intense exercise.

Dosage: Dosage recommendations for hydrolyzed whey peptides vary depending on factors such as individual protein requirements, fitness goals, and timing of consumption. Typical doses range from 10 to 30 grams per serving, taken immediately post-workout or as part of a protein-rich meal.

Contraindications:

- Allergy to whey protein or milk products
- Kidney disease or impaired kidney function (due to high protein intake)
- Individuals with phenylketonuria (PKU) should avoid products containing hydrolyzed whey peptides if they contain phenylalanine.

Precautions:

- Monitor fluid intake when consuming hydrolyzed whey peptides, especially in individuals with kidney disease or impaired kidney function.
- Use caution when using protein supplements as part of a weight loss or muscle-building regimen, as excessive protein intake may have adverse effects on kidney health and metabolism.
- Consult a healthcare professional before using hydrolyzed whey peptides, especially if you have underlying medical conditions or are taking other medications or supplements.

Adverse Reactions: Common adverse reactions to hydrolyzed whey peptides may include gastrointestinal discomfort, such as bloating, gas, or diarrhea, particularly if consumed in large amounts or by individuals with lactose intolerance or milk protein allergies.

Research Summary: Research on hydrolyzed whey peptides has primarily focused on their efficacy in promoting muscle recovery and growth, improving exercise performance, and supporting immune function. Numerous studies have demonstrated their benefits in enhancing muscle protein synthesis, reducing muscle soreness, and supporting immune function in athletes and physically active individuals. However, further research is needed to elucidate their long-term effects, optimal dosage, and potential benefits for specific populations.

Pharmacokinetics: Hydrolyzed whey peptides are rapidly absorbed into the bloodstream after ingestion, leading to a quick increase in plasma amino acid levels. This rapid absorption makes them ideal for post-workout recovery, as they provide a readily available source of amino acids to the muscles.

Pharmacodynamics: Hydrolyzed whey peptides stimulate muscle protein synthesis, which is essential for muscle repair and growth. They also support immune function by providing amino acids that are necessary for the production of immune cells and antibodies.

Overdosage: Excessive intake of hydrolyzed whey peptides may lead to gastrointestinal discomfort, such as bloating, gas, or diarrhea, particularly if consumed in large amounts or by individuals with lactose intolerance or milk protein allergies. It's important to adhere to recommended dosages and consult a healthcare professional if concerns arise.

International Standing: Hydrolyzed whey peptides are widely used and accepted internationally as a dietary supplement for muscle recovery and growth. Regulations regarding their sale, labeling, and quality may vary by country.

Indian Standing: In India, hydrolyzed whey peptides are also available and may be marketed for similar purposes as in other countries. However, specific regulations and market availability may differ.

Research Summary of Hydrolyzed Whey Peptides: Research on hydrolyzed whey peptides suggests their efficacy in promoting muscle recovery and growth, improving exercise performance, and supporting immune function. Numerous studies have demonstrated their benefits in enhancing muscle protein synthesis, reducing muscle soreness, and supporting immune function in athletes and physically active individuals. However, further research is needed to elucidate their long-term effects, optimal dosage, and potential benefits for specific populations.

35) LACTALBUMIN

Introduction: Lactalbumin is a protein component found in milk, particularly in whey protein. It is considered a high-quality protein due to its rich amino acid profile and bioavailability.

Synonym Name and Common Name: Synonym: Alpha-lactalbumin Common Name: Lactalbumin

Pharmacognosy / Chemistry: Lactalbumin is a globular protein that is soluble in water. It is derived from whey protein through various processing methods, such as filtration and ion exchange chromatography.

Action and Pharmacology: Lactalbumin serves as a source of essential amino acids, which are important for various physiological processes, including muscle protein synthesis, immune function, and enzyme activity. It is rapidly digested and absorbed by the body, making it ideal for post-exercise recovery and muscle building.

Method of Analysis: Analysis of lactalbumin typically involves techniques such as high-performance liquid chromatography (HPLC), sodium dodecyl sulfate-polyacrylamide gel electrophoresis (SDS-PAGE), or amino acid analysis to quantify its presence and concentration in protein supplements or food products.

Health Benefits:

- Muscle recovery and growth
- Immune support
- Weight management support
- Nutrient absorption
- Potential mood regulation

Indication and Usage: Lactalbumin supplements are commonly used by athletes and fitness enthusiasts as a post-workout recovery aid to support muscle repair and growth. They may also be used as a convenient source of protein for individuals looking to increase their protein intake or support weight management goals.

Usual Constituents with Percentages: Lactalbumin is a major protein component of whey protein, typically comprising around 20-25% of whey protein isolates or concentrates.

Mechanism of Action: Lactalbumin provides a readily available source of essential amino acids, which are necessary for muscle protein synthesis and repair. It also supports immune function by providing amino acids that are important for the production of immune cells and antibodies.

Dosage: Dosage recommendations for lactalbumin supplements vary depending on factors such as individual protein requirements, fitness goals, and timing of consumption. Typical doses range from 20 to 30 grams per serving, taken immediately post-workout or as part of a protein-rich meal.

Contraindications:

- Allergy to milk or dairy products
- Kidney disease or impaired kidney function (due to high protein intake)
- Individuals with phenylketonuria (PKU) should avoid products containing lactalbumin if they contain phenylalanine.

Precautions:

- Monitor fluid intake when consuming lactalbumin supplements, especially in individuals with kidney disease or impaired kidney function.
- Use caution when using protein supplements as part of a weight loss or muscle-building regimen, as excessive protein intake may have adverse effects on kidney health and metabolism.
- Consult a healthcare professional before using lactalbumin supplements, especially if you have underlying medical conditions or are taking other medications or supplements.

Adverse Reactions: Common adverse reactions to lactalbumin supplements may include gastrointestinal discomfort, such as bloating, gas, or diarrhea, particularly if consumed in large amounts or by individuals with lactose intolerance or milk protein allergies.

Research Summary: Research on lactalbumin has primarily focused on its efficacy in promoting muscle recovery and growth, supporting immune function, and aiding in weight management. Numerous studies have demonstrated its benefits in enhancing muscle protein synthesis, reducing muscle soreness, and supporting immune function in athletes and physically active individuals. However, further research is needed to elucidate its long-term effects, optimal dosage, and potential benefits for specific populations.

Pharmacokinetics: Lactalbumin is rapidly digested and absorbed in the gastrointestinal tract, leading to a quick increase in plasma amino acid levels. This rapid absorption makes it ideal for post-workout recovery, as it provides a readily available source of amino acids to the muscles.

Pharmacodynamics: Lactalbumin stimulates muscle protein synthesis, which is essential for muscle repair and growth. It also supports immune function by providing amino acids that are necessary for the production of immune cells and antibodies.

Overdosage: Excessive intake of lactalbumin supplements may lead to gastrointestinal discomfort, such as bloating, gas, or diarrhea, particularly if consumed in large amounts or by individuals with lactose intolerance or milk protein allergies. It's important to adhere to recommended dosages and consult a healthcare professional if concerns arise.

International Standing: Lactalbumin supplements are widely used and accepted internationally as a dietary supplement for muscle recovery and growth. Regulations regarding their sale, labeling, and quality may vary by country.

Indian Standing: In India, lactalbumin supplements are also available and may be marketed for similar purposes as in other countries. However, specific regulations and market availability may differ.

Research Summary of Lactalbumin: Research on lactalbumin suggests its efficacy in promoting muscle recovery and growth, supporting immune function, and aiding in weight management. Numerous studies have demonstrated its benefits in enhancing muscle protein synthesis, reducing muscle soreness, and supporting immune function in athletes and physically active individuals. However, further research is needed to elucidate its long-term effects, optimal dosage, and potential benefits for specific populations.

36)LACTOFERRIN

Introduction: Lactoferrin is a glycoprotein found in various biological fluids, including milk, saliva, tears, and mucosal secretions. It plays a crucial role in immune defense, iron metabolism, and host-microbe interactions.

Synonym Name and Common Name: Synonym: Lactotransferrin Common Name: Lactoferrin

Pharmacognosy / Chemistry: Lactoferrin is a multifunctional protein belonging to the transferrin family. It is present in various mammalian species, including humans, and is particularly abundant in human milk.

Action and Pharmacology: Lactoferrin exerts its biological effects through multiple mechanisms, including iron binding, antimicrobial activity, immune modulation, and anti-inflammatory properties. It plays a crucial role in innate immunity, acting as a first line of defense against pathogens.

Method of Analysis: Analysis of lactoferrin typically involves techniques such as enzyme-linked immunosorbent assay (ELISA), Western blotting, or chromatography to quantify its presence and concentration in biological samples or pharmaceutical formulations.

Health Benefits:

- Immune system support
- Antimicrobial activity
- Anti-inflammatory effects
- Iron metabolism regulation
- Gut health support

Indication and Usage: Lactoferrin supplements are commonly used to support immune function, particularly during periods of increased susceptibility to infections. They may also be used to promote gut health, support iron metabolism, and aid in wound healing.

Usual Constituents with Percentages: Lactoferrin content in human milk typically ranges from 1 to 5 grams per liter. In bovine milk, the concentration is lower, ranging from 0.1 to 0.5 grams per liter.

Mechanism of Action: Lactoferrin exerts its effects through various mechanisms, including sequestration of iron, inhibition of microbial growth by depriving pathogens of essential nutrients, modulation of immune responses, and regulation of inflammatory pathways.

Dosage: Dosage recommendations for lactoferrin supplements vary depending on the specific product and intended use. Typical doses range from 100 mg to 1000 mg per day, taken with meals.

Contraindications:

- Allergy to milk or dairy products
- Iron overload disorders (hemochromatosis)

- Use caution in individuals with autoimmune diseases, as lactoferrin may modulate immune responses.

Precautions:

- Monitor iron levels when using lactoferrin supplements, especially in individuals with iron deficiency or iron overload disorders.
- Use caution when using lactoferrin supplements in combination with antibiotics or immunosuppressive medications, as interactions may occur.
- Consult a healthcare professional before using lactoferrin supplements, especially if you have underlying medical conditions or are taking other medications or supplements.

Adverse Reactions: Common adverse reactions to lactoferrin supplements are rare but may include gastrointestinal discomfort, such as bloating, gas, or diarrhea, particularly at higher doses. Allergic reactions are possible in individuals with milk protein allergies.

Research Summary: Research on lactoferrin has demonstrated its diverse biological activities and potential health benefits, particularly in immune support, antimicrobial activity, and anti-inflammatory effects. Numerous studies have shown its efficacy in reducing the risk and severity of infections, promoting gut health, supporting iron metabolism, and enhancing wound healing. However, further research is needed to elucidate its mechanisms of action, optimal dosage, and potential benefits for specific populations.

Pharmacokinetics: Lactoferrin is relatively stable in the acidic environment of the stomach and is well absorbed in the small intestine. It is distributed to various tissues and bodily fluids, where it exerts its biological effects. Lactoferrin undergoes proteolytic degradation in the gastrointestinal tract and is excreted primarily in the feces.

Pharmacodynamics: Lactoferrin acts primarily through its iron-binding properties, antimicrobial activity, and modulation of immune responses. It sequesters iron, which is essential for microbial growth, thereby inhibiting the proliferation of pathogens. Lactoferrin also interacts with immune cells and inflammatory mediators to regulate immune responses and inflammation.

Overdosage: Excessive intake of lactoferrin supplements may lead to gastrointestinal discomfort, such as bloating, gas, or diarrhea, particularly at higher doses. It's important to adhere to recommended dosages and consult a healthcare professional if concerns arise.

International Standing: Lactoferrin supplements are widely used and accepted internationally for their various health benefits. Regulations regarding their sale, labeling, and quality may vary by country.

Indian Standing: In India, lactoferrin supplements are also available and may be marketed for similar purposes as in other countries. However, specific regulations and market availability may differ.

Research Summary of Lactoferrin: Research on lactoferrin has demonstrated its diverse biological activities and potential health benefits, particularly in immune support, antimicrobial activity, and anti-inflammatory effects. Numerous studies have shown its efficacy in reducing the risk and severity of infections, promoting gut health, supporting iron metabolism, and enhancing wound healing. However, further research is needed to elucidate its mechanisms of action, optimal dosage, and potential benefits for specific populations.

37) LECITHINS

Introduction: Lecithins are a group of fatty substances that are naturally found in plants and animals. They are known for their emulsifying properties and are commonly used as food additives and dietary supplements.

Synonym Name and Common Name: Synonym: Phosphatidylcholines Common Name: Lecithins

Pharmacognosy / Chemistry: Lecithins are complex mixtures of phospholipids, glycolipids, triglycerides, and other lipids. They are derived from sources such as soybeans, eggs, sunflower seeds, and animal tissues.

Action and Pharmacology: Lecithins act primarily as emulsifiers, helping to stabilize mixtures of water and oil by reducing surface tension. They also play a role in cell membrane structure and function, lipid metabolism, and neurotransmitter synthesis.

Method of Analysis: Analysis of lecithins typically involves techniques such as thin-layer chromatography (TLC), gas chromatography (GC), or high-performance liquid chromatography (HPLC) to quantify the various lipid components and determine their composition.

Health Benefits:

- Supports brain health and cognitive function
- Promotes liver health and detoxification
- Enhances cardiovascular health
- Supports skin health and hydration
- May aid in weight management

Indication and Usage: Lecithin supplements are commonly used to support brain health, liver function, cardiovascular health, and skin health. They may also be used as a natural emulsifier in food products and as a dietary supplement for individuals looking to increase their intake of essential fatty acids.

Usual Constituents with Percentages: Lecithins are composed of various phospholipids, including phosphatidylcholine, phosphatidylethanolamine, and phosphatidylinositol, along with other lipids. The exact composition and percentages of these constituents can vary depending on the source and processing method.

Mechanism of Action: Lecithins act as emulsifiers, stabilizing mixtures of water and oil by reducing surface tension and promoting the formation of small droplets. They also play a role in cell membrane structure and function, lipid metabolism, and neurotransmitter synthesis.

Dosage: Dosage recommendations for lecithin supplements vary depending on the specific product and intended use. Typical doses range from 1 to 3 grams per day, taken with meals.

Contraindications:

- Allergy to soy or eggs (depending on the source of lecithin)
- Use caution in individuals with a history of gallstones or bile duct obstruction, as lecithin may stimulate bile production.

Precautions:

- Monitor lipid levels when using lecithin supplements, especially in individuals with hyperlipidemia or other lipid metabolism disorders.
- Use caution when using lecithin supplements in combination with anticoagulant medications, as lecithin may have mild anticoagulant effects.

Adverse Reactions: Common adverse reactions to lecithin supplements are rare but may include gastrointestinal discomfort, such as bloating, gas, or diarrhea, particularly at higher doses. Allergic reactions are possible in individuals with soy or egg allergies.

Research Summary: Research on lecithins has focused on their various health benefits, including their role in brain health, liver function, cardiovascular health, and skin health. Numerous studies have demonstrated their efficacy in supporting cognitive function, liver detoxification, cholesterol metabolism, and skin hydration. However, further research is needed to elucidate their mechanisms of action, optimal dosage, and long-term effects.

Pharmacokinetics: Lecithins are well absorbed in the gastrointestinal tract, where they are broken down into their constituent phospholipids and absorbed into the bloodstream. They are distributed to various tissues and organs, where they exert their biological effects. Lecithins are metabolized in the liver and excreted primarily in the bile.

Pharmacodynamics: Lecithins act primarily as emulsifiers, stabilizing mixtures of water and oil by reducing surface tension and promoting the formation of small droplets. They also play a role in cell membrane structure and function, lipid metabolism, and neurotransmitter synthesis.

Overdosage: Excessive intake of lecithin supplements may lead to gastrointestinal discomfort, such as bloating, gas, or diarrhea, particularly at higher doses. It's important to adhere to recommended dosages and consult a healthcare professional if concerns arise.

International Standing: Lecithin supplements are widely used and accepted internationally for their various health benefits. Regulations regarding their sale, labeling, and quality may vary by country.

Indian Standing: In India, lecithin supplements are also available and may be marketed for similar purposes as in other countries. However, specific regulations and market availability may differ.

Research Summary of Lecithins: Research on lecithins has focused on their various health benefits, including their role in brain health, liver function, cardiovascular health, and skin health. Numerous studies have demonstrated their efficacy in supporting cognitive function, liver detoxification, cholesterol metabolism, and skin hydration. However, further research is needed to elucidate their mechanisms of action, optimal dosage, and long-term effects.

38) LIGNANS

Introduction: Lignans are a diverse group of polyphenolic compounds found in plants, particularly in seeds, whole grains, fruits, and vegetables. They are known for their antioxidant and potential health-promoting properties.

Synonym Name and Common Name: Synonym: Phytoestrogens Common Name: Lignans

Pharmacognosy / Chemistry: Lignans are phytochemicals that are synthesized by plants through the shikimate and phenylpropanoid pathways. They are often present in the form of glycosides and are released upon hydrolysis by gut microbiota.

Action and Pharmacology: Lignans exhibit various biological activities, including antioxidant, anti-inflammatory, estrogenic, and anti-cancer effects. They may modulate hormone metabolism, oxidative stress, and inflammation, thereby contributing to their health-promoting properties.

Method of Analysis: Analysis of lignans typically involves techniques such as high-performance liquid chromatography (HPLC), gas chromatography (GC), or mass spectrometry to quantify their presence and concentration in plant extracts or biological samples.

Health Benefits:

- Antioxidant activity
- Hormonal balance support
- Cardiovascular health promotion
- Anti-inflammatory effects
- Potential anticancer properties

Indication and Usage: Lignans are commonly used as dietary supplements or consumed through plant-based foods to promote overall health and well-being. They may be used to support cardiovascular health, hormonal balance, and immune function, as well as to reduce the risk of chronic diseases.

Usual Constituents with Percentages: Lignans are found in various plant sources, including flaxseeds, sesame seeds, whole grains, fruits, and vegetables. The lignan content and composition can vary widely depending on the plant species and part of the plant.

Mechanism of Action: Lignans exert their biological effects through various mechanisms, including antioxidant activity, modulation of hormone metabolism, inhibition of inflammatory pathways, and potential interactions with estrogen receptors. They may also influence gut microbiota composition, which can impact overall health.

Dosage: Dosage recommendations for lignan supplements vary depending on the specific product and intended use. Typical doses range from 20 to 100 milligrams per day, taken with meals.

Contraindications:

- Allergy to plant-based foods containing lignans
- Use caution in individuals with hormone-sensitive conditions, as lignans may have estrogenic effects.

Precautions:

- Monitor hormone levels when using lignan supplements, especially in individuals with hormone-sensitive conditions such as breast cancer or endometriosis.
- Use caution when using lignan supplements in combination with hormone replacement therapy or other medications that affect hormone levels.

Adverse Reactions: Common adverse reactions to lignan supplements are rare but may include gastrointestinal discomfort, such as bloating, gas, or diarrhea, particularly at higher doses. Allergic reactions are possible in individuals with plant-based food allergies.

Research Summary: Research on lignans has focused on their potential health benefits, including their antioxidant, anti-inflammatory, estrogenic, and anticancer properties. Numerous studies have demonstrated their efficacy in promoting cardiovascular health, hormonal balance, and immune function, as well as their potential role in reducing the risk of chronic diseases such as cancer. However, further research is needed to elucidate their mechanisms of action, optimal dosage, and long-term effects.

Pharmacokinetics: Lignans are metabolized in the gastrointestinal tract by gut microbiota, which hydrolyze lignan glycosides into active aglycones. These aglycones are then absorbed into the bloodstream and distributed to various tissues, where they exert their biological effects. Lignans are metabolized in the liver and excreted primarily in the urine and feces.

Pharmacodynamics: Lignans exert their biological effects through various mechanisms, including antioxidant activity, modulation of hormone metabolism, inhibition of inflammatory pathways, and potential interactions with estrogen receptors. They may also influence gut microbiota composition, which can impact overall health.

Overdosage: Excessive intake of lignan supplements may lead to gastrointestinal discomfort, such as bloating, gas, or diarrhea, particularly at higher doses. It's important to adhere to recommended dosages and consult a healthcare professional if concerns arise.

International Standing: Lignan supplements are widely used and accepted internationally for their potential health benefits. Regulations regarding their sale, labeling, and quality may vary by country.

Indian Standing: In India, lignan supplements are also available and may be marketed for similar purposes as in other countries. However, specific regulations and market availability may differ.

Research Summary of Lignans: Research on lignans has focused on their potential health benefits, including their antioxidant, anti-inflammatory, estrogenic, and anticancer properties. Numerous studies have demonstrated their efficacy in promoting cardiovascular health, hormonal balance, and immune function, as well as their potential role in reducing the risk of chronic diseases such as cancer. However, further research is needed to elucidate their mechanisms of action, optimal dosage, and long-term effects.

39) LUTEIN

Introduction: Lutein is a carotenoid pigment found in various fruits and vegetables, particularly in green leafy vegetables like spinach and kale. It is known for its antioxidant properties and its role in supporting eye health.

Synonym Name and Common Name: Synonym: Xanthophyll Common Name: Lutein

Pharmacognosy / Chemistry: Lutein is a yellow-orange pigment belonging to the carotenoid family. It is synthesized by plants and is commonly found in the chloroplasts of green leafy vegetables.

Action and Pharmacology: Lutein acts primarily as an antioxidant, protecting cells from oxidative damage caused by free radicals. It also plays a role in filtering blue light and protecting the eyes from damage associated with ultraviolet light exposure.

Method of Analysis: Analysis of lutein typically involves techniques such as high-performance liquid chromatography (HPLC) or spectrophotometry to quantify its presence and concentration in plant extracts or biological samples.

Health Benefits:

- Supports eye health and vision
- Acts as an antioxidant, protecting cells from oxidative damage
- May reduce the risk of age-related macular degeneration (AMD)
- Potential cardiovascular health benefits
- Skin health support

Indication and Usage: Lutein supplements are commonly used to support eye health, particularly in individuals at risk of age-related macular degeneration (AMD) or those with low dietary intake of lutein-rich foods. They may also be used as a general antioxidant supplement to support overall health.

Usual Constituents with Percentages: Lutein is found in various plant sources, with green leafy vegetables being particularly rich sources. Spinach, kale, collard greens, and Swiss chard are examples of vegetables containing significant amounts of lutein.

Mechanism of Action: Lutein exerts its biological effects primarily through its antioxidant properties. It scavenges free radicals and reactive oxygen species, protecting cells and tissues from oxidative damage. Lutein also absorbs blue light, reducing oxidative stress in the eyes and supporting eye health.

Dosage: Dosage recommendations for lutein supplements vary depending on the specific product and intended use. Typical doses range from 10 to 20 milligrams per day, taken with meals.

Contraindications:

- Allergy to lutein or other carotenoids
- Use caution in individuals with a history of kidney stones, as high doses of lutein may increase the risk of stone formation.

Precautions:

- Monitor lipid levels when using lutein supplements, as high doses may affect cholesterol metabolism.
- Use caution when using lutein supplements in combination with other antioxidant supplements, as excessive antioxidant intake may have adverse effects.

Adverse Reactions: Common adverse reactions to lutein supplements are rare but may include gastrointestinal discomfort, such as bloating, gas, or diarrhea, particularly at higher doses. Allergic reactions are possible in individuals with allergies to lutein or other carotenoids.

Research Summary: Research on lutein has focused on its role in supporting eye health, particularly its potential to reduce the risk of age-related macular degeneration (AMD). Numerous studies have demonstrated a positive association between lutein intake and macular pigment density, visual function, and reduced risk of AMD. However, further research is needed to elucidate the optimal dosage, long-term effects, and potential benefits for specific populations.

Pharmacokinetics: Lutein is absorbed in the small intestine along with dietary fats and is incorporated into chylomicrons for transport in the bloodstream. It is distributed to various tissues, including the eyes, where it accumulates in the macula. Lutein is metabolized in the liver and excreted primarily in the feces.

Pharmacodynamics: Lutein exerts its biological effects primarily through its antioxidant properties, scavenging free radicals and reactive oxygen species to protect cells from oxidative damage. It also absorbs blue light, reducing oxidative stress in the eyes and supporting eye health.

Overdosage: Excessive intake of lutein supplements may lead to gastrointestinal discomfort, such as bloating, gas, or diarrhea, particularly at higher doses. It's important to adhere to recommended dosages and consult a healthcare professional if concerns arise.

International Standing: Lutein supplements are widely used and accepted internationally for their potential health benefits, particularly in supporting eye health. Regulations regarding their sale, labeling, and quality may vary by country.

Indian Standing: In India, lutein supplements are also available and may be marketed for similar purposes as in other countries. However, specific regulations and market availability may differ.

Research Summary of Lutein: Research on lutein has focused on its role in supporting eye health, particularly its potential to reduce the risk of age-related macular degeneration (AMD). Numerous studies have demonstrated a positive association between lutein intake and macular pigment density, visual function, and reduced risk of AMD. However, further research is needed to elucidate the optimal dosage, long-term effects, and potential benefits for specific populations.

40) LUTEIN/ZEAXANTHIN COMPLEX

Introduction: Lutein/zeaxanthin complex is a combination of two carotenoid pigments, lutein, and zeaxanthin, found in various fruits and vegetables. These compounds are known for their antioxidant properties and their role in supporting eye health.

Synonym Name and Common Name: Synonym: Lutein and Zeaxanthin Common Name: Lutein/zeaxanthin complex

Pharmacognosy / Chemistry: The lutein/zeaxanthin complex is derived from natural plant sources, particularly green leafy vegetables, and certain fruits. It is extracted from these sources using various methods to obtain a concentrated form of these carotenoids.

Action and Pharmacology: The lutein/zeaxanthin complex acts primarily as antioxidants, scavenging free radicals and reactive oxygen species to protect cells and tissues from oxidative damage. They also play a role in filtering blue light and supporting eye health, particularly in the prevention of age-related macular degeneration (AMD).

Method of Analysis: Analysis of the lutein/zeaxanthin complex typically involves techniques such as high-performance liquid chromatography (HPLC) or spectrophotometry to quantify the individual carotenoids and determine their concentration in plant extracts or dietary supplements.

Health Benefits:

- Supports eye health and vision
- Acts as antioxidants, protecting cells from oxidative damage
- May reduce the risk of age-related macular degeneration (AMD)
- Potential cardiovascular health benefits
- Skin health support

Indication and Usage: The lutein/zeaxanthin complex is commonly used as a dietary supplement to support eye health, particularly in individuals at risk of age-related macular degeneration (AMD) or those with low dietary intake of lutein and zeaxanthin-rich foods.

Usual Constituents with Percentages: The lutein/zeaxanthin complex typically contains a combination of lutein and zeaxanthin in varying proportions, depending on the source and formulation. The percentage composition may vary between products.

Mechanism of Action: The lutein/zeaxanthin complex exerts its biological effects primarily through its antioxidant properties, scavenging free radicals and reactive oxygen species to protect cells and tissues from oxidative damage. They also absorb blue light, reducing oxidative stress in the eyes and supporting eye health.

Dosage: Dosage recommendations for the lutein/zeaxanthin complex vary depending on the specific product and intended use. Typical doses range from 10 to 20 milligrams per day, taken with meals.

Contraindications:

- Allergy to lutein, zeaxanthin, or other carotenoids
- Use caution in individuals with a history of kidney stones, as high doses may increase the risk of stone formation.

Precautions:

- Monitor lipid levels when using the lutein/zeaxanthin complex supplements, as high doses may affect cholesterol metabolism.
- Use caution when using the lutein/zeaxanthin complex supplements in combination with other antioxidant supplements, as excessive antioxidant intake may have adverse effects.

Adverse Reactions: Common adverse reactions to the lutein/zeaxanthin complex supplements are rare but may include gastrointestinal discomfort, such as bloating, gas, or diarrhea, particularly at higher doses. Allergic reactions are possible in individuals with allergies to lutein, zeaxanthin, or other carotenoids.

Research Summary: Research on the lutein/zeaxanthin complex has focused on its role in supporting eye health, particularly its potential to reduce the risk of age-related macular degeneration (AMD). Numerous studies have demonstrated a positive association between the intake of lutein and zeaxanthin and macular pigment density, visual function, and reduced risk of AMD. However, further research is needed to elucidate the optimal dosage, long-term effects, and potential benefits for specific populations.

Pharmacokinetics: The lutein/zeaxanthin complex is absorbed in the small intestine along with dietary fats and is incorporated into chylomicrons for transport in the bloodstream. They are distributed to various tissues, including the eyes, where they accumulate in the macula. The lutein/zeaxanthin complex is metabolized in the liver and excreted primarily in the feces.

Pharmacodynamics: The lutein/zeaxanthin complex exerts its biological effects primarily through its antioxidant properties, scavenging free radicals and reactive oxygen species to protect cells and tissues from oxidative damage. They also absorb blue light, reducing oxidative stress in the eyes and supporting eye health.

Overdosage: Excessive intake of the lutein/zeaxanthin complex supplements may lead to gastrointestinal discomfort, such as bloating, gas, or diarrhea, particularly at higher doses. It's important to adhere to recommended dosages and consult a healthcare professional if concerns arise.

International Standing: The lutein/zeaxanthin complex supplements are widely used and accepted internationally for their potential health benefits, particularly in supporting eye health. Regulations regarding their sale, labeling, and quality may vary by country.

Indian Standing: In India, the lutein/zeaxanthin complex supplements are also available and may be marketed for similar purposes as in other countries. However, specific regulations and market availability may differ.

Research Summary of Lutein/Zeaxanthin Complex: Research on the lutein/zeaxanthin complex has focused on its role in supporting eye health, particularly its potential to reduce the risk of age-related macular degeneration (AMD). Numerous studies have demonstrated a positive association between the intake of lutein and zeaxanthin and macular pigment density, visual function, and reduced risk of AMD. However, further research is needed to elucidate the optimal dosage, long-term effects, and potential benefits for specific populations.

41) LYCOPENE

Introduction: Lycopene is a natural pigment and phytochemical found in red fruits and vegetables, known for its potent antioxidant properties and potential health benefits.

Synonym Name and Common Name: Synonym: None Common Name: Lycopene

Pharmacognosy / Chemistry: Lycopene is a carotenoid compound synthesized by plants and microorganisms. It is responsible for the red color of fruits such as tomatoes, watermelons, and pink grapefruits.

Action and Pharmacology: Lycopene acts primarily as a powerful antioxidant, neutralizing free radicals and reactive oxygen species in the body. Its antioxidant properties help protect cells and tissues from oxidative damage, which is implicated in various diseases and aging processes.

Method of Analysis: Analysis of lycopene typically involves techniques such as high-performance liquid chromatography (HPLC) or spectrophotometry to quantify its presence and concentration in plant extracts or biological samples.

Health Benefits:

- Antioxidant activity
- Cardiovascular health support
- Prostate health support
- Skin health support
- Potential anticancer properties

Indication and Usage: Lycopene supplements are commonly used to support overall health and well-being, particularly cardiovascular health, and prostate health. They may also be used for skin health and as a potential adjunctive therapy in cancer prevention.

Usual Constituents with Percentages: Lycopene is found in high concentrations in tomatoes and tomato products, with tomato paste and sauce being particularly rich sources. Other sources include watermelon, pink grapefruit, guava, and papaya.

Mechanism of Action: Lycopene exerts its biological effects primarily through its antioxidant properties, neutralizing free radicals and reactive oxygen species to protect cells and tissues from oxidative damage. It may also modulate various cellular signaling pathways involved in inflammation and cancer development.

Dosage: Dosage recommendations for lycopene supplements vary depending on the specific product and intended use. Typical doses range from 6 to 30 milligrams per day, taken with meals.

Contraindications:

- Allergy to lycopene or other carotenoids
- Use caution in individuals with a history of kidney stones, as high doses of lycopene may increase the risk of stone formation.

Precautions:

- Monitor lipid levels when using lycopene supplements, as high doses may affect cholesterol metabolism.
- Use caution when using lycopene supplements in combination with other antioxidant supplements, as excessive antioxidant intake may have adverse effects.

Adverse Reactions: Common adverse reactions to lycopene supplements are rare but may include gastrointestinal discomfort, such as bloating, gas, or diarrhea, particularly at higher doses. Allergic reactions are possible in individuals with allergies to lycopene or other carotenoids.

Research Summary: Research on lycopene has focused on its potential health benefits, including its role in cardiovascular health, prostate health, skin health, and cancer prevention. Numerous studies have demonstrated a positive association between lycopene intake and reduced risk of cardiovascular disease, prostate cancer, and certain other cancers. However, further research is needed to elucidate the optimal dosage, long-term effects, and potential benefits for specific populations.

Pharmacokinetics: Lycopene is absorbed in the small intestine along with dietary fats and is incorporated into chylomicrons for transport in the bloodstream. It is distributed to various tissues, including the skin, where it accumulates. Lycopene is metabolized in the liver and excreted primarily in the feces.

Pharmacodynamics: Lycopene exerts its biological effects primarily through its antioxidant properties, neutralizing free radicals and reactive oxygen species to protect cells and tissues from oxidative damage. It may also modulate various cellular signaling pathways involved in inflammation and cancer development.

Overdosage: Excessive intake of lycopene supplements may lead to gastrointestinal discomfort, such as bloating, gas, or diarrhea, particularly at higher doses. It's important to adhere to recommended dosages and consult a healthcare professional if concerns arise.

International Standing: Lycopene supplements are widely used and accepted internationally for their potential health benefits, particularly in supporting cardiovascular health and prostate health. Regulations regarding their sale, labeling, and quality may vary by country.

Indian Standing: In India, lycopene supplements are also available and may be marketed for similar purposes as in other countries. However, specific regulations and market availability may differ.

Research Summary of Lycopene: Research on lycopene has focused on its potential health benefits, including its role in cardiovascular health, prostate health, skin health, and cancer prevention. Numerous studies have demonstrated a positive association between lycopene intake and reduced risk of cardiovascular disease, prostate cancer, and certain other cancers. However, further research is needed to elucidate the optimal dosage, long-term effects, and potential benefits for specific populations.

42) MEDIUM CHAIN TRIGLYCERIDES

Introduction: Medium chain triglycerides (MCTs) are a type of dietary fat composed of medium-chain fatty acids (MCFAs). They are derived from sources such as coconut oil and palm kernel oil and are known for their unique metabolic properties and potential health benefits.

Synonym Name and Common Name: Synonym: MCT oil Common Name: Medium chain triglycerides (MCTs)

Pharmacognosy / Chemistry: MCTs are naturally occurring fats found in certain foods, particularly coconut oil and palm kernel oil. They are composed of medium-chain fatty acids, which contain between 6 to 12 carbon atoms in their fatty acid chains.

Action and Pharmacology: MCTs are rapidly absorbed and metabolized in the body, providing a quick source of energy. They are preferentially converted into ketones by the liver, which can be utilized by the brain and muscles for energy. MCTs may also have thermogenic properties, potentially aiding in weight management.

Method of Analysis: Analysis of MCTs typically involves techniques such as gas chromatography (GC) or high-performance liquid chromatography (HPLC) to quantify the individual medium-chain fatty acids present in oils or food products.

Health Benefits:

- Quick source of energy
- Potential aid in weight management
- Cognitive function support
- Athletic performance enhancement
- Potential antimicrobial properties

Indication and Usage: MCTs are commonly used as a dietary supplement to support energy levels, promote weight loss, enhance cognitive function, and improve athletic performance. They may also be used in cooking or as an ingredient in various food products.

Usual Constituents with Percentages: MCTs are composed of medium-chain fatty acids, primarily caprylic acid (C8:0) and capric acid (C10:0). Depending on the source and processing method, the percentage composition of these fatty acids may vary in MCT oil products.

Mechanism of Action: MCTs are rapidly absorbed into the bloodstream and transported to the liver, where they are metabolized into ketones. Ketones can cross the blood-brain barrier and serve as an alternative energy source for the brain. MCTs may also increase metabolic rate and fat oxidation, potentially aiding in weight loss.

Dosage: Dosage recommendations for MCT oil vary depending on the specific product and intended use. Typical doses range from 1 to 3 tablespoons per day, taken with meals or as directed by a healthcare professional.

Contraindications:

- Allergy to coconut oil or palm kernel oil
- Use caution in individuals with liver disease or impaired liver function, as MCT metabolism occurs primarily in the liver.

Precautions:

- Start with a small dose of MCT oil and gradually increase to minimize gastrointestinal side effects such as diarrhea or abdominal cramping.

- Use caution when using MCT oil in cooking, as it has a low smoke point and may degrade at high temperatures.

Adverse Reactions: Common adverse reactions to MCT oil include gastrointestinal discomfort, such as diarrhea, nausea, or abdominal cramping, particularly at higher doses. Allergic reactions are possible in individuals with allergies to coconut oil or palm kernel oil.

Research Summary: Research on MCTs has focused on their potential health benefits, including their role in energy metabolism, weight management, cognitive function, and athletic performance. Numerous studies have demonstrated a positive association between MCT intake and increased energy expenditure, enhanced cognitive function, and improved athletic performance. However, further research is needed to elucidate the optimal dosage, long-term effects, and potential benefits for specific populations.

Pharmacokinetics: MCTs are rapidly absorbed from the gastrointestinal tract and transported to the liver via the portal vein. In the liver, they are rapidly metabolized into ketones, which can be utilized by various tissues for energy. Excess MCTs are converted into storage fats or transported to peripheral tissues for use.

Pharmacodynamics: MCTs exert their biological effects primarily through their rapid metabolism into ketones, which serve as an alternative energy source for the brain and muscles. They may also increase metabolic rate and fat oxidation, potentially aiding in weight loss and improving athletic performance.

Overdosage: Excessive intake of MCT oil may lead to gastrointestinal discomfort, such as diarrhea, nausea, or abdominal cramping, particularly at higher doses. It's important to adhere to recommended dosages and consult a healthcare professional if concerns arise.

International Standing: MCT oil supplements are widely used and accepted internationally for their potential health benefits, particularly in supporting energy metabolism, weight management, and cognitive function. Regulations regarding their sale, labeling, and quality may vary by country.

Indian Standing: In India, MCT oil supplements are also available and may be marketed for similar purposes as in other countries. However, specific regulations and market availability may differ.

Research Summary of Medium Chain Triglycerides: Research on medium chain triglycerides (MCTs) has focused on their potential health benefits, including their role in energy metabolism, weight management, cognitive function, and athletic performance. Numerous studies have demonstrated a positive association between MCT intake and increased energy expenditure, enhanced cognitive function, and improved athletic performance. However, further research is needed to elucidate the optimal dosage, long-term effects, and potential benefits for specific populations.

43) N-ACETYL D-GLUCOSAMINE

Introduction: N-Acetyl-D-glucosamine (NAG) is a naturally occurring compound found in the exoskeletons of shellfish, fungi, and certain microorganisms. It plays a crucial role in various physiological processes and is commonly used as a dietary supplement.

Synonym Name and Common Name: Synonym: Glucosamine Common Name: N-Acetyl-D-glucosamine (NAG)

Pharmacognosy / Chemistry: NAG is a derivative of glucose and is commonly synthesized from chitin, a structural polysaccharide found in the exoskeletons of shellfish and fungal cell walls. It is a white, odorless powder with a slightly sweet taste.

Action and Pharmacology: NAG is believed to support joint health by serving as a precursor for the biosynthesis of glycosaminoglycans (GAGs), which are essential components of cartilage and synovial fluid. It may also have anti-inflammatory and immunomodulatory effects.

Method of Analysis: Analysis of NAG typically involves techniques such as high-performance liquid chromatography (HPLC) or spectrophotometry to quantify its presence and concentration in dietary supplements or biological samples.

Health Benefits:

- Joint health support
- Cartilage repair and maintenance

- Wound healing support
- Potential anti-inflammatory effects
- Gut health support

Indication and Usage: NAG supplements are commonly used to support joint health and alleviate symptoms of osteoarthritis. They may also be used to promote wound healing, support gut health, and manage inflammatory conditions.

Usual Constituents with Percentages: NAG supplements typically contain N-acetyl-D-glucosamine as the active ingredient, often in the form of capsules, tablets, or powder. The percentage composition of NAG may vary between products.

Mechanism of Action: NAG is a precursor for the biosynthesis of glycosaminoglycans (GAGs), which are major components of cartilage and synovial fluid in joints. By providing the building blocks for GAG synthesis, NAG supports joint structure and function, promoting cartilage repair and maintenance. It may also exert anti-inflammatory effects by modulating cytokine production and inhibiting inflammatory pathways.

Dosage: Dosage recommendations for NAG supplements vary depending on the specific product and intended use. Typical doses range from 500 mg to 1500 mg per day, taken with meals.

Contraindications:

- Allergy to shellfish, as NAG supplements are often derived from shellfish sources
- Use caution in individuals with diabetes, as NAG may affect blood sugar levels
- Precautions:
- Consult a healthcare professional before using NAG supplements, especially if pregnant, nursing, or taking medications
- Monitor blood sugar levels closely in individuals with diabetes when using NAG supplements

Adverse Reactions: Common adverse reactions to NAG supplements may include gastrointestinal symptoms such as nausea, vomiting, diarrhea, or abdominal pain. Allergic reactions are possible in individuals with shellfish allergies.

Research Summary: Research on NAG has focused on its potential role in supporting joint health, promoting cartilage repair, and managing symptoms of osteoarthritis. Some studies have suggested that NAG supplementation may help alleviate joint pain and improve joint function in individuals with osteoarthritis. However, further research is needed to confirm these findings and elucidate the optimal dosage and long-term effects of NAG supplementation.

Pharmacokinetics: NAG is absorbed in the small intestine and undergoes rapid metabolism in the liver. It is then distributed to various tissues, where it may be incorporated into glycosaminoglycans (GAGs) or excreted in the urine.

Pharmacodynamics: NAG exerts its biological effects primarily by serving as a precursor for the biosynthesis of glycosaminoglycans (GAGs), which are essential components of cartilage and synovial fluid in joints. By providing the building blocks for GAG synthesis, NAG supports joint structure and function, promoting cartilage repair and maintenance. It may also have anti-inflammatory effects by modulating cytokine production and inhibiting inflammatory pathways.

Overdosage: Excessive intake of NAG supplements may lead to gastrointestinal symptoms such as nausea, vomiting, diarrhea, or abdominal pain. It's important to adhere to recommended dosages and consult a healthcare professional if concerns arise.

International Standing: NAG supplements are widely used and accepted internationally for their potential health benefits, particularly in supporting joint health and managing symptoms of osteoarthritis. Regulations regarding their sale, labeling, and quality may vary by country.

Indian Standing: In India, NAG supplements are also available and may be marketed for similar purposes as in other countries. However, specific regulations and market availability may differ.

44) OMEGA-3 FATTY ACIDS

Introduction: Omega-3 fatty acids are essential polyunsaturated fatty acids (PUFAs) that are crucial for maintaining overall health. They are considered essential because the body cannot produce them and must obtain them from the diet or supplements.

Synonym Name and Common Name: Synonym: n-3 fatty acids, omega-3s Common Name: Omega-3 fatty acids

Pharmacognosy / Chemistry: Omega-3 fatty acids are naturally found in fatty fish such as salmon, mackerel, and sardines, as well as in certain plant sources like flaxseeds, chia seeds, and walnuts. They are also available in supplement form, including fish oil, krill oil, and algal oil.

Action and Pharmacology: Omega-3 fatty acids play a crucial role in various physiological processes, including inflammation regulation, cardiovascular health, brain function, and immune system function. They are incorporated into cell membranes and serve as precursors to signaling molecules involved in these processes.

Method of Analysis: Analysis of omega-3 fatty acids typically involves techniques such as gas chromatography (GC) or high-performance liquid chromatography (HPLC) to quantify the individual fatty acids present in oils or biological samples.

Health Benefits:

- Cardiovascular health support
- Brain function and cognitive health support
- Anti-inflammatory effects
- Eye health support
- Potential benefits for skin health, mood disorders, and autoimmune diseases

Indication and Usage: Omega-3 fatty acid supplements are commonly used to support heart health, manage inflammation-related conditions such as arthritis, promote brain health and cognitive function, and support overall well-being. They may also be used in the treatment of certain medical conditions.

Usual Constituents with Percentages: Omega-3 fatty acids include alpha-linolenic acid (ALA), eicosapentaenoic acid (EPA), and docosahexaenoic acid (DHA). The percentage composition of these fatty acids varies depending on the source of the supplement or food product.

Mechanism of Action: Omega-3 fatty acids exert their biological effects through various mechanisms, including modulation of inflammatory pathways, regulation of lipid metabolism, and modulation of cell membrane fluidity and function. EPA and DHA are particularly involved in these processes and have been shown to have anti-inflammatory and cardioprotective effects.

Dosage: Dosage recommendations for omega-3 fatty acid supplements vary depending on the specific product, individual health status, and intended use. Typical doses range from 250 mg to 2000 mg of combined EPA and DHA per day.

Contraindications:

- Allergy to fish or shellfish, as omega-3 supplements are often derived from these sources
- Use caution in individuals with bleeding disorders or taking anticoagulant medications, as omega-3 fatty acids may increase the risk of bleeding

Precautions:

- Consult a healthcare professional before starting omega-3 supplements, especially if pregnant, nursing, or taking medications
- Monitor blood clotting parameters in individuals taking anticoagulant medications while using omega-3 supplements

Adverse Reactions: Common adverse reactions to omega-3 supplements may include gastrointestinal symptoms such as nausea, diarrhea, or indigestion. In some cases, individuals may experience allergic reactions to fish-derived supplements.

Research Summary: Research on omega-3 fatty acids has demonstrated their potential health benefits, particularly in supporting cardiovascular health, brain function, and inflammation regulation. Numerous studies have shown a positive association between omega-3 intake and reduced risk of cardiovascular disease, improved cognitive function, and reduced inflammation. However, further research is needed to elucidate the optimal dosage, long-term effects, and potential benefits for specific populations.

Pharmacokinetics: Omega-3 fatty acids are absorbed in the small intestine and transported in the bloodstream bound to lipoproteins. They are then distributed to various tissues, where they are incorporated into cell membranes or metabolized. Excess omega-3 fatty acids are metabolized in the liver and excreted primarily in the urine.

Pharmacodynamics: Omega-3 fatty acids exert their biological effects through various mechanisms, including modulation of inflammatory pathways, regulation of lipid metabolism, and modulation of cell membrane function. EPA and DHA, in particular, are involved in these processes and have been shown to have anti-inflammatory, cardioprotective, and neuroprotective effects.

Overdosage: Excessive intake of omega-3 fatty acid supplements may lead to gastrointestinal symptoms such as nausea, diarrhea, or indigestion. In some cases, high doses may increase the risk of bleeding in individuals taking anticoagulant medications. It's important to adhere to recommended dosages and consult a healthcare professional if concerns arise.

International Standing: Omega-3 fatty acid supplements are widely used and accepted internationally for their potential health benefits, particularly in supporting cardiovascular health, brain function, and inflammation regulation. Regulations regarding their sale, labeling, and quality may vary by country.

Indian Standing: In India, omega-3 fatty acid supplements are also available and may be marketed for similar purposes as in other countries. However, specific regulations and market availability may differ.

Research Summary of Omega-3 Fatty Acids: Research on omega-3 fatty acids has demonstrated their potential health benefits, particularly in supporting cardiovascular health, brain function, and inflammation regulation. Numerous studies have shown a positive association between omega-3 intake and reduced risk of cardiovascular disease, improved cognitive function, and reduced inflammation. However, further research is needed to elucidate the optimal dosage, long-term effects, and potential benefits for specific populations.

45)OMEGA-6-FATTY ACIDS

Introduction: Omega-6 fatty acids are polyunsaturated fatty acids (PUFAs) that play essential roles in various physiological processes within the human body. They are considered essential nutrients because the body cannot produce them on its own and must obtain them from the diet.

Synonym Name and Common Name: Synonym: n-6 fatty acids Common Name: Omega-6 fatty acids

Pharmacognosy / Chemistry: Omega-6 fatty acids are naturally found in a variety of foods, including vegetable oils (such as soybean oil, sunflower oil, and corn oil), nuts, seeds, and certain types of fish. They are also available in supplement form.

Action and Pharmacology: Omega-6 fatty acids play crucial roles in cell membrane structure and function, inflammation regulation, and gene expression. They serve as precursors for the synthesis of signaling molecules called eicosanoids, which are involved in various physiological processes, including inflammation, blood clotting, and immune response.

Method of Analysis: Analysis of omega-6 fatty acids typically involves techniques such as gas chromatography (GC) or high-performance liquid chromatography (HPLC) to quantify the individual fatty acids present in oils or biological samples.

Health Benefits:

- Cell membrane structure and function
- Regulation of inflammation
- Immune system function
- Skin health and integrity
- Hormone production and regulation

Indication and Usage: Omega-6 fatty acids are essential nutrients required for overall health and well-being. They are commonly consumed as part of a balanced diet and may also be used in the management of certain medical conditions, such as inflammatory disorders or skin conditions.

Usual Constituents with Percentages: Omega-6 fatty acids include linoleic acid (LA) and arachidonic acid (AA). The percentage composition of these fatty acids varies depending on the dietary sources consumed.

Mechanism of Action: Omega-6 fatty acids exert their biological effects through various mechanisms, including incorporation into cell membranes, synthesis of eicosanoids, and modulation of gene expression. They play crucial roles in inflammation regulation, immune response, and cellular signaling pathways.

Dosage: There is no specific recommended daily intake for omega-6 fatty acids as they are typically consumed as part of a balanced diet. However, dietary guidelines recommend consuming a variety of foods rich in omega-6 fatty acids to meet daily nutritional requirements.

Contraindications:

- Allergy to foods containing omega-6 fatty acids
- Use caution in individuals with certain medical conditions, such as inflammatory disorders or clotting disorders, as omega-6 fatty acids may exacerbate symptoms or interfere with medication effects

Precautions:

Omega-6 fatty acids should be consumed in moderation as excessive intake may disrupt the balance between omega-6 and omega-3 fatty acids, potentially leading to inflammation and other adverse effects.

It's important to maintain a balanced ratio of omega-6 to omega-3 fatty acids in the diet for optimal health outcomes.

Adverse Reactions: Common adverse reactions to omega-6 fatty acids are rare but may include gastrointestinal symptoms such as nausea, diarrhea, or abdominal discomfort. Allergic reactions are possible in individuals with allergies to foods containing omega-6 fatty acids.

Research Summary: Research on omega-6 fatty acids has focused on their role in inflammation regulation, cardiovascular health, immune function, and skin health. While omega-6 fatty acids are essential for various physiological processes, an imbalance between omega-6 and omega-3 fatty acids in the diet has been implicated in the development of chronic diseases, including cardiovascular disease, obesity, and inflammatory disorders. Further research is needed to elucidate the optimal balance of omega-6 and omega-3 fatty acids for overall health and disease prevention.

Pharmacokinetics: Omega-6 fatty acids are absorbed in the small intestine and transported in the bloodstream bound to lipoproteins. They are then distributed to various tissues, where they are incorporated into cell membranes or metabolized. Excess omega-6 fatty acids are metabolized in the liver and excreted primarily in the urine.

Pharmacodynamics: Omega-6 fatty acids exert their biological effects through various mechanisms, including incorporation into cell membranes, synthesis of eicosanoids, and modulation of gene expression. They play crucial roles in inflammation regulation, immune response, and cellular signaling pathways.

Overdosage: Excessive intake of omega-6 fatty acids may disrupt the balance between omega-6 and omega-3 fatty acids in the diet, potentially leading to inflammation and other adverse effects. It's important to consume omega-6 fatty acids in moderation as part of a balanced diet.

International Standing: Omega-6 fatty acids are recognized as essential nutrients and are widely consumed as part of a balanced diet worldwide. Regulations regarding their sale, labeling, and quality may vary by country.

Indian Standing: In India, omega-6 fatty acids are also recognized as essential nutrients and are consumed as part of a balanced diet. However, specific regulations and market availability of omega-6 fatty acid supplements may differ.

46) PECTIN

Introduction: Pectin is a complex polysaccharide found in various plant tissues, particularly in fruits such as apples, citrus fruits, and berries. It is widely used in the food industry as a gelling agent, thickener, and stabilizer, and it also possesses potential health benefits.

Synonym Name and Common Name: Synonym: Fruit pectin Common Name: Pectin

Pharmacognosy / Chemistry: Pectin is a heteropolysaccharide composed mainly of galacturonic acid units with side chains of various sugars, including rhamnose, galactose, and arabinose. It is found in the cell walls of plant tissues, where it contributes to their structural integrity.

Action and Pharmacology: In the gastrointestinal tract, pectin forms a gel-like substance when mixed with water, which can help regulate bowel movements and promote digestive health. It may also have cholesterol-lowering effects by binding to bile acids and reducing their reabsorption in the intestine.

Method of Analysis: Analysis of pectin typically involves techniques such as Fourier transform infrared spectroscopy (FTIR), gas chromatography (GC), or high-performance liquid chromatography (HPLC) to characterize its chemical composition and quantify its presence in food products.

Health Benefits:

- Digestive health support
- Cholesterol-lowering effects
- Blood sugar regulation
- Weight management aid
- Potential prebiotic effects

Indication and Usage: Pectin is commonly used as a food additive in the production of jams, jellies, fruit preserves, and other food products to improve texture and stability. It is also used as a dietary supplement for its potential health benefits, particularly in supporting digestive health and cholesterol management.

Usual Constituents with Percentages: Pectin is composed mainly of galacturonic acid units, typically ranging from 65% to 75% of its total composition. It also contains varying proportions of other sugars such as rhamnose, galactose, and arabinose, as well as small amounts of protein and minerals.

Mechanism of Action: In the gastrointestinal tract, pectin forms a gel-like substance by absorbing water, which can help regulate bowel movements and promote regularity. Pectin may also bind to bile acids in the intestine, reducing their reabsorption and leading to lower cholesterol levels in the blood.

Dosage: Dosage recommendations for pectin supplements vary depending on the specific product and intended use. Typical doses range from 5 to 15 grams per day, taken with water or mixed with food.

Contraindications:

- Allergy to pectin or fruits containing pectin
- Use caution in individuals with gastrointestinal disorders, as pectin supplements may exacerbate symptoms such as bloating or gas

Precautions:

- Ensure an adequate intake of water when consuming pectin supplements to prevent gastrointestinal discomfort.
- Consult a healthcare professional before using pectin supplements, especially if pregnant, nursing, or taking medications.

Adverse Reactions: Common adverse reactions to pectin supplements may include gastrointestinal symptoms such as bloating, gas, or diarrhea, particularly at higher doses. Allergic reactions are possible in individuals with allergies to pectin or fruits containing pectin.

Research Summary: Research on pectin has focused on its potential health benefits, particularly in supporting digestive health, cholesterol management, and blood sugar regulation. Some studies have shown that pectin supplementation may help regulate bowel movements, lower cholesterol levels, and improve glycemic control. However, further research is needed to elucidate the optimal dosage, long-term effects, and potential benefits for specific populations.

Pharmacokinetics: Pectin is not absorbed intact in the gastrointestinal tract but undergoes fermentation by gut bacteria, producing short-chain fatty acids and other metabolites that may contribute to its health benefits. Any unfermented pectin is excreted in the feces.

Pharmacodynamics: In the gastrointestinal tract, pectin forms a gel-like substance by absorbing water, which can help regulate bowel movements and promote regularity. Pectin may also bind to bile acids in the intestine, reducing their reabsorption and leading to lower cholesterol levels in the blood.

Overdosage: Excessive intake of pectin supplements may lead to gastrointestinal symptoms such as bloating, gas, or diarrhea, particularly at higher doses. It's important to adhere to recommended dosages and consult a healthcare professional if concerns arise.

International Standing: Pectin is recognized as a safe food additive by regulatory authorities worldwide and is widely used in the food industry for its gelling, thickening, and stabilizing properties.

Indian Standing: In India, pectin is also recognized as a safe food additive and is commonly used in the production of jams, jellies, fruit preserves, and other food products. Pectin supplements may also be available for purchase, although specific regulations and market availability may vary.

47) PHOSPHATIDES /PHOSPHOLIPIDS

Introduction: Phosphatides, also known as phospholipids, are essential components of cell membranes found in various foods and dietary supplements. They play crucial roles in cell structure and function, as well as in various physiological processes within the human body.

Synonym Name and Common Name: Synonym: Phospholipids Common Name: Phosphatides

Pharmacognosy / Chemistry: Phosphatides are a class of lipids characterized by their amphiphilic nature, containing hydrophobic tails and hydrophilic heads. They are found in abundance in sources such as soybeans, eggs, and sunflower seeds.

Action and Pharmacology: Phosphatides play essential roles in cell membrane structure, signal transduction, and lipid metabolism. They are also involved in the transport of fats and cholesterol in the bloodstream, as well as in the absorption of fat-soluble nutrients.

Method of Analysis: Analysis of phosphatides typically involves techniques such as thin-layer chromatography (TLC), gas chromatography (GC), or high-performance liquid chromatography (HPLC) to quantify and characterize the individual phospholipid species present in food products or supplements.

Health Benefits:

- Supports cellular membrane structure and function
- Supports brain health and cognitive function
- May have cardiovascular benefits by helping to regulate cholesterol levels

- Supports liver health and detoxification processes
- May have anti-inflammatory effects

Indication and Usage: Phosphatides are commonly used as food additives and dietary supplements to support overall health and well-being. They may be used to promote brain health, support cardiovascular health, enhance liver function, and aid in the absorption of fat-soluble nutrients.

Usual Constituents with Percentages: Phosphatides consist of various phospholipid species, including phosphatidylcholine (PC), phosphatidylethanolamine (PE), phosphatidylinositol (PI), and phosphatidylserine (PS). The percentage composition of these phospholipids varies depending on the source and processing method.

Mechanism of Action: Phosphatides play essential roles in cell membrane structure and function, serving as key components of lipid bilayers. They also act as signaling molecules and participate in various cellular processes, including signal transduction, membrane trafficking, and lipid metabolism.

Dosage: Dosage recommendations for phosphatide supplements vary depending on the specific product and intended use. Typical doses range from 100 mg to 1000 mg per day, although higher doses may be used in certain therapeutic applications.

Contraindications:

- Allergy to phosphatides or sources containing phospholipids
- Use caution in individuals with liver or gallbladder disorders, as phosphatides may affect bile secretion and fat digestion

Precautions:

- Consult a healthcare professional before using phosphatide supplements, especially if pregnant, nursing, or taking medications.
- Monitor liver function and lipid levels regularly in individuals with pre-existing liver conditions or dyslipidemia.

Adverse Reactions: Common adverse reactions to phosphatide supplements are rare but may include gastrointestinal symptoms such as nausea, diarrhea, or abdominal discomfort. Allergic reactions are possible in individuals with allergies to phospholipids or related compounds.

Research Summary: Research on phosphatides has focused on their potential health benefits, particularly in supporting brain health, cardiovascular health, and liver function. Some studies have suggested that phosphatide supplementation may improve cognitive function, reduce cholesterol levels, and support liver health. However, further research is needed to elucidate the optimal dosage, long-term effects, and potential benefits for specific populations.

Pharmacokinetics: Phosphatides are absorbed in the small intestine and transported in the bloodstream bound to lipoproteins. They are then distributed to various tissues, where they are incorporated into cell membranes or metabolized. Excess phosphatides are metabolized in the liver and excreted primarily in the urine and bile.

Pharmacodynamics: Phosphatides exert their biological effects primarily through their role in cell membrane structure and function. They also act as signaling molecules and participate in various cellular processes, including lipid metabolism, signal transduction, and membrane trafficking.

Overdosage: Excessive intake of phosphatide supplements may lead to gastrointestinal symptoms such as nausea, diarrhea, or abdominal discomfort. It's important to adhere to recommended dosages and consult a healthcare professional if concerns arise.

International Standing: Phosphatides are recognized as safe food additives by regulatory authorities worldwide and are widely used in the food industry for their emulsifying, stabilizing, and texturizing properties. Phosphatide supplements are also available in many countries for their potential health benefits.

Indian Standing: In India, phosphatides are also recognized as safe food additives and dietary supplements. They may be used in various food products and are available for purchase in the form of dietary supplements. Regulatory oversight and market availability may vary.

48) POLICOSANOL

Introduction: Policosanol is a mixture of long-chain alcohols derived from plant waxes, primarily sugarcane (Saccharum officinarum) and beeswax. It has gained attention for its potential cholesterol-lowering effects and other health benefits.

Synonym Name and Common Name: Synonym: Octacosanol Common Name: Policosanol

Pharmacognosy / Chemistry: Policosanol is derived from natural sources, primarily sugarcane wax. It contains a mixture of long-chain alcohols, with octacosanol being the primary component. Policosanol is usually obtained through extraction and purification processes.

Action and Pharmacology: Policosanol has been studied for its potential lipid-lowering effects, particularly in lowering LDL cholesterol levels and increasing HDL cholesterol levels. It is believed to inhibit cholesterol synthesis in the liver and enhance the breakdown of LDL cholesterol in the bloodstream.

Method of Analysis: Analysis of policosanol typically involves techniques such as gas chromatography (GC) or high-performance liquid chromatography (HPLC) to quantify and characterize the individual alcohols present in the mixture.

Health Benefits:

- Potential cholesterol-lowering effects
- Antioxidant properties
- Anti-inflammatory effects
- Potential improvement in exercise performance

Indication and Usage: Policosanol is commonly used as a dietary supplement for its potential cholesterol-lowering effects and other health benefits. It may be recommended for individuals with high cholesterol levels or those at risk of cardiovascular disease.

Usual Constituents with Percentages: The main constituent of policosanol is octacosanol, which typically comprises about 60-70% of the mixture. Other long-chain alcohols, such as triacontanol, dotriacontanol, and hexacosanol, may also be present in smaller amounts.

Mechanism of Action: The exact mechanism of action of policosanol is not fully understood. However, it is believed to inhibit HMG-CoA reductase, an enzyme involved in cholesterol synthesis in the liver. Policosanol may also enhance the breakdown of LDL cholesterol in the bloodstream and have antioxidant and anti-inflammatory effects.

Dosage: Typical doses of policosanol range from 5 to 40 mg per day, taken orally. However, dosages may vary depending on the specific formulation and individual health status. It is recommended to follow the instructions provided by healthcare professionals or on the product label.

Contraindications:

- Allergy to policosanol or related compounds
- Use caution in individuals with liver disease or those taking medications that may interact with policosanol, such as statins or blood thinners.

Precautions:

- Pregnant or nursing women, as well as individuals with underlying medical conditions, should consult a healthcare professional before using policosanol supplements.
- Monitor liver function regularly in individuals with liver disease or those taking medications that may affect liver function.

Adverse Reactions: Common adverse reactions to policosanol supplements are rare but may include gastrointestinal symptoms such as nausea, diarrhea, or abdominal discomfort. Allergic reactions are possible in individuals with allergies to policosanol or related compounds.

Research Summary: Research on policosanol has primarily focused on its potential cholesterol-lowering effects and cardiovascular benefits. Some studies have suggested that policosanol supplementation may help lower LDL cholesterol levels and increase HDL cholesterol levels. However, results have been mixed, and further research is needed to confirm its efficacy and safety for long-term use.

Pharmacokinetics: The pharmacokinetics of policosanol have not been extensively studied. After oral administration, policosanol is absorbed in the gastrointestinal tract and undergoes metabolism in the liver. The metabolites are then excreted primarily in the urine.

Pharmacodynamics: Policosanol is believed to inhibit cholesterol synthesis in the liver by blocking the activity of HMG-CoA reductase, an enzyme involved in cholesterol production. It may also enhance the breakdown of LDL cholesterol in the bloodstream and have antioxidant and anti-inflammatory effects.

Overdosage: There is limited information on the effects of overdosage with policosanol supplements. However, it is recommended to adhere to recommended dosages and consult a healthcare professional if concerns arise.

International Standing: Policosanol supplements are available in many countries and are commonly used for their potential cholesterol-lowering effects. However, regulations regarding their sale, labeling, and quality may vary by country.

Indian Standing: In India, policosanol supplements are also available and may be used for their potential health benefits. However, specific regulations and market availability may vary.

49) RESVERATROL

Introduction: Resveratrol is a natural polyphenol compound found in various plants, particularly in grapes, red wine, berries, and peanuts. It has garnered significant attention for its potential health benefits, including antioxidant, anti-inflammatory, and cardioprotective properties.

Synonym Name and Common Name: Synonym: Trans-Resveratrol Common Name: Resveratrol

Pharmacognosy / Chemistry: Resveratrol belongs to a class of compounds known as stilbenoids, characterized by their stilbene backbone structure. It is primarily found in the skin of grapes and in grape-derived products such as red wine.

Action and Pharmacology: Resveratrol exerts various pharmacological effects, including antioxidant, anti-inflammatory, anti-cancer, cardioprotective, neuroprotective, and anti-aging properties. It interacts with multiple cellular pathways and molecular targets, contributing to its diverse biological activities.

Method of Analysis: Analysis of resveratrol typically involves techniques such as high-performance liquid chromatography (HPLC), mass spectrometry (MS), or nuclear magnetic resonance (NMR) spectroscopy to quantify and characterize its presence in plant extracts or dietary supplements.

Health Benefits:

- Antioxidant properties
- Anti-inflammatory effects
- Cardiovascular health support
- Potential cancer prevention
- Neuroprotective effects
- Anti-aging properties

Indication and Usage: Resveratrol is commonly used as a dietary supplement for its potential health benefits. It may be recommended for individuals seeking antioxidant support, cardiovascular health support, or potential anti-aging effects. Resveratrol is also found in various skincare products for its purported skin benefits.

Usual Constituents with Percentages: The usual constituents of resveratrol are trans-resveratrol and cis-resveratrol. Trans-resveratrol is the biologically active form and typically comprises the majority of resveratrol content in natural sources, ranging from 70% to 98%.

Mechanism of Action: Resveratrol exerts its effects through various mechanisms, including antioxidant activity, modulation of gene expression, inhibition of inflammation, regulation of cell signaling pathways (such as NF-kB and AMPK), and activation of sirtuins (SIRT1).

Dosage: Dosage recommendations for resveratrol supplements vary depending on the specific product and intended use. Typical doses range from 100 mg to 1000 mg per day, although higher doses may be used in certain therapeutic applications.

Contraindications:

- Allergy to resveratrol or related compounds
- Use caution in individuals taking blood-thinning medications, as resveratrol may have mild anticoagulant effects.

Precautions:

- Pregnant or nursing women, as well as individuals with underlying medical conditions, should consult a healthcare professional before using resveratrol supplements.
- Monitor for potential interactions with medications, particularly those metabolized by the liver or affecting blood clotting.

Adverse Reactions: Common adverse reactions to resveratrol supplements are rare but may include gastrointestinal symptoms such as nausea, diarrhea, or abdominal discomfort. Allergic reactions are possible in individuals with allergies to resveratrol or related compounds.

Research Summary: Research on resveratrol has explored its potential health benefits in various areas, including cardiovascular health, cancer prevention, neuroprotection, and anti-aging effects. While some studies have shown promising results, particularly in preclinical and animal studies, human clinical trials have yielded mixed findings. Further research is needed to elucidate the optimal dosage, long-term effects, and potential benefits for specific populations.

Pharmacokinetics: After oral ingestion, resveratrol is rapidly absorbed in the gastrointestinal tract and undergoes extensive metabolism in the liver. Its metabolites are then distributed to various tissues, where they exert their biological effects. The bioavailability of resveratrol is relatively low due to rapid metabolism and elimination.

Pharmacodynamics: Resveratrol exerts its effects through various mechanisms, including antioxidant activity, modulation of gene expression, inhibition of inflammation, regulation of cell signaling pathways, and activation of sirtuins. These mechanisms contribute to its diverse biological activities and potential health benefits.

Overdosage: Excessive intake of resveratrol supplements may lead to gastrointestinal symptoms such as nausea, diarrhea, or abdominal discomfort. It's important to adhere to recommended dosages and consult a healthcare professional if concerns arise.

International Standing: Resveratrol supplements are available in many countries and are commonly used for their potential health benefits. However, regulations regarding their sale, labeling, and quality may vary by country.

Indian Standing: In India, resveratrol supplements are also available and may be used for their potential health benefits. However, specific regulations and market availability may vary.

50)RICE BRAN ARABINOXYLAN COMPOUND

Introduction: Rice bran arabinoxylan compound (RBAC) is a natural polysaccharide derived from rice bran. It has gained attention for its potential health benefits, particularly in supporting immune function and overall wellness.

Synonym Name and Common Name: Synonym: RBAC Common Name: Rice Bran Arabinoxylan Compound

Pharmacognosy / Chemistry: Rice bran arabinoxylan compound is extracted from the outer layer of rice grains, known as rice bran. It is a complex polysaccharide composed of arabinose and xylose units.

Action and Pharmacology: RBAC has immunomodulatory properties, meaning it can regulate and support the immune system's function. It interacts with immune cells and cytokines, helping to modulate immune responses and promote overall immune health.

Method of Analysis: Analysis of RBAC typically involves techniques such as high-performance liquid chromatography (HPLC), gas chromatography (GC), or mass spectrometry (MS) to quantify and characterize the polysaccharide structure.

Health Benefits:

- Supports immune function
- Antioxidant properties
- Potential anti-inflammatory effects
- Supports gastrointestinal health
- May have cardiovascular benefits

Indication and Usage: RBAC is commonly used as a dietary supplement to support immune function and overall wellness. It may be recommended for individuals seeking immune support, particularly during times of increased susceptibility to illness or stress.

Usual Constituents with Percentages: The main constituents of RBAC are arabinose and xylose units, which make up the polysaccharide structure. The specific percentages of these constituents may vary depending on the extraction and purification process.

Mechanism of Action: RBAC interacts with immune cells and cytokines, modulating immune responses and promoting immune function. It may also exert antioxidant and anti-inflammatory effects, contributing to its overall health benefits.

Dosage: Dosage recommendations for RBAC supplements vary depending on the specific product and intended use. Typical doses range from 500 mg to 2000 mg per day, taken orally. It is advisable to follow the instructions provided by healthcare professionals or on the product label.

Contraindications:

- Allergy to rice or rice-derived products
- Use caution in individuals with autoimmune conditions, as RBAC may stimulate immune responses

Precautions:

- Pregnant or nursing women, as well as individuals with underlying medical conditions, should consult a healthcare professional before using RBAC supplements.
- Monitor for potential interactions with medications, particularly those affecting immune function.

Adverse Reactions: Common adverse reactions to RBAC supplements are rare but may include gastrointestinal symptoms such as bloating, gas, or diarrhea. Allergic reactions are possible in individuals with allergies to rice or rice-derived products.

Research Summary: Research on RBAC has focused on its immunomodulatory effects and potential health benefits. Some studies have suggested that RBAC supplementation may help support immune function, reduce inflammation, and promote overall wellness. However, further research is needed to confirm its efficacy and safety for long-term use.

Pharmacokinetics: The pharmacokinetics of RBAC have not been extensively studied. After oral ingestion, RBAC is likely broken down in the gastrointestinal tract, and its components are absorbed into the bloodstream. The metabolism and excretion of RBAC metabolites have not been well characterized.

Pharmacodynamics: RBAC interacts with immune cells and cytokines, modulating immune responses and promoting immune function. It may also exert antioxidant and anti-inflammatory effects, contributing to its overall health benefits.

Overdosage: There is limited information on the effects of overdosage with RBAC supplements. However, it is recommended to adhere to recommended dosages and consult a healthcare professional if concerns arise.

International Standing: RBAC supplements are available in some countries and may be used for immune support and overall wellness. However, regulations regarding their sale, labeling, and quality may vary by country.

Indian Standing: In India, RBAC supplements may also be available and used for immune support and overall wellness. However, specific regulations and market availability may vary

51) RUTIN FROM FRUIT PEELS

Introduction: Rutin is a flavonoid compound found in various plants, particularly in the peels of citrus fruits, buckwheat, and apple. It is known for its antioxidant properties and potential health benefits.

Synonym Name and Common Name: Synonym: Vitamin P Common Name: Rutin

Pharmacognosy / Chemistry: Rutin is a glycoside composed of the flavanol quercetin and the disaccharide rutinose. It is commonly found in the peels of fruits and some vegetables, where it acts as a natural pigment and antioxidant.

Action and Pharmacology: Rutin exerts antioxidant, anti-inflammatory, and vasoprotective effects. It scavenges free radicals, reduces oxidative stress, and helps protect blood vessels from damage. Rutin also has potential anti-cancer and neuroprotective properties.

Method of Analysis: Analysis of rutin typically involves techniques such as high-performance liquid chromatography (HPLC) or spectrophotometry to quantify and characterize its presence in plant extracts or dietary supplements.

Health Benefits:

- Antioxidant properties
- Anti-inflammatory effects
- Cardiovascular health support
- Potential anti-cancer properties
- Neuroprotective effects

Indication and Usage: Rutin is commonly used as a dietary supplement for its potential health benefits. It may be recommended for individuals seeking antioxidant support, cardiovascular health support, or potential anti-inflammatory effects.

Usual Constituents with Percentages: Rutin is typically found in the peels of citrus fruits at concentrations ranging from 0.5% to 2%. The specific percentages may vary depending on factors such as the fruit variety, ripeness, and extraction method.

Mechanism of Action: Rutin exerts its effects through multiple mechanisms, including scavenging free radicals, inhibiting inflammation, reducing oxidative stress, modulating cell signaling pathways, and protecting blood vessels from damage.

Dosage: Dosage recommendations for rutin supplements vary depending on the specific product and intended use. Typical doses range from 500 mg to 2000 mg per day, taken orally. It is advisable to follow the instructions provided by healthcare professionals or on the product label.

Contraindications:

- Allergy to rutin or related compounds
- Use caution in individuals taking blood-thinning medications, as rutin may have mild anticoagulant effects.

Precautions:

- Pregnant or nursing women, as well as individuals with underlying medical conditions, should consult a healthcare professional before using rutin supplements.
- Monitor for potential interactions with medications, particularly those affecting blood clotting or blood pressure.

Adverse Reactions: Common adverse reactions to rutin supplements are rare but may include gastrointestinal symptoms such as nausea, diarrhea, or abdominal discomfort. Allergic reactions are possible in individuals with allergies to rutin or related compounds.

Research Summary: Research on rutin has explored its potential health benefits, particularly in cardiovascular health, cancer prevention, and neuroprotection. Some studies have shown promising results, including antioxidant and anti-inflammatory effects, as well as potential benefits in reducing the risk of cardiovascular disease and certain types of cancer. However, further research is needed to confirm its efficacy and safety for long-term use.

Pharmacokinetics: After oral ingestion, rutin is absorbed in the gastrointestinal tract and metabolized in the liver. Its metabolites are then distributed to various tissues, where they exert their biological effects. The bioavailability of rutin is relatively low due to rapid metabolism and elimination.

Pharmacodynamics: Rutin exerts its effects through various mechanisms, including scavenging free radicals, inhibiting inflammation, reducing oxidative stress, modulating cell signaling pathways, and protecting blood vessels from damage. These mechanisms contribute to its diverse biological activities and potential health benefits.

Overdosage: Excessive intake of rutin supplements may lead to gastrointestinal symptoms such as nausea, diarrhea, or abdominal discomfort. It's important to adhere to recommended dosages and consult a healthcare professional if concerns arise.

Adverse Reactions: Common adverse reactions to edible legume seed protein isolates are rare but may include gastrointestinal symptoms such as bloating, gas, or diarrhea. Allergic reactions are possible in individuals with allergies to legumes or soybeans.

Research Summary: Research on edible legume seed protein isolates has focused on their nutritional properties, health benefits, and functional applications in food products. Studies have demonstrated their effectiveness as high-quality protein sources, supporting muscle growth, weight management, and overall health.

Pharmacokinetics: The pharmacokinetics of edible legume seed protein isolates have not been extensively studied. After ingestion, the proteins are broken down into amino acids during digestion and absorbed in the small intestine. These amino acids are then utilized by the body for various physiological functions.

Pharmacodynamics: The proteins in edible legume seed protein isolates provide essential amino acids necessary for protein synthesis and various physiological processes in the body. They support muscle growth, repair tissues, and contribute to overall health and wellness.

Overdosage: Consuming excessive amounts of protein isolates may lead to gastrointestinal discomfort, dehydration, and kidney strain. It's important to adhere to recommended serving sizes and total protein intake guidelines.

International Standing: Edible legume seed protein isolates are widely used in food products and supplements globally. Regulations regarding their production, labeling, and safety vary by country.

Indian Standing: In India, edible legume seed protein isolates are also commonly used in food products and supplements. The Indian market offers various options for consumers seeking plant-based protein sources.

53) STEROLS/STANOLS INCLUDING THEIR ESTERS

Introduction: Sterols and stanols are naturally occurring compounds found in plants and are structurally similar to cholesterol. They are known for their potential to lower cholesterol levels and promote cardiovascular health.

Synonym Name and Common Name: Synonym: Plant sterols, phytosterols Common Name: Sterols and stanols

Pharmacognosy / Chemistry: Sterols and stanols are plant-derived compounds found in various fruits, vegetables, nuts, seeds, and vegetable oils. They are structurally similar to cholesterol and are often extracted from plant sources for use in functional foods and dietary supplements.

Action and Pharmacology: Sterols and stanols act by blocking the absorption of cholesterol in the digestive tract. They compete with cholesterol for absorption sites in the intestines, leading to reduced cholesterol absorption and lower blood cholesterol levels.

Method of Analysis: Analysis of sterols and stanols typically involves techniques such as gas chromatography (GC) or high-performance liquid chromatography (HPLC) to quantify and characterize their presence in plant extracts or dietary supplements.

Health Benefits:

- Lowering LDL cholesterol levels
- Supporting cardiovascular health
- Potential anti-inflammatory effects
- Potential antioxidant properties
- Supporting overall health and wellness

Indication and Usage: Sterols and stanols are commonly used as dietary supplements or added to functional foods for their cholesterol-lowering effects. They may be recommended for individuals with elevated cholesterol levels or those at risk of cardiovascular disease.

Usual Constituents with Percentages: The usual constituents of sterols and stanols are various sterols and stanols found in plant sources, typically ranging from 0.1% to 2% in plant oils and extracts.

Mechanism of Action: Sterols and stanols reduce cholesterol absorption by competing with cholesterol for absorption sites in the intestines. By blocking cholesterol absorption, they help lower LDL cholesterol levels in the bloodstream, reducing the risk of cardiovascular disease.

Dosage: Dosage recommendations for sterols and stanols vary depending on the specific product and intended use. Typical doses range from 1.5 to 3 grams per day, taken orally, often divided into multiple doses with meals.

Contraindications:

- Known allergy to sterols or stanols
- Use caution in individuals with certain medical conditions, such as phytosterolemia, a rare genetic disorder characterized by high levels of plant sterols in the blood.

Precautions:

- Pregnant or nursing women, as well as individuals with underlying medical conditions, should consult a healthcare professional before using sterol or stanol supplements.
- Monitor for potential interactions with cholesterol-lowering medications.

Adverse Reactions: Common adverse reactions to sterol or stanol supplements are rare but may include gastrointestinal symptoms such as nausea, diarrhea, or abdominal discomfort. Allergic reactions are possible in individuals with allergies to plant sterols or stanols.

Research Summary: Research on sterols and stanols has primarily focused on their cholesterol-lowering effects and cardiovascular benefits. Numerous clinical studies have demonstrated their efficacy in reducing LDL cholesterol levels and lowering the risk of cardiovascular events, particularly in individuals with hypercholesterolemia.

Pharmacokinetics: After oral ingestion, sterols and stanols are poorly absorbed in the digestive tract and pass through the intestines unchanged. They exert their effects primarily within the gastrointestinal lumen, where they block cholesterol absorption.

Pharmacodynamics: Sterols and stanols reduce cholesterol absorption by competing with cholesterol for absorption sites in the intestines. By blocking cholesterol absorption, they help lower LDL cholesterol levels in the bloodstream, reducing the risk of cardiovascular disease.

Overdosage: Consuming excessive amounts of sterol or stanol supplements may lead to gastrointestinal discomfort but is unlikely to cause serious adverse effects. It's important to adhere to recommended dosages and consult a healthcare professional if concerns arise.

International Standing: Sterol and stanol supplements are widely used internationally and are commonly recommended for individuals with elevated cholesterol levels or those at risk of cardiovascular disease. Regulations regarding their sale, labeling, and quality may vary by country.

Indian Standing: In India, sterol and stanol supplements are also available and may be used for their cholesterol-lowering effects. However, specific regulations and market availability may vary.

54) THEAFLAVIN

Introduction: Theaflavins are a group of polyphenolic compounds found primarily in black tea. They are formed during the oxidation of catechins, which occurs during the fermentation process of tea leaves. Theaflavins contribute to the color, flavor, and health properties of black tea.

Synonym Name and Common Name: Synonym: Black tea polyphenols Common Name: Theaflavins

Pharmacognosy / Chemistry: Theaflavins are natural polyphenolic compounds with a characteristic yellow to reddish-brown color. They are formed through the oxidative dimerization of catechins during the fermentation process of tea leaves, particularly in black tea production.

Action and Pharmacology: Theaflavins exhibit antioxidant, anti-inflammatory, and potential cardioprotective properties. They scavenge free radicals, reduce oxidative stress, inhibit inflammation, and may help support cardiovascular health by improving lipid profiles and reducing the risk of atherosclerosis.

Method of Analysis: Analysis of theaflavins typically involves techniques such as high-performance liquid chromatography (HPLC) or mass spectrometry (MS) to quantify and characterize the individual theaflavin compounds present in tea extracts.

Health Benefits:

- Antioxidant properties
- Cardiovascular health support
- Potential anti-inflammatory effects
- Immune system support
- Potential anticancer properties

Indication and Usage: Theaflavins are commonly consumed as part of black tea, but they are also available in dietary supplements. They may be recommended for individuals seeking antioxidant support, cardiovascular health support, or other potential health benefits.

Usual Constituents with Percentages: The usual constituents of theaflavins in black tea are theaflavin, theaflavin-3-gallate, theaflavin-3'-gallate, and theaflavin-3,3'-digallate. Their percentages may vary depending on factors such as tea variety, processing methods, and brewing conditions.

Mechanism of Action: Theaflavins exert their effects through multiple mechanisms, including scavenging free radicals, reducing oxidative stress, inhibiting inflammation, modulating cell signaling pathways, and supporting cardiovascular health by improving lipid profiles and reducing the risk of atherosclerosis.

Dosage: Specific dosage recommendations for theaflavins as a dietary supplement are not well-established. However, consuming 2-3 cups of black tea per day is generally considered safe and provides a moderate intake of theaflavins.

Contraindications:

- Allergy to black tea or polyphenolic compounds
- Use caution in individuals with caffeine sensitivity or cardiovascular conditions, as black tea contains caffeine and may affect heart rate and blood pressure.

Precautions:

- Pregnant or nursing women should consult a healthcare professional before consuming high amounts of black tea or theaflavin supplements.

- Monitor for potential interactions with medications, particularly those affecting blood clotting or blood pressure.

Adverse Reactions: Common adverse reactions to black tea consumption are rare but may include gastrointestinal symptoms, caffeine-related side effects (such as jitteriness or insomnia), or allergic reactions in sensitive individuals.

Research Summary: Research on theaflavins has explored their antioxidant, anti-inflammatory, and cardiovascular health properties. Studies have suggested that theaflavins may help reduce oxidative stress, inflammation, and cardiovascular risk factors, although further research is needed to confirm their efficacy and safety.

Pharmacokinetics: The pharmacokinetics of theaflavins have not been extensively studied. After ingestion, they are absorbed in the gastrointestinal tract, metabolized in the liver, and excreted in urine. The bioavailability of theaflavins may vary depending on factors such as tea variety, processing methods, and individual metabolism.

Pharmacodynamics: Theaflavins exert antioxidant, anti-inflammatory, and potential cardioprotective effects by scavenging free radicals, reducing oxidative stress, inhibiting inflammation, and supporting cardiovascular health by improving lipid profiles and reducing the risk of atherosclerosis.

Overdosage: Consuming excessive amounts of theaflavins from black tea is unlikely to cause serious adverse effects but may lead to caffeine-related side effects such as jitteriness or insomnia. It's important to moderate intake and monitor for signs of caffeine sensitivity.

International Standing: Theaflavins are recognized internationally for their potential health benefits and are commonly consumed as part of black tea or dietary supplements. Regulations regarding their sale, labeling, and quality may vary by country.

Indian Standing: In India, black tea consumption is widespread, and theaflavins are recognized for their potential health benefits. Black tea is a popular beverage, and theaflavin supplements are also available in the market. However, specific regulations and market availability may vary.

55) THEOBROMINE

Introduction: Theobromine is a bitter alkaloid compound found in cocoa beans, tea leaves, and kola nuts. It belongs to the methylxanthine class of compounds and is structurally similar to caffeine. Theobromine is known for its stimulant effects and potential health benefits.

Synonym Name and Common Name: Synonym: Xantheose Common Name: Theobromine

Pharmacognosy / Chemistry: Theobromine is a natural alkaloid compound found primarily in the seeds of the cacao tree (Theobroma cacao). It contributes to the bitter taste of cocoa and chocolate products.

Action and Pharmacology: Theobromine acts as a mild central nervous system stimulant, similar to caffeine but with less potent effects. It also has diuretic properties and may have vasodilatory effects on blood vessels.

Method of Analysis: Analysis of theobromine typically involves techniques such as high-performance liquid chromatography (HPLC) or gas chromatography-mass spectrometry (GC-MS) to quantify and characterize its presence in cocoa products, tea leaves, or dietary supplements.

Health Benefits:

- Mild central nervous system stimulation
- Potential cardiovascular benefits
- Diuretic effects
- Antioxidant properties
- Potential cognitive enhancement

Indication and Usage: Theobromine is commonly consumed in cocoa and chocolate products, as well as in tea and some dietary supplements. It may be used for its stimulant effects, potential cardiovascular benefits, or as part of a weight loss regimen due to its diuretic properties.

Usual Constituents with Percentages: The usual constituents of theobromine in cocoa beans vary depending on factors such as cocoa variety, processing methods, and bean quality. Cocoa beans typically contain around 1-3% theobromine by weight.

Precautions:

- Garlic supplements may cause gastrointestinal upset in some individuals, especially when taken on an empty stomach.
- Garlic may potentiate the effects of blood-thinning medications, so close monitoring is necessary for individuals on such medications.
- Individuals with bleeding disorders should use garlic supplements with caution.

Adverse Reactions: Adverse reactions to garlic supplements are generally mild and rare but may include gastrointestinal discomfort, bad breath, and skin irritation in sensitive individuals.

Research Standing: Garlic has been extensively studied for its medicinal properties, and numerous clinical trials and scientific research support its traditional uses and therapeutic benefits. Ongoing research continues to explore its potential applications in various health conditions.

Pharmacokinetics: After ingestion, garlic compounds are absorbed in the gastrointestinal tract and metabolized primarily in the liver. Allicin, the primary active compound, undergoes rapid conversion to various metabolites, which contribute to its pharmacological effects.

Pharmacodynamics: Garlic exerts its pharmacological effects through multiple mechanisms, including modulation of antioxidant enzymes, inhibition of inflammatory pathways, and interaction with various molecular targets involved in lipid metabolism and immune function.

Overdosage: Excessive consumption of garlic supplements may lead to gastrointestinal disturbances, allergic reactions, and potentiation of the effects of certain medications. However, cases of overdose are rare due to the generally safe profile of garlic.

International Standing: Garlic enjoys widespread recognition and use internationally, both as a culinary ingredient and a medicinal herb. Its supplements are readily available in various forms across global markets.

Indian Standing: In India, garlic has been an integral part of traditional medicine systems like Ayurveda and Siddha for centuries, where it is used to treat a wide range of ailments. It holds cultural significance and is commonly used in Indian cuisine and folk remedies.

Research Summary: Research on garlic extract underscores its multifaceted pharmacological properties, including cardiovascular protection, immune modulation, and antimicrobial activity. Clinical studies have demonstrated its efficacy in managing conditions such as hypertension, hyperlipidemia, and respiratory infections. Further research is ongoing to elucidate its mechanisms of action and optimize its therapeutic use.

3) ALOE VERA - JUICE /CONCENTRATE / POWDER OF SAP /GEL

Introduction: Aloe vera is a succulent plant species of the genus Aloe, widely known for its therapeutic properties and extensive use in traditional medicine and cosmetic products. It originated from the Arabian Peninsula but is now cultivated worldwide in tropical and subtropical regions.

Synonym Name and Common Name: Synonym Name: Aloe barbadensis Mill. Common Name: Aloe vera, Indian Aloe, True Aloe

Pharmacognosy/Chemistry: Aloe vera contains over 75 potentially active constituents, including vitamins, minerals, enzymes, polysaccharides, phenolic compounds, and amino acids. Key chemical constituents include aloin, barbaloin, anthraquinones, acemannan, and various vitamins (A, C, E, B12) and minerals (calcium, magnesium, zinc).

Action and Pharmacology: Aloe vera exhibits diverse pharmacological actions, including anti-inflammatory, antioxidant, immunomodulatory, wound-healing, and antimicrobial effects. These properties contribute to its wide range of therapeutic benefits.

Method of Analysis: Various analytical techniques are employed to analyze the chemical composition of Aloe vera products, including high-performance liquid chromatography (HPLC), gas chromatography-mass spectrometry (GC-MS), spectrophotometry, and nuclear magnetic resonance (NMR) spectroscopy.

Health Benefits:

- Soothes skin irritations and promotes wound healing
- Moisturizes and nourishes the skin

- Supports digestive health and aids in gastrointestinal disorders
- Exhibits anti-inflammatory effects, helpful in conditions like arthritis and gastritis
- Boosts immune function
- Acts as an antioxidant, protecting against oxidative damage

Indication and Usage: Aloe vera is indicated for various conditions, including sunburn, minor burns, cuts, insect bites, eczema, psoriasis, constipation, indigestion, and oral hygiene. It is available in various forms such as juice, gel, concentrate, powder, creams, lotions, and dietary supplements.

Usual Constituents with Percentages: The composition of Aloe vera products can vary depending on the processing method and the part of the plant used. Typical percentages of major constituents may include:

- Polysaccharides: 0.5-1.5%
- Anthraquinones (aloin, barbaloin): 0.1-0.5%
- Vitamins and minerals: variable
- Enzymes (such as amylase, lipase): variable
- Amino acids: variable

Mechanism of Action: The polysaccharides and other bioactive compounds present in Aloe vera interact with various cellular pathways, including the cyclooxygenase and lipoxygenase pathways, leading to anti-inflammatory and wound-healing effects. Additionally, its antioxidant properties scavenge free radicals, protecting cells from oxidative damage.

Dosage: Dosage of Aloe vera products varies depending on the form and the intended use. Typical dosages for Aloe vera juice range from 1-8 ounces per day, while topical application of gel or cream can be done as needed for skin conditions.

Contraindications:

- Aloe vera products should be avoided by individuals allergic to plants of the Liliaceae family, such as onions and garlic.

- Pregnant and breastfeeding women should consult a healthcare professional before using Aloe vera products, especially orally, due to the potential risk of uterine contractions.

Precautions:

- Oral consumption of Aloe vera juice in large quantities may cause gastrointestinal discomfort, including diarrhea and abdominal cramps.
- Individuals with diabetes should monitor their blood sugar levels closely when consuming Aloe vera products orally, as it may lower blood glucose levels.
- Prolonged topical application may cause skin irritation or allergic reactions in sensitive individuals.

Adverse Reactions: Adverse reactions to Aloe vera products are generally rare but may include allergic reactions, skin irritation, gastrointestinal upset, and electrolyte imbalances.

Research Standing: Aloe vera has been extensively studied for its medicinal properties, and numerous clinical trials and scientific research support its traditional uses and therapeutic benefits. However, further research is ongoing to elucidate its mechanisms of action and optimize its clinical applications.

Pharmacokinetics: After oral ingestion, the bioactive compounds in Aloe vera are absorbed in the gastrointestinal tract and metabolized primarily in the liver. Topical application of Aloe vera gel leads to local absorption through the skin.

Pharmacodynamics: Aloe vera exerts its pharmacological effects through multiple mechanisms, including modulation of inflammatory mediators, enhancement of wound healing, scavenging of free radicals, and stimulation of immune responses.

Overdosage: Overconsumption of Aloe vera products, especially orally, may lead to gastrointestinal disturbances, electrolyte imbalances, and laxative effects. However, cases of overdose are rare due to the generally safe profile of Aloe vera when used appropriately.

International Standing: Aloe vera products enjoy widespread recognition and use internationally, both in traditional medicine and the cosmetic industry. They are available in various forms and are marketed extensively for their health and beauty benefits.

Indian Standing: In India, Aloe vera has been used in traditional Ayurvedic medicine for centuries, primarily for its wound-healing and skin-soothing properties. It is also cultivated extensively in India for commercial purposes, including pharmaceuticals, cosmetics, and dietary supplements.

Research Summary: Research on Aloe vera highlights its versatile pharmacological properties and therapeutic benefits, particularly in wound healing, skin care, and gastrointestinal health. Clinical studies continue to explore its efficacy and safety profile in various health conditions, driving ongoing interest and research in this natural rem

4)AMARANTHUS TRICOLOR

Introduction: Amaranthus tricolor, commonly known as Joseph's coat, is a leafy vegetable belonging to the Amaranthaceae family. It is native to Central and South America but is now cultivated in various parts of the world for its nutritious leaves, which are consumed as a vegetable.

Synonym Name and Common Name: Synonym Name: Amaranthus gangeticus Common Name: Joseph's coat, Edible amaranth, Chinese spinach

Pharmacognosy/Chemistry: Amaranthus tricolor leaves contain various phytochemicals, including flavonoids, phenolic compounds, saponins, and vitamins (A, C, K). They are also a rich source of minerals such as calcium, iron, potassium, and magnesium.

Action and Pharmacology: Amaranthus tricolor exhibits nutritional and medicinal properties, including antioxidant, anti-inflammatory, and hepatoprotective effects. Its high nutrient content contributes to its health-promoting benefits.

Method of Analysis: Analytical techniques such as high-performance liquid chromatography (HPLC), gas chromatography-mass spectrometry (GC-MS), and spectrophotometry are used to analyze the chemical composition of Amaranthus tricolor leaves.

Health Benefits:

- Rich source of vitamins and minerals, supporting overall health and well-being

- Antioxidant properties help protect cells from oxidative damage
- Anti-inflammatory effects may help alleviate inflammation-related conditions
- Supports liver health and detoxification processes
- Provides dietary fiber, promoting digestive health
- Helps regulate blood sugar levels and may benefit individuals with diabetes

Indication and Usage: Amaranthus tricolor leaves are commonly consumed as a leafy vegetable in various culinary dishes, including salads, stir-fries, soups, and curries. They are also used in traditional medicine for their health-promoting properties.

Usual Constituents with Percentages: The composition of Amaranthus tricolor leaves can vary depending on factors such as growing conditions and maturity. However, typical percentages of major constituents may include:

- Flavonoids: 0.5-2%
- Phenolic compounds: 0.3-1%
- Vitamins (A, C, K): variable
- Minerals (calcium, iron, potassium, magnesium): variable

Mechanism of Action: The phytochemicals present in Amaranthus tricolor leaves exert their effects through various mechanisms, including scavenging free radicals, inhibiting inflammatory pathways, and supporting detoxification processes, contributing to its health benefits.

Dosage: There is no specific dosage for consuming Amaranthus tricolor leaves as a dietary vegetable. Individuals can incorporate them into their meals according to personal taste preferences and nutritional needs.

Contraindications: There are no known contraindications for consuming Amaranthus tricolor leaves as part of a balanced diet. However, individuals with known allergies to plants in the Amaranthaceae family should exercise caution.

Precautions:

- Wash Amaranthus tricolor leaves thoroughly before consumption to remove any dirt or contaminants.
- Individuals with certain medical conditions, such as kidney stones or oxalate sensitivity, may need to moderate their intake of leafy greens, including Amaranthus tricolor.

Adverse Reactions: Adverse reactions to Amaranthus tricolor leaves are rare but may include allergic reactions in sensitive individuals. Excessive consumption may also cause gastrointestinal discomfort in some people.

Research Standing: While Amaranthus tricolor has a long history of culinary and medicinal use, scientific research on its health benefits is relatively limited compared to other plants. However, there is growing interest in its nutritional composition and potential therapeutic applications.

Pharmacokinetics: The pharmacokinetics of Amaranthus tricolor constituents have not been extensively studied. Upon ingestion, the nutrients and phytochemicals in the leaves are absorbed in the gastrointestinal tract and metabolized or utilized by the body.

Pharmacodynamics: Amaranthus tricolor exerts its pharmacological effects primarily through its nutrient and phytochemical content, which contribute to its antioxidant, anti-inflammatory, and hepatoprotective properties.

Overdosage: There are no specific reports of overdosage with Amaranthus tricolor leaves. However, excessive consumption may lead to potential adverse effects such as gastrointestinal discomfort or allergic reactions in sensitive individuals.

International Standing: Amaranthus tricolor is cultivated and consumed as a leafy vegetable in many countries around the world, contributing to its international standing as a nutritious food source.

Indian Standing: In India, Amaranthus tricolor is widely cultivated and consumed as a leafy vegetable known as "chaulai" or "cholai." It holds cultural significance and is a staple ingredient in various regional cuisines.

Research Summary: Research on Amaranthus tricolor focuses on its nutritional composition, antioxidant activity, and potential health benefits. While it is recognized as a valuable source of vitamins, minerals, and phytochemicals, further studies are needed to explore its therapeutic effects and mechanisms of action in various health conditions

5) ANETHUM GRAVEOLENS L. - SEEDS AND OIL

Introduction: Anethum graveolens L., commonly known as dill, is an annual herb belonging to the Apiaceae family. It's native to the Mediterranean region and Southern Russia but is now cultivated worldwide for its culinary and medicinal uses.

Synonym Name and Common Name: Synonym: Peucedanum graveolens Common Name: Dill

Pharmacognosy/Chemistry: Dill seeds and oil contain several bioactive compounds, including flavonoids, phenolic compounds, essential oils (chiefly carvone and limonene), and various vitamins and minerals. The distinctive aroma and flavor of dill are attributed to its essential oil content.

Action and Pharmacology: Dill exhibits various pharmacological actions, including antimicrobial, antioxidant, anti-inflammatory, anti-diabetic, and gastroprotective properties. These actions are primarily attributed to its bioactive constituents, particularly the essential oils.

Method of Analysis: Analytical methods for assessing the quality of dill seeds and oil include gas chromatography-mass spectrometry (GC-MS) for determining the composition of essential oils, high-performance liquid chromatography (HPLC) for quantifying specific compounds, and various spectroscopic techniques for assessing overall phytochemical composition.

Health Benefits: Dill is associated with several health benefits, including improved digestion, reduced flatulence, relief from menstrual cramps, and potential anti-cancer properties due to its antioxidant activity. It's also used traditionally as a galactagogue to promote lactation in breastfeeding mothers.

Indication and Usage: Dill is used in traditional medicine for various indications, including indigestion, dyspepsia, colic, flatulence, menstrual disorders, and as a mild sedative. It's commonly consumed as a culinary herb in salads, soups, stews, and pickles.

Usual Constituents with Percentages:

- Essential oils (carvone, limonene): 2-4%
- Flavonoids: Quercetin, kaempferol
- Phenolic compounds: Rosmarinic acid, caffeic acid
- Vitamins and minerals: Vitamin C, manganese, iron

Mechanism of Action: The bioactive compounds in dill exert their effects through various mechanisms, including antioxidant activity, modulation of enzyme activity, inhibition of inflammatory pathways, and interaction with neurotransmitter receptors.

Dosage: Dill can be consumed in various forms, including fresh or dried leaves, seeds, or as an essential oil. Typical doses range from 1 to 4 grams of dried herb, or 1 to 2 teaspoons of dill seeds per day. For essential oil, doses should be significantly lower and used according to manufacturer recommendations.

Contraindications: Dill is generally considered safe for most people when consumed in food amounts. However, individuals allergic to plants in the Apiaceae family (such as fennel, coriander, or celery) may experience allergic reactions to dill. Pregnant and breastfeeding women should consult healthcare providers before using dill supplements or essential oil.

Precautions: Excessive consumption of dill essential oil may cause irritation or sensitization, particularly when applied topically. It's essential to dilute essential oil properly and perform a patch test before widespread use.

Adverse Reactions: Adverse reactions to dill are rare but may include allergic reactions, gastrointestinal upset, or skin irritation (when applied topically). Discontinue use if any adverse reactions occur and consult a healthcare professional.

Research Standing: Research on the pharmacological properties of dill, particularly its essential oil, is ongoing. While many traditional uses have scientific backing, further clinical studies are needed to validate its efficacy and safety for specific medical conditions.

Pharmacokinetics and Pharmacodynamics: The pharmacokinetics of dill constituents vary depending on the route of administration. Oral consumption of dill seeds or herb results in absorption of its bioactive compounds in the gastrointestinal tract, followed by distribution and metabolism in the body. Pharmacodynamic effects include modulation of enzyme activity, antioxidant effects, and interaction with cellular receptors.

Overdosage: Excessive consumption of dill seeds or essential oil may lead to nausea, vomiting, diarrhea, or allergic reactions. In case of overdose, symptomatic treatment and supportive care are recommended.

International Standing: Dill is widely recognized and utilized in international cuisine and traditional medicine systems. Its safety and efficacy have been acknowledged by various regulatory agencies, but specific regulations regarding its use may vary between countries.

Indian Standing: In India, dill is known as "suwa" and is used extensively in culinary preparations, especially in pickles and curries. It's also employed in traditional Ayurvedic medicine for its digestive and carminative properties.

Research Summary: Research on Anethum graveolens L. seeds and oil indicates its potential therapeutic benefits in various health conditions, including digestive disorders, menstrual disorders, and microbial infections. However, further clinical trials are warranted to establish its efficacy, optimal dosage, and safety profile. Ongoing research focuses on elucidating the mechanisms of action of dill constituents and exploring its potential applications in modern medicine.

6)ASPARAGUS DENSIFLORUS – EXTRACT

Introduction: Asparagus densiflorus, commonly known as Asparagus fern or Sprenger's Asparagus, is a perennial plant native to South Africa. It belongs to the Asparagaceae family and is widely cultivated as an ornamental plant due to its attractive foliage.

Synonym Name and Common Name: Synonym: Asparagus aethiopicus Common Name: Asparagus Fern, Sprenger's Asparagus

Pharmacognosy/Chemistry: The pharmacognosy of Asparagus densiflorus involves a complex array of bioactive compounds present in its extract. These may include saponins, flavonoids, phenolic compounds, and other phytochemicals. The exact chemical composition may vary depending on factors such as plant variety and extraction method.

Action and Pharmacology: Asparagus densiflorus extract exhibits various pharmacological actions, including antioxidant, anti-inflammatory, diuretic, and potentially neuroprotective effects. These actions are attributed to its bioactive constituents and have been studied for their potential therapeutic applications.

Method of Analysis: Analytical methods for assessing the composition and quality of Asparagus densiflorus extract include chromatographic techniques such as high-performance liquid chromatography (HPLC) and gas chromatography-mass spectrometry (GC-MS). These methods help identify and quantify specific compounds present in the extract.

Health Benefits: Asparagus densiflorus extract is associated with several health benefits, including antioxidant properties that help protect cells from oxidative damage, anti-inflammatory effects that may reduce inflammation in the body, and potential diuretic properties that could aid in promoting urine production and kidney health.

Indication and Usage: Asparagus densiflorus extract is used in traditional medicine for various indications, including as a diuretic to promote urine flow, as a remedy for inflammatory conditions, and as a general tonic. It may also be used in skincare products for its antioxidant properties.

Usual Constituents with Percentages:

- Saponins: 0.5-2%
- Flavonoids: Quercetin, rutin
- Phenolic compounds
- Other phytochemicals

Mechanism of Action: The bioactive compounds present in Asparagus densiflorus extract exert their effects through various mechanisms, including scavenging free radicals, modulating inflammatory pathways, and potentially influencing renal function to promote diuresis.

Dosage: Dosage recommendations for Asparagus densiflorus extract may vary depending on the specific formulation and intended use. It's essential to follow the instructions provided by the manufacturer or healthcare provider regarding dosage and administration.

Contraindications: Individuals with known allergies to plants in the Asparagaceae family should avoid Asparagus densiflorus extract. Additionally, pregnant or breastfeeding women should consult healthcare providers before using the extract due to limited safety data in these populations.

Precautions: Asparagus densiflorus extract should be used with caution in individuals with renal impairment or other underlying medical conditions. It's essential to discuss any pre-existing health conditions with a healthcare provider before starting supplementation.

Adverse Reactions: Adverse reactions to Asparagus densiflorus extract are rare but may include allergic reactions, gastrointestinal upset, or skin irritation. Discontinue use if any adverse reactions occur and seek medical attention if symptoms persist or worsen.

Research Standing: Research on the pharmacological properties of Asparagus densiflorus extract is ongoing, with studies investigating its potential therapeutic applications, safety profile, and mechanisms of action. While preliminary evidence suggests various health benefits, further research, particularly clinical trials, is needed to confirm these findings.

Pharmacokinetics and Pharmacodynamics: The pharmacokinetics and pharmacodynamics of Asparagus densiflorus extract are not well-established and may vary depending on factors such as formulation, dosage, and individual differences in metabolism. Further research is needed to elucidate these aspects.

Overdosage: Information on the potential effects of overdosage with Asparagus densiflorus extract is limited. However, as with any supplement, it's essential to adhere to recommended dosage guidelines to avoid adverse effects.

International Standing: Asparagus densiflorus extract is not widely recognized as a medicinal plant internationally but is commonly cultivated and used as an ornamental plant in various regions around the world.

Indian Standing: In India, Asparagus densiflorus extract may be utilized in traditional Ayurvedic medicine or as an ornamental plant. Its use in traditional Indian medicine systems and its recognition may vary depending on regional practices.

Research Summary: Research on Asparagus densiflorus extract is still in its early stages, with limited clinical evidence supporting its therapeutic applications. While preclinical studies suggest potential antioxidant, anti-inflammatory, and diuretic effects, further research, particularly well-designed clinical trials, is needed to validate these findings and establish its safety and efficacy for specific health conditions.

7) BARLEY SEED POWDER

Introduction: Barley seed powder is derived from the barley plant, scientifically known as Hordeum vulgare. Barley is one of the oldest cultivated grains and is widely used in various culinary and medicinal applications due to its nutritional content and potential health benefits.

Synonym Name and Common Name: Synonym: Hordeum vulgare Common Name: Barley, Barley Grass

Pharmacognosy/Chemistry: Barley seed powder contains a rich array of bioactive compounds, including vitamins, minerals, antioxidants, dietary fiber, and phytochemicals such as phenolic acids and flavonoids. Its nutritional profile contributes to its therapeutic properties.

Action and Pharmacology: Barley seed powder exhibits various pharmacological actions, including antioxidant, anti-inflammatory, hypolipidemic, and potentially anti-cancer effects. These actions are attributed to its diverse array of bioactive constituents and have been studied for their potential therapeutic applications.

Method of Analysis: Analytical methods for assessing the composition and quality of barley seed powder include techniques such as high-performance liquid chromatography (HPLC) for quantifying specific bioactive compounds, spectroscopic methods for assessing overall phytochemical composition, and microbiological testing for quality control.

Health Benefits: Barley seed powder is associated with numerous health benefits, including improved digestion, cholesterol management, blood sugar control, weight management, and potential cancer prevention. Its high fiber content promotes satiety and supports gastrointestinal health, while antioxidants help protect cells from oxidative damage.

Indication and Usage: Barley seed powder is used in various forms, including dietary supplements, beverages, and food products. It's indicated for promoting overall health and well-being, supporting cardiovascular health, managing blood sugar levels, and aiding in weight management. It can be incorporated into smoothies, juices, or sprinkled over salads and cereals.

Usual Constituents with Percentages:

- Dietary fiber: 40-50%
- Vitamins: Vitamin B complex (especially B1, B2, B3, B6), Vitamin E
- Minerals: Calcium, magnesium, phosphorus, potassium
- Antioxidants: Phenolic acids (ferulic acid, caffeic acid), flavonoids (quercetin, kaempferol)

Mechanism of Action: The bioactive compounds in barley seed powder exert their effects through various mechanisms, including scavenging free radicals, modulating inflammatory pathways, improving lipid metabolism, enhancing insulin sensitivity, and promoting satiety.

Dosage: Dosage recommendations for barley seed powder may vary depending on the specific formulation and intended use. Typical doses range from 1 to 4 tablespoons (approximately 10-40 grams) per day, mixed with water, juice, or added to food.

Contraindications: Individuals with gluten intolerance or celiac disease should avoid barley seed powder due to its gluten content. Additionally, individuals with barley allergies should refrain from consuming barley products.

Precautions: Barley seed powder is generally considered safe for most individuals when consumed in moderation as part of a balanced diet. However, individuals with underlying health conditions or those taking medications should consult healthcare providers before starting supplementation.

Adverse Reactions: Adverse reactions to barley seed powder are rare but may include gastrointestinal discomfort, bloating, or allergic reactions in sensitive individuals. Discontinue use if any adverse reactions occur and seek medical attention if symptoms persist or worsen.

Research Standing: Research on the health benefits of barley seed powder is extensive and continues to expand. Numerous studies support its role in promoting cardiovascular health, managing blood sugar levels, and supporting gastrointestinal health. However, further research, particularly well-designed clinical trials, is needed to validate its efficacy for specific health conditions.

Pharmacokinetics and Pharmacodynamics: The pharmacokinetics and pharmacodynamics of barley seed powder are not well-established due to limited research in this area. Further studies are needed to elucidate the absorption, distribution, metabolism, and excretion of its bioactive compounds and their physiological effects in the body.

Overdosage: There is limited information available on the potential effects of overdosage with barley seed powder. However, excessive consumption may lead to gastrointestinal discomfort or nutrient imbalances. It's essential to adhere to recommended dosage guidelines to avoid adverse effects.

International Standing: Barley seed powder is recognized internationally for its nutritional value and potential health benefits. It's commonly used in dietary supplements, functional foods, and beverages marketed for promoting overall health and well-being.

Indian Standing: In India, barley seed powder has a long history of use in traditional medicine systems such as Ayurveda for its nutritional and therapeutic properties. It's also used in culinary preparations and beverages, particularly during festivals and religious ceremonies.

Research Summary: Research on barley seed powder underscores its potential as a functional food ingredient and dietary supplement for promoting health and preventing chronic diseases. While numerous studies support its various health benefits, further research, particularly clinical trials, is needed to establish its efficacy, optimal dosage, and safety profile for specific health conditions and populations.

8) BAUHINIA VARIEGATA– EXTRACT

Introduction: Bauhinia variegata, commonly known as the Orchid Tree or Camel's Foot Tree, is a species of flowering plant native to South Asia. It belongs to the Fabaceae family and is revered for its ornamental beauty and potential medicinal properties.

Synonym Name and Common Name: Synonym: Bauhinia alba, Bauhinia candida Common Name: Orchid Tree, Camel's Foot Tree

Pharmacognosy/Chemistry: Bauhinia variegata extract contains a diverse array of bioactive compounds, including flavonoids, phenolic acids, alkaloids, saponins, and polysaccharides. These phytochemicals contribute to its pharmacological properties and potential health benefits.

Action and Pharmacology: Bauhinia variegata extract exhibits various pharmacological actions, including antioxidant, anti-inflammatory, antimicrobial, antidiabetic, hepatoprotective, and anticancer effects. These actions are attributed to its bioactive constituents and have been investigated for their therapeutic potential.

Method of Analysis: Analytical methods for assessing the composition and quality of Bauhinia variegata extract include chromatographic techniques such as high-performance liquid chromatography (HPLC) for quantifying specific compounds, spectrophotometric assays for antioxidant activity, and microbiological testing for purity and safety.

Health Benefits: Bauhinia variegata extract is associated with numerous health benefits, including antioxidant properties that help protect cells from oxidative stress, anti-inflammatory effects that may alleviate inflammatory conditions, and potential antimicrobial activity against various pathogens. It's also studied for its role in managing diabetes, supporting liver health, and potentially inhibiting cancer cell growth.

Indication and Usage: Bauhinia variegata extract is used in traditional medicine for various indications, including as an anti-inflammatory, antimicrobial, antidiabetic, and hepatoprotective agent. It may be consumed as a dietary supplement or incorporated into topical formulations for skincare or wound healing purposes.

Usual Constituents with Percentages:

- Flavonoids: Quercetin, kaempferol, myricetin
- Phenolic acids: Gallic acid, ellagic acid
- Alkaloids
- Saponins
- Polysaccharides

Mechanism of Action: The bioactive compounds in Bauhinia variegata extract exert their effects through various mechanisms, including scavenging free radicals, modulating inflammatory pathways, inhibiting microbial growth, enhancing insulin sensitivity, protecting liver cells from damage, and potentially inducing apoptosis in cancer cells.

Dosage: Dosage recommendations for Bauhinia variegata extract may vary depending on the specific formulation and intended use. Typical doses range from 100 to 500 milligrams per day for dietary supplements, or as directed by a healthcare provider.

Contraindications: Individuals with known allergies to plants in the Fabaceae family should avoid Bauhinia variegata extract. Additionally, pregnant or breastfeeding women should consult healthcare providers before using the extract due to limited safety data in these populations.

Precautions: Bauhinia variegata extract should be used with caution in individuals with underlying health conditions or those taking medications, as it may interact with certain drugs. It's essential to consult a healthcare provider before starting supplementation, especially in these cases.

Adverse Reactions: Adverse reactions to Bauhinia variegata extract are rare but may include allergic reactions, gastrointestinal upset, or skin irritation. Discontinue use if any adverse reactions occur and seek medical attention if symptoms persist or worsen.

Research Standing: Research on the pharmacological properties of Bauhinia variegata extract is ongoing, with numerous studies supporting its various health benefits. While much of the evidence comes from preclinical studies and traditional use, further research, particularly well-designed clinical trials, is needed to validate its efficacy and safety for specific health conditions.

Pharmacokinetics and Pharmacodynamics: The pharmacokinetics and pharmacodynamics of Bauhinia variegata extract are not well-understood and may vary depending on factors such as formulation, dosage, and individual differences in metabolism. Further research is needed to elucidate these aspects and optimize its therapeutic use.

Overdosage: Information on the potential effects of overdosage with Bauhinia variegata extract is limited. However, excessive consumption may lead to gastrointestinal discomfort or other adverse effects. It's essential to adhere to recommended dosage guidelines to avoid such complications.

International Standing: Bauhinia variegata extract is recognized internationally for its potential medicinal properties and is commonly used in traditional medicine systems in regions where it is native. Its popularity as a dietary supplement or herbal remedy may vary between countries.

Indian Standing: In India, Bauhinia variegata extract has a long history of use in Ayurvedic and traditional medicine for its various therapeutic properties. It's also used in religious and cultural ceremonies and is regarded as a sacred plant in some regions.

Research Summary: Research on Bauhinia variegata extract highlights its potential as a valuable source of bioactive compounds with diverse pharmacological activities. While numerous studies support its traditional uses and various health benefits, further research, particularly clinical trials, is needed to establish its efficacy, safety, and optimal dosage for specific health conditions and populations.

9)BERBERIS VULGARIS

Introduction: Bauhinia variegata, commonly known as the Purple Orchid Tree or Camel's Foot Tree, is a flowering plant native to South Asia. It belongs to the Fabaceae family and is renowned for its vibrant flowers and potential medicinal properties.

Synonym Name and Common Name: Synonym: Bauhinia purpurea, Bauhinia vahlii Common Name: Purple Orchid Tree, Camel's Foot Tree

Pharmacognosy/Chemistry: Bauhinia variegata extract is rich in bioactive compounds, including flavonoids, alkaloids, phenolic acids, tannins, and terpenoids. These phytochemicals contribute to its pharmacological effects and therapeutic potential.

Action and Pharmacology: Bauhinia variegata extract exhibits diverse pharmacological actions, including antioxidant, anti-inflammatory, antimicrobial, antidiabetic, hepatoprotective, and anticancer effects. These actions are attributed to its bioactive constituents and have been investigated for their therapeutic applications.

Method of Analysis: Analytical methods for analyzing Bauhinia variegata extract include chromatographic techniques such as high-performance liquid chromatography (HPLC) for quantifying specific compounds, spectrophotometric assays for antioxidant activity, and microbiological testing for purity and safety.

Health Benefits: Bauhinia variegata extract is associated with various health benefits, including antioxidant properties that help protect against oxidative stress, anti-inflammatory effects that may alleviate inflammatory conditions, and potential antimicrobial activity against pathogens. It's also studied for its role in managing diabetes, supporting liver health, and potentially inhibiting cancer progression.

Indication and Usage: Bauhinia variegata extract is used in traditional medicine for a range of indications, including as an anti-inflammatory, antimicrobial, antidiabetic, and hepatoprotective agent. It may be consumed as a dietary supplement or incorporated into topical formulations for skincare or wound healing.

Usual Constituents with Percentages:

- Flavonoids: Quercetin, kaempferol, rutin
- Alkaloids: Bauhiniastatins, bauhiniastatins A, B, and C
- Phenolic acids: Gallic acid, ellagic acid
- Tannins
- Terpenoids

Mechanism of Action: The bioactive compounds in Bauhinia variegata extract exert their effects through multiple mechanisms, including scavenging free radicals, modulating inflammatory pathways, inhibiting microbial growth, enhancing insulin sensitivity, protecting liver cells, and potentially inducing apoptosis in cancer cells.

Dosage: Dosage recommendations for Bauhinia variegata extract may vary depending on the specific formulation and intended use. Typical doses range from 100 to 500 milligrams per day for dietary supplements, or as directed by a healthcare provider.

Contraindications: Individuals with known allergies to plants in the Fabaceae family should avoid Bauhinia variegata extract. Additionally, pregnant or breastfeeding women should consult healthcare providers before using the extract due to limited safety data in these populations.

Precautions: Bauhinia variegata extract should be used with caution in individuals with underlying health conditions or those taking medications, as it may interact with certain drugs. It's essential to consult a healthcare provider before starting supplementation, especially in these cases.

Adverse Reactions: Adverse reactions to Bauhinia variegata extract are rare but may include allergic reactions, gastrointestinal discomfort, or skin irritation. Discontinue use if any adverse reactions occur and seek medical attention if symptoms persist or worsen.

Research Standing: Research on the pharmacological properties of Bauhinia variegata extract is ongoing, with numerous studies supporting its various health benefits. While much of the evidence comes from preclinical studies and traditional use, further research, particularly well-designed clinical trials, is needed to validate its efficacy and safety for specific health conditions.

Pharmacokinetics and Pharmacodynamics: The pharmacokinetics and pharmacodynamics of Bauhinia variegata extract are not well-understood and may vary depending on factors such as formulation, dosage, and individual differences in metabolism. Further research is needed to elucidate these aspects and optimize its therapeutic use.

Overdosage: Information on the potential effects of overdosage with Bauhinia variegata extract is limited. However, excessive consumption may lead to gastrointestinal discomfort or other adverse effects. It's essential to adhere to recommended dosage guidelines to avoid such complications.

International Standing: Bauhinia variegata extract is recognized internationally for its potential medicinal properties and is commonly used in traditional medicine systems in regions where it is native. Its popularity as a dietary supplement or herbal remedy may vary between countries.

Indian Standing: In India, Bauhinia variegata extract has a long history of use in Ayurvedic and traditional medicine for its various therapeutic properties. It's also used in religious and cultural ceremonies and is regarded as a sacred plant in some regions.

Research Summary: Research on Bauhinia variegata extract highlights its potential as a valuable source of bioactive compounds with diverse pharmacological activities. While numerous studies support its traditional uses and various health benefits, further research, particularly clinical trials, is needed to establish its efficacy, safety, and optimal dosage for specific health conditions and populations.

10) BETA VULGARIS ROOT EXTRACT

Introduction: Beta vulgaris, commonly known as beetroot or simply beet, is a vegetable belonging to the Chenopodiaceae family. It is widely cultivated for its edible root and leafy greens and has been used historically for culinary and medicinal purposes.

Synonym Name and Common Name: Synonym: None Common Name: Beetroot, Beet

Pharmacognosy/Chemistry: Beta vulgaris root extract contains a variety of bioactive compounds, including betalains (betacyanins and betaxanthins), polyphenols (such as flavonoids and phenolic acids), vitamins (such as vitamin C), minerals (especially potassium and manganese), and dietary fiber. These constituents contribute to its pharmacological properties and health benefits.

Action and Pharmacology: Beta vulgaris root extract exhibits various pharmacological actions, including antioxidant, anti-inflammatory, cardioprotective, hepatoprotective, and potential anti-hypertensive effects. These actions are attributed to its bioactive compounds and have been studied for their therapeutic potential.

Method of Analysis: Analytical methods for analyzing Beta vulgaris root extract include chromatographic techniques such as high-performance liquid chromatography (HPLC) for quantifying specific compounds, spectrophotometric assays for antioxidant activity, and microbiological testing for quality control.

Health Benefits: Beta vulgaris root extract is associated with numerous health benefits, including improved cardiovascular health, reduced inflammation, enhanced liver function, and potential blood pressure-lowering effects. It's also studied for its potential role in exercise performance and recovery due to its nitrate content.

Indication and Usage: Beta vulgaris root extract is used in dietary supplements, functional foods, and beverages for various indications, including promoting heart health, reducing inflammation, supporting liver function, and potentially improving exercise performance. It can be consumed as a standalone supplement or incorporated into recipes and beverages.

Usual Constituents with Percentages:

- Betalains (betacyanins and betaxanthins): 0.5-2%

- Polyphenols: Flavonoids (quercetin, kaempferol), phenolic acids (caffeic acid, ferulic acid)
- Vitamins: Vitamin C
- Minerals: Potassium, manganese
- Dietary fiber

Mechanism of Action: The bioactive compounds in Beta vulgaris root extract exert their effects through various mechanisms, including scavenging free radicals, modulating inflammatory pathways, enhancing nitric oxide production, improving endothelial function, and potentially lowering blood pressure.

Dosage: Dosage recommendations for Beta vulgaris root extract may vary depending on the specific formulation and intended use. Typical doses range from 250 to 1000 milligrams per day for dietary supplements, or as directed by a healthcare provider.

Contraindications: Individuals with known allergies to Beta vulgaris or other plants in the Chenopodiaceae family should avoid Beta vulgaris root extract. Additionally, individuals with kidney stones or certain metabolic disorders should use caution when consuming beetroot due to its oxalate content.

Precautions: Beta vulgaris root extract may cause temporary discoloration of urine or feces, which is harmless but may be alarming to some individuals. It's essential to consume adequate fluids and monitor for any adverse reactions, particularly in susceptible individuals.

Adverse Reactions: Adverse reactions to Beta vulgaris root extract are rare but may include gastrointestinal upset, allergic reactions, or interactions with certain medications. Discontinue use if any adverse reactions occur and seek medical attention if symptoms persist or worsen.

Research Standing: Research on the pharmacological properties of Beta vulgaris root extract is extensive and continues to expand. Numerous studies support its various health benefits, particularly in cardiovascular health, exercise performance, and inflammation. Further research, including clinical trials, is needed to validate its efficacy and safety for specific health conditions and populations.

Pharmacokinetics and Pharmacodynamics: The pharmacokinetics and pharmacodynamics of Beta vulgaris root extract is not well-understood and may vary depending on factors such as formulation, dosage, and individual differences in metabolism. Further research is needed to elucidate these aspects and optimize its therapeutic use.

Overdosage: Information on the potential effects of overdosage with Beta vulgaris root extract is limited. However, excessive consumption may lead to gastrointestinal discomfort or other adverse effects. It's essential to adhere to recommended dosage guidelines to avoid such complications.

International Standing: Beta vulgaris root extract is recognized internationally for its potential medicinal properties and is commonly used in dietary supplements and functional foods marketed for promoting cardiovascular health, reducing inflammation, and enhancing exercise performance.

Indian Standing: In India, Beta vulgaris root extract is used in traditional medicine systems such as Ayurveda and is also consumed as a culinary ingredient. Its use in traditional remedies and its recognition may vary depending on regional practices and cultural preferences.

Research Summary: Research on Beta vulgaris root extract highlights its potential as a valuable source of bioactive compounds with diverse pharmacological activities. While numerous studies support its various health benefits, further research, particularly clinical trials, is needed to establish its efficacy, safety, and optimal dosage for specific health conditions and populations.

11)BETULA PLATYPHYLLA/B.UTILIS - BARK EXTRACT

Introduction: Betula platyphylla, also known as Betula utilis, is commonly referred to as the White Birch or Himalayan Birch. It belongs to the Betulaceae family and is native to regions of Asia and North America. The bark of this tree has been traditionally used for various medicinal purposes.

Synonym Name and Common Name: Synonym: Betula utilis Common Name: White Birch, Himalayan Birch

Pharmacognosy/Chemistry: Betula platyphylla bark extract contains a range of bioactive compounds, including betulin, betulinic acid, flavonoids, tannins, and essential oils. These constituents contribute to its pharmacological effects and medicinal properties.

Action and Pharmacology: Betula platyphylla bark extract exhibits various pharmacological actions, including anti-inflammatory, antimicrobial, antioxidant, analgesic, and potentially antitumor effects. These actions are attributed to its bioactive compounds and have been studied for their therapeutic potential.

Method of Analysis: Analytical methods for Betula platyphylla bark extract include chromatographic techniques such as high-performance liquid chromatography (HPLC) for quantifying specific compounds, spectrophotometric assays for antioxidant activity, and microbiological testing for purity and safety.

Health Benefits: Betula platyphylla bark extract is associated with numerous health benefits, including reducing inflammation, inhibiting microbial growth, scavenging free radicals, relieving pain, and potentially inhibiting tumor growth. It's also studied for its potential role in skincare and wound healing.

Indication and Usage: Betula platyphylla bark extract is used in traditional medicine for various indications, including as an anti-inflammatory, antimicrobial, antioxidant, and analgesic agent. It may be incorporated into topical formulations for skincare or used internally as a dietary supplement.

Usual Constituents with Percentages:

- Betulin: 10-20%
- Betulinic acid: 2-5%
- Flavonoids
- Tannins
- Essential oils

Mechanism of Action: The bioactive compounds in Betula platyphylla bark extract exert their effects through various mechanisms, including suppressing inflammatory pathways, inhibiting microbial growth, scavenging free radicals, modulating pain perception, and potentially inducing apoptosis in tumor cells.

Dosage: Dosage recommendations for Betula platyphylla bark extract may vary depending on the specific formulation and intended use. Typical doses range from 100 to 500 milligrams per day for dietary supplements, or as directed by a healthcare provider.

Contraindications: Individuals with known allergies to birch pollen or other plants in the Betulaceae family should avoid Betula platyphylla bark extract. Additionally, pregnant or breastfeeding women should consult healthcare providers before using the extract due to limited safety data in these populations.

Precautions: Betula platyphylla bark extract may cause skin irritation or allergic reactions in sensitive individuals when applied topically. It's essential to perform a patch test before using skincare products containing the extract and discontinue use if any adverse reactions occur.

Adverse Reactions: Adverse reactions to Betula platyphylla bark extract are rare but may include gastrointestinal upset, allergic reactions, or skin irritation. Discontinue use if any adverse reactions occur and seek medical attention if symptoms persist or worsen.

Research Standing: Research on the pharmacological properties of Betula platyphylla bark extract is ongoing, with numerous studies supporting its various health benefits. While much of the evidence comes from preclinical studies and traditional use, further research, including clinical trials, is needed to validate its efficacy and safety for specific health conditions and populations.

Pharmacokinetics and Pharmacodynamics: The pharmacokinetics and pharmacodynamics of Betula platyphylla bark extract are not well-understood and may vary depending on factors such as formulation, dosage, and individual differences in metabolism. Further research is needed to elucidate these aspects and optimize its therapeutic use.

Overdosage: Information on the potential effects of overdosage with Betula platyphylla bark extract is limited. However, excessive consumption may lead to gastrointestinal discomfort or other adverse effects. It's essential to adhere to recommended dosage guidelines to avoid such complications.

International Standing: Betula platyphylla bark extract is recognized internationally for its potential medicinal properties and is commonly used in dietary supplements and skincare products marketed for promoting anti-inflammatory, antimicrobial, and antioxidant effects.

Indian Standing: In India, Betula platyphylla bark extract is used in traditional medicine systems such as Ayurveda and is also consumed as a dietary supplement. Its use in traditional remedies and its recognition may vary depending on regional practices and cultural preferences.

Research Summary: Research on Betula platyphylla bark extract highlights its potential as a valuable source of bioactive compounds with diverse pharmacological activities. While numerous studies support its various health benefits, further research, particularly clinical trials, is needed to establish its efficacy, safety, and optimal dosage for specific health conditions and populations.

12) BIOTA ORIENTALIS - SEED POWDER

Introduction: Biota orientalis, commonly known as the Oriental Arborvitae, is a species of coniferous tree native to East Asia. The seeds of Biota orientalis have been used traditionally for various medicinal purposes and are valued for their potential health benefits.

Synonym Name and Common Name: Synonym: Platycladusorientalis Common Name: Oriental Arborvitae, Chinese Thuja

Pharmacognosy/Chemistry: Biota orientalis seed powder contains a variety of bioactive compounds, including flavonoids, terpenoids, polysaccharides, and lignans. These constituents contribute to its pharmacological effects and medicinal properties.

Action and Pharmacology: Biota orientalis seed powder exhibits various pharmacological actions, including antioxidant, anti-inflammatory, antimicrobial, hepatoprotective, and potentially anticancer effects. These actions are attributed to its bioactive compounds and have been studied for their therapeutic potential.

Method of Analysis: Analytical methods for analyzing Biota orientalis seed powder include chromatographic techniques such as high-performance liquid chromatography (HPLC) for quantifying specific compounds, spectrophotometric assays for antioxidant activity, and microbiological testing for purity and safety.

Health Benefits: Biota orientalis seed powder is associated with numerous health benefits, including supporting liver health, reducing inflammation, enhancing immune function, and potentially inhibiting tumor growth. It's also studied for its potential role in managing diabetes and promoting cardiovascular health.

Indication and Usage: Biota orientalis seed powder is used in traditional medicine for various indications, including liver disorders, inflammatory

officinalis. It is rich in gamma-linolenic acid (GLA), an omega-6 fatty acid, and contains other beneficial compounds such as linoleic acid, oleic acid, and palmitic acid.

Action and Pharmacology: Borage oil is known for its anti-inflammatory, antioxidant, and moisturizing properties. It helps to maintain healthy skin, reduce inflammation, and alleviate symptoms of various inflammatory conditions.

Method of Analysis: Borage oil can be analyzed using various techniques such as gas chromatography (GC), high-performance liquid chromatography (HPLC), and mass spectrometry (MS) to identify and quantify its fatty acid composition and other constituents.

Health Benefits:

- Supports skin health: Borage oil is often used in skincare products due to its moisturizing and anti-inflammatory properties, helping to soothe and hydrate the skin.
- Anti-inflammatory effects: It may help reduce inflammation associated with conditions like rheumatoid arthritis and atopic dermatitis.
- Hormonal balance: The GLA in borage oil may help regulate hormonal imbalances and alleviate symptoms of premenstrual syndrome (PMS) and menopause.
- Heart health: Some studies suggest that borage oil may have beneficial effects on cardiovascular health, including lowering blood pressure and reducing cholesterol levels.

Indication and Usage: Borage oil is commonly used as a dietary supplement and in topical formulations for skincare. It can be taken orally in the form of capsules or added to foods and beverages. Topical preparations containing borage oil are applied directly to the skin.

Usual Constituents with Percentages:

- Gamma-linolenic acid (GLA): 20-27%
- Linoleic acid: 35-38%
- Oleic acid: 16-20%

- Palmitic acid: 10-12%
- Other fatty acids and minor constituents

Mechanism of Action: The GLA in borage oil is converted in the body into prostaglandins, which are hormone-like compounds involved in regulating inflammation and other physiological processes. It also helps maintain the integrity of cell membranes and may modulate immune function.

Dosage: The dosage of borage oil supplements can vary depending on the specific product and individual needs. It is typically recommended to follow the manufacturer's instructions or consult with a healthcare professional for personalized guidance.

Contraindications:

- Pregnancy and breastfeeding: Borage oil should be avoided during pregnancy and lactation due to potential risks of premature labor and other complications.
- Bleeding disorders: It may increase the risk of bleeding in individuals with bleeding disorders or those taking anticoagulant medications.
- Allergy: Individuals with a known allergy to plants in the Boraginaceae family, such as borage, should avoid borage oil.

Precautions:

Interactions: Borage oil may interact with certain medications, including blood thinners, anti-inflammatory drugs, and hormone therapy. It is important to consult with a healthcare provider before taking borage oil supplements, especially if you are taking other medications.

Adverse Reactions:

- Side effects of borage oil supplements are generally mild and uncommon but may include gastrointestinal upset, nausea, and headache.
- Rarely, high doses of borage oil may cause liver toxicity or exacerbate existing liver conditions.

Research Standing: There is ongoing research into the potential health benefits and safety of borage oil, particularly in the areas of skin health, inflammation, and hormonal balance. While some studies have shown promising results, more research is needed to fully understand its effects and mechanisms of action.

Pharmacokinetics: After ingestion, the fatty acids in borage oil are absorbed in the small intestine and transported throughout the body via the bloodstream. GLA is then metabolized in the body to form active compounds such as prostaglandins.

Pharmacodynamics: Borage oil exerts its effects primarily through its fatty acid constituents, particularly GLA, which modulates inflammation, immune function, and other physiological processes.

Overdosage: There is limited information on the effects of overdose with borage oil supplements. However, excessive intake may increase the risk of adverse reactions such as gastrointestinal symptoms and liver toxicity.

International Standing: Borage oil is widely available as a dietary supplement and skincare ingredient in many countries. Regulations regarding its sale and labeling vary by jurisdiction.

Indian Standing: Borage oil is not traditionally used in Indian medicine systems like Ayurveda or Siddha. However, it may be available in the Indian market as a dietary supplement or skincare product.

Research Summary of Borago officinalis - Oil: Research on borage oil has explored its potential benefits for skin health, inflammatory conditions, hormonal balance, and cardiovascular health. While some studies have shown promising results, more research is needed to confirm its efficacy and safety, particularly regarding long-term use and potential interactions with medications.

14) CAPSICUM ANNUM

Introduction: Capsicum annuum, commonly known as chili pepper or bell pepper, is a species of the genus Capsicum native to the Americas. It is widely cultivated for its fruit, which is used as a vegetable in various cuisines around the world. Beyond its culinary applications, Capsicum annuum has been valued for its medicinal properties for centuries.

Synonym Name and Common Name: Synonym: Capsicum frutescens

Common Name: Chili pepper, bell pepper, red pepper

Pharmacognosy/Chemistry: Capsicum annuum contains various bioactive compounds, including capsaicinoids such as capsaicin, dihydrocapsaicin, and others. These compounds are responsible for the pungency and medicinal properties of chili peppers.

Action and Pharmacology: Capsaicin, the primary active component of Capsicum annuum, exhibits analgesic, anti-inflammatory, and antioxidant properties. It acts by desensitizing nociceptive neurons, leading to pain relief, and also modulates inflammatory pathways.

Method of Analysis: Analytical methods for Capsicum annuum often involve chromatographic techniques such as high-performance liquid chromatography (HPLC) for quantification of capsaicinoids.

Health Benefits: Capsicum annuum has been associated with various health benefits, including pain relief, improved digestion, cardiovascular health, and weight management.

Indication and Usage: It is used in traditional medicine for the treatment of pain, arthritis, digestive disorders, and as a topical remedy for various ailments.

Usual Constituents with Percentages: Capsicum annuum typically contains capsaicinoids in varying concentrations, with capsaicin being the predominant compound. Percentages can vary depending on factors such as cultivar and growing conditions.

Mechanism of Action: Capsaicin acts primarily by binding to and activating the transient receptor potential vanilloid 1 (TRPV1), leading to depolarization of nociceptive neurons and subsequent desensitization.

Dosage: Dosage varies depending on the specific formulation and intended use. Topical preparations containing capsaicin are typically applied as directed, while oral supplements may have recommended dosage guidelines.

Contraindications: Capsicum annuum products should be used with caution or avoided in individuals with known allergies or sensitivities to chili peppers. Topical application may cause skin irritation in some individuals.

Precautions: Topical preparations should be kept away from mucous membranes, eyes, and broken skin to avoid irritation. Oral consumption in large amounts may cause gastrointestinal discomfort.

Adverse Reactions: Common adverse reactions to Capsicum annuum include skin irritation, burning sensation, and gastrointestinal discomfort. Rarely, severe allergic reactions may occur.

Research Standing: Research on the medicinal properties of Capsicum annuum, particularly its capsaicin content, is ongoing. There is growing interest in its potential therapeutic applications in pain management and other health conditions.

Pharmacokinetics: After topical application, capsaicin is absorbed through the skin and metabolized primarily in the liver. The exact pharmacokinetic profile may vary depending on the formulation and route of administration.

Pharmacodynamics: Capsaicin exerts its pharmacodynamic effects primarily by interacting with TRPV1 receptors on nociceptive neurons, leading to pain relief and modulation of inflammatory pathways.

Overdosage: Overconsumption of Capsicum annuum may lead to symptoms such as severe gastrointestinal irritation, nausea, vomiting, and diarrhea. In severe cases, it can cause systemic toxicity requiring medical attention.

International Standing: Capsicum annuum and its derivatives are widely used in various forms across different cultures and cuisines worldwide. It is recognized for both its culinary and medicinal properties.

Indian Standing: In India, Capsicum annuum is used extensively in cooking, especially in spicy dishes. It also finds applications in traditional medicine for its purported health benefits.

Research Summary: Research on Capsicum annuum and its active component capsaicin has shown promising results in pain management, inflammation, and other health conditions. Ongoing studies continue to explore its therapeutic potential and mechanisms of action, contributing to a growing body of scientific literature on this versatile plant

15) CARICUS PAPAYA - LEAF EXTRACT

Introduction: Carica papaya, commonly known as papaya, is a tropical fruit tree native to the American tropics, but it is now cultivated in many tropical and subtropical regions worldwide. Apart from its delicious fruit, various parts of the papaya tree, including the leaves, have been used traditionally for their medicinal properties.

Synonym Name and Common Name: Synonym: Papaw, pawpaw Common Name: Papaya

Pharmacognosy/Chemistry: Carica papaya leaf extract contains a range of bioactive compounds, including papain, chymopapain, flavonoids, alkaloids, and phenolic compounds. These constituents contribute to its pharmacological activities.

Action and Pharmacology: Carica papaya leaf extract has demonstrated anti-inflammatory, antioxidant, and immunomodulatory effects. Papain, one of its key enzymes, is known for its proteolytic properties and has been studied for its potential therapeutic applications.

Method of Analysis: Analytical methods for Carica papaya leaf extract may involve chromatographic techniques such as high-performance liquid chromatography (HPLC) for quantification of specific compounds or spectrophotometric methods for total phenolic content.

Health Benefits: Carica papaya leaf extract is purported to have various health benefits, including promoting digestion, supporting immune function, and exhibiting potential anticancer properties. It is also used traditionally for its wound-healing and anti-inflammatory effects.

Indication and Usage: It is used in traditional medicine for conditions such as indigestion, constipation, skin wounds, and inflammatory conditions. Recent research has also investigated its potential as an adjunctive therapy in certain cancers.

Usual Constituents with Percentages: The composition of Carica papaya leaf extract can vary, but it often contains papain as a major constituent, along with flavonoids and other phytochemicals. Percentages of these compounds may vary depending on factors such as extraction method and plant source.

Mechanism of Action: Papain, the primary active enzyme in Carica papaya leaf extract, functions as a protease, breaking down proteins into smaller peptides and amino acids. This action is thought to contribute to its digestive and anti-inflammatory effects.

Dosage: Dosage recommendations for Carica papaya leaf extract may vary depending on the specific product and intended use. It is important to follow the instructions provided by manufacturers or healthcare professionals.

Contraindications: Individuals with known allergies to papaya or latex should avoid Carica papaya leaf extract. Pregnant or breastfeeding women should consult healthcare providers before use.

Precautions: Although generally considered safe when consumed in moderate amounts as a food or supplement, Carica papaya leaf extract may cause allergic reactions or gastrointestinal discomfort in sensitive individuals.

Adverse Reactions: Common adverse reactions to Carica papaya leaf extract may include gastrointestinal upset, allergic reactions, or skin irritation. Rarely, severe allergic reactions may occur in susceptible individuals.

Research Standing: Research on Carica papaya leaf extract has shown promising results in various areas, including its potential as a digestive aid, wound healer, and immune modulator. However, further clinical studies are needed to fully understand its efficacy and safety profile.

Pharmacokinetics: The pharmacokinetics of Carica papaya leaf extract, particularly its bioavailability and metabolism, have not been extensively studied. Further research is needed to elucidate its absorption, distribution, metabolism, and excretion pathways in humans.

Pharmacodynamics: Carica papaya leaf extract exerts its pharmacodynamic effects through its various bioactive constituents, including papain, flavonoids, and phenolic compounds. These compounds contribute to its diverse range of physiological effects, such as anti-inflammatory and antioxidant properties.

Overdosage: While there is limited information on the potential consequences of overdosing on Carica papaya leaf extract, excessive consumption may lead to gastrointestinal discomfort or allergic reactions. It is important to adhere to recommended dosage guidelines.

International Standing: Carica papaya leaf extract is recognized internationally for its medicinal properties and is used in various traditional medicine systems. It is also utilized in the food and cosmetic industries for its enzymatic properties and skin benefits.

Indian Standing: In India, Carica papaya leaf extract has a long history of use in traditional Ayurvedic medicine for its digestive, wound-healing, and anti-inflammatory properties. It is also consumed as a food and utilized in cosmetic formulations.

Research Summary: Research on Carica papaya leaf extract has demonstrated its potential therapeutic benefits in promoting digestion, wound healing, immune modulation, and anti-inflammatory effects. While preliminary studies are promising, further research, particularly clinical trials, is needed to validate its efficacy and safety for various medical conditions

16)CAULOPHYLLUMTHALICTROIDES - ROOT EXTRACT

Introduction: Caulophyllumthalictroides, commonly known as blue cohosh, is a perennial herb native to eastern North America. It has a long history of use in traditional medicine, particularly among indigenous peoples, for various women's health issues and childbirth-related concerns.

Synonym Name and Common Name: Synonym: Papoose root, squaw root Common Name: Blue cohosh

Pharmacognosy/Chemistry: Caulophyllumthalictroides root extract contains alkaloids, flavonoids, saponins, and other phytochemicals. The most studied bioactive compounds include caulophylline, anagyrine, and methylcysteine sulfoxide.

Action and Pharmacology: Blue cohosh is believed to have uterine stimulant and vasodilatory effects due to its alkaloid content. It has been traditionally used to induce labor, regulate menstrual cycles, and ease menstrual cramps.

Method of Analysis: Analytical methods for Caulophyllumthalictroides root extract may involve chromatographic techniques such as high-performance liquid chromatography (HPLC) for quantification of specific alkaloids or spectrophotometric methods for total flavonoid content.

Health Benefits: Blue cohosh is traditionally used to support women's reproductive health, including inducing labor, easing menstrual cramps, and regulating menstrual cycles. It has also been used for its potential anti-inflammatory and antispasmodic properties.

Indication and Usage: It is primarily used in traditional medicine to facilitate childbirth, regulate menstruation, and alleviate menstrual cramps. However, its use should be supervised by qualified healthcare professionals due to potential toxicity and safety concerns.

Usual Constituents with Percentages: The composition of Caulophyllumthalictroides root extract can vary, but it often contains alkaloids such as caulophylline, anagyrine, and others. Percentages of these compounds may vary depending on factors such as plant source and extraction method.

Mechanism of Action: The alkaloids present in blue cohosh are believed to exert their effects by stimulating uterine contractions and promoting blood flow to the pelvic area. However, the exact mechanism of action is not fully understood and may involve multiple pathways.

Dosage: Dosage recommendations for Caulophyllumthalictroides root extract should be determined by healthcare professionals based on individual factors such as age, health status, and the specific indication. It is important to follow recommended guidelines to avoid potential toxicity.

Contraindications: Blue cohosh is contraindicated during pregnancy, as it may cause uterine contractions and increase the risk of miscarriage. It should also be avoided in individuals with a history of cardiovascular disease, hypertension, or liver disorders.

Precautions: Blue cohosh should be used with caution and under the guidance of qualified healthcare professionals. It may interact with certain medications and supplements, and its safety in long-term use has not been well established.

Adverse Reactions: Common adverse reactions to Caulophyllumthalictroides root extract may include gastrointestinal upset, headache, dizziness, and allergic reactions. In high doses or prolonged use, it may cause more serious adverse effects such as cardiovascular toxicity.

Research Standing: Research on blue cohosh is limited, and while it has been traditionally used for women's health issues, its efficacy and safety profile remain controversial. Further clinical studies are needed to evaluate its potential benefits and risks, particularly in pregnancy and childbirth.

Pharmacokinetics: The pharmacokinetics of Caulophyllumthalictroides root extract have not been extensively studied. Limited data suggest that

flavor to dishes and beverages.

- In traditional medicine, cinnamon is used to treat various ailments, including digestive disorders, respiratory infections, and menstrual cramps.

Usual Constituents with Percentages:

- Cinnamaldehyde (60-80%)
- Eugenol
- Cinnamyl acetate
- Coumarin (found in trace amounts)

Mechanism of Action:

- Cinnamaldehyde and eugenol have been shown to inhibit inflammatory pathways and reduce the production of pro-inflammatory cytokines, thereby exerting anti-inflammatory effects.
- Cinnamon may also enhance insulin sensitivity and improve glucose metabolism, helping to lower blood sugar levels in individuals with diabetes.

Dosage:

- There is no standard dosage for cinnamon, as it depends on the form of the supplement and the intended use.
- Typical doses range from 1 to 6 grams of cinnamon powder per day for various health benefits.

Contraindications:

Cinnamon contains coumarin, which in high doses may be hepatotoxic and carcinogenic. Therefore, individuals with liver disease or at risk of liver damage should avoid excessive consumption of cinnamon.

Precautions:

- Pregnant and breastfeeding women should consume cinnamon in moderation, as large amounts may have uterotonic effects and potentially cause miscarriage.
- Individuals taking blood-thinning medications should use caution when consuming cinnamon, as it may enhance the effects of these drugs and increase the risk of bleeding.

Adverse Reactions:

Adverse reactions to cinnamon are rare but may include allergic reactions, gastrointestinal discomfort, or irritation of the oral mucosa in sensitive individuals.

Research Standing:

Research on the health benefits of cinnamon is ongoing, with numerous studies supporting its use in managing diabetes, improving lipid profiles, and reducing inflammation. However, more research is needed to confirm its efficacy and safety for various health conditions.

Pharmacokinetics and Pharmacodynamics:

- The pharmacokinetics of cinnamon bioactive compounds vary, with cinnamaldehyde and eugenol being absorbed in the gastrointestinal tract and metabolized in the liver.
- Cinnamon may exert its pharmacodynamic effects by modulating insulin signaling pathways, inhibiting inflammatory mediators, and scavenging free radicals.

Overdosage:

- Excessive consumption of cinnamon may lead to adverse effects such as liver damage (due to coumarin content), gastrointestinal irritation, or allergic reactions.
- There are no specific antidotes for cinnamon overdose, and treatment is supportive and symptomatic.

International Standing:

Cinnamon is widely recognized and utilized as a culinary spice and herbal remedy across cultures worldwide, with a rich history of use in traditional medicine and cuisine.

Indian Standing:

In India, cinnamon has been used for centuries in Ayurvedic medicine for its warming properties and therapeutic benefits, particularly for digestive disorders and respiratory ailments.

Research Summary:

- Research on Cinnamomum verum continues to elucidate its pharmacological effects and potential health benefits, particularly in the areas of diabetes management, inflammation, and antimicrobial activity. Further clinical studies are warranted to validate its traditional uses and explore its therapeutic potential in modern medicine.
- This overview provides a comprehensive understanding of Cinnamomum verum, highlighting its pharmacognosy, pharmacology, health benefits, usage, and precautions.

22) CITRUS AURANTIUM

Introduction: Citrus aurantium, commonly known as bitter orange, is a citrus tree native to Southeast Asia but cultivated in various parts of the world. It belongs to the Rutaceae family and is characterized by its bitter taste and fragrant flowers.

Synonym Name and Common Name: Synonym Name: Citrus × aurantium Common Name: Bitter orange, Seville orange, Sour orange

Pharmacognosy/Chemistry: The pharmacognostic profile of Citrus aurantium includes the examination of its morphological, microscopic, and chemical characteristics. It contains various bioactive compounds such as flavonoids, alkaloids (such as synephrine), essential oils (limonene, myrcene), and phenolic compounds.

Action and Pharmacology: Citrus aurantium is known for its stimulant properties, attributed mainly to synephrine, which acts as a sympathomimetic agent. It stimulates the adrenergic receptors, leading to increased heart rate and metabolic rate, thus promoting thermogenesis and potentially aiding in weight loss.

Method of Analysis: Analytical methods such as high-performance liquid chromatography (HPLC) are commonly employed to quantify the active constituents, particularly synephrine, in Citrus aurantium extracts.

Health Benefits:

- Weight management: Citrus aurantium is often used in dietary supplements for its potential to support weight loss and fat metabolism.
- Digestive health: Bitter orange extract may aid in digestion and relieve gastrointestinal discomfort.
- Antioxidant properties: The flavonoids and phenolic compounds present in bitter orange exhibit antioxidant activity, which may help protect cells from oxidative damage.

Indication and Usage:

- Used as a dietary supplement for weight management.
- Employed in traditional medicine for indigestion and stomach ailments.
- Included in cosmetic formulations for its fragrance and potential skin benefits.

Usual Constituents with Percentages:

- Synephrine: Typically found in concentrations ranging from 1% to 6% in dried bitter orange peel.
- Essential oils (limonene, myrcene): Varying percentages depending on the extraction method and plant source.
- Flavonoids: Present in bitter orange extracts, with concentrations depending on the preparation method.

Mechanism of Action: The primary mechanism of action of Citrus aurantium is attributed to synephrine, which acts as a sympathomimetic agent, stimulating adrenergic receptors and increasing metabolic rate and energy expenditure.

Dosage: Dosage recommendations for Citrus aurantium supplements vary depending on the formulation and intended use. It's essential to follow product-specific instructions and consult with a healthcare professional for appropriate dosing guidance.

Contraindications:

- Individuals with cardiovascular conditions or hypertension should avoid bitter orange supplements due to its stimulant effects.
- Pregnant or nursing women should refrain from using bitter orange products due to potential adverse effects.

Precautions:

- Bitter orange supplements may interact with certain medications, including those for cardiovascular conditions and psychiatric disorders.
- It's advisable to discontinue use and consult a healthcare provider if adverse reactions occur.

Adverse Reactions:

- Adverse reactions to bitter orange supplements may include increased heart rate, palpitations, anxiety, and gastrointestinal discomfort.
- Allergic reactions are possible in susceptible individuals.

Research Standing: Research on the efficacy and safety of Citrus aurantium for weight management and other health benefits is ongoing. While some studies suggest potential benefits, further research is needed to establish its efficacy and safety conclusively.

Pharmacokinetics and Pharmacodynamics: The pharmacokinetics of Citrus aurantium constituents, particularly synephrine, involve absorption from the gastrointestinal tract, metabolism in the liver, and elimination via urine. Pharmacodynamics include its sympathomimetic effects on adrenergic receptors.

Overdosage: Overconsumption of Citrus aurantium supplements, particularly those containing high concentrations of synephrine, can lead to adverse effects such as increased heart rate, hypertension, and cardiac arrhythmias. It's crucial to adhere to recommended dosages and avoid excessive intake.

International Standing: Citrus aurantium and its extracts are commonly used in dietary supplements and herbal preparations worldwide. Regulations regarding its use vary among countries, with some imposing restrictions on synephrine content due to safety concerns.

Indian Standing: In India, Citrus aurantium is recognized for its medicinal properties and is used in traditional Ayurvedic and Unani medicine systems for various purposes, including digestive support and weight management.

Research Summary: Research on Citrus aurantium, particularly its active constituent synephrine, primarily focuses on its potential role in weight management and metabolic health. While some studies suggest beneficial effects, further research is needed to elucidate its mechanisms of action, efficacy, and long-term safety profile. Additionally, investigations into its traditional uses and pharmacological properties continue to contribute to our understanding of its therapeutic potential

23)SYZYGUM AROMATICUM

Introduction: Syzygium aromaticum, commonly known as cloves, is a flowering plant native to the Maluku Islands in Indonesia. It belongs to the Myrtaceae family and is renowned for its aromatic flower buds, which are used as a spice and for medicinal purposes.

Synonym Name and Common Name: Synonym Name: Eugenia aromaticum Common Name: Cloves

Pharmacognosy/Chemistry: The pharmacognostic profile of Syzygium aromaticum involves the examination of its morphological, microscopic, and chemical characteristics. Cloves contain various bioactive compounds, including eugenol, eugenol acetate, and beta-caryophyllene, which contribute to their medicinal properties.

Action and Pharmacology: Syzygium aromaticum exhibits analgesic, anti-inflammatory, antimicrobial, and antioxidant properties. These pharmacological actions are primarily attributed to its bioactive constituents, particularly eugenol, which acts on various biochemical pathways in the body.

Method of Analysis: Analytical methods such as gas chromatography-mass spectrometry (GC-MS) and high-performance liquid chromatography (HPLC) are commonly used to identify and quantify the active compounds in clove extracts, including eugenol and its derivatives.

Health Benefits:

- Pain relief: Cloves have been used traditionally for their analgesic properties, providing relief from toothaches and other types of pain.
- Antimicrobial activity: Clove extracts exhibit antimicrobial effects against bacteria, fungi, and viruses, making them valuable for oral hygiene and combating infections.
- Digestive health: Cloves may aid digestion and alleviate gastrointestinal discomfort, thanks to their carminative properties.

Indication and Usage:

- Used topically for toothache relief by applying clove oil directly to the affected area.
- Consumed as a spice in culinary dishes for flavor enhancement and potential health benefits.
- Included in herbal preparations and oral care products for its antimicrobial properties.

Usual Constituents with Percentages:

- Eugenol: Typically comprises 70% to 90% of the essential oil extracted from cloves.
- Eugenol acetate: Present in smaller percentages, usually ranging from 5% to 15%.
- Beta-caryophyllene: Found in trace amounts but contributes to the overall pharmacological profile of cloves.

Mechanism of Action: The analgesic and anti-inflammatory effects of Syzygium aromaticum are primarily attributed to eugenol, which acts as a local anesthetic and inhibits inflammatory mediators such as prostaglandins and leukotrienes. Additionally, its antimicrobial activity is due to disruption of microbial cell membranes and inhibition of essential enzymes.

Dosage: Dosage recommendations for clove products vary depending on the intended use and formulation. For topical application, a small amount of clove oil can be applied directly to the affected area. When consumed orally as a spice or supplement, moderation is key to avoid potential adverse effects.

Contraindications:

- Individuals with hypersensitivity or allergic reactions to cloves or eugenol should avoid using clove products.
- Pregnant or nursing women should consult a healthcare professional before using clove supplements or essential oil due to potential risks.

Precautions:

- Topical application of clove oil should be done with caution to avoid skin irritation or allergic reactions.
- Oral consumption of clove supplements in large amounts may lead to gastrointestinal upset or other adverse effects.

Adverse Reactions:

- Skin irritation: Topical application of undiluted clove oil may cause irritation, redness, or burning sensation in sensitive individuals.
- Allergic reactions: Some individuals may experience allergic reactions to cloves or eugenol, manifesting as skin rashes, itching, or respiratory symptoms.

Research Standing: Research on the medicinal properties of Syzygium aromaticum continues to uncover its potential health benefits, particularly in pain management, oral health, and antimicrobial therapy. While traditional uses are well-established, ongoing studies aim to elucidate its mechanisms of action and explore novel therapeutic applications.

Pharmacokinetics and Pharmacodynamics: The pharmacokinetics of clove compounds such as eugenol involve absorption from the gastrointestinal tract, metabolism in the liver, and elimination via urine and feces. Pharmacodynamics include their interactions with cellular receptors and enzymes, leading to various physiological effects.

Overdosage: Excessive consumption or topical application of clove products, especially concentrated clove oil, can lead to overdose symptoms such as nausea, vomiting, abdominal pain, and dizziness. It's crucial to adhere to recommended dosages and seek medical attention if overdose occurs.

International Standing: Clove is widely recognized and utilized internationally as a spice and medicinal herb. It is included in pharmacopeias and traditional medicine systems of various countries, reflecting its global importance and cultural significance.

Indian Standing: In India, cloves have a long history of use in Ayurvedic medicine and traditional culinary practices. They are valued for their therapeutic properties and are incorporated into numerous herbal formulations for various health conditions.

Research Summary: Research on Syzygium aromaticum, particularly its main constituent eugenol, spans various fields including pharmacology, dentistry, and microbiology. Studies continue to explore its efficacy and safety for pain management, oral health, and antimicrobial therapy, contributing to our understanding of its traditional uses and potential clinical applications.

24) CNICUSBENEDICTUS

Introduction: Cnicusbenedictus, commonly known as blessed thistle, is a thistle-like plant native to the Mediterranean region and parts of Asia. It belongs to the Asteraceae family and has a long history of use in traditional medicine for various health conditions.

Synonym Name and Common Name: Synonym Name: Carduus benedictus Common Name: Blessed thistle, Holy thistle

Pharmacognosy/Chemistry: The pharmacognostic profile of Cnicusbenedictus involves the study of its morphological, microscopic, and chemical characteristics. Blessed thistle contains several bioactive compounds, including sesquiterpene lactones (such as cnicin), flavonoids, tannins, and essential oils.

Action and Pharmacology: Cnicusbenedictus exhibits various pharmacological actions, including anti-inflammatory, antioxidant, and digestive stimulant properties. These actions are attributed to its bioactive constituents, particularly sesquiterpene lactones and flavonoids.

Method of Analysis: Analytical methods such as high-performance liquid chromatography (HPLC) and gas chromatography-mass spectrometry (GC-MS) are commonly used to identify and quantify the active compounds in blessed thistle extracts, including cnicin and flavonoids.

Health Benefits:

- Digestive health: Blessed thistle is traditionally used to stimulate appetite, improve digestion, and alleviate gastrointestinal discomfort.
- Galactagogue: It may promote lactation in nursing mothers when used as an herbal remedy.
- Anti-inflammatory: Blessed thistle extracts have shown anti-inflammatory activity in preclinical studies, suggesting potential benefits for inflammatory conditions.

Indication and Usage:

- Used in herbal medicine to support digestive health and stimulate appetite.
- Employed as a galactagogue to promote milk production in breastfeeding women.
- Included in herbal formulations for its purported anti-inflammatory and antioxidant effects.

Usual Constituents with Percentages:

- Cnicin: Typically found in concentrations ranging from 0.5% to 2% in dried blessed thistle herb.
- Flavonoids: Present in varying percentages depending on the plant source and extraction method.
- Tannins: Found in blessed thistle extracts, contributing to their astringent properties.

Mechanism of Action: The pharmacological effects of Cnicusbenedictus are attributed to its bioactive compounds, particularly cnicin, which exerts anti-inflammatory effects by inhibiting pro-inflammatory mediators and oxidative stress pathways. Additionally, its bitter constituents stimulate digestive secretions and enhance appetite.

Dosage: Dosage recommendations for blessed thistle supplements or herbal preparations vary depending on the intended use and formulation. It's advisable to follow product-specific instructions and consult with a healthcare professional for personalized dosing guidance.

Contraindications:

- Individuals with known allergies to plants in the Asteraceae family, such as ragweed or daisies, may be at risk of allergic reactions to blessed thistle.
- Pregnant or nursing women should exercise caution when using blessed thistle due to limited safety data.

Precautions:

- Blessed thistle may interact with certain medications or exacerbate existing health conditions. It's essential to consult a healthcare provider before using it, especially if you have underlying medical conditions or are taking medications.
- Individuals with gastrointestinal disorders should use blessed thistle with caution, as it may exacerbate symptoms in some cases.

Adverse Reactions:

- Allergic reactions: Some individuals may experience allergic reactions to blessed thistle, manifesting as skin rashes, itching, or respiratory symptoms.
- Gastrointestinal discomfort: High doses of blessed thistle may cause gastrointestinal upset, including nausea, vomiting, or diarrhea, in sensitive individuals.

Research Standing: Research on the medicinal properties of Cnicusbenedictus is ongoing, with studies exploring its potential health benefits, safety profile, and mechanisms of action. While traditional uses are well-established, further research is needed to validate its efficacy and safety in clinical settings.

Pharmacokinetics and Pharmacodynamics: The pharmacokinetics of blessed thistle compounds involve absorption from the gastrointestinal tract, metabolism in the liver, and elimination via urine and feces. Pharmacodynamics include interactions with cellular receptors and signaling pathways, leading to various physiological effects.

Overdosage: Overconsumption of blessed thistle supplements may lead to adverse effects such as gastrointestinal upset, allergic reactions, or interactions with medications. It's crucial to adhere to recommended dosages and seek medical attention if overdose symptoms occur.

International Standing: Blessed thistle is recognized and utilized in herbal medicine traditions worldwide, although regulations regarding its use may vary among countries. It is commonly available as a dietary supplement or herbal remedy in international markets.

Indian Standing: In India, blessed thistle may be used in traditional Ayurvedic or Unani medicine systems for its purported health benefits, although its use may not be as widespread as in some other regions.

Research Summary: Research on Cnicusbenedictus, particularly its bioactive compound cnicin, continues to uncover its potential therapeutic applications and mechanisms of action. While traditional uses suggest various health benefits, further clinical studies are needed to validate its efficacy, safety, and optimal dosage regimens for specific health conditions.

25)THEOBROMA CACAO

Introduction: Theobroma cacao, commonly known as cocoa or cacao, is a tropical evergreen tree native to the Americas. It belongs to the Malvaceae family and is primarily cultivated for its seeds, which are used to produce cocoa powder, cocoa butter, and chocolate.

Synonym Name and Common Name: Synonym Name: Cocoa tree Common Name: Cacao, Cocoa

Pharmacognosy/Chemistry: The pharmacognostic profile of Theobroma cacao involves the study of its morphological, microscopic, and chemical characteristics. Cocoa beans contain various bioactive compounds, including theobromine, caffeine, flavonoids (such as catechins and procyanidins), and polyphenols.

Action and Pharmacology: Theobroma cacao exhibits several pharmacological actions, including antioxidant, anti-inflammatory, and cardiovascular effects. These actions are primarily attributed to its bioactive constituents, particularly flavonoids and theobromine.

Method of Analysis: Analytical methods such as high-performance liquid chromatography (HPLC) and gas chromatography-mass spectrometry (GC-MS) are commonly used to identify and quantify the active compounds in cocoa products, including theobromine, caffeine, and flavonoids.

Health Benefits:

- Cardiovascular health: Cocoa flavonoids have been associated with improved cardiovascular function, including reduced risk of heart disease and improved blood flow.
- Antioxidant properties: The polyphenols in cocoa exhibit antioxidant activity, helping to protect cells from oxidative damage and reduce inflammation.
- Mood enhancement: Cocoa consumption has been linked to improved mood and cognitive function, attributed partly to its caffeine and theobromine content.

Indication and Usage:

- Consumption of cocoa and chocolate products for enjoyment and as a source of antioxidants and bioactive compounds.
- Incorporation of cocoa powder or cocoa extracts into dietary supplements and functional foods for potential health benefits.

Usual Constituents with Percentages:

- Theobromine: Typically comprises around 1-3% of cocoa beans.

- Caffeine: Present in smaller percentages, usually around 0.1-0.2%.
- Flavonoids (catechins, procyanidins): Varying percentages depending on the cocoa bean variety and processing method.

Mechanism of Action: The pharmacological effects of Theobroma cacao are mediated through its bioactive compounds, particularly theobromine and flavonoids. These compounds exert antioxidant, anti-inflammatory, and vasodilatory effects, contributing to cardiovascular health and other physiological functions.

Dosage: Dosage recommendations for cocoa products vary depending on the desired health outcome and individual tolerance. Moderate consumption of cocoa or dark chocolate, typically 20-30 grams per day, is considered safe and may provide health benefits.

Contraindications:

- Individuals with caffeine sensitivity or cardiovascular conditions should moderate their cocoa consumption or consult a healthcare professional.
- Pregnant or nursing women should limit their intake of cocoa products due to their caffeine content.

Precautions:

- Excessive consumption of cocoa or chocolate products high in sugar and fat may contribute to weight gain and other adverse health effects.
- Some individuals may experience allergic reactions to cocoa or chocolate, although this is relatively rare.

Adverse Reactions:

- Side effects of excessive cocoa consumption may include gastrointestinal discomfort, insomnia, jitteriness, and palpitations due to its caffeine and theobromine content.
- Allergic reactions to cocoa or chocolate, such as skin rashes or respiratory symptoms, may occur in susceptible individuals.

Research Standing: Research on the health effects of Theobroma cacao and its bioactive compounds is extensive and ongoing, with studies investigating its potential benefits for cardiovascular health, cognitive function, mood, and other physiological processes. While much evidence supports its positive effects, further research is needed to elucidate optimal dosage regimens and long-term effects.

Pharmacokinetics and Pharmacodynamics: The pharmacokinetics of cocoa compounds involve absorption from the gastrointestinal tract, metabolism in the liver, and distribution to various tissues. Pharmacodynamics include their interactions with cellular receptors and signaling pathways, leading to physiological effects such as antioxidant activity and vasodilation.

Overdosage: Overconsumption of cocoa or chocolate products high in caffeine and theobromine may lead to adverse effects such as insomnia, nervousness, gastrointestinal upset, and increased heart rate. It's essential to moderate consumption and avoid excessive intake.

International Standing: Cocoa and chocolate products derived from Theobroma cacao are widely consumed and recognized internationally for their culinary and potential health benefits. They are traded globally and incorporated into various food and beverage products.

Indian Standing: In India, cocoa and chocolate products are consumed and enjoyed, although they may not have the same cultural significance as in some other regions. Cocoa is also used in traditional Ayurvedic formulations for its potential health benefits.

Research Summary: Research on Theobroma cacao and its bioactive compounds continues to explore its potential health benefits and mechanisms of action. While cocoa consumption is generally regarded as safe and may provide various health advantages, further studies are needed to establish optimal dosage regimens, assess long-term effects, and elucidate potential interactions with other dietary factors or medications.

26) COCCINIA GRANDIS (L.) VOIGT

Introduction: Coccinia grandis, commonly known as ivy gourd or scarlet gourd, is a tropical vine belonging to the Cucurbitaceae family. It is native to Asia and Africa and is cultivated for its edible fruits and medicinal properties.

Synonym Name and Common Name: Synonym Name: Coccinia indica, Coccinia cordifolia Common Name: Ivy gourd, Scarlet gourd, Tindora

Pharmacognosy/Chemistry: The pharmacognostic profile of Coccinia grandis involves the study of its morphological, microscopic, and chemical characteristics. Ivy gourd contains various bioactive compounds, including alkaloids, flavonoids, saponins, and glycosides.

Action and Pharmacology: Coccinia grandis exhibits several pharmacological actions, including hypoglycemic, antioxidant, anti-inflammatory, and antimicrobial effects. These actions are attributed to its bioactive constituents and contribute to its traditional medicinal uses.

Method of Analysis: Analytical methods such as high-performance liquid chromatography (HPLC) and gas chromatography-mass spectrometry (GC-MS) are commonly used to identify and quantify the active compounds in ivy gourd extracts, including alkaloids, flavonoids, and other phytochemicals.

Health Benefits:

- Diabetes management: Ivy gourd is traditionally used for its hypoglycemic effects, helping to regulate blood sugar levels in individuals with diabetes.
- Antioxidant properties: The flavonoids and other phytochemicals in ivy gourd exhibit antioxidant activity, helping to neutralize free radicals and reduce oxidative stress.
- Digestive health: Ivy gourd is believed to support digestive function and relieve gastrointestinal discomfort, including constipation and indigestion.

Indication and Usage:

- Consumed as a vegetable in culinary dishes in various cuisines, particularly in Asian cooking.
- Used in traditional medicine systems for its purported health benefits, including diabetes management and digestive support.
- Included in dietary supplements and herbal formulations for its hypoglycemic and antioxidant properties.

Usual Constituents with Percentages:

- Alkaloids: Present in varying percentages depending on the plant source and extraction method.
- Flavonoids: Found in ivy gourd extracts, with concentrations varying among different parts of the plant and environmental factors.

Mechanism of Action: The hypoglycemic effects of Coccinia grandis are attributed to its ability to enhance insulin secretion, improve insulin sensitivity, and inhibit carbohydrate digestion and absorption in the intestines. Additionally, its antioxidant and anti-inflammatory actions contribute to overall health benefits.

Dosage: Dosage recommendations for ivy gourd supplements or herbal preparations may vary depending on the formulation and intended use. It's advisable to follow product-specific instructions and consult with a healthcare professional for personalized dosing guidance.

Contraindications:

- Individuals with known allergies to plants in the Cucurbitaceae family, such as cucumber or melon, may be at risk of allergic reactions to ivy gourd.
- Pregnant or nursing women should exercise caution when using ivy gourd due to limited safety data.

Precautions:

- Ivy gourd may interact with certain medications or exacerbate existing health conditions. It's essential to consult a healthcare provider before using it, especially if you have underlying medical conditions or are taking medications.
- Some individuals may experience gastrointestinal discomfort or allergic reactions to ivy gourd, although adverse effects are relatively rare.

Adverse Reactions:

- Allergic reactions: Some individuals may experience allergic reactions to ivy gourd, manifesting as skin rashes, itching, or respiratory symptoms.

- Gastrointestinal discomfort: High doses of ivy gourd or its extracts may cause gastrointestinal upset, including nausea, vomiting, or diarrhea, in sensitive individuals.

Research Standing: Research on the medicinal properties of Coccinia grandis is ongoing, with studies investigating its potential health benefits, safety profile, and mechanisms of action. While traditional uses are well-established, further research is needed to validate its efficacy and safety in clinical settings.

Pharmacokinetics and Pharmacodynamics: The pharmacokinetics of ivy gourd compounds involve absorption from the gastrointestinal tract, metabolism in the liver, and distribution to various tissues. Pharmacodynamics include their interactions with cellular receptors and signaling pathways, leading to physiological effects such as hypoglycemic and antioxidant actions.

Overdosage: Excessive consumption of ivy gourd or its extracts may lead to adverse effects such as gastrointestinal upset or allergic reactions. It's crucial to adhere to recommended dosages and seek medical attention if overdose symptoms occur.

International Standing: Ivy gourd is recognized and utilized in traditional medicine systems and culinary practices in various countries, particularly in Asia and Africa. Its cultivation and consumption as a vegetable and medicinal plant are widespread.

Indian Standing: In India, Coccinia grandis has a long history of use in Ayurvedic and traditional medicine systems for its hypoglycemic and digestive properties. It is also consumed as a vegetable in Indian cuisine, known locally as "tindora" or "kundru."

Research Summary: Research on Coccinia grandis, particularly its hypoglycemic effects and antioxidant properties, continues to advance our understanding of its potential health benefits and mechanisms of action. While traditional uses are well-documented, further clinical studies are needed to validate its efficacy, safety, and optimal dosage regimens for specific health conditions.

27)CRATAEVANURVALA - EXTRACT

Introduction: Crataevanurvala, commonly known as Varuna or Three-leaved caper, is a medicinal plant native to the Indian subcontinent. It has been traditionally used in Ayurvedic medicine for its various health benefits.

Synonym Name and Common Name: Synonym Name: Cratevanurvala Buch. -Ham. ex D.Don Common Name: Varuna, Three-leaved caper

Pharmacognosy/Chemistry: Crataevanurvala contains various bioactive compounds such as lupeol, β-sitosterol, quercetin, kaempferol, and rutin. Its pharmacognostic characteristics include distinctive leaf morphology and the presence of phytochemicals like alkaloids, flavonoids, and tannins.

Action and Pharmacology: Crataevanurvala exhibits diuretic, anti-inflammatory, antioxidant, and hepatoprotective properties. Its pharmacological actions involve modulation of renal function, anti-inflammatory effects through inhibition of pro-inflammatory cytokines, and scavenging of free radicals.

Method of Analysis: Analytical methods such as high-performance liquid chromatography (HPLC) and gas chromatography-mass spectrometry (GC-MS) are commonly employed to quantify the phytoconstituents present in Crataevanurvala extracts.

Health Benefits: Crataevanurvala is traditionally used for urinary disorders, kidney stones, liver ailments, and inflammatory conditions. It is also believed to promote digestive health and overall well-being.

Indication and Usage: It is indicated for conditions like urinary tract infections, nephrolithiasis (kidney stones), liver disorders, and inflammatory diseases. Crataevanurvala is often consumed as a decoction or in the form of herbal supplements.

Usual Constituents with Percentages:

- Lupeol: 0.5-1%
- β-sitosterol: 0.2-0.5%
- Quercetin: 0.1-0.3%
- Kaempferol: 0.1-0.2%

- Rutin: 0.2-0.4% (Percentages may vary depending on the source and extraction method)

Mechanism of Action: The diuretic effect of Crataevanurvala is attributed to its ability to enhance renal blood flow and inhibit the reabsorption of water and electrolytes in the kidneys. Its anti-inflammatory and antioxidant actions involve the suppression of pro-inflammatory mediators and scavenging of reactive oxygen species (ROS).

Dosage: The typical dosage of Crataevanurvala extract is 500-1000 mg per day, divided into two or three doses. However, it is advisable to consult a healthcare professional for appropriate dosage recommendations.

Contraindications: Crataevanurvala should be avoided in pregnant and breastfeeding women unless recommended by a healthcare provider. Individuals with known allergies to plants in the Capparidaceae family should also avoid its use.

Precautions: Caution should be exercised when using Crataevanurvala alongside diuretic medications or other herbs with diuretic properties, as it may potentiate their effects and lead to electrolyte imbalances.

Adverse Reactions: Although rare, allergic reactions such as rash, itching, or gastrointestinal discomfort may occur in sensitive individuals. Prolonged use or high doses may also lead to electrolyte disturbances.

Research Standing: Research on the medicinal properties of Crataevanurvala extract is ongoing, with several studies supporting its traditional uses and exploring its potential therapeutic applications in modern medicine.

Pharmacokinetics and Pharmacodynamics: The pharmacokinetics of Crataevanurvala extract have not been extensively studied. Its pharmacodynamic effects are primarily attributed to the modulation of renal function and inflammatory pathways.

Overdosage: Excessive consumption of Crataevanurvala extract may lead to gastrointestinal upset, electrolyte imbalances, or allergic reactions. In case of overdose, symptomatic treatment and supportive care are recommended.

International Standing: Crataevanurvala extract is recognized in traditional medicine systems worldwide and is gaining interest as a natural remedy for various health conditions. However, its regulatory status may vary across different countries.

Indian Standing: In India, Crataevanurvala holds a prominent place in Ayurvedic medicine, where it is used for its diuretic, anti-inflammatory, and hepatoprotective properties. It is included in various herbal formulations and is widely available in the form of supplements.

Research Summary: Research on Crataevanurvala extract highlights its potential therapeutic benefits in urinary disorders, kidney stones, liver diseases, and inflammatory conditions. Its bioactive constituents and pharmacological actions continue to be investigated, contributing to its growing popularity as a natural health supplement.

28)CRUSTACEAN SHELLS

Introduction: Crustacean shells, commonly referred to as shellfish exoskeletons, are the rigid outer coverings of various marine arthropods like crabs, lobsters, and shrimp. These shells have been used in traditional medicine systems and modern pharmaceuticals for their therapeutic properties.

Synonym Name and Common Name: Synonym Name: Exoskeletons of Crustacea Common Name: Shellfish shells, Crab shell extract

Pharmacognosy/Chemistry: Crustacean shells contain primarily chitin, a complex polysaccharide, along with minerals such as calcium carbonate and proteins. Chitin is the major component and contributes to the shells' structural integrity and therapeutic properties.

Action and Pharmacology: The pharmacological actions of crustacean shells include wound healing, anti-inflammatory, antimicrobial, and immunomodulatory effects. These actions are attributed to the presence of chitin and other bioactive compounds in the shells.

Method of Analysis: Analytical methods such as Fourier-transform infrared spectroscopy (FTIR) and scanning electron microscopy (SEM) are commonly used to characterize the chemical composition and microstructure of crustacean shells.

Health Benefits: Crustacean shell extracts are known for their potential benefits in wound healing, bone health, and skincare. They may also have applications in the treatment of inflammatory conditions and as dietary supplements for calcium intake.

Indication and Usage: Crustacean shell extracts are indicated for wounds, burns, and inflammatory skin conditions like eczema and dermatitis. They are also used in bone health supplements and as a source of dietary calcium.

Usual Constituents with Percentages:

- Chitin: 60-90%
- Calcium carbonate: 5-20%
- Proteins: 1-10% (Percentages may vary depending on the species and processing methods)

Mechanism of Action: The mechanism of action of crustacean shell extracts involves the stimulation of fibroblast activity, collagen synthesis, and angiogenesis, promoting wound healing. Chitin also exhibits immunomodulatory effects by modulating inflammatory responses.

Dosage: Dosage forms of crustacean shell extracts include topical creams, ointments, and oral supplements. Recommended dosages vary depending on the specific product and indication. It is advisable to follow the instructions provided by healthcare professionals or product labels.

Contraindications: Individuals with known allergies to shellfish should avoid the use of crustacean shell extracts due to the risk of allergic reactions. Caution is also advised in patients with hypersensitivity to any of the components present in the extracts.

Precautions: Crustacean shell extracts should be used with caution in individuals with compromised immune function or chronic medical conditions. Topical application may cause skin irritation in sensitive individuals, and oral supplements should be taken under medical supervision.

Adverse Reactions: Adverse reactions to crustacean shell extracts may include allergic reactions such as itching, rash, swelling, or difficulty breathing in susceptible individuals. Topical application may also cause local skin irritation or redness.

Research Standing: Research on the therapeutic properties of crustacean shell extracts is ongoing, with studies focusing on their wound healing, anti-inflammatory, and immunomodulatory effects. Clinical trials are exploring their efficacy and safety in various medical applications.

Pharmacokinetics and Pharmacodynamics: The pharmacokinetics of crustacean shell extracts have not been extensively studied. Their pharmacodynamic effects are primarily attributed to the bioactive components like chitin, which interact with the immune system and promote tissue regeneration.

Overdosage: Overdosage of crustacean shell extracts is unlikely to occur with topical application. However, excessive oral intake may lead to gastrointestinal discomfort or allergic reactions in sensitive individuals. Adherence to recommended dosages is advised.

International Standing: Crustacean shell extracts are recognized for their therapeutic potential in traditional medicine systems worldwide. They are also used as dietary supplements and functional ingredients in various pharmaceutical and cosmetic products.

Indian Standing: In India, crustacean shell extracts are utilized in Ayurvedic medicine and traditional wound healing practices. They are incorporated into topical formulations and dietary supplements for their beneficial effects on skin health and overall well-being.

Research Summary: Research on crustacean shell extracts underscores their potential as natural remedies for wound healing, inflammatory conditions, and bone health. Their rich chitin content and diverse pharmacological actions continue to be explored, contributing to their growing importance in modern healthcare and pharmaceutical industries.

29)CUMINUM CYMINUM L

Introduction: Cuminum cyminum L., commonly known as cumin, is a flowering plant belonging to the Apiaceae family. It is cultivated for its aromatic seeds, which are widely used as a spice and traditional medicine in various cuisines and cultures around the world.

Synonym Name and Common Name: Synonym Name: Cumin, Cummin Common Name: Jeera (in Hindi), Jeerakam (in Malayalam)

Pharmacognosy/Chemistry: Cuminum cyminum seeds contain essential oils, cuminaldehyde, cumuninic alcohol, and various phenolic compounds. These compounds contribute to the characteristic aroma and therapeutic properties of cumin.

Action and Pharmacology: Cumin exhibits antioxidant, antimicrobial, anti-inflammatory, and digestive-stimulating properties. Its pharmacological actions are attributed to the bioactive compounds present in the seeds.

Method of Analysis: Analytical methods such as gas chromatography-mass spectrometry (GC-MS) and high-performance liquid chromatography (HPLC) are commonly used to analyze the chemical composition of cumin seeds and quantify their major constituents.

Health Benefits: Cumin is traditionally used for its digestive benefits, including relieving indigestion, bloating, and flatulence. It is also believed to have anti-inflammatory effects and may support immune function due to its antioxidant properties.

Indication and Usage: Cumin is indicated for digestive disorders such as dyspepsia, flatulence, and diarrhea. It is commonly used as a culinary spice and is also consumed in the form of teas, decoctions, or capsules for its medicinal benefits.

Usual Constituents with Percentages:

- Essential oils (cuminaldehyde, etc.): 2-4%
- Cumuninic alcohol: 1-2%
- Phenolic compounds: 0.5-1% (Percentages may vary depending on the source and processing methods)

Mechanism of Action: The carminative and digestive-stimulating effects of cumin are attributed to its ability to enhance digestive enzyme secretion, promote bile production, and reduce intestinal spasms. Its anti-inflammatory and antioxidant actions involve the modulation of pro-inflammatory pathways and scavenging of free radicals.

Dosage: The typical dosage of cumin seeds is 1-2 teaspoons (2-4 grams) per day, either consumed directly or infused in hot water as a tea. Higher doses may be used in traditional medicine formulations under the guidance of a healthcare professional.

Contraindications: Cumin is generally safe for most individuals when consumed in culinary amounts. However, individuals with known allergies to plants in the Apiaceae family, such as celery or carrot, should avoid cumin due to the risk of cross-reactivity.

Precautions: Cumin may potentiate the effects of anticoagulant medications due to its potential antiplatelet activity. Patients taking blood thinners should use cumin cautiously and consult with their healthcare provider.

Adverse Reactions: Adverse reactions to cumin are rare but may include allergic reactions such as skin rash, itching, or gastrointestinal discomfort in sensitive individuals. Prolonged use of high doses may also lead to liver toxicity in susceptible individuals.

Research Standing: Research on the therapeutic properties of cumin continues to expand, with studies investigating its potential benefits for digestion, inflammation, metabolic health, and immune function. Clinical trials are underway to explore its efficacy and safety in various medical applications.

Pharmacokinetics and Pharmacodynamics: The pharmacokinetics of cumin constituents have been studied in animal models, showing absorption in the gastrointestinal tract and metabolism in the liver. Its pharmacodynamic effects involve modulation of digestive enzyme activity and inflammatory pathways.

Overdosage: Overconsumption of cumin seeds may lead to gastrointestinal upset, including nausea, vomiting, or diarrhea. Adherence to recommended doses is advisable to avoid adverse effects.

International Standing: Cumin is recognized internationally as a popular culinary spice and traditional medicine ingredient. It is widely used in Middle Eastern, Indian, and Latin American cuisines and is also valued for its medicinal properties in traditional medicine systems worldwide.

Indian Standing: In India, cumin holds a prominent place in Ayurvedic and Unani medicine, where it is used for its digestive, carminative, and anti-inflammatory properties. It is a common ingredient in Indian cuisine and is also consumed as a tea or decoction for its health benefits.

Research Summary: Research on Cuminum cyminum L. highlights its diverse pharmacological properties and therapeutic potential in digestive disorders, inflammation, and immune modulation. Its bioactive constituents continue to be investigated, contributing to its widespread use in both culinary and medicinal applications globally.

30)CURCUMA LONGA

Introduction: Curcuma longa, commonly known as turmeric, is a perennial herbaceous plant belonging to the ginger family, Zingiberaceae. It is native to the Indian subcontinent and Southeast Asia and has been used for centuries in traditional medicine and culinary practices.

Synonym Name and Common Name: Synonym Name: Turmeric, Haldi Common Name: Indian saffron, Jiang huang (in Chinese)

Pharmacognosy/Chemistry: Curcuma longa contains bioactive compounds called curcuminoids, with curcumin being the most abundant and pharmacologically active compound. Other curcuminoids include demethoxycurcumin and bisdemethoxycurcumin. These compounds contribute to turmeric's characteristic yellow color and medicinal properties.

Action and Pharmacology: Turmeric exhibits antioxidant, anti-inflammatory, antimicrobial, and anticancer properties. Its pharmacological actions are primarily attributed to curcumin, which modulates various signaling pathways involved in inflammation, oxidative stress, and cell proliferation.

Method of Analysis: Analytical methods such as high-performance liquid chromatography (HPLC), spectrophotometry, and gas chromatography-mass spectrometry (GC-MS) are commonly used to analyze the chemical composition of turmeric extracts and quantify the curcuminoid content.

Health Benefits: Turmeric is renowned for its numerous health benefits, including promoting joint health, supporting digestion, boosting immune function, and improving skin health. It is also studied for its potential neuroprotective and cardiovascular effects.

Indication and Usage: Turmeric is indicated for inflammatory conditions such as arthritis, gastrointestinal disorders like dyspepsia and irritable bowel syndrome (IBS), and skin conditions like eczema and psoriasis. It is consumed in various forms, including as a spice in cooking, as a dietary supplement, or applied topically.

Usual Constituents with Percentages:

- Curcumin: 2-5%
- Demethoxycurcumin: 0.3-0.5%

- Bisdemethoxycurcumin: 0.2-0.4% (Percentages may vary depending on the source and processing methods)

Mechanism of Action: The mechanism of action of turmeric is primarily attributed to curcumin's ability to inhibit inflammatory enzymes, suppress oxidative stress, and modulate gene expression involved in cell proliferation and apoptosis. It also interacts with various molecular targets involved in disease pathogenesis.

Dosage: The typical dosage of turmeric extract standardized to contain 95% curcuminoids is 500-2000 mg per day. For culinary use, turmeric powder can be added to dishes in moderate amounts. Dosages may vary based on the specific health condition and individual response.

Contraindications: Turmeric supplements are generally safe for most individuals when consumed in recommended doses. However, individuals with gallbladder disease, bile duct obstruction, or those taking anticoagulant medications should use turmeric with caution due to its potential blood-thinning effects.

Precautions: Turmeric may potentiate the effects of anticoagulant and antiplatelet medications, increasing the risk of bleeding. It is advisable to consult with a healthcare professional before starting turmeric supplementation, especially for individuals with underlying medical conditions or those undergoing surgery.

Adverse Reactions: Adverse reactions to turmeric supplements are rare but may include gastrointestinal discomfort, such as nausea, diarrhea, or abdominal pain, in sensitive individuals. Allergic reactions to turmeric are also possible but uncommon.

Research Standing: Turmeric has been extensively studied for its pharmacological properties and therapeutic potential in various health conditions, including inflammation, cancer, cardiovascular disease, and neurodegenerative disorders. Ongoing research continues to explore its mechanisms of action and clinical applications.

Pharmacokinetics and Pharmacodynamics: Curcumin is poorly absorbed in the gastrointestinal tract and rapidly metabolized in the liver, leading to low systemic bioavailability. Strategies to enhance curcumin bioavailability, such as combining it with black pepper extract (piperine) or lipid-based formulations, are being investigated.

Overdosage: Overconsumption of turmeric is unlikely to cause serious adverse effects. However, high doses may lead to gastrointestinal symptoms or allergic reactions in sensitive individuals. Adherence to recommended dosages is advisable to prevent overdosage.

International Standing: Turmeric is widely recognized and utilized internationally as both a culinary spice and a traditional medicine ingredient. Its popularity has led to its incorporation into various food products, dietary supplements, and cosmetic formulations worldwide.

Indian Standing: In India, turmeric holds a revered place in Ayurvedic medicine and traditional healing practices. It is considered sacred and is used in rituals and ceremonies. Turmeric is also a staple ingredient in Indian cuisine, adding flavor and color to dishes.

Research Summary: Research on Curcuma longa, particularly its major bioactive compound curcumin, underscores its diverse pharmacological properties and therapeutic potential in managing various health conditions. Continued investigation into its mechanisms of action, formulation strategies, and clinical efficacy is driving the ongoing interest in turmeric as a natural remedy and functional food ingredient.

31) CURCUMINOIDS -SOFT EXTRACT

Introduction: Curcuminoids-oft extract is a standardized extract derived from Curcuma longa, commonly known as turmeric. It is renowned for its potent medicinal properties and is widely used in traditional medicine and modern healthcare.

Synonym Name and Common Name: Synonym Name: Curcumin extract Common Name: Turmeric extract, Curcuminoids extract

Pharmacognosy/Chemistry: Curcuminoids-oft extract primarily consists of curcumin, demethoxycurcumin, and bisdemethoxycurcumin. These curcuminoids are polyphenolic compounds responsible for turmeric's characteristic yellow color and therapeutic effects.

Action and Pharmacology: Curcuminoids-oft extract exhibits antioxidant, anti-inflammatory, antimicrobial, and anticancer properties. Its pharmacological actions are attributed to the modulation of various signaling pathways involved in inflammation, oxidative stress, and cell proliferation.

Method of Analysis: Analytical methods such as high-performance liquid chromatography (HPLC) and spectrophotometry are commonly used to analyze the chemical composition of curcuminoids-oft extract and quantify the curcuminoid content.

Health Benefits: Curcuminoids-oft extract is known for its diverse health benefits, including promoting joint health, supporting digestion, boosting immune function, and improving skin health. It is also studied for its potential neuroprotective and cardiovascular effects.

Indication and Usage: Curcuminoids-oft extract is indicated for inflammatory conditions such as arthritis, gastrointestinal disorders like dyspepsia and irritable bowel syndrome (IBS), and skin conditions like eczema and psoriasis. It is consumed as a dietary supplement or added to topical formulations for its medicinal benefits.

Usual Constituents with Percentages:

- Curcumin: 60-70%
- Demethoxycurcumin: 15-25%
- Bisdemethoxycurcumin: 5-15% (Percentages may vary depending on the source and extraction method)

Mechanism of Action: The mechanism of action of curcuminoids-oft extract is primarily attributed to the ability of curcumin to inhibit inflammatory enzymes, suppress oxidative stress, and modulate gene expression involved in cell proliferation and apoptosis. It also interacts with various molecular targets implicated in disease pathogenesis.

Dosage: The typical dosage of curcuminoids-oft extract is 500-1500 mg per day, standardized to contain 95% curcuminoids. Dosages may vary based on the specific health condition and individual response. It is advisable to consult with a healthcare professional for personalized recommendations.

Contraindications: Curcuminoids-oft extract is generally safe for most individuals when consumed in recommended doses. However, individuals with gallbladder disease, bile duct obstruction, or those taking anticoagulant medications should use curcuminoids-oft extract with caution due to its potential blood-thinning effects.

Precautions: Curcuminoids-oft extract may potentiate the effects of anticoagulant and antiplatelet medications, increasing the risk of bleeding. It is advisable to consult with a healthcare professional before starting supplementation, especially for individuals with underlying medical conditions or those undergoing surgery.

Adverse Reactions: Adverse reactions to curcuminoids-oft extract are rare but may include gastrointestinal discomfort, such as nausea, diarrhea, or abdominal pain, in sensitive individuals. Allergic reactions to curcuminoids are also possible but uncommon.

Research Standing: Curcuminoids-oft extract has been extensively researched for its pharmacological properties and therapeutic potential in various health conditions, including inflammation, cancer, cardiovascular disease, and neurodegenerative disorders. Ongoing research continues to explore its mechanisms of action and clinical applications.

Pharmacokinetics and Pharmacodynamics: Curcuminoids-oft extract is poorly absorbed in the gastrointestinal tract and rapidly metabolized in the liver, leading to low systemic bioavailability. Strategies to enhance curcumin bioavailability, such as combining it with black pepper extract (piperine) or lipid-based formulations, are being investigated.

Overdosage: Overconsumption of curcuminoids-oft extract may lead to gastrointestinal symptoms or allergic reactions in sensitive individuals. Adherence to recommended dosages is advisable to prevent overdosage.

International Standing: Curcuminoids-oft extract is recognized and utilized internationally as a dietary supplement and functional food ingredient. Its popularity has led to its incorporation into various health products and formulations worldwide.

Indian Standing: In India, curcuminoids-oft extract holds a revered place in Ayurvedic medicine and traditional healing practices. It is considered a potent natural remedy for various ailments and is incorporated into dietary supplements, cosmetics, and topical formulations.

Research Summary: Research on curcuminoids-oft extract underscores its diverse pharmacological properties and therapeutic potential in managing various health conditions. Continued investigation into its mechanisms of action, formulation strategies, and clinical efficacy is driving the ongoing interest in curcuminoids-oft extract as a natural remedy and functional food ingredient.

32)CYPERUS ROTUNDUS– EXTRACT

Introduction: Cyperus rotundus, commonly known as nutgrass or purple nutsedge, is a perennial weed native to Africa, Asia, and Australia. It has a long history of use in traditional medicine systems for its various health benefits.

Synonym Name and Common Name: Synonym Name: Nutgrass, Purple nutsedge Common Name: Musta (in Ayurveda), Nagarmotha (in Hindi)

Pharmacognosy/Chemistry: Cyperus rotundus extract contains bioactive compounds such as flavonoids, terpenoids, alkaloids, and phenolic acids. Its pharmacognostic characteristics include tuberous rhizomes with a distinctive aroma and taste.

Action and Pharmacology: Cyperus rotundus extract exhibits antioxidant, anti-inflammatory, antimicrobial, and analgesic properties. Its pharmacological actions involve modulation of inflammatory pathways, scavenging of free radicals, and inhibition of microbial growth.

Method of Analysis: Analytical methods such as high-performance liquid chromatography (HPLC), gas chromatography-mass spectrometry (GC-MS), and spectrophotometry are commonly used to analyze the chemical composition of Cyperus rotundus extract and quantify its bioactive constituents.

Health Benefits: Cyperus rotundus extract is traditionally used for its digestive, carminative, diuretic, and analgesic properties. It is also believed to have benefits for menstrual disorders, respiratory conditions, and skin ailments.

Indication and Usage: Cyperus rotundus extract is indicated for digestive disorders such as indigestion, flatulence, and abdominal pain. It is also used for menstrual irregularities, respiratory infections, and skin conditions like eczema and dermatitis.

Usual Constituents with Percentages:

- Flavonoids: 1-3%
- Terpenoids: 0.5-1.5%
- Alkaloids: 0.2-0.5%
- Phenolic acids: 0.3-0.7% (Percentages may vary depending on the source and extraction method)

Mechanism of Action: The mechanism of action of Cyperus rotundus extract involves the modulation of neurotransmitters, inhibition of inflammatory enzymes, and enhancement of antioxidant defenses. It also exhibits spasmolytic effects on smooth muscles, contributing to its digestive and analgesic properties.

Dosage: The typical dosage of Cyperus rotundus extract is 500-1000 mg per day, divided into two or three doses. Dosages may vary based on the specific health condition and individual response. It is advisable to consult with a healthcare professional for personalized recommendations.

Contraindications: Cyperus rotundus extract is generally safe for most individuals when consumed in recommended doses. However, individuals with known allergies to plants in the Cyperaceae family should avoid its use due to the risk of allergic reactions.

Precautions: Pregnant and breastfeeding women should use Cyperus rotundus extract with caution, as safety data in this population are limited. Individuals with underlying medical conditions or those taking medications should consult with a healthcare professional before starting supplementation.

Adverse Reactions: Adverse reactions to Cyperus rotundus extract are rare but may include gastrointestinal discomfort, allergic reactions, or skin irritation in sensitive individuals. Prolonged use or high doses may also lead to digestive disturbances in some people.

Research Standing: Research on the medicinal properties of Cyperus rotundus extract is ongoing, with studies investigating its efficacy and safety in various health conditions. Preclinical and clinical trials are exploring its potential therapeutic applications and mechanisms of action.

Pharmacokinetics and Pharmacodynamics: The pharmacokinetics of Cyperus rotundus extract have not been extensively studied. Its pharmacodynamic effects involve modulation of neurotransmitter release, inflammatory pathways, and smooth muscle contraction.

Overdosage: Overconsumption of Cyperus rotundus extract may lead to gastrointestinal symptoms such as nausea, vomiting, or diarrhea. Adherence to recommended dosages is advisable to prevent overdosage.

International Standing: Cyperus rotundus extract is recognized internationally as a traditional medicine ingredient and is used in various herbal formulations and dietary supplements. Its popularity is growing due to its perceived health benefits and low risk of adverse effects.

Indian Standing: In India, Cyperus rotundus extract is highly valued in Ayurvedic and Unani medicine for its therapeutic properties. It is considered a versatile herb with applications in digestive disorders, menstrual irregularities, respiratory ailments, and skin conditions.

Research Summary: Research on Cyperus rotundus extract highlights its potential as a natural remedy for various health conditions, including digestive disorders, menstrual irregularities, and inflammatory conditions. Continued investigation into its pharmacological properties and clinical efficacy is needed to fully elucidate its therapeutic potential and optimize its use in modern medicine.

33)DIOSCOREA BULBIFERA– EXTRACT

Introduction: Dioscorea bulbifera, commonly known as air potato or aerial yam, is a perennial vine belonging to the Dioscoreaceae family. It is native to tropical regions of Asia, Africa, and Australia. Dioscorea bulbifera extract is derived from the bulbils or aerial tubers of the plant and is utilized for its medicinal properties.

Synonym Name and Common Name: Synonym Name: Aerial yam, Air potato Common Name: Varahi Kand (in Ayurveda), Kanishta (in Hindi)

Pharmacognosy/Chemistry: Dioscorea bulbifera extract contains bioactive compounds such as diosgenin, alkaloids, saponins, and flavonoids. Its pharmacognostic characteristics include bulbils with a starchy texture and a bitter taste.

Action and Pharmacology: Dioscorea bulbifera extract exhibits antioxidant, anti-inflammatory, antidiabetic, and hepatoprotective properties. Its pharmacological actions involve modulation of oxidative stress, inflammation, and metabolic pathways.

Method of Analysis: Analytical methods such as high-performance liquid chromatography (HPLC), gas chromatography-mass spectrometry (GC-MS), and spectrophotometry are commonly used to analyze the chemical composition of Dioscorea bulbifera extract and quantify its bioactive constituents.

Health Benefits: Dioscorea bulbifera extract is traditionally used for its digestive, expectorant, and diuretic properties. It is also believed to have benefits for respiratory ailments, skin conditions, and diabetes management.

Indication and Usage: Dioscorea bulbifera extract is indicated for digestive disorders such as indigestion, flatulence, and constipation. It is also used for respiratory conditions like cough, asthma, and bronchitis, as well as for managing diabetes and promoting liver health.

Usual Constituents with Percentages:

- Diosgenin: 0.5-1.5%
- Alkaloids: 0.2-0.5%
- Saponins: 1-2%
- Flavonoids: 0.5-1% (Percentages may vary depending on the source and extraction method)

Mechanism of Action: The mechanism of action of Dioscorea bulbifera extract involves the modulation of oxidative stress, inflammation, and metabolic pathways. Diosgenin, a steroidal saponin found in the extract, exhibits antidiabetic effects by enhancing insulin sensitivity and glucose uptake.

Dosage: The typical dosage of Dioscorea bulbifera extract is 500-1500 mg per day, divided into two or three doses. Dosages may vary based on the specific health condition and individual response. It is advisable to consult with a healthcare professional for personalized recommendations.

Contraindications: Dioscorea bulbifera extract is generally safe for most individuals when consumed in recommended doses. However, individuals with known allergies to plants in the Dioscoreaceae family should avoid its use due to the risk of allergic reactions.

Precautions: Pregnant and breastfeeding women should use Dioscorea bulbifera extract with caution, as safety data in this population are limited. Individuals with underlying medical conditions or those taking medications should consult with a healthcare professional before starting supplementation.

Adverse Reactions: Adverse reactions to Dioscorea bulbifera extract are rare but may include gastrointestinal discomfort, allergic reactions, or skin irritation in sensitive individuals. Prolonged use or high doses may also lead to digestive disturbances in some people.

Research Standing: Research on the medicinal properties of Dioscorea bulbifera extract is ongoing, with studies investigating its efficacy and safety in various health conditions. Preclinical and clinical trials are exploring its potential therapeutic applications and mechanisms of action.

Pharmacokinetics and Pharmacodynamics: The pharmacokinetics of Dioscorea bulbifera extract have not been extensively studied. Its pharmacodynamic effects involve modulation of oxidative stress, inflammation, and metabolic pathways implicated in disease pathogenesis.

Overdosage: Overconsumption of Dioscorea bulbifera extract may lead to gastrointestinal symptoms such as nausea, vomiting, or diarrhea. Adherence to recommended dosages is advisable to prevent overdosage.

International Standing: Dioscorea bulbifera extract is recognized internationally as a traditional medicine ingredient and is used in various herbal formulations and dietary supplements. Its popularity is growing due to its perceived health benefits and low risk of adverse effects.

Indian Standing: In India, Dioscorea bulbifera extract is highly valued in Ayurvedic medicine for its therapeutic properties. It is considered a versatile herb with applications in digestive disorders, respiratory ailments, and diabetes management. Dioscorea bulbifera extract is also utilized in traditional healing practices and rituals.

Research Summary: Research on Dioscorea bulbifera extract highlights its potential as a natural remedy for various health conditions, including digestive disorders, respiratory ailments, and diabetes. Continued investigation into its pharmacological properties and clinical efficacy is needed to fully elucidate its therapeutic potential and optimize its use in modern medicine.

34) EMBLICA OFFICINALIS

Introduction: Emblica officinalis, commonly known as Indian gooseberry or amla, is a fruit-bearing tree native to the Indian subcontinent. It holds a significant place in traditional Ayurvedic medicine and is celebrated for its numerous health benefits.

Synonym Name and Common Name: Synonym Name: Phyllanthus emblica,

Amlaki Common Name: Indian gooseberry, Amla

Pharmacognosy/Chemistry: Emblica officinalis contains a rich array of bioactive compounds, including vitamin C, tannins, flavonoids, and polyphenols. Its pharmacognostic characteristics include small, greenish-yellow fruits with a sour taste.

Action and Pharmacology: Emblica officinalis exhibits antioxidant, anti-inflammatory, immunomodulatory, hepatoprotective, and anti-aging properties. Its pharmacological actions involve scavenging free radicals, modulating immune responses, and protecting against cellular damage.

Method of Analysis: Analytical methods such as high-performance liquid chromatography (HPLC), spectrophotometry, and gas chromatography-mass spectrometry (GC-MS) are commonly used to analyze the chemical composition of Emblica officinalis and quantify its bioactive constituents.

Health Benefits: Emblica officinalis is renowned for its numerous health benefits, including boosting immunity, promoting digestion, enhancing skin health, supporting cardiovascular function, and improving hair growth. It is also valued for its anti-aging properties.

Indication and Usage: Emblica officinalis is indicated for various health conditions, including colds, coughs, digestive disorders, skin ailments, and hair problems. It is consumed fresh, dried, or in the form of juice, powder, or supplements for its medicinal benefits.

Usual Constituents with Percentages:

- Vitamin C: 700-900 mg/100g
- Tannins: 5-10%
- Flavonoids: 0.5-1%
- Polyphenols: 1-2% (Percentages may vary depending on the ripeness and processing of the fruit)

Mechanism of Action: The mechanism of action of Emblica officinalis involves its rich antioxidant content, particularly vitamin C, which scavenges free radicals and protects cells from oxidative damage. Tannins and flavonoids contribute to its anti-inflammatory and immunomodulatory effects.

Dosage: The typical dosage of Emblica officinalis varies depending on the form of administration. For fresh fruit consumption, 1-2 amla fruits per day are recommended. For supplements or dried powder, dosages typically range from 500 mg to 2 grams per day.

Contraindications: Emblica officinalis is generally safe for most individuals when consumed in recommended doses. However, individuals with a history of oxalate-containing kidney stones should use caution, as amla is high in oxalates and may exacerbate the condition.

Precautions: Pregnant and breastfeeding women should consult with a healthcare professional before using Emblica officinalis supplements. Individuals with underlying medical conditions or those taking medications should also seek advice before supplementation.

Adverse Reactions: Adverse reactions to Emblica officinalis are rare but may include gastrointestinal discomfort, such as diarrhea or stomach upset, in sensitive individuals. Allergic reactions to amla are uncommon but possible in susceptible individuals.

Research Standing: Emblica officinalis has been extensively researched for its pharmacological properties and therapeutic potential. Numerous studies have investigated its effects on immunity, digestion, skin health, hair growth, and chronic diseases. Overall, research supports its traditional use and validates its health benefits.

Pharmacokinetics and Pharmacodynamics: The pharmacokinetics of Emblica officinalis constituents, particularly vitamin C, have been well studied. Its pharmacodynamic effects involve modulation of antioxidant enzymes, immune cell function, and inflammatory pathways.

Overdosage: Overconsumption of Emblica officinalis may lead to gastrointestinal discomfort or diarrhea due to its high fiber content. Adherence to recommended dosages is advisable to prevent adverse effects.

International Standing: Emblica officinalis is recognized internationally for its medicinal properties and is increasingly utilized in dietary supplements, herbal formulations, and cosmetic products. Its popularity is growing due to its perceived health benefits and safety profile.

Indian Standing: In India, Emblica officinalis holds a revered place in Ayurvedic medicine and is considered a Rasayana or rejuvenating herb. It is incorporated into various Ayurvedic formulations, including Chyawanprash, Triphala, and herbal teas. Amla is also consumed fresh and used in culinary preparations.

Research Summary: Research on Emblica officinalis underscores its significant therapeutic potential and validates its traditional use in promoting health and well-being. Continued investigation into its pharmacological properties, mechanisms of action, and clinical efficacy is essential for further understanding and optimizing its medicinal applications.

35)OENOTHERA BIENNIS

Introduction: Oenothera biennis, commonly known as evening primrose, is a flowering plant native to North America. It has a long history of medicinal use, particularly for its oil extracted from its seeds, which is rich in gamma-linolenic acid (GLA) and other bioactive compounds.

Synonym Name and Common Name: Synonym Name: Evening primrose oil, Evening star Common Name: Sundrop, Night willow-herb

Pharmacognosy/Chemistry: Oenothera biennis contains bioactive compounds such as gamma-linolenic acid (GLA), linoleic acid, oleic acid, and various flavonoids and phenolic compounds. Its pharmacognostic characteristics include yellow flowers that bloom in the evening, giving rise to its common name.

Action and Pharmacology: Evening primrose oil exhibits anti-inflammatory, antioxidant, and moisturizing properties when applied topically. When taken orally, it may have anti-inflammatory effects and support skin health, hormonal balance, and cardiovascular function.

Method of Analysis: Analytical methods such as gas chromatography (GC), high-performance liquid chromatography (HPLC), and mass spectrometry (MS) are commonly used to analyze the chemical composition of evening primrose oil and quantify its fatty acid content, particularly GLA.

Health Benefits: Evening primrose oil is known for its various health benefits, including relieving symptoms of premenstrual syndrome (PMS), menopause, eczema, and rheumatoid arthritis. It is also used for promoting healthy skin, hair, and nails.

Indication and Usage: Evening primrose oil is indicated for conditions such as PMS, menopausal symptoms, eczema, dry skin, and inflammatory conditions. It is available in oral supplement form and as a topical oil for skin and hair care.

Usual Constituents with Percentages:

- Gamma-linolenic acid (GLA): 8-10%
- Linoleic acid: 65-75%
- Oleic acid: 6-10% (Percentages may vary depending on the source and extraction method)

Mechanism of Action: The mechanism of action of evening primrose oil is attributed to its high content of GLA, an omega-6 fatty acid. GLA is converted in the body into anti-inflammatory compounds that help regulate inflammation, hormonal balance, and skin barrier function.

Dosage: The typical dosage of evening primrose oil supplements ranges from 500 to 3000 mg per day, standardized to contain around 8-10% GLA. Dosages may vary based on the specific health condition and individual response.

Contraindications: Evening primrose oil supplements are generally safe for most individuals when taken in recommended doses. However, individuals with a history of seizures, bleeding disorders, or those taking blood-thinning medications should use caution or consult with a healthcare professional before use.

Precautions: Pregnant and breastfeeding women should consult with a healthcare professional before taking evening primrose oil supplements. Individuals with underlying medical conditions or those taking medications should also seek advice before supplementation.

Adverse Reactions: Adverse reactions to evening primrose oil supplements are rare but may include gastrointestinal discomfort, headaches, or allergic reactions in sensitive individuals. Prolonged use or high doses may also increase the risk of bleeding in some people.

Research Standing: Evening primrose oil has been the subject of numerous studies investigating its efficacy in various health conditions, including PMS, menopausal symptoms, eczema, and rheumatoid arthritis. While some studies show promising results, more research is needed to fully understand its therapeutic potential and mechanisms of action.

Pharmacokinetics and Pharmacodynamics: The pharmacokinetics of evening primrose oil constituents, particularly GLA, have been studied to a limited extent. Its pharmacodynamic effects involve modulation of inflammation, hormonal balance, and skin barrier function.

Overdosage: Overconsumption of evening primrose oil supplements may lead to gastrointestinal symptoms such as nausea, diarrhea, or stomach upset. Adherence to recommended dosages is advisable to prevent adverse effects.

International Standing: Evening primrose oil supplements are widely available internationally and are recognized for their potential health benefits, particularly for women's health issues such as PMS and menopausal symptoms. It is commonly used as a dietary supplement and in skincare products.

Indian Standing: In India, evening primrose oil supplements are available and used for various health conditions, particularly for women's health concerns. It is also utilized in Ayurvedic and traditional medicine practices for its potential therapeutic effects.

Research Summary: Research on evening primrose oil continues to explore its potential health benefits and mechanisms of action. While some studies support its use for conditions like PMS, menopausal symptoms, and inflammatory skin conditions, further research is needed to fully elucidate its efficacy and safety profile.

36)FAGOPYRUM ESCULENTUM

Introduction: Fagopyrum esculentum, commonly known as buckwheat, is a nutritious pseudocereal belonging to the Polygonaceae family. Originating from Central Asia, buckwheat has gained popularity worldwide for its health benefits and culinary versatility.

Synonym Name and Common Name: Synonym Name: Common buckwheat Common Name: Buckwheat, Kuttu (in Hindi), Kutti (in Tamil)

Pharmacognosy/Chemistry: Buckwheat is rich in bioactive compounds such as flavonoids, phenolic acids, vitamins, minerals, and dietary fiber. Its pharmacognostic characteristics include triangular seeds or grains with a dark outer hull.

Action and Pharmacology: Buckwheat exhibits antioxidant, anti-inflammatory, hypolipidemic, and hypoglycemic properties. Its pharmacological actions involve scavenging free radicals, reducing inflammation, lowering cholesterol levels, and regulating blood sugar levels.

Method of Analysis: Analytical methods such as high-performance liquid chromatography (HPLC), gas chromatography-mass spectrometry (GC-MS), and spectrophotometry are commonly used to analyze the chemical composition of buckwheat and quantify its bioactive constituents.

Health Benefits: Buckwheat is known for its numerous health benefits, including promoting heart health, aiding digestion, supporting weight management, and managing diabetes. It is also valued for its gluten-free nature and high nutritional content.

Indication and Usage: Buckwheat is indicated for conditions such as high cholesterol, diabetes, obesity, constipation, and digestive disorders. It is consumed in various forms, including as whole grains, flour, noodles, and as an ingredient in baked goods and breakfast cereals.

Usual Constituents with Percentages:

- Rutin (flavonoid): 0.5-1.5%
- Quercetin (flavonoid): 0.2-0.5%
- Fiber: 10-15%
- Protein: 10-15% (Percentages may vary depending on the variety and processing of buckwheat)

Mechanism of Action: The mechanism of action of buckwheat's bioactive compounds involves reducing oxidative stress, inflammation, and cholesterol absorption. Rutin and quercetin contribute to its antioxidant and anti-inflammatory effects, while dietary fiber and protein aid in digestion and weight management.

Dosage: There is no standard dosage for buckwheat as it is consumed as a food rather than a medicinal supplement. Incorporating buckwheat into the diet on a regular basis can provide its health benefits.

Contraindications: Buckwheat is generally safe for most individuals when consumed in food amounts. However, individuals with known allergies to buckwheat should avoid its consumption due to the risk of allergic reactions, which can be severe in some cases.

Precautions: Individuals with digestive disorders or those following special diets should be cautious when incorporating buckwheat into their diet, as it may cause digestive discomfort in some people. It is advisable to consume buckwheat in moderate amounts initially to assess tolerance.

Adverse Reactions: Adverse reactions to buckwheat are rare but may include gastrointestinal discomfort, such as bloating or gas, in sensitive individuals. Allergic reactions to buckwheat proteins can occur in individuals with buckwheat allergy, leading to symptoms ranging from mild itching to severe anaphylaxis.

Research Standing: Research on the health effects of buckwheat is ongoing, with studies investigating its potential benefits for cardiovascular health, metabolic syndrome, gastrointestinal disorders, and diabetes management. While some research supports its therapeutic potential, more studies are needed to confirm its efficacy and mechanisms of action.

Pharmacokinetics and Pharmacodynamics: The pharmacokinetics and pharmacodynamics of buckwheat's bioactive compounds have not been extensively studied. However, its high content of rutin and quercetin suggests potential antioxidant and anti-inflammatory effects, while its fiber and protein content may influence digestive processes and metabolic regulation.

Overdosage: There are no reports of overdosage with buckwheat when consumed as a food. However, excessive consumption may lead to gastrointestinal discomfort or allergic reactions in sensitive individuals.

International Standing: Buckwheat is widely recognized and consumed internationally for its nutritional value and health benefits. It is utilized in various cuisines and food products, particularly in gluten-free and health-focused diets.

Indian Standing: In India, buckwheat is known as Kuttu or Kutti and is commonly consumed during fasting periods, particularly during Navratri. It is used to prepare dishes such as Kuttu ki roti (buckwheat flatbread) and Kuttu kepakode (buckwheat fritters). Buckwheat flour is also used in traditional Indian sweets and snacks.

Research Summary: Research on buckwheat highlights its potential as a nutritious food with various health benefits, including cardiovascular protection, blood sugar regulation, and digestive health. While more studies are needed to fully elucidate its mechanisms of action and clinical efficacy, buckwheat's role in promoting overall health and well-being is increasingly recognized and valued.

37)FISH OIL

Introduction: Fish oil is a dietary supplement derived from the tissues of oily fish, such as salmon, mackerel, and sardines. It is rich in omega-3 fatty acids, particularly eicosapentaenoic acid (EPA) and docosahexaenoic acid (DHA), which are essential for various physiological functions in the body.

Synonym Name and Common Name: Synonym Name: Omega-3 fatty acid supplements Common Name: Fish oil

Pharmacognosy/Chemistry: Fish oil contains omega-3 fatty acids, primarily EPA and DHA, along with smaller amounts of other fatty acids such as alpha-linolenic acid (ALA) and docosapentaenoic acid (DPA). It may also contain fat-soluble vitamins such as vitamin A and vitamin D.

Action and Pharmacology: Fish oil exerts various health effects, including anti-inflammatory, cardioprotective, neuroprotective, and mood-regulating actions. EPA and DHA play essential roles in cell membrane structure, gene expression, and the production of signaling molecules involved in inflammation and immune responses.

Method of Analysis: Analytical methods such as gas chromatography (GC) and high-performance liquid chromatography (HPLC) are commonly used to analyze the fatty acid composition of fish oil supplements and quantify the levels of EPA and DHA.

Health Benefits: Fish oil is associated with numerous health benefits, including reducing the risk of heart disease, lowering blood pressure, improving cognitive function, alleviating joint pain, and supporting eye health. It is also used in the management of inflammatory conditions such as arthritis and inflammatory bowel disease.

Indication and Usage: Fish oil supplements are indicated for individuals with inadequate dietary intake of omega-3 fatty acids, as well as those at risk of or with existing cardiovascular disease, cognitive decline, arthritis, depression, or inflammatory conditions. It is typically consumed orally in the form of capsules or liquid.

Usual Constituents with Percentages:

- EPA (Eicosapentaenoic acid): 10-20%
- DHA (Docosahexaenoic acid): 10-20%
- Other omega-3 fatty acids: <5% (Percentages may vary depending on the source and processing of the fish oil)

Mechanism of Action: The omega-3 fatty acids EPA and DHA in fish oil exert their effects through multiple mechanisms, including modulation of inflammatory pathways, regulation of lipid metabolism, improvement of endothelial function, and enhancement of neurotransmitter signaling in the brain.

Dosage: The recommended dosage of fish oil supplements varies depending on the individual's health status and the specific health condition being targeted. Typically, doses range from 500 mg to 3000 mg of combined EPA and DHA per day, divided into two or three doses.

Contraindications: Fish oil supplements are generally safe for most individuals when taken at recommended doses. However, individuals with fish or seafood allergies, bleeding disorders, or those taking blood-thinning medications should use caution or consult with a healthcare professional before use.

Precautions: Pregnant and breastfeeding women should consult with a healthcare professional before taking fish oil supplements to ensure appropriate dosage and safety. Individuals with underlying medical conditions or those taking medications should also seek advice before supplementation.

Adverse Reactions: Adverse reactions to fish oil supplements are rare but may include gastrointestinal discomfort, such as nausea, diarrhea, or fishy burps, particularly at higher doses. Allergic reactions in individuals with fish allergies may also occur in some cases.

Research Standing: Fish oil supplements have been extensively studied for their health effects, and numerous clinical trials and meta-analyses support their efficacy in various health conditions, particularly cardiovascular disease, cognitive function, and inflammatory disorders. Research continues to explore their potential benefits and optimal dosages.

Pharmacokinetics and Pharmacodynamics: The pharmacokinetics of EPA and DHA in fish oil supplements have been well studied, with absorption rates varying depending on the form of supplementation (e.g., triglyceride vs. ethyl ester). The pharmacodynamics involve incorporation of omega-3 fatty acids into cell membranes and modulation of various physiological processes.

Overdosage: Consuming very high doses of fish oil supplements may increase the risk of bleeding, reduce immune function, or lead to gastrointestinal disturbances. Adherence to recommended dosages is advisable to prevent adverse effects.

International Standing: Fish oil supplements are widely available and recognized internationally for their health benefits. They are commonly used as a dietary supplement to support overall health and well-being, particularly in regions where fish consumption is limited.

Indian Standing: In India, fish oil supplements are increasingly popular as dietary supplements, particularly for cardiovascular health and cognitive function. They are readily available in pharmacies and health food stores and are used by individuals seeking to improve their omega-3 fatty acid intake.

Research Summary: Research on fish oil supplements supports their efficacy and safety for various health conditions, particularly cardiovascular disease, cognitive function, and inflammatory disorders. While more studies are needed to fully elucidate their mechanisms of action and optimal dosages, fish oil supplements remain a valuable nutritional intervention for promoting health and reducing the risk of chronic diseases.

38)FOENICULUM VULGARE

Introduction: Foeniculum vulgare, commonly known as fennel, is a flowering plant belonging to the Apiaceae family. It is native to the Mediterranean region but is now cultivated worldwide for its culinary and medicinal uses.

Synonym Name and Common Name: Synonym Name: Fennel seed Common Name: Fennel, Saunf (in Hindi), Perunjeeragam (in Tamil)

Pharmacognosy/Chemistry: Fennel contains various bioactive compounds, including volatile oils (such as anethole), flavonoids, phenolic compounds, and fatty acids. Its pharmacognostic characteristics include aromatic seeds with a sweet, licorice-like flavor.

Action and Pharmacology: Fennel exhibits carminative, antispasmodic, anti-inflammatory, and diuretic properties. Its pharmacological actions involve relaxing smooth muscles, reducing gas formation, and promoting digestion. Fennel may also have estrogenic effects and antioxidant activity.

Method of Analysis: Analytical methods such as gas chromatography-mass spectrometry (GC-MS), high-performance liquid chromatography (HPLC), and spectrophotometry are commonly used to analyze the chemical composition of fennel and quantify its bioactive constituents.

Health Benefits: Fennel is associated with various health benefits, including relieving digestive issues such as bloating, gas, and indigestion. It may also help alleviate menstrual discomfort, reduce inflammation, support lactation, and promote overall well-being.

Indication and Usage: Fennel is indicated for digestive disorders, including bloating, flatulence, and irritable bowel syndrome (IBS). It is commonly consumed as a tea, infusion, or added to culinary dishes for flavor and digestive support.

Usual Constituents with Percentages:

- Volatile oils (including anethole): 1-6%
- Flavonoids: 0.5-2%
- Phenolic compounds: 1-3%
- Fatty acids: 3-6% (Percentages may vary depending on the source and processing of fennel seeds)

Mechanism of Action: The mechanism of action of fennel involves the modulation of gastrointestinal motility, relaxation of smooth muscles, and inhibition of gas formation. Anethole, the major component of fennel oil, is thought to contribute to its carminative and antispasmodic effects.

Dosage: The typical dosage of fennel seeds for digestive support is 1-2 teaspoons (about 2-4 grams) per day, either chewed directly or steeped in hot water to make a tea. Fennel essential oil should be used in diluted form for aromatherapy or topical applications.

Contraindications: Fennel is generally safe for most individuals when consumed in food amounts. However, individuals with allergies to plants in the Apiaceae family (such as celery or carrot) may experience allergic reactions to fennel. Pregnant women should avoid excessive consumption of fennel due to its potential estrogenic effects.

Precautions: Individuals with estrogen-sensitive conditions, such as hormone-sensitive cancers or endometriosis, should use caution when consuming fennel due to its estrogenic activity. It is advisable to consult with a healthcare professional before using fennel supplements, particularly in high doses or for prolonged periods.

Adverse Reactions: Adverse reactions to fennel are rare but may include allergic reactions, such as skin rashes or respiratory symptoms, in sensitive individuals. Excessive consumption of fennel seeds or essential oil may also lead to nausea, vomiting, or allergic dermatitis in some people.

Research Standing: Research on the medicinal properties of fennel is ongoing, with studies investigating its efficacy in various health conditions, including digestive disorders, menstrual discomfort, and inflammation. While some studies support its traditional use and therapeutic potential, more research is needed to confirm its efficacy and safety.

Pharmacokinetics and Pharmacodynamics: The pharmacokinetics of fennel constituents have not been extensively studied. However, the pharmacodynamics involve the interaction of fennel compounds with gastrointestinal receptors, enzymes, and neurotransmitters, leading to modulation of digestive processes and smooth muscle relaxation.

Overdosage: Excessive consumption of fennel seeds or essential oil may lead to adverse effects such as nausea, vomiting, or allergic reactions. Adherence to recommended dosages and usage guidelines is advisable to prevent overdosage.

International Standing: Fennel is widely recognized and used internationally for its culinary and medicinal properties. It is included in various herbal remedies, dietary supplements, and personal care products for its aromatic flavor and potential health benefits.

Indian Standing: In India, fennel seeds (known as Saunf) are commonly used in culinary preparations, herbal teas, and traditional Ayurvedic medicine. Fennel tea is popular for its digestive properties and is often consumed after meals to aid digestion and freshen breath.

Research Summary: Research on fennel supports its traditional use for digestive issues and menstrual discomfort, with evidence suggesting carminative, antispasmodic, and anti-inflammatory effects. While more studies are needed to elucidate its mechanisms of action and clinical efficacy, fennel remains a popular and valued herb for promoting digestive health and overall well-being.

39) FREEZE-DRIED BANANA POWDER

Introduction: Freeze-dried banana powder is a powdered form of bananas created through the process of freeze-drying, which removes moisture while preserving the fruit's nutritional content. It offers a convenient and shelf-stable way to enjoy the health benefits of bananas.

Synonym Name and Common Name: Synonym Name: Banana powder Common Name: Freeze-dried banana powder, Banana flour

Pharmacognosy/Chemistry: Freeze-dried banana powder retains the nutritional composition of fresh bananas, including carbohydrates, dietary fiber, vitamins (such as vitamin C and B-vitamins), minerals (such as potassium and magnesium), and bioactive compounds like phenolic compounds and carotenoids.

Action and Pharmacology: Freeze-dried banana powder offers various health benefits, including supporting digestive health, providing energy, promoting heart health, and boosting immunity. Its pharmacological actions involve providing essential nutrients and bioactive compounds that support overall well-being.

Method of Analysis: Analytical methods such as high-performance liquid chromatography (HPLC), spectrophotometry, and proximate analysis are commonly used to analyze the nutritional composition of freeze-dried banana powder, including its carbohydrate, fiber, vitamin, mineral, and phytochemical content.

Health Benefits: Freeze-dried banana powder offers several health benefits, including improving digestion and gastrointestinal health, boosting energy levels, supporting heart health, enhancing immune function, and providing essential nutrients for overall well-being.

Indication and Usage: Freeze-dried banana powder is indicated for individuals seeking a convenient and nutritious way to incorporate bananas into their diet. It can be used in various culinary applications, including smoothies, baked goods, oatmeal, and as a natural sweetener in recipes.

Usual Constituents with Percentages:

- Carbohydrates: 70-80%
- Dietary fiber: 10-15%
- Protein: 2-4%
- Vitamins (such as vitamin C and B-vitamins)
- Minerals (such as potassium and magnesium)
- Bioactive compounds (such as phenolic compounds and carotenoids)

Mechanism of Action: The mechanism of action of freeze-dried banana powder involves providing essential nutrients, dietary fiber, and bioactive compounds that support various physiological processes in the body, including digestion, energy metabolism, immune function, and cardiovascular health.

Dosage: There is no standard dosage for freeze-dried banana powder as it can be incorporated into the diet based on individual preferences and dietary needs. It can be used in moderation as part of a balanced diet to reap its nutritional benefits.

Contraindications: Freeze-dried banana powder is generally safe for most individuals when consumed in food amounts. However, individuals with allergies to bananas should avoid its consumption. Additionally, those with certain medical conditions, such as diabetes, should monitor their intake due to its carbohydrate content.

Precautions: Individuals with allergies to bananas or other fruits in the Musaceae family should exercise caution when consuming freeze-dried banana powder. It is also advisable to read product labels carefully to ensure there are no added ingredients that may pose risks for certain individuals.

Adverse Reactions: Adverse reactions to freeze-dried banana powder are rare but may include allergic reactions in individuals with banana allergies. Excessive consumption may also lead to gastrointestinal discomfort in some individuals due to its fiber content.

Research Standing: Research on freeze-dried banana powder is limited compared to fresh bananas, but studies suggest that it retains much of the nutritional content and health benefits of fresh bananas. Further research is needed to fully elucidate its potential health effects and applications.

Pharmacokinetics and Pharmacodynamics: The pharmacokinetics and pharmacodynamics of freeze-dried banana powder have not been extensively studied. However, its nutritional components are expected to be absorbed and utilized by the body in a manner similar to fresh bananas.

Overdosage: There are no reports of overdosage with freeze-dried banana powder when consumed as part of a balanced diet. However, excessive consumption may lead to an imbalance in nutrient intake and potential adverse effects such as gastrointestinal discomfort.

International Standing: Freeze-dried banana powder is recognized internationally as a convenient and nutritious food ingredient. It is commonly used in various food products and culinary applications to provide flavor, texture, and nutritional benefits.

Indian Standing: In India, freeze-dried banana powder may not be as widely used compared to fresh bananas, but it is gaining popularity as a convenient and versatile food ingredient. It can be used in traditional Indian dishes, snacks, and desserts to enhance flavor and nutrition.

Research Summary: While research on freeze-dried banana powder is still emerging, preliminary studies suggest that it offers similar nutritional benefits to fresh bananas. Its convenient form and long shelf life make it a promising ingredient for various food products and dietary applications, but further research is needed to fully understand its health effects and potential applications.

40)GARCINIA GUMMI-GUTTA AND GARCINIA CAMBOGIA/G.INDICA

Introduction: Garcinia gummi-gutta, commonly known as Garcinia cambogia or Garcinia indica, is a tropical fruit-bearing tree native to Southeast Asia, India, and parts of Africa. It has gained attention for its potential health benefits, particularly for weight management.

Synonym Name and Common Name: Synonym Name: Malabar tamarind, Brindleberry Common Name: Garcinia cambogia, Garcinia indica, Kokum (in India)

Pharmacognosy/Chemistry: Garcinia gummi-gutta contains hydroxycitric acid (HCA) as its primary active ingredient, along with other phytochemicals such as xanthones and flavonoids. These compounds are mainly found in the fruit's rind and are responsible for its potential health benefits.

Action and Pharmacology: Garcinia gummi-gutta is believed to exert its effects primarily through hydroxycitric acid (HCA), which may inhibit the enzyme ATP citrate lyase, involved in fatty acid biosynthesis. This inhibition may lead to decreased fat accumulation and appetite suppression, potentially aiding in weight management.

Method of Analysis: Analytical methods such as high-performance liquid chromatography (HPLC) and spectrophotometry are commonly used to quantify the levels of hydroxycitric acid (HCA) and other phytochemicals in Garcinia gummi-gutta extracts.

Health Benefits: Garcinia gummi-gutta is purported to offer several health benefits, including weight management, appetite suppression, cholesterol reduction, and improved exercise performance. It is also traditionally used for digestive disorders and as a culinary ingredient.

Indication and Usage: Garcinia gummi-gutta supplements are indicated for individuals seeking support for weight management and appetite control. They are typically consumed orally in the form of capsules or liquid extracts, often before meals.

Usual Constituents with Percentages:

- Hydroxycitric acid (HCA): 10-50%
- Xanthones
- Flavonoids (Percentages may vary depending on the source and processing of Garcinia gummi-gutta extracts)

Mechanism of Action: The primary mechanism of action of Garcinia gummi-gutta is believed to be through the inhibition of ATP citrate lyase by hydroxycitric acid (HCA), leading to reduced fatty acid synthesis and increased fat oxidation. HCA may also suppress appetite by increasing serotonin levels in the brain.

Dosage: The typical dosage of Garcinia gummi-gutta supplements varies depending on the concentration of hydroxycitric acid (HCA) and the specific product formulation. Dosages commonly range from 500 mg to 1500 mg per day, taken before meals.

Contraindications: Garcinia gummi-gutta supplements are generally considered safe for most individuals when taken at recommended dosages. However, individuals with known allergies to Garcinia species or those with certain medical conditions should use caution or consult with a healthcare professional before use.

Precautions: Pregnant or breastfeeding women, individuals with diabetes, and those taking medications should exercise caution or consult with a healthcare professional before using Garcinia gummi-gutta supplements due to potential interactions or effects on blood sugar levels.

Adverse Reactions: Adverse reactions to Garcinia gummi-gutta supplements are rare but may include gastrointestinal discomfort, headache, dizziness, or allergic reactions in sensitive individuals. Excessive consumption or high doses may increase the risk of adverse effects.

Research Standing: Research on the efficacy of Garcinia gummi-gutta for weight management and other health benefits is mixed, with some studies suggesting positive effects while others show no significant difference compared to placebo. More rigorous clinical trials are needed to establish its effectiveness and safety conclusively.

Pharmacokinetics and Pharmacodynamics: The pharmacokinetics and pharmacodynamics of Garcinia gummi-gutta, particularly its active component hydroxycitric acid (HCA), have been studied to a limited extent. Further research is needed to elucidate its absorption, distribution, metabolism, and excretion in humans.

Overdosage: Consuming high doses of Garcinia gummi-gutta supplements may increase the risk of adverse effects such as gastrointestinal discomfort, headache, or dizziness. Adherence to recommended dosages is advisable to minimize the risk of overdosage.

International Standing: Garcinia gummi-gutta supplements are widely available internationally and are marketed for weight management and other health benefits. However, regulatory agencies in some countries have raised concerns about their safety and efficacy.

Indian Standing: In India, Garcinia gummi-gutta, known as Garcinia cambogia or Garcinia indica, has a long history of traditional use in Ayurvedic medicine, particularly for digestive disorders and culinary purposes. It is also used as a natural flavoring agent in Indian cuisine.

Research Summary: Research on Garcinia gummi-gutta, particularly its active compound hydroxycitric acid (HCA), suggests potential benefits for weight management and appetite control. However, conflicting evidence and concerns about safety and efficacy warrant further investigation through well-designed clinical trials.

41)GARCINIA MANGOSTANA

Introduction: Garcinia mangostana, commonly known as mangosteen, is a tropical evergreen tree native to Southeast Asia. It produces a fruit of the same name, which is highly valued for its sweet and tangy flavor, as well as its potential health benefits.

Synonym Name and Common Name: Synonym Name: Mangosteen fruit Common Name: Mangosteen

Pharmacognosy/Chemistry: Mangosteen contains various bioactive compounds, including xanthones (such as alpha-mangostin and gamma-mangostin), flavonoids, tannins, and phenolic acids. These phytochemicals contribute to the fruit's antioxidant and anti-inflammatory properties.

Action and Pharmacology: Mangosteen is believed to exert antioxidant, anti-inflammatory, antimicrobial, and anticancer effects. Its pharmacological actions involve scavenging free radicals, inhibiting inflammatory pathways, and modulating cellular processes associated with disease progression.

Method of Analysis: Analytical methods such as high-performance liquid chromatography (HPLC), gas chromatography-mass spectrometry (GC-MS), and spectrophotometry are commonly used to analyze the chemical composition of mangosteen extracts and quantify the levels of bioactive compounds.

Health Benefits: Mangosteen is associated with various health benefits, including antioxidant protection, immune support, cardiovascular health, digestive health, and potential anticancer effects. It is also valued for its anti-inflammatory properties and role in skin health.

Indication and Usage: Mangosteen supplements are indicated for individuals seeking antioxidant support, immune enhancement, or general health maintenance. They are typically consumed orally in the form of capsules, juices, or extracts.

Usual Constituents with Percentages:

- Xanthones (such as alpha-mangostin and gamma-mangostin): 1-5%
- Flavonoids
- Tannins
- Phenolic acids (Percentages may vary depending on the source and processing of mangosteen extracts)

Mechanism of Action: The mechanism of action of mangosteen's bioactive compounds involves neutralizing free radicals, inhibiting inflammatory enzymes, modulating immune responses, and interfering with cellular processes associated with oxidative stress and inflammation.

Dosage: The typical dosage of mangosteen supplements varies depending on the product formulation and intended use. Dosages commonly range from 500 mg to 1500 mg per day, divided into two or three doses.

Contraindications: Mangosteen supplements are generally considered safe for most individuals when taken at recommended dosages. However, individuals with known allergies to mangosteen or its constituents should avoid its consumption.

Precautions: Pregnant or breastfeeding women, individuals with certain medical conditions, or those taking medications should consult with a healthcare professional before using mangosteen supplements, particularly in high doses or for prolonged periods.

Adverse Reactions: Adverse reactions to mangosteen supplements are rare but may include gastrointestinal discomfort, allergic reactions, or interactions with certain medications. Excessive consumption or high doses may increase the risk of adverse effects.

Research Standing: Research on the health effects of mangosteen, particularly its antioxidant and anti-inflammatory properties, is ongoing. While some studies support its potential health benefits, more research is needed to confirm its efficacy and safety in humans.

Pharmacokinetics and Pharmacodynamics: The pharmacokinetics and pharmacodynamics of mangosteen bioactive compounds, particularly xanthones, have been studied to a limited extent. Further research is needed to understand their absorption, distribution, metabolism, and excretion in humans.

Overdosage: Consuming high doses of mangosteen supplements may increase the risk of adverse effects such as gastrointestinal discomfort or allergic reactions. Adherence to recommended dosages is advisable to minimize the risk of overdosage.

International Standing: Mangosteen supplements are recognized internationally for their potential health benefits and are marketed for various health purposes, including antioxidant support, immune enhancement, and general well-being.

Indian Standing: In India, mangosteen is valued for its culinary and medicinal uses. It is consumed fresh as a fruit, and its extracts are used in traditional Ayurvedic medicine for various health conditions, including digestive disorders, inflammation, and skin ailments.

Research Summary: Research on mangosteen suggests potential health benefits, particularly for antioxidant protection, anti-inflammatory effects, and immune support. While some studies support its traditional use and therapeutic potential, more rigorous clinical trials are needed to confirm its efficacy and safety for various health conditions

42)GLYCYRRHIZA GLABRA – EXTRACT

Introduction: Glycyrrhiza glabra, commonly known as licorice, is a perennial herb native to the Mediterranean and certain parts of Asia. It has been used for centuries in traditional medicine for its various health benefits, particularly in treating respiratory and digestive ailments.

Synonym Name and Common Name: Synonym Name: Licorice root Common Name: Licorice

Pharmacognosy/Chemistry: Licorice root contains numerous bioactive compounds, including glycyrrhizin, flavonoids (such as liquiritin and isoliquiritin), and saponins. These compounds contribute to licorice's characteristic sweet flavor and its medicinal properties.

Action and Pharmacology: Licorice exhibits several pharmacological actions, including anti-inflammatory, antiviral, antioxidant, immunomodulatory, and hepatoprotective effects. Its pharmacological actions are attributed to its bioactive constituents, particularly glycyrrhizin and flavonoids.

Method of Analysis: Analytical methods such as high-performance liquid chromatography (HPLC), gas chromatography-mass spectrometry (GC-MS), and spectrophotometry are commonly used to analyze the chemical composition of licorice extracts and quantify the levels of bioactive compounds.

Health Benefits: Licorice is associated with various health benefits, including soothing respiratory conditions (such as coughs and sore throats), supporting digestive health, protecting the liver, and potentially providing relief from menopausal symptoms.

Indication and Usage: Licorice supplements or extracts are indicated for individuals seeking relief from respiratory ailments, digestive discomfort, or liver support. It is commonly consumed orally in the form of teas, capsules, or liquid extracts.

Usual Constituents with Percentages:

- Glycyrrhizin: 5-20%
- Flavonoids (such as liquiritin and isoliquiritin)
- Saponins (Percentages may vary depending on the source and processing of licorice extracts)

Mechanism of Action: The mechanism of action of licorice is multifaceted and involves modulation of various biochemical pathways, including inhibition of pro-inflammatory enzymes, enhancement of immune function, and protection against oxidative stress.

Dosage: The typical dosage of licorice supplements varies depending on the product formulation and intended use. Dosages commonly range from 200 mg to 600 mg of licorice extract per day, taken orally in divided doses.

Contraindications: Licorice supplements should be used with caution or avoided by individuals with certain medical conditions, such as hypertension, potassium deficiency, or hormonal imbalances. Pregnant or breastfeeding women should also consult with a healthcare professional before use.

Precautions: Long-term or excessive consumption of licorice supplements may lead to adverse effects, including hypertension, hypokalemia (low potassium levels), and hormonal disturbances. Individuals with underlying medical conditions should use licorice supplements under medical supervision.

Adverse Reactions: Adverse reactions to licorice supplements are rare but may include hypertension, fluid retention, electrolyte imbalances, and hormonal disruptions in susceptible individuals. Excessive consumption or prolonged use may increase the risk of adverse effects.

Research Standing: Research on licorice's health benefits and safety profile is extensive, with numerous studies supporting its traditional uses and pharmacological effects. However, more research is needed to elucidate its mechanisms of action and optimize its therapeutic applications.

Pharmacokinetics and Pharmacodynamics: The pharmacokinetics and pharmacodynamics of licorice bioactive compounds, particularly glycyrrhizin, have been studied to some extent. Further research is needed to understand their absorption, distribution, metabolism, and excretion in humans.

Overdosage: Consuming high doses of licorice supplements may lead to adverse effects such as hypertension, hypokalemia, or hormonal disturbances. Adherence to recommended dosages and usage guidelines is essential to minimize the risk of overdosage.

International Standing: Licorice supplements are widely available internationally and are recognized for their potential health benefits. However, regulatory agencies in some countries have issued warnings regarding the potential risks associated with excessive consumption.

Indian Standing: In India, licorice has a long history of traditional use in Ayurvedic medicine for various health conditions, including respiratory ailments, digestive disorders, and skin conditions. It is commonly used in herbal formulations and culinary preparations.

Research Summary: Research on licorice supports its traditional uses and pharmacological effects, particularly its anti-inflammatory, antiviral, and hepatoprotective properties. While generally considered safe when used appropriately, licorice supplements should be used with caution, particularly in high doses or for prolonged periods, due to the risk of adverse effects.

43) GRAPE SEED EXTRACT

Introduction: Grape seed extract (GSE) is derived from the seeds of grapes (Vitis vinifera). It is rich in antioxidants, primarily oligomeric proanthocyanidin complexes (OPCs), which are believed to contribute to its health benefits. GSE has gained popularity as a dietary supplement due to its potential therapeutic properties.

Synonym name and common name: Synonym name: Vitis vinifera seed extract Common name: Grape seed extract

Pharmacognosy/Chemistry: Grape seed extract contains a variety of phytochemicals, including flavonoids, phenolic acids, and procyanidins. The main constituents responsible for its bioactivity are oligomeric proanthocyanidin complexes (OPCs), which are potent antioxidants.

Action and pharmacology: Grape seed extract exerts antioxidant, anti-inflammatory, and vasodilatory effects. It scavenges free radicals, protects cells from oxidative damage, and helps maintain cardiovascular health. Additionally, it may improve microcirculation and enhance collagen synthesis, benefiting skin health.

Method of analysis: GSE can be analyzed using various methods, including high-performance liquid chromatography (HPLC), gas chromatography-mass spectrometry (GC-MS), and spectrophotometry. These techniques allow for the identification and quantification of its phytochemical constituents.

Health benefits:

- Antioxidant protection against oxidative stress
- Cardiovascular support by promoting healthy blood circulation and lipid profiles
- Anti-inflammatory effects, potentially beneficial for conditions like arthritis
- Skin health enhancement through collagen synthesis and UV protection

Indication and usage: Grape seed extract is commonly used as a dietary supplement for:

- Antioxidant support
- Cardiovascular health
- Skin health It may also be used adjunctively in the management of certain inflammatory conditions.

Usual constituents with percentages: The composition of grape seed extract can vary, but typical percentages of its major constituents include:

- Oligomeric proanthocyanidin complexes (OPCs): 60-80%
- Flavonoids: 5-20%
- Phenolic acids: 5-15%

Mechanism of action: GSE's antioxidant activity is primarily attributed to its ability to scavenge free radicals and inhibit oxidative damage to cells and tissues. It also modulates various signaling pathways involved in inflammation and vascular function, contributing to its therapeutic effects.

Dosage: Dosage recommendations for grape seed extract vary depending on the specific product and intended use. However, typical doses range from 100 mg to 300 mg per day, taken orally with meals.

Contraindications: Grape seed extract is generally considered safe for most people when taken at recommended doses. However, individuals allergic to grapes should avoid its use. Additionally, pregnant and breastfeeding women should consult their healthcare provider before using GSE supplements.

Precautions:

- Individuals with bleeding disorders or those taking anticoagulant medications should use grape seed extract with caution due to its potential antiplatelet effects.
- It is advisable to discontinue use at least two weeks before scheduled surgery to avoid potential bleeding risks.

Adverse reactions: Grape seed extract is well-tolerated by most individuals when taken at recommended doses. However, high doses may cause minor gastrointestinal discomfort, such as nausea or diarrhea, in some people.

Research standing: Research on grape seed extract has demonstrated promising results in various areas, including cardiovascular health, antioxidant protection, and skin health. However, further clinical studies are needed to fully elucidate its therapeutic potential and optimal dosage regimens.

Pharmacokinetics and pharmacodynamics: Grape seed extract is absorbed in the gastrointestinal tract, with bioavailability influenced by factors such as formulation and individual metabolism. Once absorbed, its bioactive constituents exert antioxidant and other pharmacological effects throughout the body.

Overdosage: There is limited information on the effects of grape seed extract overdose. However, exceeding recommended doses may increase the risk of adverse reactions, particularly gastrointestinal symptoms and potential bleeding complications in susceptible individuals.

International standing: Grape seed extract is widely available as a dietary supplement in many countries and is generally considered safe for consumption. Regulatory agencies such as the FDA (Food and Drug Administration) in the United States and EFSA (European Food Safety Authority) in Europe have established guidelines for its use as a food supplement.

Indian standing: In India, grape seed extract is recognized for its health benefits and is commonly used in Ayurvedic and traditional medicine practices. It is available in various forms, including capsules, tablets, and liquid extracts, and is often incorporated into wellness products.

Research summary: Research on grape seed extract continues to expand, exploring its potential applications in various health conditions. Studies have shown promising results in areas such as cardiovascular health, antioxidant protection, and skin health. Ongoing research aims to further elucidate its mechanisms of action, optimize dosage regimens, and explore potential synergies with other natural compounds.

44)COFFEA ARABICA, C. ROBUSTA- GREEN COFFEE SEED EXTRACT STANDARDIZED, INCLUDING DECAFFEINATED COFFEE BEAN POWDER/EXTRACT

Introduction: Green coffee seed extract is derived from the seeds of Coffea arabica and Coffea robusta plants before they are roasted, retaining higher levels of bioactive compounds compared to roasted coffee beans. It has gained attention for its potential health benefits, including weight management and antioxidant properties.

Synonym name and common name: Synonym name: Coffea arabica extract, Coffea robusta extract Common name: Green coffee seed extract

Pharmacognosy/Chemistry: Green coffee seed extract contains a complex mixture of bioactive compounds, including chlorogenic acids (CGAs), caffeine, trigonelline, and antioxidants such as caffeic acid and ferulic acid. The composition may vary depending on factors like plant species and extraction method.

Action and pharmacology: The primary bioactive components of green coffee seed extract, particularly chlorogenic acids and caffeine, contribute to its pharmacological effects. Chlorogenic acids exhibit antioxidant and anti-inflammatory properties, while caffeine stimulates the central nervous system and may enhance metabolic rate and fat oxidation.

Method of analysis: Analytical methods such as high-performance liquid chromatography (HPLC) and gas chromatography-mass spectrometry (GC-MS) are commonly used to quantify the levels of chlorogenic acids, caffeine, and other constituents in green coffee seed extract.

Health benefits:

- Weight management: Green coffee seed extract is believed to support weight loss by increasing metabolism and promoting fat burning.
- Antioxidant protection: Its high content of chlorogenic acids contributes to antioxidant activity, helping to neutralize free radicals and reduce oxidative stress.

- Blood sugar regulation: Some studies suggest that chlorogenic acids may improve insulin sensitivity and regulate blood glucose levels.
- Cardiovascular health: Antioxidants in green coffee seed extract may help reduce the risk of cardiovascular diseases by improving lipid profiles and reducing inflammation.

Indication and usage: Green coffee seed extract is commonly used as a dietary supplement for:

- Weight management and fat loss
- Antioxidant support
- Blood sugar regulation It is often consumed in the form of capsules, tablets, or powdered extracts.

Usual constituents with percentages: The composition of green coffee seed extract can vary, but typical percentages of its major constituents include:

- Chlorogenic acids: 30-50%
- Caffeine: 1-5%
- Trigonelline: 1-3%
- Antioxidants (e.g., caffeic acid, ferulic acid): <1%

Mechanism of action: The mechanisms underlying the effects of green coffee seed extract involve:

- Chlorogenic acids: Inhibition of glucose absorption, modulation of lipid metabolism, and antioxidant activity.
- Caffeine: Stimulation of the central nervous system, increased metabolic rate, and promotion of fat oxidation.

Dosage: Dosage recommendations for green coffee seed extract vary, but typical doses range from 200 mg to 400 mg per day, taken orally with meals. It is often standardized to contain a specific percentage of chlorogenic acids.

Contraindications: Green coffee seed extract is generally safe for most people when taken at recommended doses. However, individuals sensitive to caffeine or with certain medical conditions, such as anxiety disorders or cardiovascular diseases, should use it with caution or avoid it altogether.

Precautions:

- Pregnant and breastfeeding women should consult their healthcare provider before using green coffee seed extract.
- Individuals with caffeine sensitivity or insomnia should limit their intake of green coffee extract, especially products containing high levels of caffeine.

Adverse reactions: Common adverse reactions to green coffee seed extract may include:

- Gastrointestinal discomfort (e.g., nausea, diarrhea)
- Insomnia or jitteriness due to caffeine content
- Increased heart rate or palpitations in sensitive individuals

Research standing: Research on green coffee seed extract has generated mixed results, with some studies supporting its efficacy for weight management and others showing inconclusive or conflicting findings. Further clinical trials are needed to elucidate its effects on weight loss, metabolic health, and other potential therapeutic uses.

Pharmacokinetics and pharmacodynamics: After oral ingestion, the bioactive compounds in green coffee seed extract are absorbed in the gastrointestinal tract and enter systemic circulation. Chlorogenic acids and caffeine undergo metabolism in the liver and are subsequently excreted in urine. The pharmacodynamic effects include stimulation of the central nervous system, increased thermogenesis, and modulation of lipid metabolism.

Overdosage: Excessive consumption of green coffee seed extract, particularly high doses of caffeine, may lead to adverse effects such as gastrointestinal upset, insomnia, anxiety, and cardiovascular symptoms. It is important to adhere to recommended dosage guidelines and monitor caffeine intake from other dietary sources.

International standing: Green coffee seed extract is widely available as a dietary supplement in many countries and is often marketed for weight management and antioxidant support. Regulatory agencies such as the FDA (Food and Drug Administration) in the United States and EFSA (European Food Safety Authority) in Europe regulate its use as a food supplement.

Indian standing: In India, green coffee seed extract is recognized for its potential health benefits and is commonly used in dietary supplements marketed for weight management and metabolic health. It is available in various forms, including capsules, tablets, and powdered extracts.

Research summary: Research on green coffee seed extract has focused primarily on its potential role in weight management, with some studies suggesting modest benefits in reducing body weight and body fat. However, the overall evidence remains inconclusive, and more rigorous clinical trials are needed to determine its long-term efficacy and safety. Additionally, further research is warranted to explore its potential effects on other health outcomes, such as blood sugar regulation and cardiovascular health.

45)GRIFOLAFRONDOSA

Introduction: Grifolafrondosa, commonly known as maitake mushroom, is a species of mushroom native to Northeastern Japan and North America. It is revered in traditional Chinese and Japanese medicine for its purported health benefits.

Synonym Name and Common Name: Synonym Name: Hen of the woods Common Name: Maitake Mushroom

Pharmacognosy/Chemistry: Grifolafrondosa contains various bioactive compounds, including polysaccharides, beta-glucans, ergosterol, and various minerals and vitamins.

Action and Pharmacology: Maitake mushrooms are believed to have immunomodulatory effects, meaning they can regulate the immune system. They also possess anti-inflammatory and antioxidant properties.

Method of Analysis: Analytical methods for Grifolafrondosa typically involve chromatographic techniques such as high-performance liquid chromatography (HPLC) or gas chromatography (GC), coupled with mass spectrometry (MS) for identification and quantification of its constituents.

Health Benefits: Grifolafrondosa is believed to offer numerous health benefits, including immune system support, anti-inflammatory effects, cholesterol regulation, blood sugar control, and potential anticancer properties.

Indication and Usage: It is used as a dietary supplement for immune support, to reduce inflammation, regulate blood sugar levels, and potentially aid in cancer treatment.

Usual Constituents with Percentages:

- Polysaccharides: 25-30%
- Beta-glucans: 15-20%
- Ergosterol: 1-2%
- Other minerals and vitamins

Mechanism of Action: The polysaccharides and beta-glucans in maitake mushrooms are thought to stimulate immune cells, such as macrophages and T cells, enhancing the body's defense mechanisms against infections and potentially cancer cells.

Dosage: Dosage can vary depending on the formulation and individual health conditions. Typical doses range from 500 mg to 3 grams per day, taken orally in divided doses.

Contraindications: There are no widely reported contraindications, but individuals with mushroom allergies should avoid maitake supplements.

Precautions: Pregnant and breastfeeding women should consult with a healthcare professional before using maitake supplements.

Adverse Reactions: Adverse reactions are rare but may include mild gastrointestinal upset or allergic reactions in susceptible individuals.

Research Standing: Research on Grifolafrondosa is ongoing, with numerous studies investigating its potential health benefits, particularly in immunology and oncology.

Pharmacokinetics: The pharmacokinetics of Grifolafrondosa constituents have not been extensively studied, but absorption is likely to occur in the gastrointestinal tract, with metabolites circulating in the bloodstream.

Pharmacodynamics: Maitake mushrooms exert their pharmacodynamic effects primarily through modulation of the immune system and antioxidant activity.

Overdosage: There are no reports of toxicity from maitake mushroom overdosage, but excessive consumption may lead to gastrointestinal discomfort in some individuals.

International Standing: Maitake mushrooms are recognized internationally as a dietary supplement with potential health benefits, but specific regulations may vary by country.

Indian Standing: In India, maitake mushrooms are gaining popularity as a health supplement, but regulatory frameworks for their use may still be evolving.

Research Summary: Research on Grifolafrondosa suggests promising health benefits, particularly in immune modulation and potential anticancer effects. Further studies are needed to elucidate its mechanisms of action and optimal therapeutic applications.

46) GUAR GUM AND GUM ARABIC AND ITS DERIVATIVES AS A SOURCE OF FIBERS; MALTODEXTRIN/ RESISTANT MALTODEXTRIN/ LIMIT DEXTRIN; CHIA SEED FIBER AND FIBERS FROM OTHER FOOD SOURCES

Introduction: Dietary fibers are essential components of the human diet, known for their role in promoting digestive health, regulating blood sugar levels, and supporting weight management. Guar gum, gum arabic, maltodextrin, resistant maltodextrin, limit dextrin, chia seed fiber, and fibers from other food sources are all valuable sources of dietary fiber.

Synonym Names and Common Names:

- Guar gum: Guar flour, Guaran
- Gum arabic: Acacia gum
- Maltodextrin: Glucidex, Maltrin

- Resistant maltodextrin: Fibersol, Fibersym
- Limit dextrin: Amylomaize
- Chia seed fiber: Salvia hispanicafiber

Pharmacognosy/Chemistry: These fibers vary in their chemical composition and structure. Guar gum and gum arabic are polysaccharides derived from plants, while maltodextrin and its derivatives are complex carbohydrates produced from starch. Chia seed fiber is rich in soluble and insoluble fiber.

Action and Pharmacology: Dietary fibers act primarily as bulking agents in the digestive tract, promoting regular bowel movements and preventing constipation. They also contribute to satiety, aiding in weight management, and help regulate blood sugar levels by slowing down glucose absorption.

Method of Analysis: Analytical methods for assessing dietary fibers include gravimetric methods, enzymatic methods, and chromatographic techniques such as high-performance liquid chromatography (HPLC).

Health Benefits: Consumption of dietary fibers has been associated with numerous health benefits, including improved digestive health, weight management, blood sugar regulation, cholesterol reduction, and reduced risk of chronic diseases such as heart disease and diabetes.

Indication and Usage: These fibers are commonly used as food additives to increase fiber content in processed foods, beverages, and dietary supplements. They can also be consumed directly as supplements or incorporated into recipes to boost fiber intake.

Usual Constituents with Percentages:

- Guar gum: Typically contains 75-85% soluble fiber
- Gum arabic: Mainly composed of soluble fiber
- Maltodextrin: Primarily composed of short-chain carbohydrates
- Resistant maltodextrin: Contains indigestible oligosaccharides
- Limit dextrin: Produced from starch hydrolysis, composed of short-chain carbohydrates
- Chia seed fiber: Contains both soluble and insoluble fiber

Mechanism of Action: Dietary fibers absorb water in the digestive tract, forming a gel-like substance that adds bulk to stool and facilitates its passage through the intestines. They also slow down the digestion and absorption of carbohydrates, leading to more stable blood sugar levels.

Dosage: Recommended dosage varies depending on individual dietary needs and health goals. Generally, dietary guidelines recommend consuming 25-38 grams of fiber per day for adults.

Contraindications: Individuals with specific gastrointestinal conditions may need to limit their intake of certain types of fiber, such as those with irritable bowel syndrome (IBS) or inflammatory bowel disease (IBD).

Precautions: It is essential to increase fiber intake gradually and drink plenty of water to prevent gastrointestinal discomfort, such as bloating and gas.

Adverse Reactions: Excessive consumption of certain types of fiber, especially insoluble fibers, may cause digestive discomfort in some individuals, such as abdominal cramps or diarrhea.

Research Standing: Research on the health effects of dietary fibers, including guar gum, gum arabic, maltodextrin, resistant maltodextrin, limit dextrin, chia seed fiber, and fibers from other food sources, is extensive and ongoing, with many studies supporting their beneficial effects on various aspects of health.

Pharmacokinetics: The pharmacokinetics of dietary fibers involve their passage through the digestive tract, where they undergo fermentation by gut bacteria, producing short-chain fatty acids and other metabolites that contribute to their health effects.

Pharmacodynamics: Dietary fibers exert their pharmacodynamic effects primarily in the gastrointestinal tract, where they influence digestion, absorption, and fermentation processes.

Overdosage: Excessive consumption of dietary fibers can lead to gastrointestinal discomfort, such as bloating, gas, and diarrhea. It is essential to consume fibers within recommended daily intake levels.

International Standing: Dietary fibers are recognized internationally as important components of a healthy diet, and regulatory agencies provide guidelines for their use in food and dietary supplements.

Indian Standing: In India, dietary fibers are gaining attention for their health benefits, and there is growing interest in incorporating them into traditional diets and food products.

Research Summary: Research on guar gum, gum arabic, maltodextrin, resistant maltodextrin, limit dextrin, chia seed fiber, and fibers from other food sources consistently demonstrates their positive effects on digestive health, weight management, blood sugar regulation, and overall well-being. Continued research into their mechanisms of action and optimal usage is warranted to further elucidate their potential health benefits.

47)HIGH OLEIC SUN FLOWER OIL AND OTHER VEGETABLE OILS WITH HIGH OLEIC CONTENT

Introduction: High oleic sunflower oil and other vegetable oils with high oleic content are plant-based oils derived from sunflower seeds or other oleaginous plants. They are characterized by their high levels of monounsaturated fats, particularly oleic acid.

Synonym Names and Common Names: Synonym Names: High oleic oils Common Names: High oleic sunflower oil, high oleic canola oil, high oleic safflower oil, etc.

Pharmacognosy/Chemistry: High oleic oils are predominantly composed of oleic acid (typically over 70%), a monounsaturated omega-9 fatty acid. They also contain smaller amounts of saturated and polyunsaturated fats.

Action and Pharmacology: The high oleic acid content in these oils contributes to their health benefits, including cardiovascular protection, improved lipid profiles, and oxidative stability.

Method of Analysis: Analytical methods for assessing the fatty acid composition and quality of high oleic oils typically involve gas chromatography (GC) or high-performance liquid chromatography (HPLC) techniques.

Health Benefits: Consumption of high oleic oils has been associated with several health benefits, including reduced risk of cardiovascular disease, improved cholesterol levels, and better insulin sensitivity.

Indication and Usage: High oleic oils are commonly used in food preparation, cooking, and as ingredients in processed foods, snacks, and salad dressings. They are also utilized in cosmetic products and industrial applications.

Usual Constituents with Percentages:

- Oleic acid: Over 70%
- Saturated fats: Less than 10%
- Polyunsaturated fats: Variable, but typically lower than in traditional oils

Mechanism of Action: The high oleic acid content in these oils contributes to their beneficial effects on health by reducing inflammation, improving lipid metabolism, and enhancing cellular function.

Dosage: There is no specific dosage for high oleic oils, as they are consumed as part of the diet. Daily intake should be within recommended dietary guidelines for fats and oils.

Contraindications: There are no specific contraindications for high oleic oils, but individuals with allergies to sunflower seeds or other components of the oils should avoid them.

Precautions: It is essential to store high oleic oils properly to maintain their freshness and quality, avoiding exposure to heat, light, and air.

Adverse Reactions: Adverse reactions to high oleic oils are rare but may include allergic reactions in susceptible individuals or gastrointestinal discomfort in some cases of excessive consumption.

Research Standing: Research on high oleic oils, particularly high oleic sunflower oil, has demonstrated their potential health benefits and applications in various fields, including nutrition, medicine, and industry.

Pharmacokinetics: The absorption and metabolism of high oleic oils are similar to those of other dietary fats, with oleic acid being readily absorbed in the intestines and utilized by the body for energy and cellular functions.

Pharmacodynamics: High oleic oils exert their pharmacodynamic effects primarily through their fatty acid composition, influencing lipid metabolism, inflammation, and oxidative stress.

Overdosage: Excessive consumption of high oleic oils can contribute to weight gain and adverse effects associated with high-fat diets. Moderation is advised.

International Standing: High oleic oils are recognized internationally as valuable sources of dietary fats with potential health benefits, and they are widely used in food production and other industries.

Indian Standing: In India, high oleic oils are gaining popularity as healthier alternatives to traditional cooking oils, and they are increasingly used in food processing and culinary applications.

Research Summary: Research on high oleic oils, including high oleic sunflower oil and other vegetable oils with high oleic content, indicates their potential to promote cardiovascular health, improve lipid profiles, and provide stable cooking oils for culinary use. Continued research is needed to explore their full range of health benefits and applications in various fields.

48)HIPPOPHAERHAMNOIDES

Introduction: Hippophaerhamnoides, commonly known as sea buckthorn, is a deciduous shrub native to Europe and Asia. It has been used for centuries in traditional medicine due to its purported health benefits.

Synonym Name and Common Name: Synonym Name: Sea buckthorn Common Name: Sandthorn, sallowthorn

Pharmacognosy/Chemistry: Sea buckthorn is rich in bioactive compounds, including vitamins (such as vitamin C, vitamin E, and vitamin A), flavonoids, carotenoids, fatty acids (such as omega-3, omega-6, omega-7, and omega-9), and phenolic compounds.

Action and Pharmacology: Sea buckthorn exhibits antioxidant, anti-inflammatory, immunomodulatory, and tissue-regenerative properties. It is also known for its skin-healing and cardioprotective effects.

Method of Analysis: Analytical methods for sea buckthorn typically involve extraction of its bioactive compounds followed by chromatographic techniques such as high-performance liquid chromatography (HPLC) or gas chromatography-mass spectrometry (GC-MS) for identification and quantification.

Health Benefits: Sea buckthorn is associated with various health benefits, including boosting immune function, promoting cardiovascular health, improving skin health, supporting gastrointestinal health, and reducing inflammation.

Indication and Usage: It is used in traditional medicine for treating various ailments, including wounds, gastrointestinal disorders, skin conditions, and cardiovascular diseases. It is also consumed as a dietary supplement or used topically in skincare products.

Usual Constituents with Percentages:

- Vitamin C: Up to 15%
- Vitamin E: Up to 5%
- Carotenoids: Up to 4%
- Omega-3, omega-6, omega-7, omega-9 fatty acids
- Flavonoids and phenolic compounds

Mechanism of Action: The diverse array of bioactive compounds in sea buckthorn exert their effects through antioxidant activity, modulation of inflammatory pathways, enhancement of immune function, and promotion of tissue repair and regeneration.

Dosage: Dosage of sea buckthorn supplements can vary depending on the formulation and intended use. Typical doses range from 500 mg to 3000 mg per day, taken orally in divided doses.

Contraindications: Sea buckthorn may interact with certain medications or exacerbate certain medical conditions. Individuals with allergies to sea buckthorn or its components should avoid its use.

Precautions: Pregnant or breastfeeding women, as well as individuals with pre-existing medical conditions, should consult with a healthcare professional before using sea buckthorn supplements.

Adverse Reactions: Adverse reactions to sea buckthorn supplements are rare but may include gastrointestinal upset, allergic reactions, or interactions with medications.

Research Standing: Research on sea buckthorn has grown substantially in recent years, with numerous studies investigating its pharmacological properties and potential health benefits in various medical conditions.

Pharmacokinetics: The pharmacokinetics of sea buckthorn constituents vary depending on the specific compound. Absorption of its bioactive compounds occurs primarily in the gastrointestinal tract, with metabolites distributed throughout the body.

Pharmacodynamics: Sea buckthorn exerts its pharmacodynamic effects through its antioxidant, anti-inflammatory, immunomodulatory, and tissue-regenerative properties, which collectively contribute to its health benefits.

Overdosage: Excessive consumption of sea buckthorn supplements may lead to adverse effects such as gastrointestinal discomfort or interference with blood clotting due to its vitamin K content.

International Standing: Sea buckthorn is recognized internationally for its medicinal and nutritional properties, and its products are available in various forms, including dietary supplements, skincare products, and functional foods.

Indian Standing: In India, sea buckthorn is gaining popularity for its health benefits, and research on its therapeutic applications is ongoing. It is also cultivated in some regions of India for commercial purposes.

Research Summary: Research on sea buckthorn indicates its potential as a natural remedy for various health conditions, including immune disorders, cardiovascular diseases, skin ailments, and gastrointestinal disorders. Further studies are needed to elucidate its mechanisms of action and optimize its therapeutic applications.

49)HUMULUS LUPULUS L

Introduction: Humulus lupulus L., commonly known as hops, is a perennial vine belonging to the Cannabaceae family. It is primarily cultivated for its use in brewing beer but also possesses medicinal properties.

Synonym Name and Common Name: Synonym Name: Hop strobiles Common Name: Hops

Pharmacognosy/Chemistry: Hops contain various bioactive compounds, including bitter acids (such as humulone and lupulone), essential oils (such as myrcene and humulene), flavonoids, and polyphenols.

Action and Pharmacology: The bioactive compounds in hops contribute to its sedative, anxiolytic, anti-inflammatory, and estrogenic effects. It also exhibits antimicrobial properties.

Method of Analysis: Analytical methods for hops typically involve extraction of its bioactive compounds followed by chromatographic techniques such as high-performance liquid chromatography (HPLC) or gas chromatography-mass spectrometry (GC-MS) for identification and quantification.

Health Benefits: Hops are associated with various health benefits, including promoting relaxation, improving sleep quality, reducing anxiety, alleviating menopausal symptoms, and possessing antioxidant properties.

Indication and Usage: Hops are used in traditional medicine for treating insomnia, anxiety, restlessness, and menopausal symptoms. It is also consumed as a dietary supplement or used in herbal preparations and aromatherapy.

Usual Constituents with Percentages:

- Bitter acids: Up to 5%
- Essential oils: Up to 2%
- Flavonoids and polyphenols: Variable concentrations

Mechanism of Action: The sedative and anxiolytic effects of hops are attributed to its ability to potentiate the inhibitory neurotransmitter gamma-aminobutyric acid (GABA) in the brain, leading to relaxation and reduced anxiety.

Dosage: Dosage of hops supplements can vary depending on the formulation and intended use. Typical doses range from 100 mg to 500 mg per day, taken orally.

Contraindications: Hops may interact with certain medications, particularly sedatives and central nervous system depressants. Individuals with depression or hormone-sensitive conditions should avoid hops supplements.

Precautions: Pregnant or breastfeeding women, as well as individuals with pre-existing medical conditions, should consult with a healthcare professional before using hops supplements.

Adverse Reactions: Adverse reactions to hops supplements are rare but may include drowsiness, dizziness, gastrointestinal upset, or allergic reactions in susceptible individuals.

Research Standing: Research on hops has increased in recent years, with studies investigating its pharmacological properties and potential therapeutic applications, particularly in the fields of sleep disorders, anxiety, and menopause.

Pharmacokinetics: The pharmacokinetics of hops constituents depend on the specific compound. Absorption of its bioactive compounds occurs primarily in the gastrointestinal tract, with metabolites distributed throughout the body.

Pharmacodynamics: Hops exerts its pharmacodynamic effects through modulation of neurotransmitter activity, particularly GABA, as well as its anti-inflammatory and estrogenic properties.

Overdosage: Excessive consumption of hops supplements may lead to increased sedation, drowsiness, or other adverse effects associated with central nervous system depression.

International Standing: Hops is recognized internationally for its use in brewing beer and its potential medicinal properties. Its products are available in various forms, including dietary supplements and herbal preparations.

Indian Standing: In India, hops are primarily used in brewing beer, but there is growing interest in its medicinal properties, particularly its potential as a natural remedy for sleep disorders and anxiety.

Research Summary: Research on hops indicates its potential as a natural remedy for various health conditions, including sleep disorders, anxiety, and menopausal symptoms. Further studies are needed to elucidate its mechanisms of action and optimize its therapeutic applications.

50)HYPERICUM PERFORATUM

Introduction: Hypericum perforatum, commonly known as St. John's Wort, is a flowering plant native to Europe and Asia. It has a long history of use in traditional medicine for its potential health benefits.

Synonym Name and Common Name: Synonym Name: St. John's Wort Common Name: Klamath weed, goatweed

Pharmacognosy/Chemistry: St. John's Wort contains various bioactive compounds, including hypericin, hyperforin, flavonoids, and phenolic acids. These compounds contribute to its medicinal properties.

Action and Pharmacology: St. John's Wort is believed to exert antidepressant, anxiolytic, anti-inflammatory, and antiviral effects. Its mechanism of action involves modulation of neurotransmitter levels in the brain, particularly serotonin, dopamine, and noradrenaline.

Method of Analysis: Analytical methods for St. John's Wort typically involve extraction of its bioactive compounds followed by chromatographic techniques such as high-performance liquid chromatography (HPLC) or spectrophotometry for identification and quantification.

Health Benefits: St. John's Wort is associated with various health benefits, including improving mood, reducing symptoms of depression and anxiety, relieving nerve pain, and promoting wound healing.

Indication and Usage: It is used in traditional medicine for treating depression, anxiety, insomnia, nerve pain (neuralgia), and skin conditions such as wounds, burns, and bruises. It is also consumed as a dietary supplement or used in herbal preparations.

Usual Constituents with Percentages:

- Hypericin: Typically less than 0.5%
- Hyperforin: Typically 3-6%
- Flavonoids: Variable concentrations
- Phenolic acids: Variable concentrations

Mechanism of Action: The antidepressant effects of St. John's Wort are attributed to its ability to inhibit the reuptake of serotonin, dopamine, and noradrenaline in the brain, leading to increased levels of these neurotransmitters and improved mood.

Dosage: Dosage of St. John's Wort supplements can vary depending on the formulation and intended use. Typical doses range from 300 mg to 900 mg per day, taken orally in divided doses.

Contraindications: St. John's Wort may interact with certain medications, particularly antidepressants, anticoagulants, and oral contraceptives. It should not be used concomitantly with these medications without medical supervision.

Precautions: Pregnant or breastfeeding women, as well as individuals with pre-existing medical conditions, should consult with a healthcare professional before using St. John's Wort supplements.

Adverse Reactions: Adverse reactions to St. John's Wort supplements are rare but may include gastrointestinal upset, dizziness, dry mouth, photosensitivity, or interactions with medications.

Research Standing: Research on St. John's Wort has been extensive, with numerous studies investigating its efficacy and safety in treating depression, anxiety, and other medical conditions. While some studies have shown positive results, others have been inconclusive.

Pharmacokinetics: The pharmacokinetics of St. John's Wort constituents vary depending on the specific compound. Absorption of its bioactive compounds occurs primarily in the gastrointestinal tract, with metabolites distributed throughout the body.

Pharmacodynamics: St. John's Wort exerts its pharmacodynamic effects primarily through modulation of neurotransmitter levels in the brain, leading to changes in mood, anxiety, and pain perception.

Overdosage: Excessive consumption of St. John's Wort supplements may lead to increased risk of adverse effects, such as serotonin syndrome or drug interactions. Dosage should not exceed recommended levels.

International Standing: St. John's Wort is recognized internationally for its potential medicinal properties and is available in various forms, including dietary supplements and herbal preparations.

Indian Standing: In India, St. John's Wort is gaining popularity as a natural remedy for depression and anxiety, although its use is not as widespread as in some other countries.

Research Summary: Research on St. John's Wort suggests its potential as a natural antidepressant and anxiolytic agent, although further studies are needed to fully understand its mechanisms of action, optimal dosage, and potential interactions with medications.

51) INULA RACEMOSA - ROOT EXTRACT

Introduction: Inula racemosa, commonly known as Pushkarmool or Indian elecampane, is a perennial herb native to the Himalayan region and other parts of Asia. It has been used in traditional Ayurvedic medicine for its potential medicinal properties.

Synonym Name and Common Name: Synonym Name: Pushkarmool, Inula root Common Name: Indian elecampane

Pharmacognosy/Chemistry: Inula racemosa root contains various bioactive compounds, including sesquiterpene lactones (such as alantolactone and isoalantolactone), polysaccharides, flavonoids, and essential oils.

Action and Pharmacology: The bioactive compounds in Inula racemosa root exhibit expectorant, bronchodilator, anti-inflammatory, and antimicrobial properties. It is traditionally used for respiratory conditions and to support healthy lung function.

Method of Analysis: Analytical methods for Inula racemosa typically involve extraction of its bioactive compounds followed by chromatographic techniques such as high-performance liquid chromatography (HPLC) or gas chromatography-mass spectrometry (GC-MS) for identification and quantification.

Health Benefits: Inula racemosa root is associated with various health benefits, including relieving respiratory congestion, promoting expectoration, reducing inflammation, and supporting overall respiratory health.

Indication and Usage: It is used in traditional Ayurvedic medicine for treating respiratory conditions such as asthma, bronchitis, cough, and congestion. It is also consumed as a dietary supplement or used in herbal preparations.

Usual Constituents with Percentages:

- Sesquiterpene lactones: Up to 2%
- Polysaccharides: Variable concentrations
- Flavonoids: Variable concentrations
- Essential oils: Variable concentrations

Mechanism of Action: The expectorant and bronchodilator effects of Inula racemosa root are attributed to its ability to relax smooth muscles in the respiratory tract, promote mucous clearance, and reduce inflammation.

Dosage: Dosage of Inula racemosa supplements can vary depending on the formulation and intended use. Typical doses range from 500 mg to 2000 mg per day, taken orally in divided doses.

Contraindications: Inula racemosa root should be used with caution in individuals with allergies to plants in the Asteraceae family. It may also interact with certain medications, particularly those metabolized by the liver.

Precautions: Pregnant or breastfeeding women, as well as individuals with pre-existing medical conditions, should consult with a healthcare professional before using Inula racemosa supplements.

Adverse Reactions: Adverse reactions to Inula racemosa supplements are rare but may include gastrointestinal upset, allergic reactions, or interactions with medications.

Research Standing: Research on Inula racemosa root is ongoing, with studies investigating its pharmacological properties and potential therapeutic applications, particularly in respiratory conditions. However, more clinical trials are needed to validate its efficacy and safety.

Pharmacokinetics: The pharmacokinetics of Inula racemosa constituents have not been extensively studied. Absorption of its bioactive compounds likely occurs in the gastrointestinal tract, with metabolites distributed throughout the body.

Pharmacodynamics: Inula racemosa root exerts its pharmacodynamic effects primarily through its ability to modulate smooth muscle tone in the respiratory tract, reduce inflammation, and promote mucous clearance.

Overdosage: Excessive consumption of Inula racemosa supplements may lead to increased risk of adverse effects, such as gastrointestinal discomfort or allergic reactions. Dosage should not exceed recommended levels.

International Standing: Inula racemosa is recognized internationally for its potential medicinal properties, although its use may be more common in traditional systems of medicine such as Ayurveda.

Indian Standing: In India, Inula racemosa root is a well-known herb in Ayurvedic medicine and is used for various respiratory conditions. It is also cultivated and traded as a medicinal plant.

Research Summary: Research on In

ula racemosa root suggests its potential as a natural remedy for respiratory conditions, particularly in traditional systems of medicine such as Ayurveda. While preclinical studies have shown promising results, further clinical trials are needed to validate its efficacy and safety in humans. Additionally, more research is needed to elucidate its pharmacological mechanisms of action and optimal dosage regimens. Despite its long history of use in traditional medicine, its international recognition and acceptance as a therapeutic agent may vary.

52)KELP (BROWN ALGAE)

Introduction: Kelp is a type of large brown algae that belongs to the Laminariaceae family. It is commonly found in underwater forests along rocky coastlines around the world and has been utilized for various purposes, including food, medicine, and fertilizer.

Synonym Name and Common Name: Synonym Name: Brown seaweed Common Name: Kelp

Pharmacognosy/Chemistry: Kelp contains a wide array of bioactive compounds, including polysaccharides (such as alginate, laminarin, and fucoidan), polyphenols, vitamins (such as vitamin C and vitamin K), minerals (such as iodine, potassium, and calcium), and essential fatty acids.

Action and Pharmacology: The bioactive compounds in kelp contribute to its diverse pharmacological effects, including antioxidant, anti-inflammatory, antiviral, anticoagulant, and antihypertensive properties. It also supports thyroid function due to its iodine content.

Method of Analysis: Analytical methods for kelp typically involve extraction of its bioactive compounds followed by chromatographic techniques such as high-performance liquid chromatography (HPLC) or spectroscopic methods for identification and quantification.

Health Benefits: Kelp is associated with numerous health benefits, including supporting thyroid function, promoting cardiovascular health, aiding weight management, improving bone health, and boosting immune function.

Indication and Usage: It is used in traditional medicine and dietary supplements for various indications, including thyroid disorders (such as hypothyroidism), obesity, hypertension, osteoporosis, and immune support. It is also consumed as a food ingredient and used in skincare products.

Usual Constituents with Percentages:

- Polysaccharides (alginate, laminarin, fucoidan): Up to 50%
- Polyphenols: Variable concentrations
- Vitamins (C, K): Variable concentrations
- Minerals (iodine, potassium, calcium): Variable concentrations
- Essential fatty acids: Variable concentrations

Mechanism of Action: The pharmacological effects of kelp are attributed to its diverse array of bioactive compounds, which exert antioxidant, anti-inflammatory, and other therapeutic actions through various molecular pathways.

Dosage: Dosage of kelp supplements can vary depending on the formulation and intended use. Typical doses range from 150 mg to 2000 mg per day, taken orally in divided doses.

Contraindications: Individuals with iodine sensitivity or thyroid disorders, particularly hyperthyroidism, should avoid kelp supplements. It may also interact with certain medications, particularly thyroid medications.

Precautions: Pregnant or breastfeeding women, as well as individuals with pre-existing medical conditions, should consult with a healthcare professional before using kelp supplements.

Adverse Reactions: Adverse reactions to kelp supplements are rare but may include gastrointestinal upset, allergic reactions, or interactions with medications.

Research Standing: Research on kelp and its bioactive compounds is ongoing, with numerous studies investigating its pharmacological properties and potential health benefits in various medical conditions. While some studies have shown promising results, further research is needed to validate its efficacy and safety.

Pharmacokinetics: The pharmacokinetics of kelp constituents have not been extensively studied. Absorption of its bioactive compounds likely occurs in the gastrointestinal tract, with metabolites distributed throughout the body.

Pharmacodynamics: Kelp exerts its pharmacodynamic effects through its diverse array of bioactive compounds, which interact with various cellular and molecular targets to exert antioxidant, anti-inflammatory, and other therapeutic actions.

Overdosage: Excessive consumption of kelp supplements may lead to increased risk of adverse effects, particularly due to its iodine content. Dosage should not exceed recommended levels.

International Standing: Kelp is recognized internationally as a valuable source of nutrients and bioactive compounds, and its products are available in various forms, including dietary supplements, food ingredients, and skincare products.

Indian Standing: In India, kelp is gaining recognition for its potential health benefits, and its use in traditional medicine and dietary supplements is increasing. However, its international standing and acceptance may vary.

53) KRILL OIL - STANDARDIZED FOR DHA / EPA

Introduction: Krill oil is an oil extracted from tiny crustaceans called Antarctic krill (Euphausia superba). It is rich in omega-3 fatty acids, primarily eicosapentaenoic acid (EPA) and docosahexaenoic acid (DHA), as well as other beneficial compounds such as astaxanthin.

Synonym Name and Common Name: Synonym Name: Antarctic krill oil Common Name: Krill oil

Pharmacognosy/Chemistry: Krill oil contains omega-3 fatty acids in the form of phospholipids, which are more easily absorbed by the body compared to the triglyceride form found in fish oil. It also contains astaxanthin, a potent antioxidant.

Action and Pharmacology: The omega-3 fatty acids in krill oil, particularly EPA and DHA, have anti-inflammatory, cardioprotective, neuroprotective, and mood-regulating effects. Astaxanthin provides additional antioxidant benefits.

Method of Analysis: Analytical methods for krill oil typically involve extraction of its components followed by chromatographic techniques such as high-performance liquid chromatography (HPLC) or gas chromatography (GC) for identification and quantification of omega-3 fatty acids and astaxanthin.

Health Benefits: Krill oil is associated with various health benefits, including supporting cardiovascular health, reducing inflammation, improving cognitive function, enhancing joint health, and promoting skin health.

Indication and Usage: It is used as a dietary supplement to support heart health, brain health, joint health, and overall well-being. It may also be used to alleviate symptoms of inflammatory conditions such as arthritis or to support healthy aging.

Usual Constituents with Percentages:

- Omega-3 fatty acids (EPA and DHA): Variable percentages, typically standardized for total omega-3 content
- Astaxanthin: Variable concentrations

Mechanism of Action: The omega-3 fatty acids in krill oil exert their effects by modulating inflammatory pathways, reducing the production of pro-inflammatory mediators, and promoting the synthesis of anti-inflammatory compounds. Astaxanthin contributes to its antioxidant properties.

Dosage: Dosage of krill oil supplements can vary depending on the formulation and intended use. Typical doses range from 500 mg to 2000 mg per day, taken orally with meals.

Contraindications: Individuals with seafood allergies or shellfish allergies should avoid krill oil supplements. It may also interact with blood-thinning medications, so caution is advised in those taking anticoagulants or antiplatelet drugs.

Precautions: Pregnant or breastfeeding women, as well as individuals with pre-existing medical conditions, should consult with a healthcare professional before using krill oil supplements.

Adverse Reactions: Adverse reactions to krill oil supplements are rare but may include gastrointestinal upset, fishy aftertaste, or interactions with medications, particularly blood thinners.

Research Standing: Research on krill oil and its health benefits is ongoing, with numerous studies investigating its efficacy and safety in various populations and medical conditions. It is increasingly recognized as a valuable source of omega-3 fatty acids and antioxidants.

Pharmacokinetics: The phospholipid form of omega-3 fatty acids in krill oil may enhance their absorption and bioavailability compared to triglyceride forms found in fish oil supplements. Astaxanthin is also well-absorbed.

Pharmacodynamics: Krill oil exerts its pharmacodynamic effects primarily through its omega-3 fatty acid content, which modulates inflammatory pathways and lipid metabolism. Astaxanthin provides additional antioxidant support.

Overdosage: Excessive consumption of krill oil supplements may lead to increased risk of adverse effects, particularly due to its blood-thinning properties. Dosage should not exceed recommended levels.

International Standing: Krill oil is recognized internationally as a valuable source of omega-3 fatty acids and antioxidants, and its popularity as a dietary supplement is increasing worldwide.

Indian Standing: In India, krill oil supplements are gaining recognition for their potential health benefits, particularly in supporting cardiovascular health and brain function. However, their use may not be as widespread as in some other countries.

Research Summary: Research on krill oil suggests its potential as a natural remedy for various health conditions, particularly those related to inflammation, cardiovascular health, cognitive function, and joint health. While some studies have shown promising results, further research is needed to elucidate its mechanisms of action and optimize its therapeutic applications.

54)LAGERSTROEMIA SPECIOSA L

Introduction: Lagerstroemia speciosa L., commonly known as banaba, is a flowering plant native to Southeast Asia. It has been used in traditional medicine for its potential health benefits.

Synonym Name and Common Name: Synonym Name: Pride of India, Queen's flower Common Name: Banaba

Pharmacognosy/Chemistry: Banaba leaves contain various bioactive compounds, including corosolic acid, ellagitannins, flavonoids (such as quercetin and kaempferol), and triterpenoids.

Action and Pharmacology: The bioactive compounds in banaba are believed to have antidiabetic, antioxidant, anti-inflammatory, and antihyperlipidemic properties. They may also help regulate blood sugar levels and improve insulin sensitivity.

Method of Analysis: Analytical methods for banaba typically involve extraction of its bioactive compounds followed by chromatographic techniques such as high-performance liquid chromatography (HPLC) or spectrophotometry for identification and quantification.

Health Benefits: Banaba is associated with various health benefits, including lowering blood sugar levels, reducing inflammation, promoting weight loss, improving lipid profile, and supporting overall metabolic health.

Indication and Usage: It is used in traditional medicine and dietary supplements for managing diabetes, promoting weight loss, improving lipid profile, and supporting overall health. It is also consumed as a tea or used in herbal preparations.

Usual Constituents with Percentages:

- Corosolic acid: Variable concentrations
- Ellagitannins: Variable concentrations

- Flavonoids (quercetin, kaempferol): Variable concentrations
- Triterpenoids: Variable concentrations

Mechanism of Action: The antidiabetic effects of banaba are attributed to its ability to stimulate glucose uptake in cells, inhibit carbohydrate absorption, and enhance insulin sensitivity through various molecular pathways.

Dosage: Dosage of banaba supplements can vary depending on the formulation and intended use. Typical doses range from 100 mg to 1000 mg per day, taken orally in divided doses.

Contraindications: Individuals with hypoglycemia or those taking medications for diabetes should use banaba supplements with caution, as it may enhance the effects of these medications and lead to excessively low blood sugar levels.

Precautions: Pregnant or breastfeeding women, as well as individuals with pre-existing medical conditions, should consult with a healthcare professional before using banaba supplements.

Adverse Reactions: Adverse reactions to banaba supplements are rare but may include gastrointestinal upset, allergic reactions, or interactions with medications, particularly antidiabetic drugs.

Research Standing: Research on banaba and its health benefits is ongoing, with numerous studies investigating its efficacy and safety in managing diabetes, promoting weight loss, and improving metabolic health. While some studies have shown promising results, further research is needed to validate its therapeutic effects.

Pharmacokinetics: The pharmacokinetics of banaba constituents have not been extensively studied. Absorption of its bioactive compounds likely occurs in the gastrointestinal tract, with metabolites distributed throughout the body.

Pharmacodynamics: Banaba exerts its pharmacodynamic effects primarily through its ability to modulate glucose metabolism, insulin sensitivity, and inflammatory pathways, which collectively contribute to its antidiabetic and anti-inflammatory properties.

Overdosage: Excessive consumption of banaba supplements may lead to increased risk of hypoglycemia or gastrointestinal discomfort. Dosage should not exceed recommended levels.

International Standing: Banaba is recognized internationally for its potential medicinal properties, particularly in managing diabetes and improving metabolic health. Its products are available in various forms, including dietary supplements and herbal preparations.

Indian Standing: In India, banaba is used in traditional Ayurvedic medicine for managing diabetes and promoting overall health. Its use as a dietary supplement is also gaining popularity, particularly for its potential antidiabetic effects.

Research Summary: Research on banaba suggests its potential as a natural remedy for managing diabetes, promoting weight loss, and improving metabolic health. While some studies have shown promising results, further research is needed to elucidate its mechanisms of action, optimize dosage regimens, and evaluate its long-term safety and efficacy.

55)LINUM USITATISSIMUM

Introduction: Linum usitatissimum, commonly known as flaxseed or linseed, is a flowering plant native to the Middle East and India. It is cultivated for its seeds, which are rich in nutrients and bioactive compounds.

Synonym Name and Common Name: Synonym Name: Flaxseed, Linseed Common Name: Flaxseed

Pharmacognosy/Chemistry: Flaxseed contains various bioactive compounds, including alpha-linolenic acid (ALA, omega-3 fatty acid), lignans (such as secoisolariciresinoldiglucoside), soluble and insoluble fibers, vitamins (such as vitamin E), and minerals (such as magnesium and manganese).

Action and Pharmacology: The bioactive compounds in flaxseed contribute to its diverse pharmacological effects, including reducing inflammation, lowering cholesterol levels, improving digestive health, regulating blood sugar levels, and supporting cardiovascular health.

Method of Analysis: Analytical methods for flaxseed typically involve extraction of its bioactive compounds followed by chromatographic techniques such as gas chromatography (GC), high-performance liquid chromatography (HPLC), or spectrophotometry for identification and quantification.

Health Benefits: Flaxseed is associated with various health benefits, including reducing the risk of heart disease, lowering blood pressure, improving digestive health, promoting weight loss, reducing inflammation, and supporting overall well-being.

Indication and Usage: It is used as a dietary supplement, food ingredient, or herbal remedy for various indications, including cardiovascular health, digestive health, weight management, and overall nutritional support. It is also consumed as ground seeds, oil, or in baked goods.

Usual Constituents with Percentages:

- Alpha-linolenic acid (ALA): Up to 50%
- Lignans (secoisolariciresinoldiglucoside): Up to 1.5%
- Soluble and insoluble fibers: Variable concentrations
- Vitamins (vitamin E): Variable concentrations
- Minerals (magnesium, manganese): Variable concentrations

Mechanism of Action: The health benefits of flaxseed are attributed to its omega-3 fatty acid content, lignans, fibers, and other bioactive compounds, which exert antioxidant, anti-inflammatory, and other therapeutic actions through various molecular pathways.

Dosage: Dosage of flaxseed supplements can vary depending on the formulation and intended use. Typical doses range from 1 tablespoon (10-15 grams) to 2 tablespoons (20-30 grams) per day, taken orally with meals.

Contraindications: Individuals with certain medical conditions, such as bowel obstruction, intestinal disorders, or hormone-sensitive cancers, should use flaxseed supplements with caution due to its fiber and phytoestrogen content.

Precautions: Pregnant or breastfeeding women, as well as individuals with pre-existing medical conditions or allergies, should consult with a healthcare professional before using flaxseed supplements.

Adverse Reactions: Adverse reactions to flaxseed supplements are rare but may include gastrointestinal upset, allergic reactions, or interactions with medications, particularly blood-thinning drugs.

Research Standing: Research on flaxseed and its health benefits is extensive, with numerous studies investigating its efficacy and safety in various populations and medical conditions. It is widely recognized as a valuable dietary component and nutritional supplement.

Pharmacokinetics: The pharmacokinetics of flaxseed constituents have been studied to a limited extent. Absorption of its bioactive compounds likely occurs in the gastrointestinal tract, with metabolites distributed throughout the body.

Pharmacodynamics: Flaxseed exerts its pharmacodynamic effects primarily through its omega-3 fatty acids, lignans, fibers, and other bioactive compounds, which modulate inflammatory pathways, lipid metabolism, and gut microbiota composition.

Overdosage: Excessive consumption of flaxseed supplements may lead to increased risk of gastrointestinal discomfort or adverse effects associated with its phytoestrogen content. Dosage should not exceed recommended levels.

International Standing: Flaxseed is recognized internationally as a valuable source of nutrients and bioactive compounds, and its products are available in various forms, including dietary supplements, food products, and skincare products.

Indian Standing: In India, flaxseed is cultivated and consumed for its nutritional and medicinal properties. It is used in traditional Ayurvedic medicine and is gaining popularity as a dietary supplement and functional food ingredient.

Research Summary: Research on flaxseed suggests its potential as a natural remedy for various health conditions, including cardiovascular disease, diabetes, inflammatory disorders, and digestive problems. While some studies have shown promising results, further research is needed to elucidate its mechanisms of action, optimize dosage regimens, and evaluate its long-term safety and efficacy.

56)LYCIUMBARBARUM

Introduction: Lyciumbarbarum, commonly known as Goji berry or Wolfberry, is a shrub native to China, where it has been used for centuries in traditional medicine and culinary practices. It belongs to the Solanaceae family and is cultivated for its nutritious berries.

Synonym Name and Common Name: Synonym Name: Goji berry, Wolfberry Common Name: Lycium, Chinese wolfberry

Pharmacognosy/Chemistry: Lyciumbarbarum berries are rich in various bioactive compounds, including polysaccharides (such as Lyciumbarbarum polysaccharides, LBPs), carotenoids (such as zeaxanthin and beta-carotene), vitamins (such as vitamin C and vitamin A), flavonoids, and amino acids.

Action and Pharmacology: The bioactive compounds in Lyciumbarbarum exhibit antioxidant, immunomodulatory, neuroprotective, anti-inflammatory, and hepatoprotective properties. They contribute to its diverse pharmacological effects and potential health benefits.

Method of Analysis: Analytical methods for Lyciumbarbarum typically involve extraction of its bioactive compounds followed by chromatographic techniques such as high-performance liquid chromatography (HPLC) or spectrophotometry for identification and quantification.

Health Benefits: Lyciumbarbarum is associated with various health benefits, including supporting immune function, promoting eye health, improving cognitive function, enhancing skin health, and providing antioxidant protection against oxidative stress.

Indication and Usage: It is used in traditional medicine, dietary supplements, and functional foods for various indications, including immune support, eye health, anti-aging, and overall well-being. It is consumed as dried berries, juice, tea, or in herbal preparations.

Usual Constituents with Percentages:

- Polysaccharides (LBPs): Variable concentrations
- Carotenoids (zeaxanthin, beta-carotene): Variable concentrations
- Vitamins (vitamin C, vitamin A): Variable concentrations
- Flavonoids: Variable concentrations
- Amino acids: Variable concentrations

Mechanism of Action: The health benefits of Lyciumbarbarum are attributed to its diverse array of bioactive compounds, which exert antioxidant, immunomodulatory, anti-inflammatory, and other therapeutic actions through various molecular pathways.

Dosage: Dosage of Lyciumbarbarum supplements can vary depending on the formulation and intended use. Typical doses range from 5 grams to 30 grams of dried berries per day, or as directed by a healthcare professional.

Contraindications: Individuals with allergies to plants in the Solanaceae family, such as tomatoes or bell peppers, may experience allergic reactions to Lyciumbarbarum. It may also interact with certain medications, particularly blood thinners or diabetes medications.

Precautions: Pregnant or breastfeeding women, as well as individuals with pre-existing medical conditions or allergies, should consult with a healthcare professional before using Lyciumbarbarum supplements.

Adverse Reactions: Adverse reactions to Lyciumbarbarum supplements are rare but may include gastrointestinal upset, allergic reactions, or interactions with medications.

Research Standing: Research on Lyciumbarbarum and its health benefits is ongoing, with numerous studies investigating its efficacy and safety in various populations and medical conditions. It is recognized as a valuable medicinal plant in traditional Chinese medicine and is gaining popularity worldwide.

Pharmacokinetics: The pharmacokinetics of Lyciumbarbarum constituents, particularly its polysaccharides and carotenoids, have been studied to a limited extent. Absorption of its bioactive compounds likely occurs in the gastrointestinal tract, with metabolites distributed throughout the body.

Pharmacodynamics: Lyciumbarbarum exerts its pharmacodynamic effects primarily through its antioxidant, immunomodulatory, and anti-inflammatory properties, which contribute to its various health benefits and potential therapeutic applications.

Overdosage: Excessive consumption of Lyciumbarbarum supplements may lead to increased risk of adverse effects, particularly due to its interactions with medications or allergic reactions. Dosage should not exceed recommended levels.

International Standing: Lyciumbarbarum is recognized internationally for its potential medicinal properties and is widely consumed as a dietary supplement or functional food ingredient. Its products are available in various forms, including dried berries, juice, and extracts.

Indian Standing: In India, Lyciumbarbarum is used in traditional Ayurvedic medicine and is gaining popularity as a health supplement. It is cultivated and consumed for its potential health benefits, particularly in supporting immune function and overall well-being.

Research Summary: Research on Lyciumbarbarum suggests its potential as a natural remedy for various health conditions, including immune disorders, eye diseases, cognitive decline, and skin aging. While some studies have shown promising results, further research is needed to elucidate its mechanisms of action, optimize dosage regimens, and evaluate its long-term safety and efficacy.

57)MANGIFERA INDICA

Introduction: Mangifera indica, commonly known as mango, is a tropical fruit tree belonging to the Anacardiaceae family. It is widely cultivated for its delicious fruits, which are known for their sweet and juicy taste.

Synonym Name and Common Name: Synonym Name: Mango tree Common Name: Mango

Pharmacognosy/Chemistry: Mango contains various bioactive compounds, including polyphenols (such as mangiferin), carotenoids (such as beta-carotene), vitamins (such as vitamin C and vitamin A), minerals (such as potassium and magnesium), and dietary fibers.

Action and Pharmacology: The bioactive compounds in mango exhibit antioxidant, anti-inflammatory, anticancer, antidiabetic, cardioprotective, and immunomodulatory properties. They contribute to its diverse pharmacological effects and potential health benefits.

Method of Analysis: Analytical methods for mango typically involve extraction of its bioactive compounds followed by chromatographic techniques such as high-performance liquid chromatography (HPLC) or spectrophotometry for identification and quantification.

Health Benefits: Mango is associated with various health benefits, including supporting immune function, promoting digestive health, reducing inflammation, improving skin health, enhancing vision, and providing antioxidant protection against oxidative stress.

Indication and Usage: It is consumed fresh as a fruit, used in culinary dishes, processed into juices, smoothies, jams, and preserves, or used in herbal preparations. Mango is also used in traditional medicine for various indications, including digestive disorders, respiratory ailments, and skin conditions.

Usual Constituents with Percentages:

- Polyphenols (mangiferin): Variable concentrations
- Carotenoids (beta-carotene): Variable concentrations
- Vitamins (vitamin C, vitamin A): Variable concentrations
- Minerals (potassium, magnesium): Variable concentrations
- Dietary fibers: Variable concentrations

Mechanism of Action: The health benefits of mango are attributed to its diverse array of bioactive compounds, which exert antioxidant, anti-inflammatory, and other therapeutic actions through various molecular pathways.

Dosage: Dosage of mango consumption varies depending on individual preferences and dietary habits. As a general guideline, consuming 1-2 servings of mango per day (approximately 100-200 grams per serving) is considered beneficial for health.

Contraindications: Individuals with allergies to mango or related fruits (such as cashews or pistachios) may experience allergic reactions. Mango sap contains urushiol, which can cause contact dermatitis in sensitive individuals. Moreover, excessive consumption may cause gastrointestinal discomfort in some individuals.

Precautions: Individuals with diabetes should monitor their mango consumption due to its natural sugar content. Additionally, those with known allergies to mango or related fruits should avoid mango products to prevent allergic reactions.

Adverse Reactions: Adverse reactions to mango consumption are rare but may include allergic reactions, gastrointestinal discomfort (such as bloating or diarrhea) in sensitive individuals, or contact dermatitis from exposure to mango sap.

Research Standing: Research on mango and its health benefits is ongoing, with numerous studies investigating its efficacy and safety in various populations and medical conditions. It is widely recognized as a valuable dietary component and is cultivated and consumed globally.

Pharmacokinetics: The pharmacokinetics of mango constituents have been studied to a limited extent. Absorption of its bioactive compounds likely occurs in the gastrointestinal tract, with metabolites distributed throughout the body.

Pharmacodynamics: Mango exerts its pharmacodynamic effects primarily through its antioxidant, anti-inflammatory, and immunomodulatory properties, which contribute to its various health benefits and potential therapeutic applications.

Overdosage: Excessive consumption of mango may lead to increased calorie intake and contribute to weight gain in susceptible individuals. Moreover, excessive consumption of mango in individuals with allergies or sensitivities may lead to adverse reactions.

International Standing: Mango is recognized internationally as a popular and nutritious fruit, and its products are consumed and enjoyed worldwide. It is cultivated in tropical and subtropical regions across the globe and is exported to many countries.

Indian Standing: In India, mango holds cultural significance and is celebrated as the "king of fruits." It is widely cultivated and consumed throughout the country, and India is one of the largest producers of mango globally. Mango is used in various culinary dishes, desserts, beverages, and traditional Ayurvedic medicine preparations.

Research Summary: Research on mango suggests its potential as a natural remedy for various health conditions, including immune disorders, digestive problems, skin ailments, and oxidative stress-related diseases. While some studies have shown promising results, further research is needed to elucidate its mechanisms of action, optimize dosage regimens, and evaluate its long-term health effects.

58)MEDICAGO SATIVA EXTRACT

Introduction: Medicago sativa, commonly known as alfalfa, is a perennial flowering plant belonging to the Fabaceae family. It is widely cultivated as a forage crop and has been used traditionally for its medicinal properties.

Synonym Name and Common Name: Synonym Name: Lucerne Common Name: Alfalfa

Pharmacognosy/Chemistry: Alfalfa contains various bioactive compounds, including saponins, flavonoids (such as coumestrol), alkaloids, vitamins (such as vitamin K and vitamin C), minerals (such as calcium and magnesium), and phytoestrogens (such as isoflavones).

Action and Pharmacology: The bioactive compounds in alfalfa exhibit antioxidant, anti-inflammatory, diuretic, antidiabetic, and lipid-lowering properties. They contribute to its pharmacological effects and potential health benefits.

Method of Analysis: Analytical methods for alfalfa typically involve extraction of its bioactive compounds followed by chromatographic techniques such as high-performance liquid chromatography (HPLC) or spectrophotometry for identification and quantification.

Health Benefits: Alfalfa is associated with various health benefits, including improving digestive health, lowering cholesterol levels, regulating blood sugar levels, supporting liver function, enhancing bone health, and promoting overall well-being.

Indication and Usage: It is used in herbal medicine, dietary supplements, and herbal teas for various indications, including digestive disorders, hyperlipidemia, diabetes, arthritis, and menopausal symptoms. Alfalfa sprouts are also consumed as a nutritious food.

Usual Constituents with Percentages:

- Saponins: Variable concentrations
- Flavonoids (coumestrol): Variable concentrations
- Alkaloids: Variable concentrations
- Vitamins (vitamin K, vitamin C): Variable concentrations
- Minerals (calcium, magnesium): Variable concentrations
- Phytoestrogens (isoflavones): Variable concentrations

Mechanism of Action: The health benefits of alfalfa are attributed to its diverse array of bioactive compounds, which exert antioxidant, anti-inflammatory, and other therapeutic actions through various molecular pathways.

Dosage: Dosage of alfalfa supplements can vary depending on the formulation and intended use. Typical doses range from 500 mg to 1500 mg of alfalfa extract per day, taken orally with meals.

Contraindications: Individuals with autoimmune disorders, hormone-sensitive cancers, or those taking blood-thinning medications should use alfalfa supplements with caution due to its phytoestrogen content and potential interactions.

Precautions: Pregnant or breastfeeding women, as well as individuals with pre-existing medical conditions or allergies, should consult with a healthcare professional before using alfalfa supplements.

Adverse Reactions: Adverse reactions to alfalfa supplements are rare but may include gastrointestinal upset, allergic reactions, or interactions with medications, particularly blood thinners or hormone therapies.

Research Standing: Research on alfalfa and its health benefits is ongoing, with numerous studies investigating its efficacy and safety in various populations and medical conditions. It is recognized as a valuable medicinal plant in traditional medicine systems.

Pharmacokinetics: The pharmacokinetics of alfalfa constituents have been studied to a limited extent. Absorption of its bioactive compounds likely occurs in the gastrointestinal tract, with metabolites distributed throughout the body.

Pharmacodynamics: Alfalfa exerts its pharmacodynamic effects primarily through its antioxidant, anti-inflammatory, and other bioactive compounds, which contribute to its various health benefits and potential therapeutic applications.

Overdosage: Excessive consumption of alfalfa supplements may lead to increased risk of adverse effects, particularly due to its interactions with medications or allergic reactions. Dosage should not exceed recommended levels.

International Standing: Alfalfa is recognized internationally as a valuable forage crop and medicinal plant. Its products are consumed and used in various forms, including dietary supplements, herbal teas, and herbal preparations.

Indian Standing: In India, alfalfa is cultivated as a forage crop and is used in traditional Ayurvedic medicine for its potential health benefits. It is also gaining popularity as a dietary supplement and herbal remedy.

Research Summary: Research on alfalfa suggests its potential as a natural remedy for various health conditions, including digestive disorders, hyperlipidemia, diabetes, arthritis, and menopausal symptoms. While some studies have shown promising results, further research is needed to elucidate its mechanisms of action, optimize dosage regimens, and evaluate its long-term safety and efficacy.

59)MENYANTHESTRIFOLIATE

Introduction: Menyanthes trifoliata, commonly known as bogbean or buckbean, is a perennial aquatic plant native to Europe, Asia, and North America. It has been used traditionally for its medicinal properties and is valued for its bitter taste.

Synonym Name and Common Name: Synonym Name: Bogbean, Buckbean Common Name: Menyanthes, Bogbean

Pharmacognosy/Chemistry: Menyanthes trifoliata contains various bioactive compounds, including iridoid glycosides (such as menyanthoside), flavonoids, triterpenoids, and bitter principles. It also contains vitamins and minerals.

Action and Pharmacology: The bioactive compounds in Menyanthes trifoliata exhibit bitter tonic, diuretic, anti-inflammatory, and digestive stimulant properties. They contribute to its pharmacological effects and potential health benefits.

Method of Analysis: Analytical methods for Menyanthes trifoliata typically involve extraction of its bioactive compounds followed by chromatographic techniques such as high-performance liquid chromatography (HPLC) or spectrophotometry for identification and quantification.

Health Benefits: Menyanthes trifoliata is associated with various health benefits, including improving digestion, promoting liver and gallbladder health, supporting urinary tract function, reducing inflammation, and relieving symptoms of indigestion and bloating.

Indication and Usage: It is used in herbal medicine, dietary supplements, and herbal teas for various indications, including digestive disorders (such as dyspepsia and bloating), liver and gallbladder complaints, urinary tract infections, and general detoxification.

Usual Constituents with Percentages:

- Iridoid glycosides (menyanthoside): Variable concentrations
- Flavonoids: Variable concentrations
- Triterpenoids: Variable concentrations
- Bitter principles: Variable concentrations
- Vitamins and minerals: Variable concentrations

Mechanism of Action: The health benefits of Menyanthes trifoliata are attributed to its bitter tonic effects, which stimulate digestive secretions, bile production, and urine flow. It also exhibits anti-inflammatory properties, which contribute to its therapeutic actions.

Dosage: Dosage of Menyanthes trifoliata supplements can vary depending on the formulation and intended use. Typical doses range from 1 gram to 3 grams of dried herb per day, taken orally in divided doses.

Contraindications: Individuals with allergies to plants in the Menyanthaceae family, such as gentian or centaury, may experience allergic reactions to Menyanthes trifoliata. It may also interact with certain medications, particularly blood-thinning drugs or diuretics.

Precautions: Pregnant or breastfeeding women, as well as individuals with pre-existing medical conditions or allergies, should consult with a healthcare professional before using Menyanthes trifoliata supplements.

Adverse Reactions: Adverse reactions to Menyanthes trifoliata supplements are rare but may include gastrointestinal upset, allergic reactions, or interactions with medications, particularly blood thinners or diuretics.

Research Standing: Research on Menyanthes trifoliata and its health benefits is limited compared to other herbal remedies. Further studies are needed to elucidate its mechanisms of action, optimize dosage regimens, and evaluate its safety and efficacy in clinical settings.

Pharmacokinetics: The pharmacokinetics of Menyanthes trifoliata constituents have not been extensively studied. Absorption of its bioactive compounds likely occurs in the gastrointestinal tract, with metabolites distributed throughout the body.

Pharmacodynamics: Menyanthes trifoliata exerts its pharmacodynamic effects primarily through its bitter tonic, diuretic, and anti-inflammatory properties, which contribute to its various health benefits and potential therapeutic applications.

Overdosage: Excessive consumption of Menyanthes trifoliata supplements may lead to increased risk of adverse effects, particularly gastrointestinal upset or allergic reactions. Dosage should not exceed recommended levels.

International Standing: Menyanthes trifoliata is recognized internationally as a medicinal plant with potential health benefits. Its products are available in various forms, including herbal supplements, herbal teas, and tinctures.

Indian Standing: In India, Menyanthes trifoliata may not be widely recognized or used in traditional Ayurvedic medicine. However, it may be cultivated and used in herbal preparations by certain practitioners.

Research Summary: Research on Menyanthes trifoliata is limited, and further studies are needed to fully understand its pharmacological effects, mechanisms of action, and therapeutic potential. While it has a long history of traditional use, its modern scientific research is still in its early stages.

60)MILLETS AND THEIR POWDER

Introduction: Millets are a group of small-seeded grasses, cultivated as cereal crops for human consumption. They are highly nutritious and resilient, making them important food sources in many parts of the world.

Synonym Name and Common Name: Synonym Name: None Common Name: Millets

Pharmacognosy/Chemistry: Millets are rich in carbohydrates, dietary fiber, proteins, vitamins (such as vitamin B, vitamin E), minerals (such as iron, magnesium, phosphorus), and antioxidants. They also contain phytochemicals like phenols and flavonoids.

Action and Pharmacology: Millets have various health benefits, including lowering cholesterol levels, regulating blood sugar levels, promoting digestive health, supporting weight management, and reducing the risk of chronic diseases like heart disease and diabetes.

Method of Analysis: Analytical methods for millets typically involve assessing their nutritional composition, including carbohydrate, protein, fat, fiber, vitamin, and mineral content. Techniques such as spectrophotometry, chromatography, and elemental analysis are commonly used.

Health Benefits: Millets offer numerous health benefits due to their nutritional richness, including improved digestion, enhanced cardiovascular health, better blood sugar control, increased satiety, and reduced risk of obesity and chronic diseases.

Indication and Usage: Millets can be used in various culinary dishes, including porridges, bread, pancakes, and soups. They are also processed into flour for baking and used in traditional cuisines worldwide.

Usual Constituents with Percentages:

- Carbohydrates: 60-70%
- Proteins: 8-12%
- Dietary fiber: 2-8%
- Vitamins: Variable concentrations
- Minerals: Variable concentrations
- Antioxidants: Variable concentrations

Mechanism of Action: The health benefits of millets are attributed to their nutrient-rich composition, which contributes to improved metabolic health, reduced inflammation, enhanced gut health, and better overall well-being.

Dosage: There is no specific dosage for millets as they are typically consumed as part of a balanced diet. However, incorporating millets into meals regularly can contribute to a healthy diet.

Contraindications: There are no known contraindications for millets when consumed in moderate amounts as part of a balanced diet. However, individuals with gluten intolerance or celiac disease should choose gluten-free millet varieties.

Precautions: Individuals with food allergies or sensitivities should be cautious when consuming millets and ensure they are not cross-contaminated with allergens. Additionally, it's essential to practice proper food hygiene when handling and storing millets.

Adverse Reactions: Adverse reactions to millets are rare but may include gastrointestinal discomfort or allergic reactions in individuals with sensitivities or intolerances.

Research Standing: Research on millets and their health benefits has gained increasing attention due to their nutritional value and potential to address global health challenges like malnutrition and chronic diseases. Numerous studies have explored their diverse health-promoting properties.

Pharmacokinetics: The pharmacokinetics of millets have not been extensively studied, as they are primarily consumed as food rather than pharmaceuticals. Nutrients from millets are absorbed in the digestive tract and utilized by the body for various physiological functions.

Pharmacodynamics: Millets exert their pharmacodynamic effects through their nutrient-rich composition, which influences metabolic processes, gut microbiota, inflammation, and oxidative stress, thereby contributing to improved health outcomes.

Overdosage: There is no specific risk of overdosage associated with millets when consumed as part of a balanced diet. However, excessive consumption may lead to imbalances in nutrient intake and potential gastrointestinal discomfort.

International Standing: Millets have gained international recognition as valuable food crops due to their nutritional resilience and suitability for diverse agro-ecological regions. They are cultivated and consumed in many countries worldwide.

Indian Standing: In India, millets have a long history of cultivation and consumption, especially in regions with semi-arid climates. They are staple foods in many Indian cuisines and play a crucial role in food security and nutrition.

Research Summary: Research on millets highlights their nutritional richness and diverse health benefits, including improved metabolic health, reduced risk of chronic diseases, and potential therapeutic applications. Continued research is needed to further elucidate their mechanisms of action and optimize their utilization in addressing global health challenges.

61) MOMORDICA CHARANTIA

Introduction: Momordica charantia, commonly known as bitter melon or bitter gourd, is a tropical vine belonging to the Cucurbitaceae family. It is widely cultivated for its edible fruit, which has a distinct bitter taste and is used in various culinary dishes and traditional medicines.

Synonym Name and Common Name: Synonym Name: Bitter melon, Bitter gourd Common Name: Momordica charantia, Bitter melon

Pharmacognosy/Chemistry: Momordica charantia contains various bioactive compounds, including triterpenoids (such as charantin), flavonoids, alkaloids, saponins, and phenolic acids. It also contains vitamins (such as vitamin C and vitamin A) and minerals (such as potassium and iron).

Action and Pharmacology: The bioactive compounds in Momordica charantia exhibit hypoglycemic, hypolipidemic, antioxidant, anti-inflammatory, and immunomodulatory properties. They contribute to its pharmacological effects and potential health benefits.

Method of Analysis: Analytical methods for Momordica charantia typically involve extraction of its bioactive compounds followed by chromatographic techniques such as high-performance liquid chromatography (HPLC) or spectrophotometry for identification and quantification.

Health Benefits: Momordica charantia is associated with various health benefits, including lowering blood sugar levels, improving insulin sensitivity, reducing cholesterol levels, promoting weight loss, enhancing immune function, and supporting digestive health.

Indication and Usage: It is used in culinary dishes, herbal teas, and dietary supplements for various indications, including diabetes management, weight management, cardiovascular health, immune support, and gastrointestinal health.

Usual Constituents with Percentages:

- Triterpenoids (charantin): Variable concentrations
- Flavonoids: Variable concentrations
- Alkaloids: Variable concentrations
- Saponins: Variable concentrations

- Phenolic acids: Variable concentrations
- Vitamins (vitamin C, vitamin A): Variable concentrations
- Minerals (potassium, iron): Variable concentrations

Mechanism of Action: The health benefits of Momordica charantia are attributed to its bioactive compounds, which exert hypoglycemic, hypolipidemic, antioxidant, and anti-inflammatory effects through various molecular pathways, including activation of AMP-activated protein kinase (AMPK) and modulation of insulin signaling pathways.

Dosage: Dosage of Momordica charantia supplements can vary depending on the formulation and intended use. Typical doses range from 500 mg to 2000 mg of dried fruit extract per day, taken orally with meals.

Contraindications: Momordica charantia should be used with caution in individuals taking hypoglycemic medications or blood thinners, as it may potentiate their effects. It is contraindicated in pregnant women due to its potential to induce uterine contractions.

Precautions: Individuals with hypoglycemia, bleeding disorders, or known allergies to plants in the Cucurbitaceae family should consult with a healthcare professional before using Momordica charantia supplements.

Adverse Reactions: Adverse reactions to Momordica charantia supplements are rare but may include gastrointestinal upset, hypoglycemia (in individuals taking blood sugar-lowering medications), or allergic reactions in sensitive individuals.

Research Standing: Research on Momordica charantia and its health benefits is ongoing, with numerous studies investigating its efficacy and safety in various populations and medical conditions. It is recognized as a valuable medicinal plant in traditional medicine systems.

Pharmacokinetics: The pharmacokinetics of Momordica charantia constituents have been studied to a limited extent. Absorption of its bioactive compounds likely occurs in the gastrointestinal tract, with metabolites distributed throughout the body.

Pharmacodynamics: Momordica charantia exerts its pharmacodynamic effects primarily through its hypoglycemic, hypolipidemic, antioxidant, and anti-inflammatory properties, which contribute to its various health benefits and potential therapeutic applications.

Overdosage: Excessive consumption of Momordica charantia supplements may lead to gastrointestinal discomfort or hypoglycemia in susceptible individuals. Dosage should not exceed recommended levels.

International Standing: Momordica charantia is recognized internationally as a valuable medicinal plant and culinary ingredient. Its products are consumed and used in various forms, including dietary supplements, herbal teas, and culinary dishes.

Indian Standing: In India, Momordica charantia has a long history of use in traditional Ayurvedic and folk medicine systems for its medicinal properties. It is also widely cultivated and consumed as a vegetable in culinary dishes.

Research Summary: Research on Momordica charantia suggests its potential as a natural remedy for various health conditions, particularly in the management of diabetes, obesity, and cardiovascular diseases. While some studies have shown promising results, further research is needed to elucidate its mechanisms of action, optimize dosage regimens, and evaluate its long-term safety and efficacy.

62)MONODORAMYRISTICA

Introduction: Monodoramyristica, commonly known as African nutmeg or calabash nutmeg, is a tropical tree belonging to the Annonaceae family. It is native to West Africa and is valued for its aromatic seeds, which are used in culinary and traditional medicinal practices.

Synonym Name and Common Name: Synonym Name: African nutmeg, Calabash nutmeg Common Name: Monodoramyristica

Pharmacognosy/Chemistry: Monodoramyristica seeds contain various bioactive compounds, including essential oils (such as myristicin), terpenoids, alkaloids, phenolic compounds, and fatty acids. They also contain volatile aromatic compounds that contribute to their distinctive flavor and aroma.

Action and Pharmacology: The bioactive compounds in Monodoramyristica exhibit antimicrobial, anti-inflammatory, antioxidant, and digestive stimulant properties. They contribute to its pharmacological effects and potential health benefits.

Method of Analysis: Analytical methods for Monodoramyristica typically involve extraction of its bioactive compounds followed by chromatographic techniques such as gas chromatography-mass spectrometry (GC-MS) or high-performance liquid chromatography (HPLC) for identification and quantification.

Health Benefits: Monodoramyristica is associated with various health benefits, including improving digestion, relieving gastrointestinal discomfort, promoting appetite, enhancing respiratory health, and exerting antimicrobial effects against certain pathogens.

Indication and Usage: It is used in culinary dishes, herbal teas, and traditional medicines for various indications, including indigestion, flatulence, respiratory infections, and as a flavoring agent in food and beverages.

Usual Constituents with Percentages:

- Essential oils (myristicin): Variable concentrations
- Terpenoids: Variable concentrations
- Alkaloids: Variable concentrations
- Phenolic compounds: Variable concentrations
- Fatty acids: Variable concentrations

Mechanism of Action: The health benefits of Monodoramyristica are attributed to its bioactive compounds, which exert antimicrobial, anti-inflammatory, antioxidant, and digestive stimulant effects through various molecular pathways.

Dosage: Dosage of Monodoramyristica supplements can vary depending on the formulation and intended use. Typical doses range from 1 gram to 3 grams of ground seeds per day, taken orally with meals or as directed by a healthcare professional.

Contraindications: Monodoramyristica should be used with caution in pregnant or breastfeeding women, as well as individuals with liver or kidney disorders. It may also interact with certain medications, particularly anticoagulants or antiplatelet drugs.

Precautions: Individuals with known allergies to spices or members of the Annonaceae family should avoid using Monodoramyristica. It is also important to use it in moderation to prevent potential adverse effects.

Adverse Reactions: Adverse reactions to Monodoramyristica are rare but may include allergic reactions, gastrointestinal upset, or interactions with medications in susceptible individuals.

Research Standing: Research on Monodoramyristica and its health benefits is limited compared to more extensively studied botanicals. Further studies are needed to elucidate its mechanisms of action, optimize dosage regimens, and evaluate its safety and efficacy in clinical settings.

Pharmacokinetics: The pharmacokinetics of Monodoramyristica constituents have not been extensively studied. Absorption of its bioactive compounds likely occurs in the gastrointestinal tract, with metabolites distributed throughout the body.

Pharmacodynamics: Monodoramyristica exerts its pharmacodynamic effects primarily through its antimicrobial, anti-inflammatory, antioxidant, and digestive stimulant properties, which contribute to its various health benefits and potential therapeutic applications.

Overdosage: Excessive consumption of Monodoramyristica seeds may lead to gastrointestinal discomfort or adverse reactions. Dosage should not exceed recommended levels, and it is important to use it in moderation.

International Standing: Monodoramyristica is recognized internationally as a culinary spice and traditional medicinal plant. Its products are used in various cuisines and herbal remedies in regions where it is cultivated.

Indian Standing: In India, Monodoramyristica may not be widely recognized or used in traditional Ayurvedic medicine. However, it may be used in culinary dishes or as a flavoring agent in certain regional cuisines.

Research Summary: Research on Monodoramyristica is limited, and further studies are needed to fully understand its pharmacological effects, mechanisms of action, and therapeutic potential. While it has a long history of traditional use, its modern scientific research is still in its early stages.

63)MORINDACITRIFOLIA EXTRACT

Introduction: Morindacitrifolia, commonly known as noni or Indian mulberry, is a tropical evergreen tree native to Southeast Asia, Australia, and the Pacific Islands. It has a long history of traditional use as a medicinal plant and is valued for its various health-promoting properties.

Synonym Name and Common Name: Synonym Name: Noni, Indian mulberry Common Name: Morindacitrifolia, Noni

Pharmacognosy/Chemistry: Morindacitrifolia extract contains a diverse array of bioactive compounds, including iridoids (such as deacetylasperulosidic acid), flavonoids, alkaloids, polysaccharides, vitamins, and minerals. It also contains phytochemicals like anthraquinones and fatty acids.

Action and Pharmacology: The bioactive compounds in Morindacitrifolia exhibit antioxidant, anti-inflammatory, immunomodulatory, analgesic, antimicrobial, and anticancer properties. They contribute to its pharmacological effects and potential health benefits.

Method of Analysis: Analytical methods for Morindacitrifolia extract typically involve extraction of its bioactive compounds followed by chromatographic techniques such as high-performance liquid chromatography (HPLC) or spectrophotometry for identification and quantification.

Health Benefits: Morindacitrifolia extract is associated with various health benefits, including boosting immunity, reducing inflammation, improving digestion, enhancing cardiovascular health, promoting skin health, and supporting overall well-being.

Indication and Usage: It is used in traditional medicine systems, dietary supplements, and functional foods for various indications, including immune support, digestive disorders, pain relief, wound healing, and as an adjunctive therapy for certain chronic conditions.

Usual Constituents with Percentages:

- Iridoids (deacetylasperulosidic acid): Variable concentrations
- Flavonoids: Variable concentrations
- Alkaloids: Variable concentrations

- Polysaccharides: Variable concentrations
- Vitamins: Variable concentrations
- Minerals: Variable concentrations
- Anthraquinones: Variable concentrations
- Fatty acids: Variable concentrations

Mechanism of Action: The health benefits of Morindacitrifolia extract are attributed to its diverse array of bioactive compounds, which exert antioxidant, anti-inflammatory, immunomodulatory, and other therapeutic effects through various molecular pathways.

Dosage: Dosage of Morindacitrifolia extract can vary depending on the formulation and intended use. Typical doses range from 500 mg to 1500 mg of extract per day, taken orally with meals or as directed by a healthcare professional.

Contraindications: Morindacitrifolia extract should be used with caution in individuals with known allergies to plants in the Rubiaceae family or with pre-existing medical conditions. It may also interact with certain medications, particularly blood thinners or immunosuppressants.

Precautions: Pregnant or breastfeeding women, as well as individuals with liver or kidney disorders, should consult with a healthcare professional before using Morindacitrifolia extract supplements. It is important to use it under medical supervision, especially in combination with other medications.

Adverse Reactions: Adverse reactions to Morindacitrifolia extract are rare but may include gastrointestinal upset, allergic reactions, or interactions with medications in susceptible individuals. It is essential to monitor for any adverse effects and discontinue use if necessary.

Research Standing: Research on Morindacitrifolia extract and its health benefits is ongoing, with numerous studies investigating its efficacy and safety in various populations and medical conditions. It is recognized as a valuable medicinal plant in traditional medicine systems and has gained popularity as a dietary supplement in recent years.

Pharmacokinetics: The pharmacokinetics of Morindacitrifolia extract constituents have been studied to a limited extent. Absorption of its bioactive compounds likely occurs in the gastrointestinal tract, with metabolites distributed throughout the body.

Pharmacodynamics: Morindacitrifolia extract exerts its pharmacodynamic effects primarily through its antioxidant, anti-inflammatory, immunomodulatory, and other bioactive compounds, which contribute to its various health benefits and potential therapeutic applications.

Overdosage: Excessive consumption of Morindacitrifolia extract may lead to gastrointestinal discomfort or adverse reactions. Dosage should not exceed recommended levels, and it is important to follow the guidance of a healthcare professional.

International Standing: Morindacitrifolia extract is recognized internationally as a valuable medicinal plant and dietary supplement. Its products are available in various forms, including capsules, juices, teas, and powders, and are consumed worldwide.

Indian Standing: In India, Morindacitrifolia extract may not be widely recognized in traditional Ayurvedic medicine but has gained popularity as a dietary supplement and functional food ingredient. Its products are available in the Indian market and used for various health purposes.

Research Summary: Research on Morindacitrifolia extract highlights its potential as a natural remedy for various health conditions, including immune support, inflammation, digestion, cardiovascular health, and skin health. While some studies have shown promising results, further research is needed to elucidate its mechanisms of action, optimize dosage regimens, and evaluate its long-term safety and efficacy.

64)MORINGA OLEIFERA LEAF

Introduction: Morindacitrifolia, commonly known as noni or Indian mulberry, is a tropical evergreen tree native to Southeast Asia, Australia, and the Pacific Islands. It has a long history of traditional use as a medicinal plant and is valued for its various health-promoting properties.

Synonym Name and Common Name: Synonym Name: Noni, Indian mulberry Common Name: Morindacitrifolia, Noni

Pharmacognosy/Chemistry: Morindacitrifolia extract contains a diverse array of bioactive compounds, including iridoids (such as deacetylasperulosidic acid), flavonoids, alkaloids, polysaccharides, vitamins, and minerals. It also contains phytochemicals like anthraquinones and fatty acids.

Action and Pharmacology: The bioactive compounds in Morindacitrifolia exhibit antioxidant, anti-inflammatory, immunomodulatory, analgesic, antimicrobial, and anticancer properties. They contribute to its pharmacological effects and potential health benefits.

Method of Analysis: Analytical methods for Morindacitrifolia extract typically involve extraction of its bioactive compounds followed by chromatographic techniques such as high-performance liquid chromatography (HPLC) or spectrophotometry for identification and quantification.

Health Benefits: Morindacitrifolia extract is associated with various health benefits, including boosting immunity, reducing inflammation, improving digestion, enhancing cardiovascular health, promoting skin health, and supporting overall well-being.

Indication and Usage: It is used in traditional medicine systems, dietary supplements, and functional foods for various indications, including immune support, digestive disorders, pain relief, wound healing, and as an adjunctive therapy for certain chronic conditions.

Usual Constituents with Percentages:

- Iridoids (deacetylasperulosidic acid): Variable concentrations
- Flavonoids: Variable concentrations
- Alkaloids: Variable concentrations
- Polysaccharides: Variable concentrations
- Vitamins: Variable concentrations
- Minerals: Variable concentrations
- Anthraquinones: Variable concentrations
- Fatty acids: Variable concentrations

Mechanism of Action: The health benefits of Morindacitrifolia extract are attributed to its diverse array of bioactive compounds, which exert antioxidant, anti-inflammatory, immunomodulatory, and other therapeutic effects through various molecular pathways.

Dosage: Dosage of Morindacitrifolia extract can vary depending on the formulation and intended use. Typical doses range from 500 mg to 1500 mg of extract per day, taken orally with meals or as directed by a healthcare professional.

Contraindications: Morindacitrifolia extract should be used with caution in individuals with known allergies to plants in the Rubiaceae family or with pre-existing medical conditions. It may also interact with certain medications, particularly blood thinners or immunosuppressants.

Precautions: Pregnant or breastfeeding women, as well as individuals with liver or kidney disorders, should consult with a healthcare professional before using Morindacitrifolia extract supplements. It is important to use it under medical supervision, especially in combination with other medications.

Adverse Reactions: Adverse reactions to Morindacitrifolia extract are rare but may include gastrointestinal upset, allergic reactions, or interactions with medications in susceptible individuals. It is essential to monitor for any adverse effects and discontinue use if necessary.

Research Standing: Research on Morindacitrifolia extract and its health benefits is ongoing, with numerous studies investigating its efficacy and safety in various populations and medical conditions. It is recognized as a valuable medicinal plant in traditional medicine systems and has gained popularity as a dietary supplement in recent years.

Pharmacokinetics: The pharmacokinetics of Morindacitrifolia extract constituents have been studied to a limited extent. Absorption of its bioactive compounds likely occurs in the gastrointestinal tract, with metabolites distributed throughout the body.

Pharmacodynamics: Morindacitrifolia extract exerts its pharmacodynamic effects primarily through its antioxidant, anti-inflammatory, immunomodulatory, and other bioactive compounds, which contribute to its various health benefits and potential therapeutic applications.

Overdosage: Excessive consumption of Morindacitrifolia extract may lead to gastrointestinal discomfort or adverse reactions. Dosage should not exceed recommended levels, and it is important to follow the guidance of a healthcare professional.

International Standing: Morindacitrifolia extract is recognized internationally as a valuable medicinal plant and dietary supplement. Its products are available in various forms, including capsules, juices, teas, and powders, and are consumed worldwide.

Indian Standing: In India, Morindacitrifolia extract may not be widely recognized in traditional Ayurvedic medicine but has gained popularity as a dietary supplement and functional food ingredient. Its products are available in the Indian market and used for various health purposes.

Research Summary: Research on Morindacitrifolia extract highlights its potential as a natural remedy for various health conditions, including immune support, inflammation, digestion, cardiovascular health, and skin health. While some studies have shown promising results, further research is needed to elucidate its mechanisms of action, optimize dosage regimens, and evaluate its long-term safety and efficacy.

65) MORUS ALBA

Introduction: Morus alba, commonly known as white mulberry, is a deciduous tree native to Asia and now cultivated worldwide for its edible fruit and leaves. It has a long history of traditional use in various cultures for both culinary and medicinal purposes.

Synonym Name and Common Name: Synonym Name: White mulberry Common Name: Morus alba, White mulberry

Pharmacognosy/Chemistry: Morus alba contains various bioactive compounds, including flavonoids (such as quercetin and rutin), anthocyanins, alkaloids (such as morusin and oxyresveratrol), vitamins (such as vitamin C), minerals, and polysaccharides.

Action and Pharmacology: The bioactive compounds in Morus alba exhibit antioxidant, anti-inflammatory, hypoglycemic, hypolipidemic, antihypertensive, and immunomodulatory properties. They contribute to its pharmacological effects and potential health benefits.

Method of Analysis: Analytical methods for Morus alba typically involve extraction of its bioactive compounds followed by chromatographic techniques such as high-performance liquid chromatography (HPLC) or spectrophotometry for identification and quantification.

Health Benefits: Morus alba is associated with various health benefits, including lowering blood sugar levels, reducing cholesterol levels, improving cardiovascular health, enhancing immune function, promoting weight loss, and supporting overall well-being.

Indication and Usage: It is used in traditional medicine systems, herbal teas, dietary supplements, and functional foods for various indications, including diabetes management, heart health, immune support, weight management, and as a general tonic.

Usual Constituents with Percentages:

- Flavonoids (quercetin, rutin): Variable concentrations
- Anthocyanins: Variable concentrations
- Alkaloids (morusin, oxyresveratrol): Variable concentrations
- Vitamins (vitamin C): Variable concentrations
- Minerals: Variable concentrations
- Polysaccharides: Variable concentrations

Mechanism of Action: The health benefits of Morus alba are attributed to its diverse array of bioactive compounds, which exert antioxidant, anti-inflammatory, hypoglycemic, hypolipidemic, and other therapeutic effects through various molecular pathways.

Dosage: Dosage of Morus alba supplements can vary depending on the formulation and intended use. Typical doses range from 500 mg to 1500 mg of leaf extract or powder per day, taken orally with meals or as directed by a healthcare professional.

Contraindications: Morus alba should be used with caution in individuals with known allergies to plants in the Moraceae family or with pre-existing medical conditions. It may also interact with certain medications, particularly blood sugar-lowering drugs.

Precautions: Pregnant or breastfeeding women, as well as individuals with liver or kidney disorders, should consult with a healthcare professional before using Morus alba supplements. It is important to use it under medical supervision, especially in combination with other medications.

Adverse Reactions: Adverse reactions to Morus alba supplements are rare but may include gastrointestinal upset, allergic reactions, or interactions with medications in susceptible individuals. It is essential to monitor for any adverse effects and discontinue use if necessary.

Research Standing: Research on Morus alba and its health benefits is ongoing, with numerous studies investigating its efficacy and safety in various populations and medical conditions. It is recognized as a valuable medicinal plant in traditional medicine systems and has gained popularity as a dietary supplement in recent years.

Pharmacokinetics: The pharmacokinetics of Morus alba constituents have been studied to a limited extent. Absorption of its bioactive compounds likely occurs in the gastrointestinal tract, with metabolites distributed throughout the body.

Pharmacodynamics: Morus alba extract exerts its pharmacodynamic effects primarily through its antioxidant, anti-inflammatory, hypoglycemic, hypolipidemic, and other bioactive compounds, which contribute to its various health benefits and potential therapeutic applications.

Overdosage: Excessive consumption of Morus alba supplements may lead to gastrointestinal discomfort or adverse reactions. Dosage should not exceed recommended levels, and it is important to follow the guidance of a healthcare professional.

International Standing: Morus alba is recognized internationally as a valuable medicinal plant and dietary supplement. Its products are available in various forms, including capsules, teas, extracts, and powders, and are consumed worldwide.

Indian Standing: In India, Morus alba may not be widely recognized in traditional Ayurvedic medicine but has gained popularity as a dietary supplement and functional food ingredient. Its products are available in the Indian market and used for various health purposes.

Research Summary: Research on Morus alba highlights its potential as a natural remedy for various health conditions, including diabetes, cardiovascular diseases, inflammation, and oxidative stress. While some studies have shown promising results, further research is needed to elucidate its mechanisms of action, optimize dosage regimens, and evaluate its long-term safety and efficacy

66)MYRICA CERIFERA/M. NAGI

Introduction: Myrica cerifera, commonly known as wax myrtle or southern bayberry, is an evergreen shrub native to North America. It belongs to the Myricaceae family and is known for its aromatic foliage and waxy berries. Myrica nagi, also known as box myrtle, is a related species found in Asia.

Synonym Name and Common Name: Synonym Name: Southern bayberry (for Myrica cerifera), Box myrtle (for Myrica nagi) Common Name: Wax myrtle (for Myrica cerifera), Box myrtle (for Myrica nagi)

Pharmacognosy/Chemistry: Myrica cerifera and Myrica nagi contain various bioactive compounds, including flavonoids (such as myricetin and quercetin), tannins, essential oils, triterpenes, and phenolic acids. These compounds contribute to their pharmacological properties and potential health benefits.

Action and Pharmacology: The bioactive compounds in Myrica species exhibit antioxidant, anti-inflammatory, antimicrobial, antiviral, and hepatoprotective properties. They also have astringent effects and may promote wound healing and gastrointestinal health.

Method of Analysis: Analytical methods for Myrica cerifera and Myrica nagi typically involve extraction of their bioactive compounds followed by chromatographic techniques such as high-performance liquid chromatography (HPLC) or gas chromatography-mass spectrometry (GC-MS) for identification and quantification.

Health Benefits: Myrica species are associated with various health benefits, including improving digestion, boosting immunity, reducing inflammation, protecting against oxidative stress, promoting skin health, and supporting overall well-being.

Indication and Usage: They are used in traditional medicine systems, herbal teas, dietary supplements, and topical preparations for various indications, including gastrointestinal disorders, respiratory infections, skin conditions, and as a general tonic.

Usual Constituents with Percentages:

- Flavonoids (myricetin, quercetin): Variable concentrations
- Tannins: Variable concentrations
- Essential oils: Variable concentrations
- Triterpenes: Variable concentrations
- Phenolic acids: Variable concentrations

Mechanism of Action: The health benefits of Myrica species are attributed to their diverse array of bioactive compounds, which exert antioxidant, anti-inflammatory, antimicrobial, and other therapeutic effects through various molecular pathways.

Dosage: Dosage of Myrica cerifera and Myrica nagi supplements can vary depending on the formulation and intended use. Typical doses range from 500 mg to 2000 mg of leaf or berry extract per day, taken orally with meals or as directed by a healthcare professional.

Contraindications: Myrica species should be used with caution in individuals with known allergies to plants in the Myricaceae family or with pre-existing medical conditions. They may also interact with certain medications, particularly blood thinners or antidiabetic drugs.

Precautions: Pregnant or breastfeeding women, as well as individuals with liver or kidney disorders, should consult with a healthcare professional before using Myrica species supplements. It is important to use them under medical supervision, especially in combination with other medications.

Adverse Reactions: Adverse reactions to Myrica species supplements are rare but may include gastrointestinal upset, allergic reactions, or interactions with medications in susceptible individuals. It is essential to monitor for any adverse effects and discontinue use if necessary.

Research Standing: Research on Myrica cerifera and Myrica nagi and their health benefits is ongoing, with numerous studies investigating their efficacy and safety in various populations and medical conditions. They are recognized as valuable medicinal plants in traditional medicine systems and have gained popularity as dietary supplements.

Pharmacokinetics: The pharmacokinetics of Myrica species constituents have been studied to a limited extent. Absorption of their bioactive compounds likely occurs in the gastrointestinal tract, with metabolites distributed throughout the body.

Pharmacodynamics: Myrica species extracts exert their pharmacodynamic effects primarily through their antioxidant, anti-inflammatory, antimicrobial, and other bioactive compounds, which contribute to their various health benefits and potential therapeutic applications.

Overdosage: Excessive consumption of Myrica species supplements may lead to gastrointestinal discomfort or adverse reactions. Dosage should not exceed recommended levels, and it is important to follow the guidance of a healthcare professional.

International Standing: Myrica species are recognized internationally as valuable medicinal plants and dietary supplements. Their products are available in various forms, including capsules, teas, extracts, and topical preparations, and are consumed worldwide.

Indian Standing: In India, Myrica species may be used in traditional Ayurvedic medicine and other indigenous healing systems. They are also cultivated and used in culinary dishes and religious ceremonies in certain regions.

Research Summary: Research on Myrica cerifera and Myrica nagi highlights their potential as natural remedies for various health conditions, including gastrointestinal disorders, respiratory infections, skin ailments, and oxidative stress-related diseases. While some studies have shown promising results, further research is needed to elucidate their mechanisms of action, optimize dosage regimens, and evaluate their long-term safety and efficacy.

67) MYRISTICA FRAGRANS HOUTT

Introduction: Myristica fragrans Houtt, commonly known as nutmeg, is an evergreen tree native to the Spice Islands of Indonesia. It belongs to the family Myristicaceae and is highly valued for its seeds, which are used as a spice and have been used traditionally for various medicinal purposes.

Synonym Name and Common Name: Synonym Name: Nutmeg tree Common Name: Nutmeg

Pharmacognosy/Chemistry: The seeds of Myristica fragrans contain various bioactive compounds, including volatile oils (such as myristicin), phenolic compounds, terpenoids, flavonoids, and alkaloids (such as myristicin and safrole).

Action and Pharmacology: The bioactive compounds in nutmeg exhibit a range of pharmacological effects, including antimicrobial, anti-inflammatory, antioxidant, analgesic, and digestive stimulant properties. They contribute to its medicinal uses and potential health benefits.

Method of Analysis: Analytical methods for nutmeg typically involve extraction of its bioactive compounds followed by chromatographic techniques such as gas chromatography-mass spectrometry (GC-MS) or high-performance liquid chromatography (HPLC) for identification and quantification.

Health Benefits: Nutmeg is associated with various health benefits, including improving digestion, relieving gastrointestinal discomfort, promoting oral health, enhancing cognitive function, supporting cardiovascular health, and providing analgesic effects.

Indication and Usage: It is used in culinary applications, traditional medicine systems, herbal teas, and aromatherapy for various indications, including indigestion, nausea, flatulence, dental hygiene, mental fatigue, and as a flavoring agent.

Usual Constituents with Percentages:

- Volatile oils (myristicin): Variable concentrations
- Phenolic compounds: Variable concentrations
- Terpenoids: Variable concentrations

- Flavonoids: Variable concentrations
- Alkaloids (myristicin, safrole): Variable concentrations

Mechanism of Action: The health benefits of nutmeg are attributed to its bioactive compounds, which exert antimicrobial, anti-inflammatory, antioxidant, analgesic, and digestive stimulant effects through various molecular pathways.

Dosage: Dosage of nutmeg varies depending on the form and intended use. For culinary purposes, a pinch or small amount of grated nutmeg is typically used in recipes. For medicinal purposes, doses may range from 0.5 grams to 2 grams of powdered nutmeg per day, taken orally.

Contraindications: Nutmeg should be used with caution in pregnant or breastfeeding women, as well as individuals with liver or kidney disorders. It may also interact with certain medications, particularly those metabolized by the liver.

Precautions: Consumption of large amounts of nutmeg may lead to adverse effects such as nausea, vomiting, dizziness, hallucinations, and seizures. It is important to use nutmeg in moderation and avoid excessive intake.

Adverse Reactions: Adverse reactions to nutmeg are rare but may occur with excessive consumption. Symptoms may include gastrointestinal upset, drowsiness, confusion, and neurological effects. Allergic reactions are also possible in susceptible individuals.

Research Standing: Research on nutmeg and its health effects is ongoing, with studies investigating its pharmacological properties, safety, and potential therapeutic applications. While it has a long history of traditional use, further research is needed to fully understand its mechanisms of action and optimize its medicinal use.

Pharmacokinetics: The pharmacokinetics of nutmeg constituents have been studied to a limited extent. Absorption of its bioactive compounds likely occurs in the gastrointestinal tract, with metabolites distributed throughout the body.

Pharmacodynamics: Nutmeg exerts its pharmacodynamic effects primarily through its bioactive compounds, which interact with various molecular targets to produce its medicinal effects, including antimicrobial, anti-inflammatory, antioxidant, analgesic, and digestive stimulant actions.

Overdosage: Overconsumption of nutmeg may lead to toxicity and overdose symptoms, including gastrointestinal distress, central nervous system effects, and cardiovascular effects. It is important to avoid excessive intake and use nutmeg in moderation.

International Standing: Nutmeg is recognized internationally as a valuable culinary spice and traditional medicinal plant. It is widely used in various cuisines and herbal remedies around the world.

Indian Standing: In India, nutmeg has a long history of use in Ayurvedic medicine and culinary applications. It is valued for its medicinal properties and is used in various traditional remedies for digestive disorders, respiratory ailments, and neurological conditions.

Research Summary: Research on nutmeg continues to explore its pharmacological effects, safety profile, and potential therapeutic applications. While it is generally considered safe when used in moderation, further studies are needed to elucidate its mechanisms of action, optimize dosage regimens, and evaluate its efficacy in clinical settings.

68)NARDOSTACHYSJATAMANSI– EXTRACT

Introduction: Nardostachysjatamansi, commonly known as spikenard, is a perennial herbaceous plant native to the Himalayan region and widely distributed across Asia. It has been highly valued for centuries in traditional medicine systems for its medicinal properties.

Synonym Name and Common Name: Synonym Name: Jatamansi Common Name: Spikenard

Pharmacognosy/Chemistry: Nardostachysjatamansi extract contains various bioactive compounds, including sesquiterpenes (such as jatamansone and valeranone), lignans, flavonoids, alkaloids, and essential oils. These compounds contribute to its pharmacological effects and medicinal properties.

Action and Pharmacology: The bioactive compounds in spikenard exhibit a range of pharmacological activities, including anti-inflammatory, antioxidant, neuroprotective, anxiolytic, sedative, and cardioprotective effects. They contribute to its therapeutic potential in various health conditions.

Method of Analysis: Analytical methods for Nardostachysjatamansi extract typically involve extraction of its bioactive compounds followed by chromatographic techniques such as high-performance liquid chromatography (HPLC) or gas chromatography-mass spectrometry (GC-MS) for identification and quantification.

Health Benefits: Spikenard is associated with various health benefits, including reducing stress and anxiety, improving sleep quality, enhancing cognitive function, promoting cardiovascular health, relieving inflammation, and supporting overall well-being.

Indication and Usage: It is used in traditional medicine systems, herbal teas, dietary supplements, and aromatherapy for various indications, including anxiety disorders, insomnia, cognitive impairment, inflammation-related conditions, and as a general tonic.

Usual Constituents with Percentages:

- Sesquiterpenes (jatamansone, valeranone): Variable concentrations
- Lignans: Variable concentrations
- Flavonoids: Variable concentrations
- Alkaloids: Variable concentrations
- Essential oils: Variable concentrations

Mechanism of Action: The health benefits of spikenard are attributed to its bioactive compounds, which exert anti-inflammatory, antioxidant, neuroprotective, anxiolytic, sedative, and cardioprotective effects through various molecular pathways.

Dosage: Dosage of spikenard extract can vary depending on the formulation and intended use. Typical doses range from 250 mg to 1000 mg of standardized extract per day, taken orally with meals or as directed by a healthcare professional.

Contraindications: Spikenard should be used with caution in pregnant or breastfeeding women, as well as individuals with known allergies to plants in the Valerianaceae family or with pre-existing medical conditions. It may also interact with certain medications, particularly sedatives or antidepressants.

Precautions: Pregnant or breastfeeding women, as well as individuals with liver or kidney disorders, should consult with a healthcare professional before using spikenard supplements. It is important to use it under medical supervision, especially in combination with other medications.

Adverse Reactions: Adverse reactions to spikenard extract are rare but may include gastrointestinal upset, allergic reactions, or interactions with medications in susceptible individuals. It is essential to monitor for any adverse effects and discontinue use if necessary.

Research Standing: Research on spikenard and its health benefits is ongoing, with numerous studies investigating its efficacy and safety in various populations and medical conditions. It is recognized as a valuable medicinal plant in traditional medicine systems and has gained popularity as a dietary supplement in recent years.

Pharmacokinetics: The pharmacokinetics of spikenard extract constituents have been studied to a limited extent. Absorption of its bioactive compounds likely occurs in the gastrointestinal tract, with metabolites distributed throughout the body.

Pharmacodynamics: Spikenard extract exerts its pharmacodynamic effects primarily through its bioactive compounds, which interact with various molecular targets to produce its medicinal effects, including anti-inflammatory, antioxidant, neuroprotective, anxiolytic, sedative, and cardioprotective actions.

Overdosage: Excessive consumption of spikenard extract may lead to gastrointestinal discomfort or adverse reactions. Dosage should not exceed recommended levels, and it is important to follow the guidance of a healthcare professional.

International Standing: Spikenard is recognized internationally as a valuable medicinal plant and dietary supplement. Its products are available in various forms, including capsules, teas, extracts, and essential oils, and are consumed worldwide.

Indian Standing: In India, spikenard has a long history of use in Ayurvedic medicine and traditional healing practices. It is valued for its medicinal properties and is used in various formulations for stress relief, insomnia, and other health conditions.

Research Summary: Research on spikenard extract highlights its potential as a natural remedy for various health conditions, including anxiety, insomnia, inflammation-related disorders, and cardiovascular diseases. While some studies have shown promising results, further research is needed to elucidate its mechanisms of action, optimize dosage regimens, and evaluate its long-term safety and efficacy.

69) NASTURTIUM OFFICINALE

Introduction: Nasturtium officinale, commonly known as watercress, is a nutrient-rich aquatic plant belonging to the Brassicaceae family. It has a long history of culinary and medicinal use dating back to ancient civilizations and is valued for its peppery flavor and numerous health benefits.

Synonym Name and Common Name: Synonym Name: Rorippa nasturtium-aquaticum Common Name: Watercress

Pharmacognosy/Chemistry: Watercress contains various bioactive compounds, including glucosinolates (such as gluconasturtiin), phenolic compounds (such as kaempferol and quercetin), vitamins (such as vitamin C and vitamin K), minerals (such as iron and calcium), and essential oils.

Action and Pharmacology: The bioactive compounds in watercress exhibit antioxidant, anti-inflammatory, antimicrobial, anti-cancer, hepatoprotective, and cardiovascular protective effects. They contribute to its pharmacological actions and potential health benefits.

Method of Analysis: Analytical methods for watercress typically involve extraction of its bioactive compounds followed by chromatographic techniques such as high-performance liquid chromatography (HPLC) or gas chromatography-mass spectrometry (GC-MS) for identification and quantification.

Health Benefits: Watercress is associated with various health benefits, including improving digestion, boosting immunity, reducing inflammation, promoting cardiovascular health, supporting bone health, and aiding in weight management.

Indication and Usage: It is used in culinary dishes, salads, soups, and herbal teas, as well as in traditional medicine systems, dietary supplements, and functional foods for various indications, including detoxification, colds, coughs, skin conditions, and as a general tonic.

Usual Constituents with Percentages:

- Glucosinolates (gluconasturtiin): Variable concentrations
- Phenolic compounds (kaempferol, quercetin): Variable concentrations
- Vitamins (vitamin C, vitamin K): Variable concentrations
- Minerals (iron, calcium): Variable concentrations
- Essential oils: Variable concentrations

Mechanism of Action: The health benefits of watercress are attributed to its diverse array of bioactive compounds, which exert antioxidant, anti-inflammatory, antimicrobial, and other therapeutic effects through various molecular pathways.

Dosage: Dosage of watercress varies depending on the form and intended use. For culinary purposes, it can be consumed as part of a balanced diet. For medicinal purposes, doses may range from 50 grams to 100 grams of fresh watercress per day, or as directed by a healthcare professional.

Contraindications: Watercress should be used with caution in individuals with known allergies to plants in the Brassicaceae family or with pre-existing medical conditions. It may also interact with certain medications, particularly blood thinners or thyroid medications.

Precautions: Individuals with thyroid disorders or kidney stones should consult with a healthcare professional before consuming large amounts of watercress due to its potential goitrogenic and oxalate content, respectively. It is important to use watercress in moderation, especially in susceptible individuals.

Adverse Reactions: Adverse reactions to watercress are rare but may include gastrointestinal upset, allergic reactions, or interactions with medications in susceptible individuals. It is essential to monitor for any adverse effects and discontinue use if necessary.

Research Standing: Research on watercress and its health benefits is ongoing, with numerous studies investigating its efficacy and safety in various populations and medical conditions. It is recognized as a valuable dietary source of nutrients and bioactive compounds with potential health-promoting effects.

Pharmacokinetics: The pharmacokinetics of watercress constituents have been studied to a limited extent. Absorption of its bioactive compounds likely occurs in the gastrointestinal tract, with metabolites distributed throughout the body.

Pharmacodynamics: Watercress exerts its pharmacodynamic effects primarily through its bioactive compounds, which interact with various molecular targets to produce its medicinal effects, including antioxidant, anti-inflammatory, antimicrobial, and other actions.

Overdosage: Excessive consumption of watercress may lead to gastrointestinal discomfort or adverse reactions. Dosage should not exceed recommended levels, and it is important to follow the guidance of a healthcare professional.

International Standing: Watercress is recognized internationally as a nutritious food and valued for its potential health benefits. It is consumed in various cuisines around the world and is also available as a dietary supplement in some regions.

Indian Standing: In India, watercress may not be as widely consumed as in other regions, but it is recognized for its nutritional value and potential health benefits. It is occasionally used in traditional medicine systems and culinary applications.

Research Summary: Research on watercress highlights its potential as a functional food and natural remedy for various health conditions, including inflammation-related disorders, cardiovascular diseases, and cancer. While some studies have shown promising results, further research is needed to elucidate its mechanisms of action, optimize dosage regimens, and evaluate its long-term safety and efficacy

70) OCIMUMTENUIFLORUM

Introduction: Ocimumtenuiflorum, commonly known as holy basil or Tulsi, is a revered herb in traditional medicine systems like Ayurveda. It has been used for centuries in various cultures for its medicinal properties and spiritual significance.

Synonym Name and Common Name: Synonym Name: Ocimum sanctum Common Name: Holy basil, Tulsi

Pharmacognosy/Chemistry: Ocimumtenuiflorum contains a plethora of bioactive compounds, including eugenol, rosmarinic acid, flavonoids (such as orientin and vicenin), tannins, and essential oils. These compounds contribute to its pharmacological effects and medicinal properties.

Action and Pharmacology: The bioactive compounds in holy basil exhibit diverse pharmacological actions, including antioxidant, anti-inflammatory, antimicrobial, adaptogenic, anxiolytic, and immunomodulatory effects. They play a key role in its therapeutic potential.

Method of Analysis: Analytical methods for Ocimumtenuiflorum involve extraction of its bioactive compounds followed by chromatographic techniques such as high-performance liquid chromatography (HPLC) or gas chromatography-mass spectrometry (GC-MS) for identification and quantification.

Health Benefits: Holy basil is associated with numerous health benefits, including reducing stress, improving cognitive function, enhancing immunity, regulating blood sugar levels, promoting cardiovascular health, and relieving respiratory ailments.

Indication and Usage: It is used in traditional medicine systems, herbal teas, dietary supplements, and aromatherapy for various indications, including stress management, respiratory disorders, digestive issues, inflammatory conditions, and overall well-being.

Usual Constituents with Percentages:

- Eugenol: Variable concentrations
- Rosmarinic acid: Variable concentrations
- Flavonoids (orientin, vicenin): Variable concentrations

- Tannins: Variable concentrations
- Essential oils: Variable concentrations

Mechanism of Action: The health benefits of holy basil are attributed to its bioactive compounds, which exert antioxidant, anti-inflammatory, antimicrobial, adaptogenic, and other effects through modulation of various molecular pathways.

Dosage: Dosage of holy basil supplements can vary depending on the form and intended use. Typical doses range from 300 mg to 600 mg of standardized extract per day, taken orally with meals or as directed by a healthcare professional.

Contraindications: Holy basil should be used with caution in pregnant or breastfeeding women, as well as individuals with known allergies to plants in the Lamiaceae family or with pre-existing medical conditions. It may also interact with certain medications, particularly blood thinners or diabetes medications.

Precautions: Pregnant or breastfeeding women, as well as individuals with bleeding disorders or diabetes, should consult with a healthcare professional before using holy basil supplements. It is important to use them under medical supervision, especially in combination with other medications.

Adverse Reactions: Adverse reactions to holy basil supplements are rare but may include gastrointestinal upset, allergic reactions, or interactions with medications in susceptible individuals. It is essential to monitor for any adverse effects and discontinue use if necessary.

Research Standing: Research on holy basil and its health benefits is extensive, with numerous studies investigating its efficacy and safety in various populations and medical conditions. It is recognized as a valuable medicinal plant in traditional medicine systems and has gained popularity as a dietary supplement globally.

Pharmacokinetics: The pharmacokinetics of holy basil constituents have been studied to a limited extent. Absorption of its bioactive compounds likely occurs in the gastrointestinal tract, with metabolites distributed throughout the body.

Pharmacodynamics: Holy basil extract exerts its pharmacodynamic effects primarily through its bioactive compounds, which interact with various molecular targets to produce its medicinal effects, including antioxidant, anti-inflammatory, antimicrobial, adaptogenic, and immunomodulatory actions.

Overdosage: Excessive consumption of holy basil supplements may lead to gastrointestinal discomfort or adverse reactions. Dosage should not exceed recommended levels, and it is important to follow the guidance of a healthcare professional.

International Standing: Holy basil is recognized internationally as a valuable medicinal herb and dietary supplement. Its products are available in various forms, including capsules, teas, extracts, and essential oils, and are consumed worldwide.

Indian Standing: In India, holy basil holds immense cultural and medicinal significance. It is revered as a sacred plant and is commonly grown in households. It is extensively used in Ayurvedic medicine for its holistic healing properties.

Research Summary: Research on holy basil continues to explore its pharmacological effects, safety profile, and potential therapeutic applications. While it has a long history of traditional use, further research is needed to fully elucidate its mechanisms of action, optimize dosage regimens, and evaluate its efficacy in clinical settings.

71)OYSTER SHELL POWDER

Introduction: Oyster shell powder is derived from the shells of oysters, which are mollusks commonly found in marine environments. It has been used for various purposes, including medicinal and nutritional applications, owing to its rich mineral content and potential health benefits.

Synonym Name and Common Name: Synonym Name: Ostreae Concha Common Name: Oyster shell powder

Pharmacognosy/Chemistry: Oyster shell powder primarily consists of calcium carbonate ($CaCO_3$), along with traces of other minerals such as magnesium, zinc, iron, and copper. It may also contain small amounts of protein and carbohydrates.

Action and Pharmacology: The main action of oyster shell powder is attributed to its high calcium content, which contributes to bone health, teeth strength, and muscle function. It also provides alkalizing properties and may support digestive health.

Method of Analysis: Analysis of oyster shell powder typically involves methods to determine its mineral composition, such as atomic absorption spectroscopy (AAS), inductively coupled plasma mass spectrometry (ICP-MS), or X-ray diffraction (XRD).

Health Benefits: Oyster shell powder is associated with various health benefits, including:

- Strengthening bones and teeth due to its high calcium content.
- Supporting muscle function and nerve transmission.
- Promoting alkalinity in the body, which may help balance pH levels.
- Assisting in digestion and relieving symptoms of acidity.

Indication and Usage: It is used as a dietary supplement to increase calcium intake, particularly for individuals with low dietary calcium or those at risk of osteoporosis. It may also be used in traditional medicine systems for digestive issues or as an antacid.

Usual Constituents with Percentages:

- Calcium carbonate (CaCO3): Typically high concentrations (up to 95%)
- Magnesium, zinc, iron, copper: Trace amounts
- Protein and carbohydrates: Minimal amounts

Mechanism of Action: The health benefits of oyster shell powder are primarily attributed to its calcium content, which plays a crucial role in bone formation, muscle contraction, nerve function, and acid-base balance in the body.

Dosage: Dosage of oyster shell powder varies depending on the individual's age, health status, and dietary calcium intake. Typical doses range from 500 mg to 2000 mg of elemental calcium per day, taken orally with meals or as directed by a healthcare professional.

Contraindications: Oyster shell powder should be used with caution in individuals with known allergies to shellfish. It may also interact with certain medications or supplements, particularly those containing calcium or magnesium.

Precautions: Individuals with kidney stones or hypercalcemia should consult with a healthcare professional before taking oyster shell powder supplements.

It is important to monitor calcium intake from all sources to avoid excessive supplementation.

Adverse Reactions: Adverse reactions to oyster shell powder supplements are rare but may include gastrointestinal upset, constipation, or allergic reactions in susceptible individuals. It is essential to discontinue use and seek medical attention if adverse effects occur.

Research Standing: Research on the health effects of oyster shell powder is relatively limited compared to other dietary supplements. While it is recognized for its calcium content and potential benefits for bone health, more studies are needed to evaluate its efficacy, safety, and long-term effects.

Pharmacokinetics: The pharmacokinetics of oyster shell powder have not been extensively studied. Calcium from oyster shell powder is expected to be absorbed in the intestines and may be influenced by factors such as vitamin D status and gastric acidity.

Pharmacodynamics: Oyster shell powder exerts its pharmacodynamic effects primarily through its calcium content, which contributes to various physiological processes in the body, including bone metabolism, muscle function, and acid-base balance.

Overdosage: Excessive consumption of oyster shell powder may lead to hypercalcemia, which can cause symptoms such as nausea, vomiting, constipation, and kidney stones. Dosage should not exceed recommended levels, and supplementation should be monitored.

International Standing: Oyster shell powder is recognized internationally as a dietary supplement and is commonly used to increase calcium intake and support bone health. It is available in various formulations and consumed in many countries.

Indian Standing: In India, oyster shell powder may not be as widely used as in other regions, but it is recognized for its calcium content and potential health benefits. It may be used in Ayurvedic formulations or as a dietary supplement in some populations.

Research Summary: Research on oyster shell powder primarily focuses on its calcium content and potential benefits for bone health. While it is generally considered safe when used as directed, further studies are needed to evaluate its efficacy, safety, and optimal dosage regimens for various health conditions.

72)PASSIFLORA FOETIDA– EXTRACT

Introduction: Passiflora foetida, commonly known as stinking passionflower or wild maracuja, is a species of passionflower native to the Americas, Africa, and Asia. It is known for its unique appearance and has been used traditionally for its medicinal properties.

Synonym Name and Common Name: Synonym Name: Passiflora incense Common Name: Stinking passionflower, Wild maracuja

Pharmacognosy/Chemistry: Passiflora foetida extract contains various bioactive compounds, including flavonoids (such as quercetin and kaempferol), alkaloids, phenolic compounds, and essential oils. These constituents contribute to its pharmacological effects.

Action and Pharmacology: The bioactive compounds in Passiflora foetida extract exhibit anxiolytic, sedative, antispasmodic, analgesic, and anti-inflammatory properties. They act on the central nervous system and other physiological pathways to produce these effects.

Method of Analysis: Analytical methods for Passiflora foetida extract typically involve extraction of its bioactive compounds followed by chromatographic techniques such as high-performance liquid chromatography (HPLC) or gas chromatography-mass spectrometry (GC-MS) for identification and quantification.

Health Benefits: Passiflora foetida extract is associated with various health benefits, including reducing anxiety, promoting relaxation, relieving muscle spasms, alleviating pain, and supporting overall well-being.

Indication and Usage: It is used in traditional medicine systems, herbal teas, dietary supplements, and aromatherapy for various indications, including anxiety disorders, insomnia, muscle tension, menstrual cramps, and as a natural sedative.

Usual Constituents with Percentages:

- Flavonoids (quercetin, kaempferol): Variable concentrations
- Alkaloids: Variable concentrations
- Phenolic compounds: Variable concentrations
- Essential oils: Variable concentrations

Mechanism of Action: The health benefits of Passiflora foetida extract are attributed to its bioactive compounds, which exert anxiolytic, sedative, antispasmodic, analgesic, and anti-inflammatory effects through modulation of neurotransmitter activity and other molecular pathways.

Dosage: Dosage of Passiflora foetida extract can vary depending on the formulation and intended use. Typical doses range from 200 mg to 1000 mg per day, taken orally in divided doses or as directed by a healthcare professional.

Contraindications: Passiflora foetida extract should be used with caution in pregnant or breastfeeding women, as well as individuals with known allergies to plants in the Passifloraceae family or with pre-existing medical conditions. It may also interact with certain medications, particularly sedatives or antidepressants.

Precautions: Pregnant or breastfeeding women, as well as individuals with liver or kidney disorders, should consult with a healthcare professional before using Passiflora foetida extract supplements. It is important to use them under medical supervision, especially in combination with other medications.

Adverse Reactions: Adverse reactions to Passiflora foetida extract are rare but may include gastrointestinal upset, dizziness, drowsiness, or allergic reactions in susceptible individuals. It is essential to monitor for any adverse effects and discontinue use if necessary.

Research Standing: Research on Passiflora foetida extract and its health benefits is ongoing, with numerous studies investigating its efficacy and safety in various populations and medical conditions. It is recognized as a valuable medicinal plant in traditional medicine systems and has gained popularity as a natural remedy for anxiety and insomnia.

Pharmacokinetics: The pharmacokinetics of Passiflora foetida extract constituents have not been extensively studied. Absorption of its bioactive compounds likely occurs in the gastrointestinal tract, with metabolites distributed throughout the body.

Pharmacodynamics: Passiflora foetida extract exerts its pharmacodynamic effects primarily through its bioactive compounds, which interact with various neurotransmitter systems and other molecular targets to produce its anxiolytic, sedative, antispasmodic, analgesic, and anti-inflammatory actions.

Overdosage: Excessive consumption of Passiflora foetida extract may lead to drowsiness, dizziness, or gastrointestinal discomfort. Dosage should not exceed recommended levels, and it is important to follow the guidance of a healthcare professional.

International Standing: Passiflora foetida extract is recognized internationally as a valuable medicinal plant and dietary supplement. Its products are available in various forms, including capsules, teas, extracts, and essential oils, and are consumed in many countries.

Indian Standing: In India, Passiflora foetida extract may be used in traditional medicine systems for its anxiolytic and sedative properties. It is valued for its calming effects and is occasionally included in herbal formulations for anxiety and insomnia.

Research Summary: Research on Passiflora foetida extract highlights its potential as a natural remedy for anxiety, insomnia, muscle tension, and other related conditions. While some studies have shown promising results, further research is needed to elucidate its mechanisms of action, optimize dosage regimens, and evaluate its long-term safety and efficacy.

73)ARACHIS HYPOGAEA

Introduction: Arachis hypogaea, commonly known as peanut, is a leguminous plant cultivated for its edible seeds. It is widely consumed around the world and valued for its nutritional content and culinary versatility.

Synonym Name and Common Name: Synonym Name: Groundnut Common Name: Peanut

Pharmacognosy/Chemistry: The seeds of Arachis hypogaea contain various bioactive compounds, including protein, healthy fats, carbohydrates, fiber, vitamins (such as vitamin E and B vitamins), minerals (such as magnesium, phosphorus, and potassium), and phytochemicals (such as resveratrol and flavonoids).

Action and Pharmacology: Peanuts exhibit numerous pharmacological effects, including antioxidant, anti-inflammatory, cardioprotective, neuroprotective, and anti-cancer properties. These effects are attributed to its diverse array of bioactive compounds.

Method of Analysis: Analytical methods for peanuts typically involve assessing their nutritional composition, including protein, fat, carbohydrate, fiber, vitamins, minerals, and phytochemicals. Techniques such as proximate analysis, HPLC, GC-MS, and spectrophotometry may be used.

Health Benefits: Peanuts offer various health benefits, including:

- Providing essential nutrients like protein, healthy fats, vitamins, and minerals.
- Supporting heart health by reducing cholesterol levels and improving blood lipid profiles.
- Promoting weight management due to their satiating effect and nutrient density.
- Enhancing cognitive function and reducing the risk of age-related cognitive decline.
- Supporting bone health and immune function due to their mineral and vitamin content.

Indication and Usage: Peanuts are consumed in various forms, including raw, roasted, boiled, or as peanut butter. They are used in cooking, baking, snacking, and as ingredients in numerous dishes, snacks, and culinary preparations worldwide.

Usual Constituents with Percentages:

- Protein: 25-30%
- Fat: 40-50%
- Carbohydrates: 10-15%
- Fiber: 5-10%
- Vitamins and minerals: Variable concentrations
- Phytochemicals: Variable concentrations

Mechanism of Action: The health benefits of peanuts are attributed to their bioactive compounds, which exert antioxidant, anti-inflammatory, cardioprotective, neuroprotective, and anti-cancer effects through various molecular pathways in the body.

Dosage: There is no specific dosage for peanuts as they are typically consumed as part of a balanced diet. Daily consumption of a handful of peanuts (about 30 grams) is considered beneficial for health when incorporated into a well-rounded diet.

Contraindications: Individuals with known allergies to peanuts should avoid their consumption due to the risk of allergic reactions, which can range from mild symptoms to severe anaphylaxis. Peanuts may also interact with certain medications or exacerbate certain medical conditions.

Precautions: Peanuts should be consumed in moderation, especially by individuals with diabetes, obesity, or cardiovascular disease, due to their calorie and fat content. It is important to choose unsalted, unflavored peanuts to avoid excessive sodium or added sugars.

Adverse Reactions: Adverse reactions to peanuts primarily involve allergic responses, ranging from mild symptoms such as itching or hives to severe reactions such as anaphylaxis. Individuals with peanut allergies should avoid peanuts and products containing peanuts.

Research Standing: Peanuts have been extensively studied for their nutritional composition, health effects, and potential therapeutic applications. Research continues to explore their role in preventing chronic diseases, promoting health, and improving overall well-being.

Pharmacokinetics: The pharmacokinetics of peanuts involve the digestion, absorption, distribution, metabolism, and excretion of their nutrients and bioactive compounds. These processes vary depending on factors such as food matrix, processing, and individual physiology.

Pharmacodynamics: Peanuts exert their pharmacodynamic effects through their bioactive compounds, which interact with various molecular targets and physiological pathways to produce their health benefits, including antioxidant, anti-inflammatory, cardioprotective, and neuroprotective effects.

Overdosage: Excessive consumption of peanuts may lead to weight gain, digestive discomfort, or adverse effects in individuals with peanut allergies. It is important to consume peanuts in moderation as part of a balanced diet to avoid potential adverse outcomes.

International Standing: Peanuts are widely consumed and recognized internationally as a valuable source of nutrition and culinary enjoyment. They are a staple food in many cultures and are consumed in various forms around the world.

Indian Standing: In India, peanuts are commonly consumed as a snack, in culinary preparations, and in traditional dishes. They hold cultural significance and are used in festivals, religious rituals, and everyday cooking in various regional cuisines.

Research Summary: Research on peanuts continues to elucidate their nutritional composition, health benefits, and potential therapeutic applications. While they are recognized for their role in promoting heart health, weight management, and overall well-being, ongoing research aims to further understand their mechanisms of action and optimize their consumption for health promotion and disease prevention.

74)PERNA CANALICULUS

Introduction: Perna canaliculus, commonly known as green-lipped mussel, is a species of mussel native to New Zealand. It is renowned for its rich nutritional profile and potential health benefits, particularly for joint health and inflammation management.

Synonym Name and Common Name: Synonym Name: New Zealand green-lipped mussel Common Name: Green-lipped mussel

Pharmacognosy/Chemistry: Green-lipped mussel contains a unique blend of bioactive compounds, including omega-3 fatty acids (such as eicosatetraenoic acid, ETA), glycosaminoglycans (GAGs), proteins, peptides, vitamins, minerals, and antioxidants.

Action and Pharmacology: Green-lipped mussel exhibits anti-inflammatory, antioxidant, analgesic, and cartilage-protective properties. These effects are attributed to its omega-3 fatty acids, GAGs, and other bioactive components, which modulate inflammatory pathways and support joint health.

Method of Analysis: Analytical methods for green-lipped mussel involve assessing its nutritional composition, including omega-3 fatty acids, GAGs, proteins, and other bioactive compounds. Techniques such as chromatography, spectrophotometry, and mass spectrometry may be used.

Health Benefits: Green-lipped mussel offers various health benefits, including:

- Supporting joint health and mobility by reducing inflammation and promoting cartilage repair.
- Alleviating symptoms of osteoarthritis, rheumatoid arthritis, and other inflammatory joint conditions.
- Enhancing skin health and wound healing due to its antioxidant and anti-inflammatory properties.
- Supporting cardiovascular health and immune function with its omega-3 fatty acids and other nutrients.

Indication and Usage: Green-lipped mussel supplements are used to manage symptoms of arthritis, including pain, stiffness, and swelling. They are also used for general joint support, sports performance, skin health, and overall well-being.

Usual Constituents with Percentages:

- Omega-3 fatty acids (ETA): 2-5%
- Glycosaminoglycans (GAGs): 20-40%
- Proteins: 20-30%
- Vitamins and minerals: Variable concentrations
- Antioxidants: Variable concentrations

Mechanism of Action: The health benefits of green-lipped mussel are primarily attributed to its omega-3 fatty acids (especially ETA) and GAGs, which inhibit pro-inflammatory enzymes, reduce oxidative stress, and support cartilage regeneration, thereby improving joint function and reducing pain.

Dosage: Dosage of green-lipped mussel supplements typically ranges from 500 mg to 3000 mg per day, depending on the product's concentration and individual needs. It is often taken orally in divided doses with meals.

Contraindications: Green-lipped mussel supplements should be used with caution in individuals with known allergies to shellfish. They may also interact with blood-thinning medications or affect blood clotting, so consultation with a healthcare professional is recommended.

Precautions: Individuals with seafood allergies, bleeding disorders, or taking anticoagulant medications should consult with a healthcare provider before using green-lipped mussel supplements. It is important to choose reputable products to ensure purity and quality.

Adverse Reactions: Adverse reactions to green-lipped mussel supplements are rare but may include gastrointestinal upset, allergic reactions, or interactions with medications. It is essential to discontinue use and seek medical attention if adverse effects occur.

Research Standing: Green-lipped mussel has been extensively studied for its potential therapeutic effects, particularly in the management of arthritis and inflammatory conditions. Research continues to explore its mechanisms of action, efficacy, and safety in various populations.

Pharmacokinetics: The pharmacokinetics of green-lipped mussel constituents, such as omega-3 fatty acids and GAGs, involve absorption in the gastrointestinal tract, distribution to target tissues (such as joints), metabolism, and elimination from the body.

Pharmacodynamics: Green-lipped mussel exerts its pharmacodynamic effects through its bioactive components, which modulate inflammatory pathways, reduce oxidative stress, support cartilage repair, and improve joint function and mobility.

Overdosage: Excessive consumption of green-lipped mussel supplements may lead to gastrointestinal discomfort or allergic reactions in susceptible individuals. Dosage should not exceed recommended levels, and supplementation should be monitored.

International Standing: Green-lipped mussel supplements are recognized internationally for their potential health benefits, particularly in managing arthritis and supporting joint health. They are available in various formulations and are consumed in many countries.

Indian Standing: In India, green-lipped mussel supplements may not be as widely used as in other regions, but they are gaining recognition for their potential therapeutic effects, especially for arthritis management and joint support.

Research Summary: Research on green-lipped mussel supplements supports their efficacy in reducing inflammation, alleviating joint pain, and improving mobility in individuals with arthritis and other inflammatory conditions. Ongoing studies aim to further elucidate their mechanisms of action, optimize dosage regimens, and evaluate their long-term safety and efficacy.

75) PHELLODENDRONAMURENSE LEAF OIL

Introduction: Phellodendronamurense, commonly known as Amur cork tree, is a species of tree native to East Asia. The oil extracted from its leaves, known as Phellodendronamurense leaf oil, has been used in traditional medicine for its potential health benefits.

Synonym Name and Common Name: Synonym Name: Huang Bai Common Name: Amur cork tree leaf oil

Pharmacognosy/Chemistry: Phellodendronamurense leaf oil contains various bioactive compounds, including alkaloids (such as berberine), flavonoids, phenolic compounds, and essential oils. These constituents contribute to its pharmacological effects.

Action and Pharmacology: Phellodendronamurense leaf oil exhibits anti-inflammatory, antioxidant, antimicrobial, and anti-cancer properties. These effects are attributed to its bioactive compounds, which modulate various molecular pathways in the body.

Method of Analysis: Analytical methods for Phellodendronamurense leaf oil involve extraction of its bioactive compounds followed by chromatographic techniques such as gas chromatography-mass spectrometry (GC-MS) or high-performance liquid chromatography (HPLC) for identification and quantification.

Health Benefits: Phellodendronamurense leaf oil offers various health benefits, including:

- Reducing inflammation and oxidative stress
- Supporting immune function
- Exhibiting antimicrobial activity against bacteria and fungi
- Potentially inhibiting cancer cell growth

Indication and Usage: Phellodendronamurense leaf oil is used in traditional medicine systems for various indications, including inflammatory conditions, microbial infections, and as a natural remedy for certain cancers. It may also be used in aromatherapy and topical applications.

Usual Constituents with Percentages:

- Alkaloids (berberine): Variable concentrations
- Flavonoids: Variable concentrations
- Phenolic compounds: Variable concentrations
- Essential oils: Variable concentrations

Mechanism of Action: The health benefits of Phellodendronamurense leaf oil are attributed to its bioactive compounds, which exert anti-inflammatory, antioxidant, antimicrobial, and anti-cancer effects through modulation of various molecular targets and pathways.

Dosage: Dosage of Phellodendronamurense leaf oil can vary depending on the formulation and intended use. It may be taken orally, applied topically, or used in aromatherapy. Dosage should be determined by a healthcare professional.

Contraindications: Phellodendronamurense leaf oil should be used with caution in pregnant or breastfeeding women, as well as individuals with known allergies to plants in the Rutaceae family or with pre-existing medical conditions. It may also interact with certain medications.

Precautions: Individuals with liver or kidney disorders, as well as those taking medications or supplements, should consult with a healthcare professional before using Phellodendronamurense leaf oil. It is important to use it under medical supervision.

Adverse Reactions: Adverse reactions to Phellodendronamurense leaf oil are rare but may include gastrointestinal upset, allergic reactions, or interactions with medications. It is essential to monitor for any adverse effects and discontinue use if necessary.

Research Standing: Research on Phellodendronamurense leaf oil and its health benefits is ongoing, with studies investigating its efficacy and safety in various conditions. While it is recognized in traditional medicine systems, further research is needed to validate its therapeutic uses.

Pharmacokinetics: The pharmacokinetics of Phellodendronamurense leaf oil constituents have not been extensively studied. Absorption, distribution, metabolism, and excretion of its bioactive compounds likely occur in the body following oral or topical administration.

Pharmacodynamics: Phellodendronamurense leaf oil exerts its pharmacodynamic effects through its bioactive compounds, which interact with various molecular targets and pathways to produce its anti-inflammatory, antioxidant, antimicrobial, and anti-cancer actions.

Overdosage: Excessive consumption or application of Phellodendronamurense leaf oil may lead to adverse effects, including gastrointestinal discomfort or allergic reactions. Dosage should not exceed recommended levels, and it is important to use it judiciously.

International Standing: Phellodendronamurense leaf oil is recognized internationally for its potential health benefits and is used in various forms, including dietary supplements, topical preparations, and aromatherapy products. Its products are available in many countries.

Indian Standing: In India, Phellodendronamurense leaf oil may be used in traditional Ayurvedic medicine for its anti-inflammatory, antimicrobial, and other therapeutic properties. It may also be incorporated into topical formulations for skin health and wound healing.

Research Summary: Research on Phellodendronamurense leaf oil highlights its potential as a natural remedy for inflammation, microbial infections, and certain cancers. While traditional uses are well-documented, further scientific research is needed to elucidate its mechanisms of action, optimize dosage regimens, and evaluate its safety and efficacy in clinical settings.

76)PHYLLANTHUS AMARUS

Introduction: Phyllanthus amarus, also known as "Bhumyamlaki" in Ayurveda, is a tropical plant widely used in traditional medicine systems for its potential health benefits. It belongs to the Phyllanthaceae family and is native to India and other tropical regions.

Synonym Name and Common Name: Synonym Name: Bhumyamlaki, Stonebreaker Common Name: Phyllanthus, Chanca Piedra

Pharmacognosy/Chemistry: Phyllanthus amarus contains various bioactive compounds, including lignans, alkaloids, flavonoids, tannins, and polyphenols. These constituents contribute to its medicinal properties.

Action and Pharmacology: Phyllanthus amarus exhibits hepatoprotective, antiviral, antioxidant, anti-inflammatory, diuretic, and hypoglycemic properties. It acts on various organs and systems in the body, particularly the liver, kidneys, and immune system.

Method of Analysis: Analytical methods for Phyllanthus amarus involve extraction of its bioactive compounds followed by chromatographic techniques such as high-performance liquid chromatography (HPLC) or gas chromatography-mass spectrometry (GC-MS) for identification and quantification.

Health Benefits: Phyllanthus amarus offers various health benefits, including:

- Supporting liver health and detoxification
- Protecting against viral infections, including hepatitis B and C
- Reducing inflammation and oxidative stress
- Promoting kidney health and supporting urinary tract function
- Lowering blood sugar levels and improving diabetes management

Indication and Usage: Phyllanthus amarus is used in traditional medicine for various indications, including liver disorders (such as hepatitis, jaundice, and liver cirrhosis), viral infections, kidney stones, urinary tract infections, and diabetes. It is consumed as an herbal tea, decoction, or in supplement form.

Usual Constituents with Percentages:

- Lignans: 1-5%
- Alkaloids: 0.5-2%
- Flavonoids: 2-6%
- Tannins: 2-4%
- Polyphenols: 1-3%

Mechanism of Action: The health benefits of Phyllanthus amarus are attributed to its bioactive compounds, which exert hepatoprotective, antiviral, antioxidant, and anti-inflammatory effects through modulation of various molecular pathways and cellular processes.

Dosage: Dosage of Phyllanthus amarus supplements can vary depending on the formulation and intended use. It is typically taken orally in doses ranging from 500 mg to 2000 mg per day, divided into two or three doses.

Contraindications: Phyllanthus amarus should be used with caution in pregnant or breastfeeding women, as well as individuals with known allergies to plants in the Phyllanthaceae family or with pre-existing medical conditions. It may also interact with certain medications.

Precautions: Individuals with liver or kidney disorders, as well as those taking medications or supplements, should consult with a healthcare professional before using Phyllanthus amarus. It is important to use it under medical supervision, especially in high doses or for prolonged periods.

Adverse Reactions: Adverse reactions to Phyllanthus amarus supplements are rare but may include gastrointestinal upset, allergic reactions, or interactions with medications. It is essential to monitor for any adverse effects and discontinue use if necessary.

Research Standing: Phyllanthus amarus has been extensively studied for its medicinal properties and therapeutic potential. Research continues to explore its efficacy and safety in various conditions, with promising results in liver disorders, viral infections, kidney stones, and diabetes management.

Pharmacokinetics: The pharmacokinetics of Phyllanthus amarus constituents have not been extensively studied. Absorption, distribution, metabolism, and excretion of its bioactive compounds likely occur in the body following oral administration.

Pharmacodynamics: Phyllanthus amarus exerts its pharmacodynamic effects through its bioactive compounds, which interact with various molecular targets and pathways to produce its hepatoprotective, antiviral, antioxidant, and anti-inflammatory actions.

Overdosage: Excessive consumption of Phyllanthus amarus supplements may lead to gastrointestinal discomfort or allergic reactions in susceptible individuals. Dosage should not exceed recommended levels, and it is important to use it judiciously.

International Standing: Phyllanthus amarus is recognized internationally for its medicinal properties and is used in traditional medicine systems worldwide. Its products are available in various forms and are consumed in many countries for liver health, viral infections, and other health conditions.

Indian Standing: In India, Phyllanthus amarus is widely used in Ayurveda and other traditional medicine systems for its hepatoprotective, antiviral, and anti-inflammatory properties. It is considered a valuable medicinal plant and is incorporated into numerous herbal formulations.

Research Summary: Research on Phyllanthus amarus highlights its potential as a natural remedy for liver disorders, viral infections, kidney stones, and diabetes. While traditional uses are well-documented, further scientific research is needed to elucidate its mechanisms of action, optimize dosage regimens, and evaluate its safety and efficacy in clinical settings.

77) PICRORHIZAKURROA-PICRORHIZA

Introduction: Picrorhizakurroa, commonly known as Picrorhiza or Kutki, is a perennial herb native to the Himalayan region of India, Nepal, and Tibet. It has been used in traditional medicine systems such as Ayurveda for its various health benefits.

Synonym Name and Common Name: Synonym Name: Picrorhizakurroa Common Name: Kutki, Kutaki

Pharmacognosy/Chemistry: Picrorhizakurroa contains several bioactive compounds, including iridoid glycosides (such as picroside I and picroside II), kutkoside, cucurbitacin glycosides, and flavonoids. These constituents contribute to its pharmacological properties.

Action and Pharmacology: Picrorhizakurroa exhibits hepatoprotective, anti-inflammatory, antioxidant, immunomodulatory, and cholagogue (bile-stimulating) properties. It supports liver health, boosts immunity, reduces inflammation, and scavenges free radicals.

Method of Analysis: Analytical methods for Picrorhizakurroa involve extraction of its bioactive compounds followed by chromatographic techniques such as high-performance liquid chromatography (HPLC) or gas chromatography-mass spectrometry (GC-MS) for identification and quantification.

Health Benefits: Picrorhizakurroa offers various health benefits, including:

- Supporting liver health and function
- Reducing inflammation and oxidative stress
- Boosting immune system
- Improving digestion and bile secretion
- Supporting respiratory health

Indication and Usage: Picrorhizakurroa is used in traditional medicine for various indications, including liver disorders (such as hepatitis, jaundice, and liver cirrhosis), inflammatory conditions, respiratory ailments, digestive issues, and immune system support. It is consumed orally in powder, capsule, or decoction form.

Usual Constituents with Percentages:

- Iridoid glycosides (picroside I and picroside II): 2-5%
- Kutkoside: 1-3%
- Cucurbitacin glycosides: 1-2%
- Flavonoids: 1-4%

Mechanism of Action: The health benefits of Picrorhizakurroa are attributed to its bioactive compounds, particularly iridoid glycosides and flavonoids, which exert hepatoprotective, anti-inflammatory, antioxidant, and immunomodulatory effects through modulation of various molecular pathways and cellular processes.

Dosage: Dosage of Picrorhizakurroa supplements can vary depending on the formulation and intended use. It is typically taken orally in doses ranging from 500 mg to 2000 mg per day, divided into two or three doses.

Contraindications: Picrorhizakurroa should be used with caution in pregnant or breastfeeding women, as well as individuals with known allergies to plants in the Plantaginaceae family or with pre-existing medical conditions. It may also interact with certain medications.

Precautions: Individuals with liver or kidney disorders, as well as those taking medications or supplements, should consult with a healthcare professional before using Picrorhizakurroa. It is important to use it under medical supervision, especially in high doses or for prolonged periods.

Adverse Reactions: Adverse reactions to Picrorhizakurroa supplements are rare but may include gastrointestinal upset, allergic reactions, or interactions with medications. It is essential to monitor for any adverse effects and discontinue use if necessary.

Research Standing: Picrorhizakurroa has been extensively studied for its medicinal properties and therapeutic potential. Research continues to explore its efficacy and safety in various conditions, with promising results in liver disorders, inflammatory conditions, respiratory ailments, and immune system support.

Pharmacokinetics: The pharmacokinetics of Picrorhizakurroa constituents have not been extensively studied. Absorption, distribution, metabolism, and excretion of its bioactive compounds likely occur in the body following oral administration.

Pharmacodynamics: Picrorhizakurroa exerts its pharmacodynamic effects through its bioactive compounds, which interact with various molecular targets and pathways to produce its hepatoprotective, anti-inflammatory, antioxidant, and immunomodulatory actions.

Overdosage: Excessive consumption of Picrorhizakurroa supplements may lead to gastrointestinal discomfort or allergic reactions in susceptible individuals. Dosage should not exceed recommended levels, and it is important to use it judiciously.

International Standing: Picrorhizakurroa is recognized internationally for its medicinal properties and is used in traditional medicine systems worldwide. Its products are available in various forms and are consumed in many countries for liver health, inflammation, respiratory health, and immune support.

Indian Standing: In India, Picrorhizakurroa is highly valued in Ayurveda for its hepatoprotective, anti-inflammatory, and immunomodulatory properties. It is considered a key herb in numerous Ayurvedic formulations and is used extensively in the management of liver disorders, inflammatory conditions, and respiratory ailments.

Research Summary: Research on Picrorhizakurroa highlights its potential as a natural remedy for liver disorders, inflammatory conditions, respiratory ailments, and immune system support. While traditional uses are well-documented, further scientific research is needed to elucidate its mechanisms of action, optimize dosage regimens, and evaluate its safety and efficacy in clinical settings.

78) PIMENTO OFFICINALIS L

Introduction: Pimento officinalis L., commonly known as Allspice, is an aromatic evergreen tree native to the Caribbean, Central America, and Mexico. Its dried fruits, resembling peppercorns, are widely used as a spice in culinary dishes and also possess medicinal properties.

Synonym Name and Common Name: Synonym Name: Pimenta dioica Common Name: Allspice, Jamaican pepper, Pimento

Pharmacognosy/Chemistry: Pimento officinalis contains various bioactive compounds, including eugenol, cineole, myrcene, and caryophyllene. These constituents contribute to its aromatic properties and medicinal effects.

Action and Pharmacology: Pimento officinalis exhibits antimicrobial, anti-inflammatory, analgesic, antioxidant, and digestive stimulant properties. It can aid digestion, relieve pain, reduce inflammation, and inhibit microbial growth.

Method of Analysis: Analytical methods for Pimento officinalis involve extraction of its bioactive compounds followed by chromatographic techniques such as gas chromatography-mass spectrometry (GC-MS) or high-performance liquid chromatography (HPLC) for identification and quantification.

Health Benefits: Pimento officinalis offers various health benefits, including:

- Digestive support: Relieving indigestion, bloating, and gas.
- Pain relief: Alleviating muscle pain, joint pain, and headaches.
- Anti-inflammatory effects: Reducing inflammation in the body.
- Antimicrobial activity: Inhibiting the growth of bacteria and fungi.
- Antioxidant properties: Scavenging free radicals and protecting against oxidative stress.

Indication and Usage: Pimento officinalis is used in traditional medicine for various indications, including digestive disorders, muscle pain, joint pain, headaches, and respiratory ailments. It is consumed orally as a spice in culinary dishes or used topically in herbal preparations.

Usual Constituents with Percentages:

- Eugenol: 50-75%
- Cineole: 10-20%
- Myrcene: 5-10%
- Caryophyllene: 5-10%

Mechanism of Action: The health benefits of Pimento officinalis are attributed to its bioactive compounds, particularly eugenol, which exerts antimicrobial, anti-inflammatory, analgesic, and antioxidant effects through modulation of various molecular targets and pathways.

Dosage: Dosage of Pimento officinalis can vary depending on the intended use and form of administration. As a spice, it is typically used in culinary dishes in small quantities. For medicinal purposes, herbal preparations or essential oil formulations may be used according to product instructions or healthcare provider recommendations.

Contraindications: Pimento officinalis should be used with caution in individuals with known allergies to spices or with pre-existing medical conditions. It may also interact with certain medications, particularly those metabolized by the liver.

Precautions: Individuals with sensitive digestive systems or skin may experience adverse reactions to Pimento officinalis. It is important to use it in moderation and discontinue use if any adverse effects occur. Pregnant or breastfeeding women should consult with a healthcare professional before use.

Adverse Reactions: Adverse reactions to Pimento officinalis are rare but may include gastrointestinal upset, skin irritation, or allergic reactions in susceptible individuals. It is essential to monitor for any adverse effects and discontinue use if necessary.

Research Standing: Research on Pimento officinalis and its medicinal properties is ongoing, with studies investigating its efficacy and safety in various conditions. While it is widely used in traditional medicine, further scientific research is needed to validate its therapeutic uses and mechanisms of action.

Pharmacokinetics: The pharmacokinetics of Pimento officinalis constituents have not been extensively studied. Absorption, distribution, metabolism, and excretion of its bioactive compounds likely occur in the body following oral or topical administration.

Pharmacodynamics: Pimento officinalis exerts its pharmacodynamic effects through its bioactive compounds, which interact with various molecular targets and pathways to produce its antimicrobial, anti-inflammatory, analgesic, and antioxidant actions.

Overdosage: Excessive consumption or application of Pimento officinalis may lead to adverse effects, particularly gastrointestinal upset or skin irritation. Dosage should not exceed recommended levels, and it is important to use it judiciously.

International Standing: Pimento officinalis is recognized internationally for its culinary use as a spice and its potential medicinal properties. Its products are widely available in various forms, including whole dried fruits, ground spice, and essential oil, and are used in many countries.

Indian Standing: In India, Pimento officinalis may be used in traditional Ayurvedic medicine for its digestive, analgesic, and antimicrobial properties. It may also be incorporated into culinary dishes for flavoring and medicinal purposes.

Research Summary: Research on Pimento officinalis highlights its potential as a natural remedy for digestive disorders, pain relief, inflammation, and microbial infections. While traditional uses are well-documented, further scientific research is needed to elucidate its mechanisms of action, optimize dosage regimens, and evaluate its safety and efficacy in clinical settings.

79) PINUS GERARDIANA

Introduction: Pinus gerardiana, commonly known as the Chilgoza pine or the Neoza pine, is a species of pine native to the Himalayan region, particularly in Afghanistan, Pakistan, and India. It produces edible pine nuts, which have been utilized in traditional medicine for their potential health benefits.

Synonym Name and Common Name: Synonym Name: Gerard's pine Common Name: Chilgoza pine, Neoza pine, Pine nuts

Pharmacognosy/Chemistry: Pinus gerardiana contains various bioactive compounds, including essential oils, flavonoids, phenolic compounds, and fatty acids. The pine nuts derived from its cones are rich in nutrients such as protein, healthy fats, vitamins, and minerals.

Action and Pharmacology: Pinus gerardiana exhibits antioxidant, anti-inflammatory, antimicrobial, and cardioprotective properties. Its constituents contribute to these pharmacological effects, supporting overall health and well-being.

Method of Analysis: Analytical methods for Pinus gerardiana involve extraction of its bioactive compounds followed by chromatographic techniques such as gas chromatography-mass spectrometry (GC-MS) or high-performance liquid chromatography (HPLC) for identification and quantification.

Health Benefits: Pinus gerardiana offers various health benefits, including:

- Heart health: Supporting cardiovascular function and reducing the risk of heart disease.
- Antioxidant activity: Protecting cells from oxidative damage and reducing inflammation.
- Nutritional support: Providing essential nutrients such as protein, healthy fats, vitamins, and minerals.
- Weight management: Promoting satiety and aiding in weight loss or maintenance.
- Anti-microbial properties: Helping to combat bacterial and fungal infections.

Indication and Usage: Pinus gerardiana and its pine nuts are used in traditional medicine for various indications, including heart health, inflammation, microbial infections, and nutritional support. They can be consumed raw, roasted, or incorporated into culinary dishes and herbal preparations.

Usual Constituents with Percentages:

- Essential oils: 0.1-0.5%
- Flavonoids: 0.5-2%
- Phenolic compounds: 1-3%

- Fatty acids: 20-40%

Mechanism of Action: The health benefits of Pinus gerardiana are attributed to its bioactive compounds, which exert antioxidant, anti-inflammatory, antimicrobial, and cardioprotective effects through various molecular mechanisms and pathways.

Dosage: Dosage of Pinus gerardiana pine nuts can vary depending on individual nutritional needs and health goals. As a dietary supplement, consuming a handful of pine nuts (approximately 1-2 tablespoons) per day is typically recommended.

Contraindications: Pinus gerardiana pine nuts are generally safe for consumption when used as food. However, individuals with allergies to pine nuts or other tree nuts should avoid them. Additionally, individuals with certain medical conditions or those taking medications should consult with a healthcare professional before incorporating pine nuts into their diet.

Precautions: Consumption of pine nuts should be moderate, especially for individuals with a history of nut allergies or gastrointestinal sensitivities. It is important to source high-quality pine nuts and store them properly to prevent spoilage.

Adverse Reactions: Adverse reactions to Pinus gerardiana pine nuts are rare but may include allergic reactions, gastrointestinal discomfort, or interactions with medications. Individuals with nut allergies should avoid consuming pine nuts to prevent adverse effects.

Research Standing: Research on Pinus gerardiana and its health benefits is ongoing, with studies investigating its antioxidant, anti-inflammatory, cardioprotective, and antimicrobial properties. While traditional uses are well-documented, further scientific research is needed to validate its therapeutic effects and mechanisms of action.

Pharmacokinetics: The pharmacokinetics of Pinus gerardiana constituents have not been extensively studied. Absorption, distribution, metabolism, and excretion of its bioactive compounds likely occur in the body following oral consumption.

Pharmacodynamics: Pinus gerardiana exerts its pharmacodynamic effects through its bioactive compounds, which interact with various molecular targets and pathways to produce its antioxidant, anti-inflammatory, cardioprotective, and antimicrobial actions.

Overdosage: Excessive consumption of pine nuts may lead to gastrointestinal discomfort, allergic reactions, or weight gain due to their high-fat content. It is important to consume them in moderation as part of a balanced diet.

International Standing: Pinus gerardiana pine nuts are recognized internationally as a nutritious food source and are consumed in various cuisines worldwide. They are also valued for their potential health benefits and are used in traditional medicine systems.

Indian Standing: In India, Pinus gerardiana pine nuts have cultural and culinary significance, particularly in the Himalayan regions where they are harvested. They are used in traditional dishes, sweets, and herbal preparations for their flavor and nutritional properties.

Research Summary: Research on Pinus gerardiana pine nuts highlights their potential as a nutritious food source and their health-promoting effects. While they have been used in traditional medicine for centuries, further scientific research is needed to elucidate their specific mechanisms of action, optimize dosage regimens, and evaluate their safety and efficacy in various health conditions.

80)PIPER LONGUM

Introduction: Piper longum, commonly known as long pepper, is a flowering vine native to India. It has been used for centuries in traditional medicine systems like Ayurveda, Siddha, and Unani for its various health benefits.

Synonym Name and Common Name: Synonym Name: Piper officinarum Common Name: Long pepper, Indian long pepper, Pippali

Pharmacognosy/Chemistry: Piper longum contains bioactive compounds such as piperine, piperlonguminine, piperlongumine, and sesquiterpenes. These compounds contribute to its medicinal properties.

Action and Pharmacology: Piper longum exhibits diverse pharmacological actions including antimicrobial, anti-inflammatory, antioxidant, analgesic, immunomodulatory, and digestive stimulant effects. It is also known for its bioavailability-enhancing properties.

Method of Analysis: Analytical methods for Piper longum involve extraction of its bioactive compounds followed by chromatographic techniques such as high-performance liquid chromatography (HPLC) or gas chromatography-mass spectrometry (GC-MS) for identification and quantification.

Health Benefits: Piper longum offers various health benefits, including:

- Digestive support: Improving digestion, stimulating appetite, and relieving gastrointestinal discomfort.
- Respiratory health: Alleviating cough, cold, and respiratory congestion.
- Anti-inflammatory effects: Reducing inflammation and pain associated with arthritis and other inflammatory conditions.
- Antimicrobial activity: Fighting against bacterial and fungal infections.
- Antioxidant properties: Protecting cells from oxidative damage and supporting overall health.

Indication and Usage: Piper longum is used in traditional medicine for various indications, including digestive disorders, respiratory ailments, inflammatory conditions, and microbial infections. It is consumed orally in powder, decoction, or herbal formulations.

Usual Constituents with Percentages:

- Piperine: 5-9%
- Piperlonguminine: 1-3%
- Piperlongumine: 0.5-1%
- Sesquiterpenes: 1-2%

Mechanism of Action: The health benefits of Piper longum are attributed to its bioactive compounds, particularly piperine, which enhances the bioavailability of other nutrients and drugs, as well as its antimicrobial, anti-inflammatory, and antioxidant effects through various molecular mechanisms.

Dosage: Dosage of Piper longum powder or formulations can vary depending on the intended use and individual response. Typical doses range from 1 to 3 grams of powder per day, divided into two or three doses.

Contraindications: Piper longum should be used with caution in pregnant or breastfeeding women, as well as individuals with gastroesophageal reflux disease (GERD), peptic ulcers, or other gastrointestinal disorders. It may also interact with certain medications.

Precautions: Individuals with known allergies to Piperaceae family plants or with pre-existing medical conditions should consult with a healthcare professional before using Piper longum. It is important to use it under medical supervision, especially in high doses or for prolonged periods.

Adverse Reactions: Adverse reactions to Piper longum are rare but may include gastrointestinal upset, heartburn, or allergic reactions in susceptible individuals. It is essential to monitor for any adverse effects and discontinue use if necessary.

Research Standing: Piper longum has been extensively studied for its medicinal properties and therapeutic potential. Research continues to explore its efficacy and safety in various conditions, with promising results in digestive disorders, respiratory ailments, inflammatory conditions, and microbial infections.

Pharmacokinetics: The pharmacokinetics of Piper longum constituents, particularly piperine, have been studied for their role in enhancing the absorption of nutrients and drugs. Piperine inhibits drug-metabolizing enzymes and increases the bioavailability of co-administered substances.

Pharmacodynamics: Piper longum exerts its pharmacodynamic effects through its bioactive compounds, which interact with various molecular targets and pathways to produce its digestive, respiratory, anti-inflammatory, antimicrobial, and antioxidant actions.

Overdosage: Excessive consumption of Piper longum may lead to gastrointestinal discomfort or adverse reactions in susceptible individuals. Dosage should not exceed recommended levels, and it is important to use it judiciously.

International Standing: Piper longum is recognized internationally for its medicinal properties and is used in traditional medicine systems worldwide. Its products are available in various forms and are consumed in many countries for their health benefits.

Indian Standing: In India, Piper longum holds a significant place in Ayurveda, where it is used in numerous herbal formulations for its digestive, respiratory, anti-inflammatory, and antimicrobial properties. It is considered a key herb for promoting overall health and well-being.

Research Summary: Research on Piper longum highlights its potential as a natural remedy for digestive disorders, respiratory ailments, inflammatory conditions, and microbial infections. While traditional uses are well-documented, further scientific research is needed to elucidate its specific mechanisms of action, optimize dosage regimens, and evaluate its safety and efficacy in clinical settings

81) PIPER NIGRAM

Introduction: Piper nigrum, commonly known as black pepper, is a flowering vine cultivated for its fruit, which is dried and used as a spice and seasoning worldwide. It has a long history of culinary and medicinal use in various cultures.

Synonym Name and Common Name: Synonym Name: Piper Common Name: Black pepper

Pharmacognosy/Chemistry: Piper nigrum contains bioactive compounds such as piperine, essential oils (including beta-caryophyllene), alkaloids, and flavonoids. These compounds contribute to its distinctive flavor and potential medicinal properties.

Action and Pharmacology: Piper nigrum exhibits diverse pharmacological actions, including antimicrobial, antioxidant, anti-inflammatory, analgesic, digestive stimulant, and bioavailability-enhancing effects. It also has thermogenic properties, potentially aiding in weight management.

Method of Analysis: Analytical methods for Piper nigrum involve extraction of its bioactive compounds followed by chromatographic techniques such as high-performance liquid chromatography (HPLC) or gas chromatography-mass spectrometry (GC-MS) for identification and quantification.

Health Benefits: Piper nigrum offers various health benefits, including:

- Digestive support: Improving digestion, stimulating appetite, and relieving gastrointestinal discomfort.

- Antioxidant activity: Protecting cells from oxidative damage and reducing inflammation.
- Respiratory health: Alleviating cough, cold, and respiratory congestion.
- Pain relief: Easing muscle pain, joint pain, and headaches.
- Thermogenic effects: Increasing metabolism and promoting weight loss.

Indication and Usage: Piper nigrum is used in culinary dishes as a spice and seasoning agent. Medicinally, it is utilized in herbal formulations and traditional remedies for digestive disorders, respiratory ailments, inflammatory conditions, and pain relief.

Usual Constituents with Percentages:

- Piperine: 5-9%
- Essential oils: 1-3%
- Alkaloids: 1-2%
- Flavonoids: <1%

Mechanism of Action: The health benefits of Piper nigrum are attributed to its bioactive compounds, particularly piperine, which enhances the bioavailability of other nutrients and drugs, as well as its antimicrobial, antioxidant, anti-inflammatory, analgesic, and thermogenic effects through various molecular mechanisms.

Dosage: Dosage of Piper nigrum powder or formulations can vary depending on the intended use and individual response. Typical doses range from 1 to 3 grams of powder per day, divided into two or three doses.

Contraindications: Piper nigrum should be used with caution in individuals with gastroesophageal reflux disease (GERD), peptic ulcers, or other gastrointestinal disorders. It may also interact with certain medications, particularly those metabolized by the liver.

Precautions: Individuals with known allergies to Piperaceae family plants or with pre-existing medical conditions should consult with a healthcare professional before using Piper nigrum. It is important to use it under medical supervision, especially in high doses or for prolonged periods.

Adverse Reactions: Adverse reactions to Piper nigrum are rare but may include gastrointestinal upset, heartburn, or allergic reactions in susceptible individuals. It is essential to monitor for any adverse effects and discontinue use if necessary.

Research Standing: Piper nigrum has been extensively studied for its culinary and medicinal properties. Research continues to explore its efficacy and safety in various conditions, with promising results in digestive disorders, respiratory ailments, inflammatory conditions, pain relief, and weight management.

Pharmacokinetics: The pharmacokinetics of Piper nigrum constituents, particularly piperine, have been studied for their role in enhancing the absorption of nutrients and drugs. Piperine inhibits drug-metabolizing enzymes and increases the bioavailability of co-administered substances.

Pharmacodynamics: Piper nigrum exerts its pharmacodynamic effects through its bioactive compounds, which interact with various molecular targets and pathways to produce its digestive, respiratory, anti-inflammatory, antioxidant, analgesic, and thermogenic actions.

Overdosage: Excessive consumption of Piper nigrum may lead to gastrointestinal discomfort or adverse reactions in susceptible individuals. Dosage should not exceed recommended levels, and it is important to use it judiciously.

International Standing: Piper nigrum is recognized internationally as a popular spice and seasoning, commonly used in culinary dishes worldwide. Its products are widely available in various forms and are consumed in many countries for their flavor-enhancing properties.

Indian Standing: In India, Piper nigrum has cultural, culinary, and medicinal significance. It is used in traditional Ayurvedic medicine for its digestive, respiratory, anti-inflammatory, and analgesic properties. Black pepper is a staple spice in Indian cuisine.

Research Summary: Research on Piper nigrum highlights its potential as a versatile spice and medicinal herb. While traditional uses are well-documented, further scientific research is needed to elucidate its specific mechanisms of action, optimize dosage regimens, and evaluate its safety and efficacy in clinical settings.

82)PIPER NIGRUM

Introduction: Piper nigrum, commonly known as black pepper, is a perennial flowering vine native to South India. It is widely cultivated for its fruit, which is dried and used as a spice and seasoning in cuisines around the world. Apart from its culinary uses, black pepper has a long history of medicinal use in traditional systems of medicine.

Synonym Name and Common Name: Synonym Name: Piper Common Name: Black pepper

Pharmacognosy/Chemistry: Piper nigrum contains various bioactive compounds, including piperine, essential oils (such as β-caryophyllene), alkaloids (including piperidine), flavonoids, and other volatile compounds. These constituents contribute to its flavor and therapeutic properties.

Action and Pharmacology: Black pepper exhibits diverse pharmacological actions, including antimicrobial, antioxidant, anti-inflammatory, analgesic, digestive stimulant, and hepatoprotective effects. It also enhances the bioavailability of certain drugs and nutrients.

Method of Analysis: Analytical methods for Piper nigrum involve extraction of its bioactive compounds followed by chromatographic techniques such as high-performance liquid chromatography (HPLC) or gas chromatography-mass spectrometry (GC-MS) for identification and quantification.

Health Benefits: The health benefits of black pepper include:

- Digestive support: Stimulating digestive enzymes, improving gastrointestinal motility, and relieving indigestion.
- Antioxidant activity: Scavenging free radicals and reducing oxidative stress.
- Anti-inflammatory effects: Alleviating inflammation and associated conditions like arthritis.
- Analgesic properties: Providing pain relief, particularly in musculoskeletal disorders.
- Respiratory health: Easing congestion and promoting respiratory function.

Indication and Usage: Black pepper is used both as a spice in culinary preparations and as a medicinal herb. It is employed in various traditional remedies for digestive disorders, respiratory ailments, inflammatory conditions, and pain relief.

Usual Constituents with Percentages:

- Piperine: 5-9%
- Essential oils: 1-3%
- Alkaloids: 1-2%
- Flavonoids: <1%

Mechanism of Action: The bioactive compounds in black pepper exert their effects through various mechanisms, including modulation of enzyme activity, inhibition of inflammatory pathways, and enhancement of nutrient absorption. Piperine, in particular, is known to inhibit drug-metabolizing enzymes, thereby increasing the bioavailability of co-administered substances.

Dosage: The dosage of black pepper can vary depending on the form of administration and the specific health condition. Typical doses range from 1 to 3 grams of black pepper powder per day, divided into multiple doses.

Contraindications: Black pepper should be used with caution in individuals with gastroesophageal reflux disease (GERD), peptic ulcers, or other gastrointestinal disorders. It may also interact with certain medications, particularly those metabolized by the liver.

Precautions: Individuals with known allergies to Piperaceae family plants or with pre-existing medical conditions should consult with a healthcare professional before using black pepper. It is important to use it judiciously, especially in high doses or for prolonged periods.

Adverse Reactions: Adverse reactions to black pepper are rare but may include gastrointestinal upset, heartburn, or allergic reactions in susceptible individuals. It is essential to monitor for any adverse effects and discontinue use if necessary.

Research Standing: Black pepper has been extensively studied for its culinary and medicinal properties. Research continues to explore its efficacy and safety in various conditions, with promising results in digestive disorders, respiratory ailments, inflammatory conditions, pain relief, and antioxidant activity.

Pharmacokinetics: Piperine, the major bioactive compound in black pepper, has been studied for its pharmacokinetic properties. It inhibits drug-metabolizing enzymes and increases the bioavailability of co-administered substances, thereby enhancing their therapeutic effects.

Pharmacodynamics: Black pepper exerts its pharmacodynamic effects through its bioactive compounds, which interact with various molecular targets and pathways to produce its diverse medicinal actions, including antioxidant, anti-inflammatory, analgesic, and digestive-stimulating effects.

Overdosage: Excessive consumption of black pepper may lead to gastrointestinal discomfort or adverse reactions in susceptible individuals. Dosage should not exceed recommended levels, and it is important to use it in moderation.

International Standing: Black pepper is widely recognized and utilized as a spice and seasoning in cuisines worldwide. Its medicinal properties are also acknowledged in various traditional medicine systems, contributing to its global popularity.

Indian Standing: In India, black pepper has cultural, culinary, and medicinal significance. It is an essential ingredient in Indian cuisine and is used in Ayurvedic medicine for its digestive, respiratory, and anti-inflammatory properties.

Research Summary: Research on black pepper underscores its importance as both a culinary spice and a medicinal herb. While traditional uses are well-established, further scientific investigation is warranted to elucidate its specific mechanisms of action, optimize dosage regimens, and evaluate its safety and efficacy in clinical settings.

83)PRUNUS SEROTINA

Introduction: Prunus serotina, commonly known as black cherry, is a species of cherry native to North America. It belongs to the Rosaceae family and is renowned for its dark-colored fruit, which is edible and used in various culinary applications. Black cherry has also been utilized in traditional medicine for its potential health benefits.

Synonym Name and Common Name: Synonym Name: Wild cherry Common Name: Black cherry

Pharmacognosy/Chemistry: Black cherry contains bioactive compounds such as cyanogenic glycosides (prunasin), flavonoids, phenolic acids, and antioxidants. Its bark, leaves, and fruit are rich sources of these constituents, contributing to its medicinal properties.

Action and Pharmacology: Black cherry exhibits diverse pharmacological actions, including antioxidant, anti-inflammatory, analgesic, anti-arthritic, and antitussive effects. It also has potential benefits for digestive health and may support overall well-being.

Method of Analysis: Analytical methods for Prunus serotina involve extraction of its bioactive compounds followed by chromatographic techniques such as high-performance liquid chromatography (HPLC) or gas chromatography-mass spectrometry (GC-MS) for identification and quantification.

Health Benefits: The health benefits of black cherry include:

- Antioxidant activity: Protecting cells from oxidative damage and reducing inflammation.
- Anti-inflammatory effects: Alleviating pain and inflammation associated with arthritis and other inflammatory conditions.
- Analgesic properties: Providing pain relief, particularly for musculoskeletal discomfort.
- Digestive support: Promoting gastrointestinal health and relieving digestive discomfort.
- Respiratory health: Easing cough and respiratory congestion.

Indication and Usage: Black cherry is used in various forms, including extracts, capsules, and syrups, for medicinal purposes. It is employed in traditional remedies for arthritis, gout, muscle pain, cough, and other inflammatory or respiratory conditions.

Usual Constituents with Percentages: The usual constituents of black cherry may vary, but commonly include:

- Prunasin (cyanogenic glycoside)
- Flavonoids
- Phenolic acids
- Antioxidants

Mechanism of Action: The bioactive compounds in black cherry exert their effects through multiple mechanisms, including modulation of inflammatory pathways, scavenging of free radicals, and inhibition of pain perception. Prunasin may also contribute to its therapeutic actions.

Dosage: Dosage of black cherry supplements or preparations can vary depending on the form and intended use. Typical doses may range from 500 mg to 2000 mg of black cherry extract per day, divided into multiple doses.

Contraindications: Black cherry supplements should be used with caution in individuals with known allergies to cherries or members of the Rosaceae family. It may also interact with certain medications, particularly those metabolized by the liver.

Precautions: Individuals with pre-existing medical conditions, such as liver disease or diabetes, should consult with a healthcare professional before using black cherry supplements. Pregnant or breastfeeding women should also exercise caution.

Adverse Reactions: Adverse reactions to black cherry supplements are rare but may include gastrointestinal upset, allergic reactions, or interactions with medications. It is important to monitor for any adverse effects and discontinue use if necessary.

Research Standing: Black cherry has been studied for its potential therapeutic effects, particularly in the management of inflammatory conditions and pain relief. While research is ongoing, further studies are needed to elucidate its specific mechanisms of action and evaluate its safety and efficacy in clinical settings.

Pharmacokinetics: The pharmacokinetics of black cherry constituents have not been extensively studied. However, absorption and metabolism of its bioactive compounds may vary depending on factors such as formulation and individual metabolism.

Pharmacodynamics: Black cherry exerts its pharmacodynamic effects through its bioactive compounds, which interact with various molecular targets and pathways to produce its diverse medicinal actions, including antioxidant, anti-inflammatory, and analgesic effects.

Overdosage: Excessive consumption of black cherry supplements may lead to gastrointestinal discomfort or adverse reactions in susceptible individuals. Dosage should not exceed recommended levels, and it is important to use it judiciously.

International Standing: Black cherry supplements are available internationally and are recognized for their potential health benefits. Its products are commonly consumed as dietary supplements in various countries.

Indian Standing: In India, black cherry supplements are not as widely known or utilized compared to other traditional herbs and remedies. However, interest in its potential health benefits is increasing, and it may gain recognition in the future.

Research Summary: Research on black cherry highlights its potential as a natural remedy for inflammatory conditions, pain relief, and overall health support. While traditional uses are well-documented, further scientific investigation is warranted to validate its efficacy, safety, and optimal dosage regimens.

84) PLANTAGO OVATE

Introduction: Plantago ovata, commonly known as Psyllium or Blond Psyllium, is a medicinal plant native to the Mediterranean region. It belongs to the Plantaginaceae family and has been used traditionally for its therapeutic properties. Psyllium husk, derived from the seeds of Plantago ovata, is a popular dietary supplement known for its high fiber content.

Synonym Name and Common Name: Synonym Name: Blond Psyllium Common Name: Psyllium

Pharmacognosy/Chemistry: Psyllium husk contains primarily soluble fiber, including hemicellulose, mucilage, and cellulose. It also contains small amounts of insoluble fiber. The husk is obtained by milling the seeds of Plantago ovata.

Action and Pharmacology: Psyllium husk acts as a bulk-forming laxative due to its high fiber content. It absorbs water in the digestive tract, increasing stool bulk and promoting regular bowel movements. Additionally, it may help lower cholesterol levels and improve glycemic control by slowing the absorption of sugar and cholesterol in the intestines.

Method of Analysis: Analytical methods for Psyllium husk involve determining its fiber content, moisture content, and purity. Common techniques include gravimetric analysis, spectrophotometry, and chromatography.

Health Benefits: The health benefits of Psyllium husk include:

- Improved digestive health and relief from constipation.
- Lowered cholesterol levels and improved heart health.
- Better glycemic control and management of diabetes.
- Weight management and appetite control.
- Potential relief from diarrhea and irritable bowel syndrome (IBS).

Indication and Usage: Psyllium husk is commonly used as a dietary supplement to promote regular bowel movements, relieve constipation, and support digestive health. It is also used to lower cholesterol levels, manage diabetes, and aid in weight loss.

Usual Constituents with Percentages: The usual constituents of Psyllium husk include:

- Soluble fiber (hemicellulose, mucilage): Up to 70%
- Insoluble fiber (cellulose): Up to 30%

Mechanism of Action: Psyllium husk absorbs water in the digestive tract, forming a gel-like substance that increases stool bulk and promotes peristalsis. It also slows down the absorption of sugar and cholesterol in the intestines, leading to improved glycemic control and reduced cholesterol levels.

Dosage: The recommended dosage of Psyllium husk varies depending on the individual's age, health status, and specific health goals. Generally, a typical dose ranges from 5 to 10 grams per day, mixed with water or other fluids.

Contraindications: Psyllium husk should be used with caution in individuals with intestinal blockage, fecal impaction, or difficulty swallowing. It may also interact with certain medications, so consultation with a healthcare professional is recommended.

Precautions: It is important to consume an adequate amount of water when taking Psyllium husk to prevent dehydration and ensure proper bowel function. Individuals with gastrointestinal disorders should consult with a healthcare provider before using Psyllium supplements.

Adverse Reactions: Adverse reactions to Psyllium husk are rare but may include bloating, gas, or allergic reactions in susceptible individuals. It is essential to start with a low dose and gradually increase intake to minimize gastrointestinal discomfort.

Research Standing: Psyllium husk has been extensively studied for its therapeutic effects on digestive health, cholesterol management, glycemic control, and weight management. Research continues to explore its potential applications and mechanisms of action.

Pharmacokinetics: Psyllium husk is not significantly absorbed in the gastrointestinal tract but instead absorbs water and forms a gel-like substance. It passes through the digestive system intact, contributing to its bulk-forming laxative effect.

Pharmacodynamics: Psyllium husk exerts its pharmacodynamic effects primarily by increasing stool bulk and promoting regular bowel movements. It also modulates the absorption of sugar and cholesterol in the intestines, leading to improved metabolic parameters.

Overdosage: Consuming excessive amounts of Psyllium husk may lead to gastrointestinal discomfort, bloating, or intestinal obstruction. It is important to follow dosage recommendations and drink plenty of water to prevent these adverse effects.

International Standing: Psyllium husk is recognized internationally as a dietary supplement with various health benefits. It is commonly used in Western countries as well as traditional medicine systems worldwide.

Indian Standing: In India, Psyllium husk is known as Isabgol and has been used traditionally for its laxative and digestive properties. It is widely available and used as a popular home remedy for constipation and digestive issues.

Research Summary: Research on Psyllium husk supports its efficacy in promoting digestive health, lowering cholesterol levels, improving glycemic control, and aiding in weight management. Its safety profile and potential applications continue to be investigated in both preclinical and clinical studies.

85)CUCURBITA PEPO, C. MAXIMA-PUMPKIN SEED OIL /MEAL

Introduction: Cucurbita pepo and C. maxima, commonly known as pumpkins, are members of the Cucurbitaceae family and are widely cultivated for their edible fruits and seeds. Pumpkin seed oil and meal, extracted from the seeds of these plants, have gained popularity for their potential health benefits.

Synonym Name and Common Name: Synonym Name: None Common Name: Pumpkin seed oil, Pumpkin seed meal

Pharmacognosy/Chemistry: Pumpkin seed oil and meal contain various bioactive compounds, including fatty acids (such as linoleic acid and oleic acid), phytosterols, tocopherols (vitamin E), and carotenoids. These constituents contribute to their nutritional and therapeutic properties.

Action and Pharmacology: Pumpkin seed oil and meal have demonstrated several pharmacological actions, including anti-inflammatory, antioxidant, antimicrobial, and anthelmintic properties. They may also support prostate health, lower cholesterol levels, and promote urinary tract health.

Method of Analysis: Analytical methods for pumpkin seed oil and meal involve extraction of the bioactive compounds followed by chromatographic techniques such as gas chromatography (GC) or high-performance liquid chromatography (HPLC) for qualitative and quantitative analysis.

Health Benefits: The health benefits of pumpkin seed oil and meal include:

- Prostate health support
- Heart health promotion

- Antioxidant activity
- Anti-inflammatory effects
- Urinary tract health support

Indication and Usage: Pumpkin seed oil and meal are used as dietary supplements and functional food ingredients. They are employed for various health purposes, including prostate health, cardiovascular support, and overall well-being.

Usual Constituents with Percentages: The usual constituents of pumpkin seed oil and meal may vary, but commonly include:

- Fatty acids (such as linoleic acid, oleic acid): Up to 70%
- Phytosterols
- Tocopherols (vitamin E)
- Carotenoids

Mechanism of Action: The bioactive compounds in pumpkin seed oil and meal exert their effects through multiple mechanisms, including modulation of inflammatory pathways, scavenging of free radicals, and inhibition of microbial growth. They may also influence hormonal balance and lipid metabolism.

Dosage: The dosage of pumpkin seed oil and meal varies depending on the specific health condition and individual factors. Typical doses may range from 1000 mg to 2000 mg of pumpkin seed oil per day or 30 grams of pumpkin seed meal per day.

Contraindications: Pumpkin seed oil and meal are generally considered safe for most individuals when consumed in moderate amounts. However, individuals with known allergies to pumpkin seeds should avoid their use.

Precautions: Individuals with certain medical conditions or those taking medications should consult with a healthcare professional before using pumpkin seed oil or meal supplements. Pregnant or breastfeeding women should also exercise caution.

Adverse Reactions: Adverse reactions to pumpkin seed oil and meal are rare but may include gastrointestinal discomfort, allergic reactions, or interactions with medications. It is essential to monitor for any adverse effects and discontinue use if necessary.

Research Standing: Pumpkin seed oil and meal have been extensively studied for their potential health benefits, particularly in the areas of prostate health, cardiovascular support, and antioxidant activity. Research continues to explore their therapeutic effects and mechanisms of action.

Pharmacokinetics: The pharmacokinetics of pumpkin seed oil and meal constituents have not been extensively studied. However, absorption and metabolism may vary depending on factors such as formulation and individual metabolism.

Pharmacodynamics: Pumpkin seed oil and meal exert their pharmacodynamic effects through their bioactive compounds, which interact with various molecular targets and pathways to produce their therapeutic actions, including anti-inflammatory, antioxidant, and antimicrobial effects.

Overdosage: Excessive consumption of pumpkin seed oil or meal may lead to gastrointestinal discomfort or adverse reactions in susceptible individuals. Dosage should not exceed recommended levels, and it is important to use them judiciously.

International Standing: Pumpkin seed oil and meal supplements are recognized internationally for their potential health benefits and are commonly consumed as dietary supplements or functional food ingredients.

Indian Standing: In India, pumpkin seed oil and meal are not as widely known or utilized compared to other traditional herbs and remedies. However, interest in their potential health benefits is increasing, and they may gain recognition in the future.

Research Summary: Research on pumpkin seed oil and meal highlights their potential as functional foods and dietary supplements for promoting prostate health, cardiovascular support, and overall well-being. While traditional uses are well-documented, further scientific investigation is warranted to elucidate their specific mechanisms of action and evaluate their safety and efficacy in clinical settings.

86)PUNICA GRANATUM

Introduction: Punica granatum, commonly known as pomegranate, is a fruit-bearing shrub or small tree native to the Middle East and Mediterranean region. It has been cultivated for centuries for its culinary, medicinal, and ornamental purposes.

Synonym Name and Common Name: Synonym Name: None Common Name: Pomegranate

Pharmacognosy/Chemistry: Pomegranate contains various bioactive compounds, including polyphenols (such as ellagic acid, punicalagins, and anthocyanins), flavonoids, tannins, and vitamins (such as vitamin C and vitamin K). These constituents contribute to its medicinal properties.

Action and Pharmacology: Pomegranate exhibits diverse pharmacological actions, including antioxidant, anti-inflammatory, antimicrobial, anticancer, cardioprotective, and hepatoprotective effects. It also supports digestive health, immune function, and skin health.

Method of Analysis: Analytical methods for pomegranate involve extraction of its bioactive compounds followed by qualitative and quantitative analysis using techniques such as high-performance liquid chromatography (HPLC), gas chromatography-mass spectrometry (GC-MS), and spectrophotometry.

Health Benefits: The health benefits of pomegranate include:

- Antioxidant and anti-inflammatory properties
- Cardiovascular health support
- Cancer prevention and treatment adjunct
- Digestive health promotion
- Immune system enhancement
- Skin health improvement

Indication and Usage: Pomegranate is used in various forms, including fresh fruit, juice, extract, and supplements. It is employed for numerous health purposes, including cardiovascular support, cancer prevention, gastrointestinal health, and overall well-being.

Usual Constituents with Percentages: The usual constituents of pomegranate may vary depending on the part of the plant and the preparation method. However, typical percentages of major constituents include:

- Polyphenols (such as punicalagins, ellagic acid): Up to 20%
- Flavonoids
- Tannins
- Vitamins (such as vitamin C)

Mechanism of Action: The bioactive compounds in pomegranate exert their effects through multiple mechanisms, including scavenging of free radicals, modulation of inflammatory pathways, inhibition of cancer cell proliferation, and enhancement of immune function.

Dosage: The dosage of pomegranate products varies depending on the specific health condition and formulation. Typical doses may range from 250 mg to 1000 mg of pomegranate extract per day or 8 ounces of pomegranate juice per day.

Contraindications: Pomegranate is generally safe for most individuals when consumed in moderation. However, individuals with known allergies to pomegranate or its constituents should avoid its use. It may also interact with certain medications, so consultation with a healthcare professional is advisable.

Precautions: Pomegranate supplements should be used with caution in pregnant or breastfeeding women and individuals with certain medical conditions, such as diabetes or kidney disease. It is essential to consult with a healthcare provider before starting supplementation.

Adverse Reactions: Adverse reactions to pomegranate are rare but may include gastrointestinal discomfort, allergic reactions, or interactions with medications. It is important to monitor for any adverse effects and discontinue use if necessary.

Research Standing: Pomegranate has been extensively studied for its therapeutic properties, and research continues to explore its potential applications in various health conditions. Clinical trials and preclinical studies support its efficacy in promoting health and preventing disease.

Pharmacokinetics: The pharmacokinetics of pomegranate constituents have been investigated in preclinical and clinical studies. Absorption, distribution, metabolism, and excretion may vary depending on factors such as the formulation and dosage form.

Pharmacodynamics: Pomegranate exerts its pharmacodynamic effects through its bioactive compounds, which interact with various molecular targets and pathways to produce therapeutic actions, including antioxidant, anti-inflammatory, and anticancer effects.

Overdosage: Excessive consumption of pomegranate products may lead to gastrointestinal upset or adverse reactions in susceptible individuals. Dosage should not exceed recommended levels, and it is important to use them judiciously.

International Standing: Pomegranate is recognized internationally for its nutritional and medicinal properties. It is consumed and cultivated in various countries worldwide and is commonly used in traditional medicine systems.

Indian Standing: In India, pomegranate has a long history of culinary and medicinal use. It is valued for its health-promoting properties and is a common ingredient in traditional Ayurvedic preparations.

Research Summary: Research on pomegranate has demonstrated its diverse health benefits and therapeutic potential in preventing and managing various health conditions. Clinical studies and experimental research support its efficacy in promoting cardiovascular health, preventing cancer, supporting immune function, and enhancing overall well-being. Further investigation is ongoing to elucidate its mechanisms of action and optimize its therapeutic use.

87)RAPHANUS SATIVUS VAR. NIGER

Introduction: Raphanus sativus var. niger, commonly known as black radish or Spanish radish, is a subspecies of radish belonging to the Brassicaceae family. It is cultivated and consumed for its culinary and medicinal properties.

Synonym Name and Common Name: Synonym Name: Spanish radish Common Name: Black radish

Pharmacognosy/Chemistry: Black radish contains various bioactive compounds, including glucosinolates (such as glucoraphenin), phenolic compounds, flavonoids, vitamins (such as vitamin C), minerals, and fiber. These constituents contribute to its medicinal properties.

Action and Pharmacology: Black radish exhibits pharmacological actions such as hepatoprotective, antioxidant, antimicrobial, anti-inflammatory, and digestive stimulant effects. It is traditionally used for liver and gallbladder support, detoxification, and digestive health.

Method of Analysis: Analytical methods for black radish involve extraction of its bioactive compounds followed by qualitative and quantitative analysis using techniques such as high-performance liquid chromatography (HPLC), gas chromatography-mass spectrometry (GC-MS), and spectrophotometry.

Health Benefits: The health benefits of black radish include:

- Liver and gallbladder support
- Detoxification and antioxidant activity
- Digestive health promotion
- Immune system enhancement
- Respiratory health support

Indication and Usage: Black radish is used in various forms, including fresh root, juice, extract, and supplements. It is employed for numerous health purposes, including liver support, detoxification, digestive health, and overall well-being.

Usual Constituents with Percentages: The usual constituents of black radish may vary depending on factors such as cultivation and processing methods. However, typical percentages of major constituents include:

- Glucosinolates (such as glucoraphenin): Up to 10%
- Phenolic compounds
- Flavonoids
- Vitamins (such as vitamin C)
- Minerals

Mechanism of Action: The bioactive compounds in black radish exert their effects through multiple mechanisms, including induction of phase II detoxification enzymes, scavenging of free radicals, modulation of inflammatory pathways, and enhancement of digestive function.

Dosage: The dosage of black radish supplements varies depending on the specific health condition and formulation. Typical doses may range from 500 mg to 2000 mg of black radish extract per day or consumption of fresh black radish root.

Contraindications: Black radish is generally safe for most individuals when consumed in moderation. However, individuals with known allergies to cruciferous vegetables or specific components of black radish should avoid its use.

Precautions: Black radish supplements should be used with caution in pregnant or breastfeeding women and individuals with certain medical conditions, such as thyroid disorders or gastrointestinal issues. It is essential to consult with a healthcare provider before starting supplementation.

Adverse Reactions: Adverse reactions to black radish are rare but may include gastrointestinal discomfort, allergic reactions, or interactions with medications. It is important to monitor for any adverse effects and discontinue use if necessary.

Research Standing: Black radish has been studied for its potential health benefits, particularly in the areas of liver support, detoxification, and digestive health. While traditional uses are well-documented, further scientific investigation is warranted to elucidate its specific mechanisms of action and evaluate its safety and efficacy in clinical settings.

Pharmacokinetics: The pharmacokinetics of black radish constituents have not been extensively studied. Absorption, distribution, metabolism, and excretion may vary depending on factors such as the formulation and dosage form.

Pharmacodynamics: Black radish exerts its pharmacodynamic effects through its bioactive compounds, which interact with various molecular targets and pathways to produce therapeutic actions, including hepatoprotective, antioxidant, and antimicrobial effects.

Overdosage: Excessive consumption of black radish may lead to gastrointestinal upset or adverse reactions in susceptible individuals. Dosage should not exceed recommended levels, and it is important to use them judiciously.

International Standing: Black radish is recognized internationally for its potential health benefits and is consumed and cultivated in various countries worldwide. It is commonly used as a culinary ingredient and traditional medicine remedy.

Indian Standing: In India, black radish is not as widely known or utilized compared to other traditional herbs and remedies. However, interest in its potential health benefits is increasing, and it may gain recognition in the future.

Research Summary: Research on black radish highlights its potential as a functional food and dietary supplement for promoting liver health, detoxification, and digestive function. While traditional uses are well-documented, further scientific investigation is needed to validate its efficacy, elucidate its mechanisms of action, and optimize its therapeutic use.

88)RED WINE – EXTRACT

Introduction: Red wine extract is derived from red grapes and is rich in polyphenols, flavonoids, and antioxidants. It has gained attention for its potential health benefits, particularly its cardiovascular protective effects.

Synonym Name and Common Name: Synonym Name: Grape seed extract Common Name: Red wine extract

Pharmacognosy/Chemistry: Red wine extract contains various bioactive compounds, including resveratrol, flavonoids (such as quercetin and catechins), anthocyanins, and procyanidins. These compounds contribute to its pharmacological properties.

Action and Pharmacology: Red wine extract exhibits antioxidant, anti-inflammatory, cardioprotective, neuroprotective, and anticancer properties. It is known for its ability to improve cardiovascular health, reduce oxidative stress, and enhance overall well-being.

Method of Analysis: Analytical methods for red wine extract involve extraction of its bioactive compounds followed by qualitative and quantitative analysis using techniques such as high-performance liquid chromatography (HPLC), spectrophotometry, and mass spectrometry.

Health Benefits: The health benefits of red wine extract include:

- Cardiovascular protection
- Antioxidant activity
- Anti-inflammatory effects

- Neuroprotective properties
- Potential anticancer activity

Indication and Usage: Red wine extract is used as a dietary supplement for promoting cardiovascular health, reducing oxidative stress, and supporting overall wellness. It is available in various forms, including capsules, tablets, and liquid extracts.

Usual Constituents with Percentages: The usual constituents of red wine extract may vary depending on factors such as grape variety and extraction method. However, typical percentages of major constituents include:

- Resveratrol: Up to 5%
- Flavonoids (quercetin, catechins)
- Anthocyanins
- Procyanidins

Mechanism of Action: The bioactive compounds in red wine extract exert their effects through multiple mechanisms, including scavenging of free radicals, modulation of inflammatory pathways, enhancement of endothelial function, and inhibition of cancer cell proliferation.

Dosage: The dosage of red wine extract supplements varies depending on the specific formulation and health condition. Typical doses may range from 100 mg to 1000 mg per day, taken with meals.

Contraindications: Red wine extract supplements are generally safe for most individuals when consumed in moderation. However, individuals with certain medical conditions, such as bleeding disorders or pregnancy, should consult with a healthcare provider before use.

Precautions: Red wine extract should be used with caution in individuals taking blood-thinning medications or those with known allergies to grapes or wine. It is essential to follow recommended dosage guidelines and monitor for any adverse effects.

Adverse Reactions: Adverse reactions to red wine extract supplements are rare but may include gastrointestinal upset, allergic reactions, or interactions with medications. It is important to discontinue use and seek medical attention if any adverse effects occur.

Research Standing: Red wine extract has been extensively studied for its potential health benefits, particularly in the areas of cardiovascular health, oxidative stress, and cancer prevention. While research findings are promising, further clinical trials are needed to elucidate its specific mechanisms of action and optimal therapeutic use.

Pharmacokinetics: The pharmacokinetics of red wine extract constituents, such as resveratrol, have been investigated in preclinical and clinical studies. Absorption, distribution, metabolism, and excretion may vary depending on factors such as formulation and dosage.

Pharmacodynamics: Red wine extract exerts its pharmacodynamic effects through its bioactive compounds, which interact with various molecular targets and pathways to produce therapeutic actions, including antioxidant, anti-inflammatory, and cardioprotective effects.

Overdosage: Excessive consumption of red wine extract supplements may lead to gastrointestinal discomfort or adverse reactions. Dosage should not exceed recommended levels, and it is important to use them judiciously.

International Standing: Red wine extract is recognized internationally for its potential health benefits and is available as a dietary supplement in various countries. It is commonly used as a natural remedy for cardiovascular health and overall wellness.

Indian Standing: In India, red wine extract supplements are gaining popularity due to their purported health benefits. While traditional Ayurvedic medicine does not specifically include red wine extract, interest in its therapeutic properties is increasing.

Research Summary: Research on red wine extract highlights its potential as a natural remedy for promoting cardiovascular health, reducing oxidative stress, and preventing chronic diseases such as cancer. While preclinical and clinical studies support its efficacy, further research is needed to establish optimal dosage, safety profiles, and long-term effects in diverse populations.

89)RED YEAST RICE

Introduction: Red wine extract is derived from red grapes and is rich in polyphenols, flavonoids, and antioxidants. It has gained attention for its potential health benefits, particularly its cardiovascular protective effects.

Synonym Name and Common Name: Synonym Name: Grape seed extract Common Name: Red wine extract

Pharmacognosy/Chemistry: Red wine extract contains various bioactive compounds, including resveratrol, flavonoids (such as quercetin and catechins), anthocyanins, and procyanidins. These compounds contribute to its pharmacological properties.

Action and Pharmacology: Red wine extract exhibits antioxidant, anti-inflammatory, cardioprotective, neuroprotective, and anticancer properties. It is known for its ability to improve cardiovascular health, reduce oxidative stress, and enhance overall well-being.

Method of Analysis: Analytical methods for red wine extract involve extraction of its bioactive compounds followed by qualitative and quantitative analysis using techniques such as high-performance liquid chromatography (HPLC), spectrophotometry, and mass spectrometry.

Health Benefits: The health benefits of red wine extract include:

- Cardiovascular protection
- Antioxidant activity
- Anti-inflammatory effects
- Neuroprotective properties
- Potential anticancer activity

Indication and Usage: Red wine extract is used as a dietary supplement for promoting cardiovascular health, reducing oxidative stress, and supporting overall wellness. It is available in various forms, including capsules, tablets, and liquid extracts.

Usual Constituents with Percentages: The usual constituents of red wine extract may vary depending on factors such as grape variety and extraction method. However, typical percentages of major constituents include:

- Resveratrol: Up to 5%
- Flavonoids (quercetin, catechins)
- Anthocyanins
- Procyanidins

Mechanism of Action: The bioactive compounds in red wine extract exert their effects through multiple mechanisms, including scavenging of free radicals, modulation of inflammatory pathways, enhancement of endothelial function, and inhibition of cancer cell proliferation.

Dosage: The dosage of red wine extract supplements varies depending on the specific formulation and health condition. Typical doses may range from 100 mg to 1000 mg per day, taken with meals.

Contraindications: Red wine extract supplements are generally safe for most individuals when consumed in moderation. However, individuals with certain medical conditions, such as bleeding disorders or pregnancy, should consult with a healthcare provider before use.

Precautions: Red wine extract should be used with caution in individuals taking blood-thinning medications or those with known allergies to grapes or wine. It is essential to follow recommended dosage guidelines and monitor for any adverse effects.

Adverse Reactions: Adverse reactions to red wine extract supplements are rare but may include gastrointestinal upset, allergic reactions, or interactions with medications. It is important to discontinue use and seek medical attention if any adverse effects occur.

Research Standing: Red wine extract has been extensively studied for its potential health benefits, particularly in the areas of cardiovascular health, oxidative stress, and cancer prevention. While research findings are promising, further clinical trials are needed to elucidate its specific mechanisms of action and optimal therapeutic use.

Pharmacokinetics: The pharmacokinetics of red wine extract constituents, such as resveratrol, have been investigated in preclinical and clinical studies. Absorption, distribution, metabolism, and excretion may vary depending on factors such as formulation and dosage.

Pharmacodynamics: Red wine extract exerts its pharmacodynamic effects through its bioactive compounds, which interact with various molecular targets and pathways to produce therapeutic actions, including antioxidant, anti-inflammatory, and cardioprotective effects.

Overdosage: Excessive consumption of red wine extract supplements may lead to gastrointestinal discomfort or adverse reactions. Dosage should not exceed recommended levels, and it is important to use them judiciously.

International Standing: Red wine extract is recognized internationally for its potential health benefits and is available as a dietary supplement in various countries. It is commonly used as a natural remedy for cardiovascular health and overall wellness.

Indian Standing: In India, red wine extract supplements are gaining popularity due to their purported health benefits. While traditional Ayurvedic medicine does not specifically include red wine extract, interest in its therapeutic properties is increasing.

Research Summary: Research on red wine extract highlights its potential as a natural remedy for promoting cardiovascular health, reducing oxidative stress, and preventing chronic diseases such as cancer. While preclinical and clinical studies support its efficacy, further research is needed to establish optimal dosage, safety profiles, and long-term effects in diverse populations.

90) RHODODENDRON ARBOREUM/R. CAMPANULATA - JUICE/EXTRACT

Introduction: Rhododendron arboreum and Rhododendron campanulata, commonly known as Rhododendron, are flowering plants native to the Himalayas and other mountainous regions. The juice or extract derived from these plants is used in traditional medicine for various health purposes.

Synonym Name and Common Name: Synonym Name: None Common Name: Rhododendron juice/extract

Pharmacognosy/Chemistry: Rhododendron contains various phytochemicals, including flavonoids, tannins, terpenoids, and phenolic compounds. These constituents contribute to its pharmacological properties.

Action and Pharmacology: Rhododendron exhibits antioxidant, anti-inflammatory, antimicrobial, and antiviral properties. It is used traditionally for its potential therapeutic effects on various ailments.

Method of Analysis: Analytical methods for Rhododendron extract involve extraction of its bioactive compounds followed by qualitative and quantitative analysis using techniques such as chromatography (HPLC, TLC), spectrophotometry, and mass spectrometry.

Health Benefits: The health benefits of Rhododendron juice/extract may include:

- Antioxidant activity
- Anti-inflammatory effects
- Antimicrobial and antiviral properties
- Digestive health support
- Immune system modulation

Indication and Usage: Rhododendron juice/extract is used in traditional medicine for various purposes, including improving digestion, relieving inflammation, and supporting overall well-being. It may be consumed as a beverage or used topically.

Usual Constituents with Percentages: The usual constituents of Rhododendron juice/extract may vary depending on factors such as species and extraction method. However, typical percentages of major constituents include flavonoids, tannins, and terpenoids.

Mechanism of Action: The bioactive compounds in Rhododendron exert their effects through multiple mechanisms, including scavenging of free radicals, inhibition of inflammatory pathways, and modulation of microbial growth.

Dosage: The dosage of Rhododendron juice/extract may vary depending on the specific formulation and intended use. It is essential to follow product labeling instructions or consult with a healthcare provider for appropriate dosage guidance.

Contraindications: Rhododendron juice/extract should be used with caution in individuals with known allergies to plants in the Ericaceae family. Pregnant or breastfeeding women should avoid its use due to the lack of safety data.

Precautions: Rhododendron juice/extract may cause allergic reactions or gastrointestinal upset in sensitive individuals. It is important to use it cautiously and discontinue use if any adverse effects occur.

Adverse Reactions: Adverse reactions to Rhododendron juice/extract are rare but may include allergic reactions, digestive discomfort, or skin irritation. It is advisable to discontinue use and seek medical attention if adverse effects occur.

Research Standing: Research on the pharmacological properties of Rhododendron juice/extract is limited. While traditional use suggests potential health benefits, more scientific studies are needed to validate its efficacy, safety, and optimal dosage.

Pharmacokinetics: Limited information is available on the pharmacokinetics of Rhododendron juice/extract. Absorption, distribution, metabolism, and excretion of its bioactive compounds require further investigation.

Pharmacodynamics: Rhododendron juice/extract exerts its pharmacodynamic effects through its bioactive constituents, which interact with various cellular targets and pathways to produce therapeutic actions, including antioxidant and anti-inflammatory effects.

Overdosage: Excessive consumption of Rhododendron juice/extract may lead to adverse reactions such as gastrointestinal discomfort or allergic responses. Dosage should not exceed recommended levels, and caution should be exercised when using it.

International Standing: Rhododendron juice/extract is primarily used in traditional medicine practices in regions where Rhododendron species are native. Its international standing as a therapeutic agent is limited, and more research is needed to explore its potential on a global scale.

Indian Standing: In India, Rhododendron juice/extract may be used in traditional Ayurvedic and folk medicine practices. Its use and recognition vary across different regions and communities within the country.

Research Summary: Research on Rhododendron juice/extract is ongoing, with a focus on its traditional uses and potential health benefits. While preliminary evidence suggests antioxidant, anti-inflammatory, and antimicrobial properties, further scientific investigations are warranted to establish its efficacy and safety profile.

91) RICE BRAN

Introduction: Rice bran, a byproduct of rice milling, is garnering increasing attention for its rich nutritional profile and potential health benefits. It is a valuable source of various bioactive compounds like antioxidants, vitamins, and minerals.

Synonym Name and Common Name: Synonyms: Oryza sativa bran Common Name: Rice bran

Pharmacognosy/Chemistry: Rice bran comprises various bioactive compounds, including oryzanol, tocopherols, tocotrienols, phytosterols, and polyphenols. These constituents contribute to its pharmacological properties.

Action and Pharmacology: Rice bran exhibits antioxidant, anti-inflammatory, hypocholesterolemic, and hepatoprotective actions. Its diverse bioactive compounds contribute to these pharmacological effects.

Method of Analysis: Analytical methods such as HPLC (High-Performance Liquid Chromatography) and GC-MS (Gas Chromatography-Mass Spectrometry) are commonly employed to quantify the bioactive compounds present in rice bran.

Health Benefits:

- Cardiovascular health support
- Antioxidant protection
- Digestive health improvement
- Skin health enhancement
- Weight management aid

Indication and Usage: Rice bran is indicated for:

- Hypercholesterolemia
- Oxidative stress-related conditions
- Digestive disorders
- Skin conditions
- Nutritional supplementation

Usual Constituents with Percentages:

- Oryzanol: 1-2%
- Tocopherols and tocotrienols: 0.5-1.5%
- Phytosterols: 0.1-0.5%
- Polyphenols: 0.2-1%

Mechanism of Action: The bioactive compounds in rice bran exert their effects through antioxidant activity, modulation of lipid metabolism, and anti-inflammatory actions, among others.

Dosage: Dosage varies depending on the formulation and specific health condition. Consultation with a healthcare professional is recommended for personalized dosage recommendations.

Contraindications:

- Allergy to rice or rice products
- Pregnancy and lactation (due to limited safety data)

Precautions:

- Monitor lipid levels regularly during supplementation, especially in individuals with pre-existing hyperlipidemia.
- Ensure the quality and purity of the rice bran product to avoid contaminants.

Adverse Reactions: Adverse reactions to rice bran are rare but may include allergic reactions, gastrointestinal discomfort, and potential interactions with certain medications.

Research Standing: Rice bran research is actively ongoing, with numerous studies exploring its health benefits, safety profile, and potential therapeutic applications. It is considered a promising functional food ingredient.

Pharmacokinetics: The pharmacokinetics of rice bran constituents vary depending on factors such as formulation, route of administration, and individual metabolism. Further studies are needed to elucidate specific pharmacokinetic parameters.

Pharmacodynamics: Rice bran exerts its pharmacodynamic effects through various mechanisms, including antioxidant activity, modulation of lipid metabolism, and anti-inflammatory actions, among others.

Overdosage: Limited information is available regarding the effects of rice bran overdosage. However, excessive intake may lead to gastrointestinal disturbances or allergic reactions.

International Standing: Rice bran is recognized internationally for its nutritional value and potential health benefits. It is commonly used as a functional food ingredient in various culinary and dietary applications.

Indian Standing: In India, rice bran is utilized in traditional medicine systems like Ayurveda for its purported health benefits. It is also incorporated into culinary practices and dietary supplements.

Research Summary of Rice Bran: Research on rice bran continues to expand, with a focus on elucidating its bioactive compounds, pharmacological effects, and potential therapeutic applications. Studies highlight its role in promoting cardiovascular health, antioxidant protection, and digestive wellness, among other benefits. Further research is warranted to fully understand its mechanisms of action, optimize dosage regimens, and explore its therapeutic potential across various health conditions.

92)ROSE HIPS

Introduction: Rose hips are the fruit of the rose plant, known for their vibrant color and potent nutritional profile. They have been used traditionally for centuries due to their medicinal properties and are gaining popularity in modern herbal medicine.

Synonym Name and Common Name: Synonym: Rose haw, rose hep Common Name: Rose hips

Pharmacognosy/Chemistry: Rose hips contain a variety of bioactive compounds, including vitamin C, flavonoids, carotenoids, phenolic acids, and essential fatty acids. These constituents contribute to their pharmacological properties.

Action and Pharmacology: Rose hips exhibit antioxidant, anti-inflammatory, immunomodulatory, and wound-healing properties. The combination of bioactive compounds contributes to these diverse pharmacological effects.

Method of Analysis: Analytical methods such as HPLC (High-Performance Liquid Chromatography) and spectrophotometry are commonly used to quantify the bioactive compounds present in rose hips.

Health Benefits:

- Immune system support
- Skin health enhancement
- Joint health improvement
- Digestive system support
- Cardiovascular health promotion

Indication and Usage: Rose hips are indicated for:

- Cold and flu prevention and treatment
- Skin rejuvenation and wound healing
- Joint pain relief
- Digestive disorders
- Cardiovascular health maintenance

Usual Constituents with Percentages:

- Vitamin C: 0.5-1.5%
- Flavonoids: 0.2-0.8%
- Carotenoids: 0.1-0.5%
- Phenolic acids: 0.2-0.6%
- Essential fatty acids: 0.1-0.5%

Mechanism of Action: The bioactive compounds in rose hips exert their effects through antioxidant activity, modulation of inflammatory pathways, enhancement of immune function, and promotion of tissue repair and regeneration.

Dosage: Dosage recommendations vary depending on the formulation and specific health condition. It is advisable to follow the instructions provided by healthcare professionals or product labels.

Contraindications:

- Allergy to roses or rose-related products
- Pregnancy and lactation (due to limited safety data)

Precautions:

- Avoid excessive intake, especially in individuals prone to kidney stones due to the high vitamin C content.
- Ensure the quality and purity of rose hip products to avoid potential contaminants.

Adverse Reactions: Adverse reactions to rose hips are rare but may include allergic reactions, gastrointestinal discomfort, and potential interactions with certain medications.

Research Standing: Rose hips have been extensively studied for their health benefits and therapeutic potential. Research indicates their efficacy in supporting immune function, promoting skin health, and alleviating inflammatory conditions. Continued research is ongoing to further explore their mechanisms of action and clinical applications.

Pharmacokinetics: The pharmacokinetics of rose hip constituents vary depending on factors such as formulation, route of administration, and individual metabolism. Further studies are needed to elucidate specific pharmacokinetic parameters.

Pharmacodynamics: Rose hips exert their pharmacodynamic effects through various mechanisms, including antioxidant activity, modulation of inflammatory pathways, and enhancement of immune function, among others.

Overdosage: Limited information is available regarding the effects of rose hip overdosage. However, excessive intake may lead to gastrointestinal disturbances or allergic reactions.

International Standing: Rose hips are recognized internationally for their nutritional value and therapeutic potential. They are commonly used in herbal medicine traditions worldwide and are increasingly incorporated into dietary supplements and functional foods.

Indian Standing: In India, rose hips are utilized in traditional Ayurvedic and Unani medicine systems for their medicinal properties. They are also used in culinary preparations and herbal remedies.

Research Summary of Rose Hips: Research on rose hips underscores their diverse health benefits and therapeutic potential. Studies highlight their antioxidant, anti-inflammatory, immunomodulatory, and wound-healing properties, supporting their traditional uses in various cultures. Continued research is warranted to elucidate their mechanisms of action, optimize dosage regimens, and explore their potential applications in preventing and treating various health conditions.

93)ROSMARINUS OFFICINALIS

Introduction: Rosmarinus officinalis, commonly known as rosemary, is a fragrant herb native to the Mediterranean region. It has been revered for centuries for its culinary, medicinal, and aromatic properties and is widely used in various cultural traditions worldwide.

Synonym Name and Common Name: Synonym: None Common Name: Rosemary

Pharmacognosy/Chemistry: Rosemary contains several bioactive compounds, including rosmarinic acid, carnosic acid, flavonoids (e.g., apigenin, luteolin), and essential oils (e.g., cineole, camphor). These constituents contribute to its pharmacological properties.

Action and Pharmacology: Rosemary exhibits antioxidant, anti-inflammatory, antimicrobial, neuroprotective, and hepatoprotective actions. The diverse array of bioactive compounds contributes to these pharmacological effects.

Method of Analysis: Analytical methods such as HPLC (High-Performance Liquid Chromatography) and GC-MS (Gas Chromatography-Mass Spectrometry) are commonly used to identify and quantify the bioactive compounds present in rosemary extracts.

Health Benefits:

- Cognitive function enhancement
- Digestive health improvement
- Hair and skin health support
- Respiratory health promotion
- Mood regulation

Indication and Usage: Rosemary is indicated for:

- Memory and cognitive function enhancement
- Digestive disorders
- Topical applications for hair and skin health
- Respiratory conditions
- Culinary use as a flavoring agent

Usual Constituents with Percentages:

- Rosmarinic acid: 0.5-2%
- Carnosic acid: 0.1-0.5%
- Flavonoids: 0.2-0.8%
- Essential oils: 1-2%

Mechanism of Action: The bioactive compounds in rosemary exert their effects through antioxidant activity, modulation of inflammatory pathways, inhibition of microbial growth, and enhancement of neurological function, among others.

Dosage: Dosage recommendations vary depending on the formulation and intended use. It is advisable to follow the instructions provided by healthcare professionals or product labels.

Contraindications:

- Allergy to rosemary or related plants (Lamiaceae family)
- Pregnancy and lactation (due to limited safety data)

Precautions:

- Avoid excessive intake, especially in individuals prone to allergic reactions.
- Use caution when applying rosemary topically, especially in concentrated forms, to avoid skin irritation or sensitization.

Adverse Reactions: Adverse reactions to rosemary are rare but may include allergic reactions, gastrointestinal discomfort, and skin irritation.

Research Standing: Rosemary has been extensively studied for its medicinal properties and potential health benefits. Research indicates its efficacy in enhancing cognitive function, supporting digestive health, promoting hair and skin health, and exerting antimicrobial and anti-inflammatory effects. Continued research is ongoing to further elucidate its mechanisms of action and explore its potential applications in various health conditions.

Pharmacokinetics: The pharmacokinetics of rosemary constituents vary depending on factors such as formulation, route of administration, and individual metabolism. Further studies are needed to elucidate specific pharmacokinetic parameters.

Pharmacodynamics: Rosemary exerts its pharmacodynamic effects through various mechanisms, including antioxidant activity, modulation of inflammatory pathways, enhancement of neurological function, and inhibition of microbial growth, among others.

Overdosage: Limited information is available regarding the effects of rosemary overdosage. However, excessive intake may lead to gastrointestinal disturbances or allergic reactions.

International Standing: Rosemary is recognized internationally for its culinary, medicinal, and aromatic properties. It is widely used in various cuisines and herbal medicine traditions worldwide and is increasingly incorporated into dietary supplements, personal care products, and aromatherapy practices.

Indian Standing: In India, rosemary is gaining popularity for its medicinal and culinary uses. It is utilized in traditional Ayurvedic and Unani medicine systems and is also used in culinary preparations and aromatherapy practices.

Research Summary of Rosemary: Research on rosemary underscores its diverse health benefits and therapeutic potential. Studies highlight its antioxidant, anti-inflammatory, antimicrobial, and neuroprotective properties, supporting its traditional uses and expanding its applications in modern medicine and wellness practices. Continued research is warranted to further elucidate its mechanisms of action, optimize dosage regimens, and explore its potential in preventing and treating various health conditions

94) ROYAL JELLY

Introduction: Royal jelly is a nutritious substance secreted by worker honey bees, primarily used to feed bee larvae and the queen bee. It is renowned for its potential health benefits and has been used for centuries in traditional medicine practices.

Synonym Name and Common Name: Synonym: Bee's milk Common Name: Royal jelly

Pharmacognosy/Chemistry: Royal jelly is composed of water, proteins, sugars, lipids, vitamins (particularly B vitamins), minerals, and various bioactive compounds such as 10-hydroxy-2-decenoic acid (10-HDA) and royalactin.

Action and Pharmacology: Royal jelly exhibits antioxidant, immunomodulatory, antimicrobial, anti-inflammatory, and wound-healing properties. Its diverse array of bioactive compounds contributes to these pharmacological effects.

Method of Analysis: Analytical methods such as HPLC (High-Performance Liquid Chromatography) and ELISA (Enzyme-Linked Immunosorbent Assay) are commonly used to identify and quantify the bioactive compounds present in royal jelly.

Health Benefits:

- Immune system support
- Skin health enhancement
- Energy and vitality boost
- Reproductive health promotion
- Cognitive function improvement

Indication and Usage: Royal jelly is indicated for:

- Boosting immune function
- Enhancing skin health and appearance
- Increasing energy and vitality
- Supporting reproductive health
- Improving cognitive function and memory

Usual Constituents with Percentages:

- Water: 50-60%
- Proteins: 10-15%
- Carbohydrates (sugars): 10-20%
- Lipids: 3-6%
- Vitamins and minerals: Trace amounts

Mechanism of Action: The bioactive compounds in royal jelly exert their effects through antioxidant activity, modulation of immune responses, promotion of tissue repair and regeneration, and regulation of hormonal pathways, among others.

Dosage: Dosage recommendations vary depending on the formulation and specific health condition. It is advisable to follow the instructions provided by healthcare professionals or product labels.

Contraindications:

- Allergy to bee products (such as honey or propolis)
- Asthma or other respiratory conditions
- Pregnancy and lactation (due to limited safety data)

Precautions:

- Use caution if allergic to bee products, as royal jelly may cause allergic reactions.
- Avoid excessive intake, especially in individuals prone to allergic reactions or with respiratory conditions.
- Ensure the quality and purity of royal jelly products to avoid potential contaminants.

Adverse Reactions: Adverse reactions to royal jelly are rare but may include allergic reactions (such as skin rash, itching, or respiratory symptoms) and gastrointestinal discomfort.

Research Standing: Royal jelly research is ongoing, with numerous studies investigating its potential health benefits and therapeutic applications. While some evidence supports its efficacy in immune support, skin health, and reproductive health, further research is needed to elucidate its mechanisms of action and optimize its clinical use.

Pharmacokinetics: The pharmacokinetics of royal jelly constituents vary depending on factors such as formulation, route of administration, and individual metabolism. Further studies are needed to elucidate specific pharmacokinetic parameters.

Pharmacodynamics: Royal jelly exerts its pharmacodynamic effects through various mechanisms, including antioxidant activity, modulation of immune responses, promotion of tissue repair and regeneration, and regulation of hormonal pathways, among others.

Overdosage: Limited information is available regarding the effects of royal jelly overdosage. However, excessive intake may lead to allergic reactions or gastrointestinal disturbances.

International Standing: Royal jelly is recognized internationally for its potential health benefits and is commonly used in dietary supplements, skincare products, and traditional medicine practices worldwide.

Indian Standing: In India, royal jelly is gaining popularity for its purported health benefits and is used in dietary supplements and skincare formulations. It is also incorporated into traditional Ayurvedic and Unani medicine practices.

Research Summary of Royal Jelly: Research on royal jelly highlights its potential health benefits, particularly in immune support, skin health, and reproductive health. While some evidence supports its efficacy, further studies are needed to elucidate its mechanisms of action, optimize dosage regimens, and explore its potential applications in various health conditions. Additionally, more research is warranted to assess its safety profile and potential adverse effects, especially in vulnerable populations.

95) SALVIA OFFICINALIS

Introduction: Salvia officinalis, commonly known as sage, is an aromatic herb native to the Mediterranean region. It has a long history of use in culinary, medicinal, and ceremonial practices and is renowned for its potential health benefits.

Synonym Name and Common Name: Synonym: Garden sage Common Name: Sage

Pharmacognosy/Chemistry: Sage contains various bioactive compounds, including phenolic acids (e.g., rosmarinic acid), flavonoids (e.g., apigenin, luteolin), essential oils (e.g., thujone, camphor), and terpenes. These constituents contribute to its pharmacological properties.

Action and Pharmacology: Sage exhibits antioxidant, anti-inflammatory, antimicrobial, antidiabetic, and cognitive-enhancing properties. Its diverse array of bioactive compounds contributes to these pharmacological effects.

Method of Analysis: Analytical methods such as HPLC (High-Performance Liquid Chromatography) and GC-MS (Gas Chromatography-Mass Spectrometry) are commonly used to identify and quantify the bioactive compounds present in sage extracts.

Health Benefits:

- Cognitive function improvement
- Digestive health promotion
- Menopausal symptom relief
- Oral health enhancement
- Antioxidant protection

Indication and Usage: Sage is indicated for:

- Enhancing cognitive function and memory
- Alleviating digestive discomfort
- Managing menopausal symptoms
- Promoting oral health
- Providing antioxidant support

Usual Constituents with Percentages:

- Phenolic acids: 1-3%
- Flavonoids: 0.5-1.5%
- Essential oils: 1-2%
- Terpenes: 0.1-0.5%

Mechanism of Action: The bioactive compounds in sage exert their effects through antioxidant activity, modulation of inflammatory pathways, inhibition of microbial growth, regulation of hormonal balance, and enhancement of cognitive function, among others.

Dosage: Dosage recommendations vary depending on the formulation and specific health condition. It is advisable to follow the instructions provided by healthcare professionals or product labels.

Contraindications:

- Allergy to sage or related plants (Lamiaceae family)
- Pregnancy and lactation (due to limited safety data)

Precautions:

- Use caution if allergic to sage or related plants.
- Avoid excessive intake, especially in pregnant or breastfeeding women.
- Consult a healthcare professional before using sage supplements, especially in individuals with pre-existing medical conditions or taking medications.

Adverse Reactions: Adverse reactions to sage are rare but may include allergic reactions, gastrointestinal discomfort, and potential interactions with certain medications.

Research Standing: Sage has been extensively studied for its medicinal properties and potential health benefits. Research indicates its efficacy in enhancing cognitive function, alleviating digestive discomfort, managing menopausal symptoms, promoting oral health, and providing antioxidant protection. Continued research is ongoing to further elucidate its mechanisms of action and explore its potential applications in various health conditions.

Pharmacokinetics: The pharmacokinetics of sage constituents vary depending on factors such as formulation, route of administration, and individual metabolism. Further studies are needed to elucidate specific pharmacokinetic parameters.

Pharmacodynamics: Sage exerts its pharmacodynamic effects through various mechanisms, including antioxidant activity, modulation of inflammatory pathways, inhibition of microbial growth, regulation of hormonal balance, and enhancement of cognitive function, among others.

Overdosage: Limited information is available regarding the effects of sage overdosage. However, excessive intake may lead to gastrointestinal disturbances or potential adverse effects due to its bioactive compounds.

International Standing: Sage is recognized internationally for its culinary, medicinal, and aromatic properties. It is widely used in various cuisines, herbal medicine traditions, and personal care products worldwide.

Indian Standing: In India, sage is gaining recognition for its potential health benefits and is used in traditional Ayurvedic and Unani medicine practices. It is also incorporated into culinary preparations, herbal remedies, and personal care products.

Research Summary of Sage: Research on sage highlights its diverse health benefits and therapeutic potential. Studies support its efficacy in enhancing cognitive function, promoting digestive health, managing menopausal symptoms, improving oral health, and providing antioxidant protection. Continued research is warranted to further elucidate its mechanisms of action, optimize dosage regimens, and explore its potential applications in preventing and treating various health conditions. Additionally, more research is needed to assess its safety profile and potential adverse effects, especially with long-term use or in vulnerable populations.

96)SAMBUCUS NIGRA

Introduction: Sambucus nigra, commonly known as elderberry, is a flowering plant native to Europe and North America. Its berries have been used for centuries in traditional medicine for their potential health benefits.

Synonym Name and Common Name: Synonym: Elderberry Common Name: Elderberry

Pharmacognosy/Chemistry: Elderberry contains various bioactive compounds, including flavonoids (e.g., quercetin, rutin), anthocyanins, phenolic acids, and vitamins (e.g., vitamin C, vitamin A). These constituents contribute to its pharmacological properties.

Action and Pharmacology: Elderberry exhibits antioxidant, anti-inflammatory, antiviral, immunomodulatory, and antihistaminic properties. Its diverse array of bioactive compounds contributes to these pharmacological effects.

Method of Analysis: Analytical methods such as HPLC (High-Performance Liquid Chromatography) and spectrophotometry are commonly used to identify and quantify the bioactive compounds present in elderberry extracts.

Health Benefits:

- Immune system support
- Cold and flu symptom relief
- Antioxidant protection
- Heart health promotion
- Digestive health improvement

Indication and Usage: Elderberry is indicated for:

- Boosting immune function
- Alleviating symptoms of cold and flu
- Providing antioxidant support
- Supporting heart health
- Enhancing digestive function

Usual Constituents with Percentages:

- Flavonoids: 1-3%
- Anthocyanins: 0.5-1.5%
- Phenolic acids: 0.5-1%
- Vitamins: Trace amounts

Mechanism of Action: The bioactive compounds in elderberry exert their effects through antioxidant activity, modulation of inflammatory pathways, inhibition of viral replication, enhancement of immune responses, and improvement of cardiovascular and digestive function, among others.

Dosage: Dosage recommendations vary depending on the formulation and specific health condition. It is advisable to follow the instructions provided by healthcare professionals or product labels.

Contraindications:

- Allergy to elderberry or related plants
- Pregnancy and lactation (due to limited safety data)

Precautions:

- Use caution if allergic to elderberry or related plants.
- Avoid excessive intake, especially in pregnant or breastfeeding women.
- Consult a healthcare professional before using elderberry supplements, especially in individuals with pre-existing medical conditions or taking medications.

Adverse Reactions: Adverse reactions to elderberry are rare but may include allergic reactions, gastrointestinal discomfort, and potential interactions with certain medications.

Research Standing: Elderberry has been extensively studied for its medicinal properties and potential health benefits. Research indicates its efficacy in supporting immune function, alleviating symptoms of cold and flu, providing antioxidant protection, promoting heart health, and improving digestive function. Continued research is ongoing to further elucidate its mechanisms of action and explore its potential applications in various health conditions.

Pharmacokinetics: The pharmacokinetics of elderberry constituents vary depending on factors such as formulation, route of administration, and individual metabolism. Further studies are needed to elucidate specific pharmacokinetic parameters.

Pharmacodynamics: Elderberry exerts its pharmacodynamic effects through various mechanisms, including antioxidant activity, modulation of inflammatory pathways, inhibition of viral replication, enhancement of immune responses, and improvement of cardiovascular and digestive function, among others.

Overdosage: Limited information is available regarding the effects of elderberry overdosage. However, excessive intake may lead to gastrointestinal disturbances or potential adverse effects due to its bioactive compounds.

International Standing: Elderberry is recognized internationally for its potential health benefits and is commonly used in dietary supplements, herbal remedies, and traditional medicine practices worldwide.

Indian Standing: In India, elderberry is gaining recognition for its medicinal properties and potential health benefits. It is used in traditional Ayurvedic medicine practices and is also incorporated into dietary supplements and herbal remedies.

Research Summary of Elderberry: Research on elderberry underscores its diverse health benefits and therapeutic potential. Studies support its efficacy in supporting immune function, alleviating symptoms of cold and flu, providing antioxidant protection, promoting heart health, and improving digestive function. Continued research is warranted to further elucidate its mechanisms of action, optimize dosage regimens, and explore its potential applications in preventing and treating various health conditions. Additionally, more research is needed to assess its safety profile and potential adverse effects, especially with long-term use or in vulnerable populations.

97)SHARK CARTILAGE /SQUALENE OIL

Introduction: Shark cartilage and squalene oil are natural substances derived from sharks, known for their potential health benefits. Shark cartilage is extracted from the skeletal tissues of sharks, while squalene oil is obtained from shark liver oil or plant sources.

Synonym Name and Common Name: Synonyms: None for shark cartilage; Squalene oil is also known as shark liver oil. Common Names:

- Shark cartilage
- Squalene oil

Pharmacognosy/Chemistry:

- Shark cartilage primarily consists of proteins, glycosaminoglycans (e.g., chondroitin sulfate), and minerals (e.g., calcium, phosphorus).
- Squalene oil contains mainly squalene, a polyunsaturated hydrocarbon, along with other lipids and fatty acids.

Action and Pharmacology:

- Shark cartilage may have anti-inflammatory, antioxidant, and potential anti-cancer properties.
- Squalene oil is known for its antioxidant, moisturizing, and skin health-enhancing effects.

Method of Analysis:

Analytical methods such as HPLC (High-Performance Liquid Chromatography) and GC-MS (Gas Chromatography-Mass Spectrometry) are commonly used to analyze the constituents of shark cartilage and squalene oil.

Health Benefits:

- Shark cartilage: Potential benefits include joint health support, wound healing, and possible anticancer effects.
- Squalene oil: Benefits may include skin hydration, antioxidant protection, and support for heart health.

Indication and Usage:

- Shark cartilage: Indicated for joint health conditions like osteoarthritis, wound healing, and as a complementary therapy for certain cancers.
- Squalene oil: Used in skincare products for moisturizing, anti-aging, and antioxidant properties, and in dietary supplements for heart health support.

Usual Constituents with Percentages:

- Shark cartilage: Variable composition, primarily proteins (approx. 60-70%), glycosaminoglycans (approx. 20-30%), and minerals (approx. 10-15%).
- Squalene oil: Predominantly squalene (approx. 70-85%), along with other lipids and fatty acids.

Mechanism of Action:

- Shark cartilage: May work through anti-inflammatory effects, inhibition of blood vessel formation (angiogenesis), and modulation of immune responses.
- Squalene oil: Likely exerts antioxidant effects, enhances skin hydration, and may modulate lipid metabolism.

Dosage:

Dosage recommendations vary widely depending on the specific product and intended use. Consultation with a healthcare professional is recommended.

Contraindications:

- Shark cartilage: Contraindicated in individuals with seafood allergies or sensitivity to shark-derived products.
- Squalene oil: Generally considered safe, but caution is advised in individuals with allergies to any components of the oil.

Precautions:

- Use caution with shark cartilage due to potential contaminants like heavy metals and toxins.
- Ensure the purity and quality of squalene oil, especially in products sourced from sharks, to avoid potential contaminants and ethical concerns.

Adverse Reactions:

- Shark cartilage: Possible adverse reactions may include gastrointestinal upset, allergic reactions, and interference with blood clotting.
- Squalene oil: Adverse reactions are rare but may include skin irritation or allergic reactions in sensitive individuals.

Research Standing:

Research on shark cartilage and squalene oil is ongoing, with studies exploring their potential health benefits and safety profiles. While some research suggests promising effects, further studies are needed to confirm efficacy and establish optimal dosages.

Pharmacokinetics:

Pharmacokinetic data for shark cartilage and squalene oil are limited. Absorption, distribution, metabolism, and excretion may vary depending on the formulation and route of administration.

Pharmacodynamics:

Shark cartilage and squalene oil likely exert their pharmacodynamic effects through various mechanisms, including anti-inflammatory, antioxidant, and immunomodulatory actions, among others.

Overdosage:

Limited information is available on the effects of overdosage for shark cartilage and squalene oil. Excessive intake may lead to adverse effects, especially gastrointestinal symptoms or allergic reactions.

International Standing:

Shark cartilage and squalene oil are recognized internationally for their potential health benefits and are used in various dietary supplements, skincare products, and pharmaceutical formulations.

Indian Standing:

In India, shark cartilage and squalene oil are available in dietary supplements and skincare products, but their usage and popularity may vary. Further research may be needed to establish their standing within traditional medicine systems.

98) SHIITAKE MUSHROOM – EXTRACT

Introduction: Shiitake mushroom extract is derived from the shiitake mushroom (Lentinula edodes), a popular edible fungus native to East Asia. It has a long history of use in traditional medicine and culinary practices and is esteemed for its potential health-promoting properties.

Synonym Name and Common Name: Synonym: Lentinula edodes extract Common Name: Shiitake mushroom extract

Pharmacognosy/Chemistry: Shiitake mushroom extract contains various bioactive compounds, including polysaccharides (such as beta-glucans), ergosterol (provitamin D2), amino acids, and minerals (such as potassium, phosphorus, and zinc).

Action and Pharmacology: Shiitake mushroom extract exhibits immunomodulatory, antioxidant, antimicrobial, anti-inflammatory, and potential anticancer properties. Its diverse array of bioactive compounds contributes to these pharmacological effects.

Method of Analysis: Analytical methods such as HPLC (High-Performance Liquid Chromatography), GC-MS (Gas Chromatography-Mass Spectrometry), and ELISA (Enzyme-Linked Immunosorbent Assay) are commonly used to identify and quantify the bioactive compounds present in shiitake mushroom extract.

HEALTH BENEFITS:

- Immune system support
- Antioxidant protection
- Cardiovascular health promotion
- Liver health support
- Anti-inflammatory effects

Indication and Usage: Shiitake mushroom extract is indicated for:

- Boosting immune function
- Providing antioxidant support
- Promoting cardiovascular health
- Supporting liver function
- Alleviating inflammation

Usual Constituents with Percentages:

- Polysaccharides (beta-glucans): 20-30%
- Ergosterol (provitamin D2): 1-5%
- Amino acids: 5-10%
- Minerals: Trace amounts

Mechanism of Action: The bioactive compounds in shiitake mushroom extract exert their effects through various mechanisms, including modulation of immune responses, scavenging of free radicals, inhibition of microbial growth, reduction of inflammation, and promotion of cardiovascular and liver health.

Dosage: Dosage recommendations vary depending on the formulation and specific health condition. It is advisable to follow the instructions provided by healthcare professionals or product labels.

Contraindications:

- Allergy to mushrooms or related fungi
- Pregnancy and lactation (due to limited safety data)

Precautions:

- Use caution if allergic to mushrooms or related fungi.
- Ensure the purity and quality of shiitake mushroom extract, especially in products sourced from reputable manufacturers.

- Consult a healthcare professional before using shiitake mushroom extract, especially in individuals with pre-existing medical conditions or taking medications.

Adverse Reactions: Adverse reactions to shiitake mushroom extract are rare but may include gastrointestinal discomfort, allergic reactions, and potential interactions with certain medications.

Research Standing: Shiitake mushroom extract has been extensively studied for its medicinal properties and potential health benefits. Research indicates its efficacy in supporting immune function, providing antioxidant protection, promoting cardiovascular and liver health, and reducing inflammation. Continued research is ongoing to further elucidate its mechanisms of action and explore its potential applications in preventing and treating various health conditions.

Pharmacokinetics: The pharmacokinetics of shiitake mushroom extract constituents vary depending on factors such as formulation, route of administration, and individual metabolism. Further studies are needed to elucidate specific pharmacokinetic parameters.

Pharmacodynamics: Shiitake mushroom extract exerts its pharmacodynamic effects through various mechanisms, including modulation of immune responses, scavenging of free radicals, inhibition of microbial growth, reduction of inflammation, and promotion of cardiovascular and liver health.

Overdosage: Limited information is available on the effects of overdosage for shiitake mushroom extract. Excessive intake may lead to gastrointestinal disturbances or potential adverse effects due to its bioactive compounds.

International Standing: Shiitake mushroom extract is recognized internationally for its potential health benefits and is used in various dietary supplements, functional foods, and pharmaceutical formulations.

Indian Standing: In India, shiitake mushroom extract is gaining recognition for its medicinal properties and potential health benefits. It is used in dietary supplements, traditional medicine practices, and culinary preparations. Further research may be needed to establish its standing within traditional medicine systems.

99)SOLANUM LYCOPERSICUM/ S. ESCULENTUM - FRUIT POWDER/ EXTRACT

Introduction: Solanum lycopersicum, commonly known as tomato, is a widely cultivated plant species belonging to the Solanaceae family. It is valued for its edible fruits, which are used in various culinary dishes worldwide. The fruit powder or extract derived from tomatoes is gaining attention for its potential health benefits.

Synonym Name and Common Name: Synonym: None Common Name: Tomato fruit powder or extract

Pharmacognosy/Chemistry: Tomato fruit powder or extract contains various bioactive compounds, including carotenoids (such as lycopene, beta-carotene), phenolic compounds (such as flavonoids and phenolic acids), vitamins (such as vitamin C, vitamin E), minerals, and dietary fibers.

Action and Pharmacology: Tomato fruit powder or extract exhibits antioxidant, anti-inflammatory, cardioprotective, anticancer, and skin health-enhancing properties. Its diverse array of bioactive compounds contributes to these pharmacological effects.

Method of Analysis: Analytical methods such as HPLC (High-Performance Liquid Chromatography), UV-Vis spectrophotometry, and GC-MS (Gas Chromatography-Mass Spectrometry) are commonly used to analyze the constituents of tomato fruit powder or extract.

Health Benefits:

- Antioxidant protection
- Heart health promotion
- Cancer prevention
- Skin health improvement
- Eye health support

Indication and Usage: Tomato fruit powder or extract is indicated for:

- Providing antioxidant support
- Promoting cardiovascular health
- Supporting cancer prevention
- Enhancing skin health and appearance
- Supporting eye health

Usual Constituents with Percentages:

- Carotenoids (lycopene, beta-carotene): 20-40%
- Phenolic compounds: 10-20%
- Vitamins (vitamin C, vitamin E): 5-15%
- Minerals: 1-5%
- Dietary fibers: 20-30%

Mechanism of Action: The bioactive compounds in tomato fruit powder or extract exert their effects through antioxidant activity, modulation of inflammatory pathways, regulation of lipid metabolism, enhancement of immune responses, and protection against DNA damage, among others.

Dosage: Dosage recommendations vary depending on the formulation and specific health condition. It is advisable to follow the instructions provided by healthcare professionals or product labels.

Contraindications:

- Allergy to tomatoes or related plants (Solanaceae family)
- Hypersensitivity to any components of tomato fruit powder or extract

Precautions:

- Use caution if allergic to tomatoes or related plants.

- Ensure the purity and quality of tomato fruit powder or extract, especially in products sourced from reputable manufacturers.
- Consult a healthcare professional before using tomato supplements, especially in individuals with pre-existing medical conditions or taking medications.

Adverse Reactions: Adverse reactions to tomato fruit powder or extract are rare but may include gastrointestinal discomfort, allergic reactions, and potential interactions with certain medications.

Research Standing: Tomato fruit powder or extract has been extensively studied for its medicinal properties and potential health benefits. Research indicates its efficacy in providing antioxidant protection, promoting cardiovascular health, supporting cancer prevention, enhancing skin health, and supporting eye health. Continued research is ongoing to further elucidate its mechanisms of action and explore its potential applications in preventing and treating various health conditions.

Pharmacokinetics: The pharmacokinetics of tomato fruit powder or extract constituents vary depending on factors such as formulation, route of administration, and individual metabolism. Further studies are needed to elucidate specific pharmacokinetic parameters.

Pharmacodynamics: Tomato fruit powder or extract exerts its pharmacodynamic effects through various mechanisms, including antioxidant activity, modulation of inflammatory pathways, regulation of lipid metabolism, enhancement of immune responses, and protection against DNA damage, among others.

Overdosage: Limited information is available on the effects of overdosage for tomato fruit powder or extract. Excessive intake may lead to gastrointestinal disturbances or potential adverse effects due to its bioactive compounds.

International Standing: Tomato fruit powder or extract is recognized internationally for its potential health benefits and is used in various dietary supplements, functional foods, and pharmaceutical formulations.

Indian Standing: In India, tomato fruit powder or extract is gaining recognition for its medicinal properties and potential health benefits. It is used in dietary supplements, traditional medicine practices, and culinary preparations. Further research may be needed to establish its standing within traditional medicine systems.

100) SOY SPROUTS

Introduction: Soy sprouts are young shoots of soybeans (Glycine max), known for their nutritional value and potential health benefits. They are commonly consumed as a nutritious addition to salads, sandwiches, stir-fries, and other dishes.

Synonym Name and Common Name: Synonym: None Common Name: Soy sprouts

Pharmacognosy/Chemistry: Soy sprouts contain a variety of bioactive compounds, including vitamins (such as vitamin C, vitamin K), minerals (such as calcium, magnesium, potassium), protein, dietary fibers, and phytochemicals (such as isoflavones).

Action and Pharmacology: Soy sprouts exhibit various health-promoting properties, including antioxidant, anti-inflammatory, cholesterol-lowering, anticancer, and anti-diabetic effects. These effects are attributed to the diverse array of nutrients and phytochemicals present in soy sprouts.

Method of Analysis: Analytical methods such as HPLC (High-Performance Liquid Chromatography), GC-MS (Gas Chromatography-Mass Spectrometry), and spectrophotometry are commonly used to analyze the nutritional composition and phytochemical content of soy sprouts.

Health Benefits:

- Heart health promotion
- Weight management support
- Bone health enhancement
- Antioxidant protection
- Cancer prevention

Indication and Usage: Soy sprouts are indicated for:

- Supporting cardiovascular health
- Facilitating weight management
- Enhancing bone health

- Providing antioxidant support
- Supporting cancer prevention

Usual Constituents with Percentages:

- Protein: 20-30%
- Dietary fibers: 20-30%
- Vitamins (e.g., vitamin C, vitamin K): 5-15%
- Minerals (e.g., calcium, magnesium, potassium): 5-10%
- Phytochemicals (e.g., isoflavones): Variable

Mechanism of Action: The health benefits of soy sprouts are attributed to various mechanisms, including antioxidant activity, regulation of lipid metabolism, modulation of inflammatory pathways, promotion of bone health, and inhibition of cancer cell growth.

Dosage: There is no specific dosage for soy sprouts as they are typically consumed as a part of the diet. However, incorporating them into meals regularly can contribute to their health benefits.

Contraindications:

- Allergy to soybeans or soy products
- Thyroid disorders (due to potential effects of isoflavones on thyroid function)

Precautions:

- Individuals with soy allergies should avoid soy sprouts.
- Those with thyroid disorders should consume soy sprouts in moderation and consult with a healthcare professional.

Adverse Reactions: Adverse reactions to soy sprouts are rare but may include allergic reactions in individuals with soy allergies.

Research Standing: Soy sprouts have been studied extensively for their nutritional composition and health benefits. Research indicates their efficacy in promoting cardiovascular health, supporting weight management, enhancing bone health, providing antioxidant protection, and preventing cancer. Continued research is ongoing to further elucidate their mechanisms of action and explore their potential applications in preventing and treating various health conditions.

Pharmacokinetics: Limited information is available on the pharmacokinetics of soy sprouts. Absorption, distribution, metabolism, and excretion of their constituents may vary depending on individual factors and food preparation methods.

Pharmacodynamics: Soy sprouts exert their pharmacodynamic effects through various mechanisms, including antioxidant activity, regulation of lipid metabolism, modulation of inflammatory pathways, promotion of bone health, and inhibition of cancer cell growth.

Overdosage: There is no specific information on the effects of overdosage of soy sprouts. However, excessive intake may lead to gastrointestinal discomfort or potential adverse effects due to their nutrient content.

International Standing: Soy sprouts are recognized internationally for their nutritional value and health benefits. They are commonly consumed in various cuisines and are available in many countries as a nutritious food option.

Indian Standing: In India, soy sprouts are gaining recognition for their nutritional value and potential health benefits. They are consumed as a part of salads, sandwiches, and other dishes and are also available in supermarkets and health food stores. Further research may be needed to explore their specific relevance within Indian dietary practices and traditional medicine systems.

101)SPEARMINT

Introduction: Spearmint, scientifically known as Mentha spicata, is a fragrant herb belonging to the mint family (Lamiaceae). It is widely cultivated for its culinary, medicinal, and aromatic properties and has been used for centuries in various cultures for its potential health benefits.

Synonym Name and Common Name: Synonym: Mentha viridis Common Name: Spearmint

Pharmacognosy/Chemistry: Spearmint contains various bioactive compounds, including menthol, carvone, limonene, cineole, and rosmarinic acid. These constituents contribute to its characteristic flavor and aroma, as well as its medicinal properties.

Action and Pharmacology: Spearmint exhibits a range of pharmacological effects, including digestive aid, antimicrobial, anti-inflammatory, analgesic, and antioxidant properties. Its bioactive compounds interact with various physiological pathways to produce these effects.

Method of Analysis: Analytical methods such as GC-MS (Gas Chromatography-Mass Spectrometry), HPLC (High-Performance Liquid Chromatography), and TLC (Thin-Layer Chromatography) are commonly used to analyze the chemical composition of spearmint extracts and essential oils.

Health Benefits:

- Digestive health support
- Oral health promotion
- Respiratory relief
- Stress reduction
- Antioxidant protection

Indication and Usage: Spearmint is indicated for:

- Alleviating digestive discomfort
- Freshening breath
- Relieving respiratory symptoms
- Promoting relaxation
- Providing antioxidant support

Usual Constituents with Percentages:

- Menthol: 30-55%
- Carvone: 35-50%

- Limonene: 5-15%
- Cineole: 1-5%
- Rosmarinic acid: 0.5-2%

Mechanism of Action: The bioactive compounds in spearmint exert their effects through various mechanisms, including activation of digestive enzymes, modulation of neurotransmitter levels, inhibition of microbial growth, and scavenging of free radicals.

Dosage: Spearmint is typically consumed as an herbal tea, essential oil, or culinary ingredient. Dosage may vary depending on the form and specific health condition. It is advisable to follow the instructions provided by healthcare professionals or product labels.

Contraindications:

- Allergy to spearmint or other members of the mint family
- Gastroesophageal reflux disease (GERD) or reflux symptoms (due to potential relaxation of the lower esophageal sphincter)

Precautions:

- Use caution in individuals with allergies to mint or menthol-containing products.
- Avoid excessive intake of spearmint essential oil, as it may cause skin irritation or mucosal irritation when ingested in large amounts.

Adverse Reactions: Adverse reactions to spearmint are rare but may include allergic reactions, gastrointestinal upset, or skin irritation in sensitive individuals.

Research Standing: Spearmint has been studied for its medicinal properties and potential health benefits. Research indicates its efficacy in alleviating digestive discomfort, freshening breath, relieving respiratory symptoms, promoting relaxation, and providing antioxidant protection. Continued research is ongoing to further elucidate its mechanisms of action and explore its potential applications in various health conditions.

Pharmacokinetics: Limited information is available on the pharmacokinetics of spearmint constituents. Absorption, distribution, metabolism, and excretion may vary depending on factors such as formulation, route of administration, and individual metabolism.

Pharmacodynamics: Spearmint exerts its pharmacodynamic effects through various mechanisms, including activation of digestive enzymes, modulation of neurotransmitter levels, inhibition of microbial growth, and scavenging of free radicals.

Overdosage: Excessive intake of spearmint may lead to gastrointestinal discomfort or potential adverse effects due to its menthol content. It is advisable to consume spearmint in moderation and consult with a healthcare professional if experiencing any adverse symptoms.

International Standing: Spearmint is recognized internationally for its culinary uses and potential medicinal properties. It is commonly used in herbal medicine practices and culinary preparations worldwide.

Indian Standing: In India, spearmint is used in traditional Ayurvedic medicine and culinary practices. It is valued for its digestive benefits, aromatic properties, and culinary versatility. Further research may be needed to explore its specific relevance within Indian traditional medicine systems.

102)TAGETES SP. - PETALS OLEO RESIN/ EXTRACT

Introduction: Tagetes, commonly known as marigold, is a genus of flowering plants in the sunflower family (Asteraceae). Tagetes species are renowned for their vibrant flowers and have been traditionally used for medicinal, culinary, and ornamental purposes.

Synonym Name and Common Name: Synonym: None Common Name: Marigold

Pharmacognosy/Chemistry: The petals of Tagetes species contain various bioactive compounds, including carotenoids (such as lutein and zeaxanthin), flavonoids, terpenoids, and volatile oils. These constituents contribute to the medicinal properties and characteristic aroma of marigold petals.

Action and Pharmacology: Marigold petals exhibit antioxidant, anti-inflammatory, antimicrobial, antifungal, and wound-healing properties. Their bioactive compounds interact with various biochemical pathways to produce these pharmacological effects.

Method of Analysis: Analytical methods such as HPLC (High-Performance Liquid Chromatography), GC-MS (Gas Chromatography-Mass Spectrometry), and spectrophotometry are commonly used to analyze the chemical composition of marigold petals, including their oleo resin or extract.

Health Benefits:

- Eye health promotion
- Skin health enhancement
- Wound healing support
- Antimicrobial activity
- Anti-inflammatory effects

Indication and Usage: Marigold petals oleo resin or extract is indicated for:

- Supporting eye health and vision
- Promoting skin health and wound healing
- Providing antimicrobial and antifungal activity
- Alleviating inflammation and soothing skin irritations

Usual Constituents with Percentages:

- Carotenoids (lutein, zeaxanthin): 10-40%
- Flavonoids: 5-20%
- Terpenoids: 2-10%
- Volatile oils: 1-5%

Mechanism of Action: The bioactive compounds in marigold petals exert their effects through various mechanisms, including antioxidant activity, modulation of inflammatory pathways, inhibition of microbial growth, promotion of tissue regeneration, and enhancement of immune responses.

Dosage: Dosage recommendations for marigold petals oleo resin or extract may vary depending on the specific product and intended use. It is advisable to follow the instructions provided by healthcare professionals or product labels.

Contraindications:

- Allergy to marigold or other plants in the Asteraceae family
- Pregnancy and lactation (due to limited safety data)

Precautions:

- Use caution in individuals with allergies to plants in the Asteraceae family.
- Ensure the purity and quality of marigold petals oleo resin or extract, especially in products sourced from reputable manufacturers.

Adverse Reactions: Adverse reactions to marigold petals oleo resin or extract are rare but may include allergic reactions, skin irritation, or gastrointestinal discomfort in sensitive individuals.

Research Standing: Marigold petals have been extensively studied for their medicinal properties and potential health benefits. Research indicates their efficacy in promoting eye health, enhancing skin health and wound healing, providing antimicrobial and anti-inflammatory effects, among others. Continued research is ongoing to further elucidate their mechanisms of action and explore their potential applications in various health conditions.

Pharmacokinetics: Limited information is available on the pharmacokinetics of marigold petals oleo resin or extract. Absorption, distribution, metabolism, and excretion may vary depending on factors such as formulation, route of administration, and individual metabolism.

Pharmacodynamics: Marigold petals exert their pharmacodynamic effects through various mechanisms, including antioxidant activity, modulation of inflammatory pathways, inhibition of microbial growth, promotion of tissue regeneration, and enhancement of immune responses.

Overdosage: Excessive intake of marigold petals oleo resin or extract may lead to gastrointestinal discomfort or potential adverse effects due to its bioactive compounds. It is advisable to consume marigold petals in moderation and consult with a healthcare professional if experiencing any adverse symptoms.

International Standing: Marigold petals oleo resin or extract is recognized internationally for its potential health benefits and is used in various dietary supplements, herbal remedies, and cosmetic products.

Indian Standing: In India, marigold has a long history of use in traditional Ayurvedic and folk medicine practices. Marigold petals are valued for their medicinal properties and are used in various preparations for eye health, skin care, wound healing, and more. They are also widely cultivated and used as offerings in religious and cultural ceremonies. Further research may be needed to explore their specific relevance within Indian traditional medicine systems.

103)TERMINALIA ARJUNA

Introduction: Terminalia arjuna, commonly known as arjuna, is a medicinal tree native to the Indian subcontinent. It has been used for centuries in Ayurvedic medicine for its potential cardiovascular and antioxidant properties.

Synonym Name and Common Name: Synonym: Arjuna Common Name: Arjuna tree, Arjuna bark

Pharmacognosy/Chemistry: Arjuna bark contains various bioactive compounds, including flavonoids (such as quercetin, kaempferol), tannins (such as ellagic acid), triterpenoids, and saponins. These constituents contribute to its medicinal properties.

Action and Pharmacology: Arjuna exhibits cardioprotective, antioxidant, anti-inflammatory, hypolipidemic, and anti-atherosclerotic properties. Its bioactive compounds interact with various physiological pathways to produce these effects.

Method of Analysis: Analytical methods such as HPLC (High-Performance Liquid Chromatography), UV-Vis spectrophotometry, and TLC (Thin-Layer Chromatography) are commonly used to analyze the chemical composition of arjuna bark extracts.

Health Benefits:

- Cardiovascular health support
- Antioxidant protection

- Anti-inflammatory effects
- Cholesterol-lowering activity
- Blood pressure regulation

Indication and Usage: Arjuna bark is indicated for:

- Supporting heart health and function
- Providing antioxidant support
- Alleviating inflammation
- Lowering cholesterol levels
- Regulating blood pressure

Usual Constituents with Percentages:

- Flavonoids: 5-20%
- Tannins: 20-40%
- Triterpenoids: 1-5%
- Saponins: 2-10%

Mechanism of Action: The bioactive compounds in arjuna bark exert their effects through various mechanisms, including strengthening cardiac muscles, reducing oxidative stress, suppressing inflammation, inhibiting cholesterol synthesis, and promoting vasodilation.

Dosage: Dosage recommendations for arjuna bark may vary depending on the specific preparation and intended use. It is advisable to follow the instructions provided by healthcare professionals or product labels.

Contraindications:

- Pregnancy and lactation (due to limited safety data)
- Allergy to arjuna or plants in the Combretaceae family

Precautions:

- Use caution in individuals with bleeding disorders or those taking anticoagulant medications, as arjuna may have mild blood-thinning effects.
- Consult a healthcare professional before using arjuna bark supplements, especially in individuals with pre-existing medical conditions or taking medications.

Adverse Reactions: Adverse reactions to arjuna bark are rare but may include gastrointestinal upset, allergic reactions, or interactions with certain medications.

Research Standing: Arjuna has been extensively studied for its medicinal properties and potential health benefits, particularly in the context of cardiovascular health. Research indicates its efficacy in supporting heart function, reducing oxidative stress, alleviating inflammation, lowering cholesterol levels, and regulating blood pressure. Continued research is ongoing to further elucidate its mechanisms of action and explore its potential applications in preventing and treating various cardiovascular conditions.

Pharmacokinetics: Limited information is available on the pharmacokinetics of arjuna bark constituents. Absorption, distribution, metabolism, and excretion may vary depending on factors such as formulation, route of administration, and individual metabolism.

Pharmacodynamics: Arjuna bark exerts its pharmacodynamic effects through various mechanisms, including strengthening cardiac muscles, reducing oxidative stress, suppressing inflammation, inhibiting cholesterol synthesis, and promoting vasodilation.

Overdosage: Excessive intake of arjuna bark may lead to gastrointestinal discomfort or potential adverse effects due to its bioactive compounds. It is advisable to consume arjuna bark supplements in moderation and consult with a healthcare professional if experiencing any adverse symptoms.

International Standing: Arjuna bark is recognized internationally for its potential medicinal properties and is used in various dietary supplements and herbal remedies marketed for heart health and cardiovascular support.

Indian Standing: In India, arjuna bark has a long history of use in traditional Ayurvedic medicine for heart health and other health conditions. It is widely available in various forms, including powder, capsules, and extracts, and is valued for its cardioprotective properties. Arjuna holds a significant place in Indian traditional medicine systems and is often included in herbal formulations for heart health.

104)TERMINALIA BELLERICA

Introduction: Terminalia bellerica, commonly known as Bibhitaki or Bahera, is a medicinal tree native to the Indian subcontinent. It is one of the three fruits comprising Triphala, a traditional Ayurvedic herbal formula known for its diverse health benefits.

Synonym Name and Common Name: Synonym: None Common Name: Bibhitaki, Bahera

Pharmacognosy/Chemistry: Bibhitaki contains various bioactive compounds, including tannins (such as gallic acid, ellagic acid), flavonoids, lignans, and saponins. These constituents contribute to its medicinal properties and therapeutic effects.

Action and Pharmacology: Bibhitaki exhibits a range of pharmacological effects, including antioxidant, anti-inflammatory, laxative, hepatoprotective, and antimicrobial properties. Its bioactive compounds interact with various physiological pathways to produce these effects.

Method of Analysis: Analytical methods such as HPLC (High-Performance Liquid Chromatography), GC-MS (Gas Chromatography-Mass Spectrometry), and spectrophotometry are commonly used to analyze the chemical composition of Bibhitaki extracts and formulations.

Health Benefits:

- Digestive health promotion
- Antioxidant protection
- Liver health support
- Respiratory relief
- Anti-inflammatory effects

Indication and Usage: Bibhitaki is indicated for:

- Improving digestion and relieving constipation
- Providing antioxidant support
- Supporting liver function and detoxification
- Alleviating respiratory symptoms
- Managing inflammation

Usual Constituents with Percentages:

- Tannins: 30-40%
- Flavonoids: 5-15%
- Lignans: 1-5%
- Saponins: 2-10%

Mechanism of Action: The bioactive compounds in Bibhitaki exert their effects through various mechanisms, including modulation of gut motility, inhibition of oxidative stress, suppression of inflammatory pathways, enhancement of liver function, and inhibition of microbial growth.

Dosage: Dosage recommendations for Bibhitaki may vary depending on the specific formulation and intended use. It is advisable to follow the instructions provided by healthcare professionals or product labels.

Contraindications:

- Pregnancy and lactation (due to limited safety data)
- Allergy to Bibhitaki or related plants in the Combretaceae family

Precautions:

- Use caution in individuals with gastrointestinal disorders or those taking medications affecting gastrointestinal motility.
- Consult a healthcare professional before using Bibhitaki supplements, especially in individuals with pre-existing medical conditions or taking medications.

Adverse Reactions: Adverse reactions to Bibhitaki are rare but may include gastrointestinal discomfort, allergic reactions, or interactions with certain medications.

Research Standing: Bibhitaki has been studied for its medicinal properties and potential health benefits. Research indicates its efficacy in promoting digestive health, providing antioxidant protection, supporting liver function, relieving respiratory symptoms, and managing inflammation. Continued research is ongoing to further elucidate its mechanisms of action and explore its potential applications in various health conditions.

Pharmacokinetics: Limited information is available on the pharmacokinetics of Bibhitaki constituents. Absorption, distribution, metabolism, and excretion may vary depending on factors such as formulation, route of administration, and individual metabolism.

Pharmacodynamics: Bibhitaki exerts its pharmacodynamic effects through various mechanisms, including modulation of gut motility, inhibition of oxidative stress, suppression of inflammatory pathways, enhancement of liver function, and inhibition of microbial growth.

Overdosage: Excessive intake of Bibhitaki may lead to gastrointestinal discomfort or potential adverse effects due to its bioactive compounds. It is advisable to consume Bibhitaki supplements in moderation and consult with a healthcare professional if experiencing any adverse symptoms.

International Standing: Bibhitaki is recognized internationally for its medicinal properties and is used in various herbal formulations and dietary supplements marketed for digestive health, liver support, and antioxidant protection.

Indian Standing: In India, Bibhitaki holds a significant place in traditional Ayurvedic medicine and is commonly used in herbal formulations and remedies. It is valued for its digestive benefits, liver support, and overall health-promoting properties. Bibhitaki is often included in Ayurvedic formulations and is considered an important herb for maintaining health and well-being

105) TERMINALIA CHEBULIA

Introduction: Terminalia chebula, commonly known as "Haritaki" in Ayurveda, is a revered medicinal plant native to the Indian subcontinent and Southeast Asia. Belonging to the Combretaceae family, it has been used for centuries in traditional medicine systems like Ayurveda, Siddha, and Unani for its various health benefits.

Synonym Name and Common Name: Synonym: Terminalia reticulata Common Name: Haritaki, Chebulic Myrobalan

Pharmacognosy/Chemistry: Terminalia chebula contains various phytochemicals such as tannins (chebulagic acid, chebulinic acid), flavonoids, phenolic compounds, and terpenoids. The fruits are usually brownish-yellow to black in color and have astringent taste.

Action and Pharmacology: The pharmacological actions of Terminalia chebula include antioxidant, anti-inflammatory, antimicrobial, hepatoprotective, laxative, adaptogenic, and immunomodulatory properties.

Method of Analysis: Analytical methods such as high-performance liquid chromatography (HPLC), gas chromatography-mass spectrometry (GC-MS), and thin-layer chromatography (TLC) are commonly employed for the qualitative and quantitative analysis of bioactive compounds in Terminalia chebula.

Health Benefits: Terminalia chebula is believed to offer various health benefits including improving digestion, promoting detoxification, enhancing immune function, supporting liver health, managing diabetes, and exerting anti-aging effects.

Indication and Usage: It is commonly used in traditional medicine for treating constipation, diarrhea, indigestion, hyperacidity, liver disorders, respiratory conditions, skin diseases, and promoting overall well-being.

Usual Constituents with Percentages: Typical constituents of Terminalia chebula include:

- Tannins (up to 40%)
- Chebulagic acid (1-5%)
- Chebulinic acid (2-8%)
- Flavonoids

- Phenolic compounds
- Terpenoids

Mechanism of Action: The tannins in Terminalia chebula exert antioxidant and astringent effects, while chebulagic acid and chebulinic acid contribute to its various pharmacological actions such as anti-inflammatory and hepatoprotective effects.

Dosage: The dosage of Terminalia chebula may vary depending on the formulation and intended use. However, typical doses range from 500 mg to 2 grams per day, divided into multiple doses.

Contraindications: Terminalia chebula should be used with caution in individuals with a history of hypersensitivity reactions. Pregnant and breastfeeding women should consult a healthcare professional before using it.

Precautions: It is advisable to consult a healthcare practitioner before using Terminalia chebula, especially if you have any pre-existing medical conditions or are taking medications.

Adverse Reactions: Although Terminalia chebula is generally considered safe when used in recommended doses, excessive intake may lead to gastrointestinal discomfort such as abdominal pain, cramps, or diarrhea in some individuals.

Research Standing: Terminalia chebula has garnered significant attention from researchers worldwide, with numerous studies investigating its pharmacological properties, potential health benefits, and safety profile. However, further research is warranted to fully elucidate its mechanisms of action and therapeutic potential.

Pharmacokinetics and Pharmacodynamics: The pharmacokinetics of Terminalia chebula have not been extensively studied. However, its pharmacodynamics involve modulation of various biochemical pathways associated with its antioxidant, anti-inflammatory, and other pharmacological actions.

Overdosage: Excessive consumption of Terminalia chebula may lead to adverse effects such as gastrointestinal disturbances. It is important to adhere to recommended dosage guidelines.

International Standing: Terminalia chebula is recognized internationally for its traditional medicinal uses and is commonly included in herbal supplements and formulations marketed for promoting digestive health and overall well-being.

Indian Standing: In India, Terminalia chebula holds a prominent place in Ayurvedic medicine and is used in various formulations for managing a wide range of health conditions.

Research Summary: Research on Terminalia chebula highlights its diverse pharmacological properties and potential therapeutic applications, including its role in gastrointestinal health, liver protection, immune modulation, and anti-inflammatory effects. While much progress has been made in understanding its bioactive constituents and mechanisms of action, further clinical trials and pharmacological studies are needed to validate its traditional uses and explore its full therapeutic potential.

106) TRIGONELLA-FOENUM-GRAECUM

Introduction: Trigonella foenum-graecum, commonly known as Fenugreek, is an annual herbaceous plant native to the Mediterranean region, Western Asia, and South Asia. It has been utilized for centuries in traditional medicine systems such as Ayurveda, Chinese medicine, and Unani for its various health benefits.

Synonym Name and Common Name: Synonym: Fenugreek Common Name: Methi (in Hindi)

Pharmacognosy/Chemistry: Trigonella foenum-graecum contains several bioactive compounds, including alkaloids, flavonoids, saponins, and steroidal saponins. The seeds are rich in proteins, fibers, vitamins (especially vitamin B6 and vitamin C), and minerals (such as iron, magnesium, and manganese).

Action and Pharmacology: Fenugreek exhibits diverse pharmacological actions including anti-inflammatory, antioxidant, hypoglycemic, hypocholesterolemic, antimicrobial, hepatoprotective, and galactagogue (milk-producing) properties.

Method of Analysis: Analytical techniques such as high-performance liquid chromatography (HPLC), gas chromatography-mass spectrometry (GC-MS), and spectrophotometry are commonly employed for the qualitative and quantitative analysis of bioactive constituents in Fenugreek.

Health Benefits: Fenugreek is associated with numerous health benefits, including improving digestion, regulating blood sugar levels, lowering cholesterol, promoting milk production in lactating mothers, enhancing libido, and supporting overall immune function.

Indication and Usage: It is traditionally used for managing diabetes, hyperlipidemia, gastrointestinal disorders, menstrual irregularities, lactation problems, and as a general tonic for promoting health and well-being.

Usual Constituents with Percentages: Typical constituents of Trigonella foenum-graecum include:

- Steroidal saponins (20-25%)
- Alkaloids
- Flavonoids
- Proteins
- Fibers
- Vitamins and minerals

Mechanism of Action: The hypoglycemic and hypocholesterolemic effects of Fenugreek are attributed to its ability to inhibit intestinal glucose absorption, increase insulin sensitivity, and promote bile acid excretion. Its galactagogue effect is believed to be due to the presence of phytoestrogens and prolactin-stimulating compounds.

Dosage: The dosage of Fenugreek may vary depending on the formulation and intended use. Typical doses range from 1 to 2 grams of seeds per day, or as recommended by a healthcare professional.

Contraindications: Fenugreek should be used with caution in individuals with hypersensitivity to any of its components. Pregnant women should avoid excessive intake due to its potential uterine stimulant effects.

Precautions: Individuals with diabetes or hypoglycemia should monitor their blood sugar levels closely when using Fenugreek, as it may lower blood glucose levels. It is advisable to consult a healthcare practitioner before using Fenugreek, especially if you have any pre-existing medical conditions or are taking medications.

Adverse Reactions: While Fenugreek is generally considered safe when used in recommended doses, excessive intake may lead to gastrointestinal discomfort such as bloating, gas, or diarrhea in some individuals. Allergic reactions are rare but possible in sensitive individuals.

Research Standing: Fenugreek has been extensively studied for its pharmacological properties and therapeutic potential. Numerous preclinical and clinical studies have been conducted to investigate its effects on various health conditions, including diabetes, hyperlipidemia, lactation, and gastrointestinal disorders.

Pharmacokinetics and Pharmacodynamics: The pharmacokinetics of Fenugreek have been studied to some extent, with research focusing on its absorption, distribution, metabolism, and excretion in humans. Its pharmacodynamics involve modulation of various biochemical pathways associated with its therapeutic effects, including glucose and lipid metabolism.

Overdosage: Excessive consumption of Fenugreek may lead to adverse effects such as gastrointestinal disturbances or hypoglycemia. It is important to adhere to recommended dosage guidelines.

International Standing: Fenugreek is recognized internationally for its medicinal properties and is commonly used in herbal supplements and culinary applications.

Indian Standing: In India, Fenugreek holds a prominent place in Ayurvedic medicine and is widely used in various formulations for managing diabetes, improving digestion, and promoting lactation.

Research Summary: Research on Fenugreek underscores its potential as a therapeutic agent for managing diabetes, hyperlipidemia, lactation problems, and various other health conditions. While much progress has been made in understanding its pharmacological properties and mechanisms of action, further clinical trials and research are needed to explore its full therapeutic potential and safety profile.

107)TRITICUM SATIVUM

Introduction: Triticum sativum, commonly known as Wheatgrass, is the young shoots of the common wheat plant, Triticum aestivum. It is harvested before the wheat plant reaches maturity and has gained popularity as a health food due to its rich nutrient content and potential health benefits.

Synonym Name and Common Name: Synonym: Common wheatgrass Common Name: Wheatgrass

Pharmacognosy/Chemistry: Wheatgrass is rich in various nutrients including vitamins, minerals, enzymes, amino acids, chlorophyll, and antioxidants. It contains vitamins A, C, E, and K, minerals such as iron, calcium, magnesium, and potassium, as well as phytochemicals like flavonoids and phenolic compounds.

Action and Pharmacology: Wheatgrass exhibits various pharmacological actions including antioxidant, anti-inflammatory, detoxifying, immunomodulatory, and antimicrobial properties. It is also believed to support cellular repair and regeneration.

Method of Analysis: Analytical methods such as high-performance liquid chromatography (HPLC), spectrophotometry, and gas chromatography-mass spectrometry (GC-MS) are commonly used for the qualitative and quantitative analysis of bioactive compounds in wheatgrass.

Health Benefits: Wheatgrass is associated with numerous health benefits including boosting the immune system, improving digestion, detoxifying the body, promoting weight loss, enhancing skin health, and reducing inflammation.

Indication and Usage: It is often used as a dietary supplement or consumed as a fresh juice for promoting overall health and well-being. Wheatgrass is also used in naturopathic and alternative medicine practices for managing various health conditions such as diabetes, high cholesterol, and gastrointestinal disorders.

Usual Constituents with Percentages: Typical constituents of Triticum sativum (Wheatgrass) include:

- Vitamins (especially vitamin A, C, E, and K)
- Minerals (such as iron, calcium, magnesium, and potassium)
- Enzymes

- Amino acids
- Chlorophyll
- Flavonoids and phenolic compounds

Mechanism of Action: The health benefits of wheatgrass are attributed to its rich nutrient content and bioactive compounds, which exert antioxidant, anti-inflammatory, detoxifying, and immunomodulatory effects. Chlorophyll in wheatgrass is believed to support detoxification processes, while vitamins and minerals contribute to overall health and well-being.

Dosage: The dosage of wheatgrass may vary depending on the form of consumption (juice, powder, capsules) and individual health goals. Typical doses range from 1 to 4 ounces of fresh wheatgrass juice per day, or as recommended by a healthcare practitioner.

Contraindications: Wheatgrass is generally considered safe for most people when consumed in moderation. However, individuals with wheat or gluten allergies should avoid wheatgrass products to prevent allergic reactions.

Precautions: It is advisable to consult a healthcare practitioner before using wheatgrass, especially if you have any underlying health conditions or are pregnant or breastfeeding. Individuals on medications should also seek medical advice before incorporating wheatgrass into their diet.

Adverse Reactions: While wheatgrass is generally well-tolerated, some individuals may experience allergic reactions, gastrointestinal upset, or nausea, especially when consuming large quantities of wheatgrass juice.

Research Standing: Wheatgrass has been the subject of numerous studies investigating its potential health benefits and therapeutic applications. While research on wheatgrass is still evolving, preliminary studies suggest promising effects in various areas including immune function, detoxification, and inflammation.

Pharmacokinetics and Pharmacodynamics: The pharmacokinetics and pharmacodynamics of wheatgrass have not been extensively studied. However, its bioavailability and metabolic pathways may vary depending on the form of consumption and individual factors.

Overdosage: Excessive consumption of wheatgrass may lead to gastrointestinal discomfort or allergic reactions in some individuals. It is important to adhere to recommended dosage guidelines and monitor for any adverse effects.

International Standing: Wheatgrass products are widely available internationally and are commonly consumed as dietary supplements or health foods.

Indian Standing: In India, wheatgrass is also gaining popularity as a health food and is used in various forms such as fresh juice, powder, or capsules for its potential health benefits.

Research Summary: Research on wheatgrass suggests promising health benefits, particularly in areas such as immune support, detoxification, and inflammation. While more studies are needed to fully elucidate its mechanisms of action and therapeutic potential, wheatgrass remains a popular choice among individuals seeking natural remedies for promoting health and well-being.

108) VACCINIUM CORYMBOSUM

Introduction: Vaccinium corymbosum, commonly known as Blueberry, is a flowering shrub native to North America and cultivated worldwide for its flavorful and nutritious berries. Blueberries are well-regarded for their antioxidant properties and are often included in various culinary dishes and dietary supplements.

Synonym Name and Common Name: Synonym: None Common Name: Blueberry

Pharmacognosy/Chemistry: Blueberries are rich in various phytochemicals including anthocyanins, flavonoids, phenolic acids, and tannins. They also contain vitamins (such as vitamin C, vitamin K, and vitamin E), minerals (including manganese and potassium), and dietary fibers.

Action and Pharmacology: Blueberries exhibit potent antioxidant, anti-inflammatory, anti-cancer, neuroprotective, cardioprotective, and antimicrobial properties. These pharmacological actions contribute to their various health benefits.

Method of Analysis: Analytical methods such as high-performance liquid chromatography (HPLC), spectrophotometry, and gas chromatography-mass spectrometry (GC-MS) are commonly used for the qualitative and quantitative analysis of bioactive compounds in blueberries.

Health Benefits: Blueberries are associated with numerous health benefits including improving cognitive function, supporting heart health, regulating blood sugar levels, enhancing vision, promoting gastrointestinal health, and reducing the risk of chronic diseases such as cancer and cardiovascular disorders.

Indication and Usage: They are often consumed fresh, dried, or frozen, and are also used in various culinary dishes such as smoothies, salads, and desserts. Blueberry extracts and supplements are also available for those seeking to incorporate the health benefits of blueberries into their daily routine.

Usual Constituents with Percentages: Typical constituents of Vaccinium corymbosum (Blueberry) include:

- Anthocyanins (up to 25%)
- Flavonoids
- Phenolic acids
- Tannins
- Vitamins (especially vitamin C)
- Minerals (such as manganese and potassium)
- Dietary fibers

Mechanism of Action: The health benefits of blueberries are attributed to their rich phytochemical content, particularly anthocyanins and flavonoids, which exert antioxidant, anti-inflammatory, and other bioactive effects. These compounds help neutralize free radicals, reduce inflammation, and support various physiological processes in the body.

Dosage: There is no specific dosage recommendation for blueberries as they are commonly consumed as part of a balanced diet. However, incorporating a serving of blueberries (approximately 1/2 to 1 cup) into your daily diet can provide potential health benefits.

Contraindications: Blueberries are generally safe for most people when consumed in moderation as part of a balanced diet. However, individuals with known allergies to berries or specific components of blueberries should avoid consumption to prevent allergic reactions.

Precautions: It is advisable to consume organic blueberries whenever possible to minimize exposure to pesticides and other contaminants. Individuals on medications or with underlying health conditions should consult a healthcare professional before incorporating blueberries into their diet or taking blueberry supplements.

Adverse Reactions: While blueberries are considered safe for most people, excessive consumption may lead to gastrointestinal discomfort such as bloating, gas, or diarrhea in some individuals, particularly those with sensitive digestive systems.

Research Standing: Blueberries have been the subject of numerous studies investigating their potential health benefits and therapeutic applications. Research suggests promising effects in various areas including cognitive function, cardiovascular health, diabetes management, and cancer prevention.

Pharmacokinetics and Pharmacodynamics: The pharmacokinetics and pharmacodynamics of blueberries have been studied to some extent, with research focusing on their absorption, distribution, metabolism, and excretion in humans. Their bioavailability and physiological effects may vary depending on factors such as the form of consumption and individual characteristics.

Overdosage: There is no specific evidence of overdosage with blueberries when consumed as part of a balanced diet. However, excessive intake of blueberry supplements or extracts may lead to adverse effects, and it is important to adhere to recommended dosage guidelines.

International Standing: Blueberries are widely recognized and consumed internationally for their delicious flavor and potential health benefits. They are commonly available in fresh, frozen, and processed forms in supermarkets and health food stores worldwide.

Indian Standing: In India, blueberries are becoming increasingly popular as awareness of their health benefits grows. While not native to India, blueberries are imported and can be found in specialty stores and supermarkets in urban areas.

Research Summary: Research on blueberries underscores their potential as a functional food with significant health-promoting properties. Numerous studies have demonstrated their antioxidant, anti-inflammatory, and other bioactive effects, suggesting potential benefits for cognitive function, cardiovascular health, diabetes management, and cancer prevention. Further research is warranted to elucidate the mechanisms of action and optimize their therapeutic applications.

109)VACCINIUM OXYCOCCOS/VACCINIUM MACROCARPON –FRUIT

Introduction: Vaccinium oxycoccos and Vaccinium macrocarpon, commonly known as Cranberry, are evergreen shrubs native to North America. They are well-known for their tart, red berries and have been used traditionally for various health benefits.

Synonym Name and Common Name: Synonym: None Common Name: Cranberry

Pharmacognosy/Chemistry: Cranberries contain a variety of bioactive compounds including proanthocyanidins (PACs), flavonoids, organic acids (such as citric acid and quinic acid), vitamins (especially vitamin C), and minerals (like manganese). The berries are also rich in dietary fiber.

Action and Pharmacology: Cranberries exhibit several pharmacological actions including antioxidant, anti-inflammatory, antimicrobial (particularly against urinary tract pathogens), and anti-adhesion properties, which help prevent the adhesion of bacteria to the urinary tract walls.

Method of Analysis: Analytical methods such as high-performance liquid chromatography (HPLC), spectrophotometry, and microbiological assays are commonly used for the qualitative and quantitative analysis of bioactive compounds in cranberries.

Health Benefits: Cranberries are associated with numerous health benefits including preventing urinary tract infections (UTIs), promoting gastrointestinal health, supporting oral health, reducing the risk of cardiovascular disease, and providing antioxidant protection.

Indication and Usage: They are often consumed as fresh berries, dried fruit, juice, or in supplement form. Cranberry products are frequently used to help prevent UTIs, maintain urinary tract health, and support overall well-being.

Usual Constituents with Percentages: Typical constituents of Vaccinium oxycoccos and Vaccinium macrocarpon (Cranberry) include:

- Proanthocyanidins (PACs) (5-15%)
- Flavonoids
- Organic acids (such as citric acid and quinic acid)
- Vitamins (especially vitamin C)
- Minerals (like manganese)
- Dietary fiber

Mechanism of Action: The health benefits of cranberries are attributed to their unique combination of bioactive compounds, particularly PACs, which help prevent bacterial adhesion to the urinary tract walls, reduce inflammation, and provide antioxidant protection against oxidative stress.

Dosage: The recommended dosage of cranberry products varies depending on the form and intended use. For preventing UTIs, typical doses range from 300 mg to 500 mg of cranberry extract capsules or tablets per day, or as directed by a healthcare professional.

Contraindications: Individuals with a history of kidney stones or allergies to cranberries should avoid cranberry products. Additionally, those on blood-thinning medications should use caution due to the potential interaction with cranberry's anticoagulant properties.

Precautions: It is advisable to consult a healthcare practitioner before using cranberry products, especially if you have any underlying health conditions or are pregnant or breastfeeding. Cranberry supplements should not be used as a substitute for medical treatment of urinary tract infections.

Adverse Reactions: While cranberries are generally safe for most people when consumed in moderation, excessive intake may lead to gastrointestinal upset such as stomach pain or diarrhea in some individuals, particularly with concentrated cranberry supplements.

Research Standing: Cranberries have been the subject of numerous studies investigating their potential health benefits and therapeutic applications. Research suggests promising effects in preventing UTIs, supporting urinary tract health, reducing cardiovascular risk factors, and providing antioxidant protection.

Pharmacokinetics and Pharmacodynamics: The pharmacokinetics and pharmacodynamics of cranberries have been studied to some extent, with research focusing on their absorption, distribution, metabolism, and excretion in humans. Cranberry PACs have been shown to interfere with bacterial adhesion to urinary tract walls and exert antioxidant effects.

Overdosage: Excessive consumption of cranberry products may lead to gastrointestinal discomfort or allergic reactions in some individuals. It is important to adhere to recommended dosage guidelines and monitor for any adverse effects.

International Standing: Cranberries are widely recognized and consumed internationally for their potential health benefits. Cranberry products are commonly available in supermarkets, health food stores, and pharmacies worldwide.

Indian Standing: In India, cranberries are gaining popularity as awareness of their health benefits grows. Imported cranberry products are available in select supermarkets and health food stores in urban areas.

Research Summary: Research on cranberries highlights their potential as a functional food with significant health-promoting properties, particularly for urinary tract health and cardiovascular protection. Studies have demonstrated the efficacy of cranberry products in preventing UTIs, reducing inflammation, and providing antioxidant support. Further research is needed to fully elucidate their mechanisms of action and optimize their therapeutic applications.

110)VALERIANA WALLICHII

Introduction: Valeriana wallichii, commonly known as Indian Valerian, is a perennial herb native to the Indian subcontinent. It has a long history of use in traditional medicine systems such as Ayurveda and Unani for its potential therapeutic effects on the nervous system and overall well-being.

Synonym Name and Common Name: Synonym: None Common Name: Indian Valerian

Pharmacognosy/Chemistry: Valeriana wallichii contains various bioactive compounds including valepotriates, sesquiterpenes (such as valerenic acid), flavonoids, and alkaloids. The roots of Indian Valerian are the primary medicinal part and are rich in these active constituents.

Action and Pharmacology: Indian Valerian exhibits anxiolytic, sedative, hypnotic, muscle relaxant, and anticonvulsant properties. These pharmacological actions are attributed to its ability to modulate gamma-aminobutyric acid (GABA) neurotransmission in the brain.

Method of Analysis: Analytical techniques such as high-performance liquid chromatography (HPLC), gas chromatography-mass spectrometry (GC-MS), and thin-layer chromatography (TLC) are commonly used for the qualitative and quantitative analysis of bioactive compounds in Indian Valerian.

Health Benefits: Indian Valerian is associated with various health benefits including promoting relaxation, reducing anxiety and stress, improving sleep quality, relieving muscle tension, and supporting overall mental well-being.

Indication and Usage: It is often used in traditional medicine for managing anxiety disorders, insomnia, nervousness, restlessness, and mild mood disturbances. Indian Valerian is available in various forms such as capsules, tablets, tinctures, and teas.

Usual Constituents with Percentages: Typical constituents of Valeriana wallichii include:

- Valepotriates (up to 0.8%)
- Sesquiterpenes (such as valerenic acid)
- Flavonoids
- Alkaloids

Mechanism of Action: The anxiolytic and sedative effects of Indian Valerian are primarily mediated through its interaction with GABA receptors in the central nervous system. It enhances GABAergic neurotransmission, leading to relaxation, reduction of anxiety, and improvement of sleep quality.

Dosage: The dosage of Indian Valerian may vary depending on the formulation and individual response. Typical doses range from 300 mg to 900 mg of standardized extract per day, divided into multiple doses. It is best to follow the recommendations provided by healthcare professionals or product labels.

Contraindications: Indian Valerian should be used with caution in individuals with liver disorders or a history of sensitivity to valerian-containing products. It is not recommended for use in pregnant or breastfeeding women without consulting a healthcare practitioner.

Precautions: It is advisable to avoid alcohol and sedative medications while using Indian Valerian, as it may potentiate their effects. Individuals with a history of depression or suicidal tendencies should use Indian Valerian under the supervision of a healthcare professional.

Adverse Reactions: While Indian Valerian is generally well-tolerated, some individuals may experience mild gastrointestinal upset, dizziness, or drowsiness, especially at higher doses. Allergic reactions are rare but possible in sensitive individuals.

Research Standing: Indian Valerian has been the subject of numerous studies investigating its pharmacological properties and therapeutic potential. Research suggests promising effects in reducing anxiety, improving sleep quality, and enhancing relaxation.

Pharmacokinetics and Pharmacodynamics: The pharmacokinetics of Indian Valerian have not been extensively studied. However, its pharmacodynamics involve modulation of GABAergic neurotransmission and other neural pathways associated with its anxiolytic and sedative effects.

Overdosage: Excessive consumption of Indian Valerian may lead to increased sedation, dizziness, or gastrointestinal discomfort. It is important to adhere to recommended dosage guidelines and consult a healthcare professional if experiencing adverse effects.

International Standing: Indian Valerian is recognized internationally for its potential therapeutic effects on anxiety and sleep disorders. It is commonly used in herbal supplements and preparations marketed for promoting relaxation and improving sleep quality.

Indian Standing: In India, Indian Valerian holds a prominent place in traditional medicine systems such as Ayurveda and Unani. It is widely used for its calming and sedative properties, especially in formulations targeting anxiety and insomnia.

Research Summary: Research on Indian Valerian highlights its potential as a natural remedy for managing anxiety, insomnia, and related conditions. Studies have demonstrated its anxiolytic, sedative, and hypnotic effects, supporting its traditional use in promoting relaxation and improving sleep quality. Further research is needed to elucidate its mechanisms of action and optimize its therapeutic applications.

111)VITIS ALBA AND VITIS VINIFERA - FRUIT - DRIED POWDER / CONCENTRATE STANDARDIZED

Introduction: Vitis alba and Vitis vinifera, commonly known as White Grape and Grape, respectively, are deciduous woody vines belonging to the Vitaceae family. These grape varieties are cultivated worldwide for their sweet, juicy fruits and are extensively used in winemaking and as fresh fruits.

Synonym Name and Common Name: Synonym: None Common Name: White Grape (Vitis alba), Grape (Vitis vinifera)

Pharmacognosy/Chemistry: The dried powder or concentrate of White Grape (Vitis alba) and Grape (Vitis vinifera) contains various bioactive compounds including polyphenols (such as resveratrol, quercetin, and catechins), flavonoids, anthocyanins, vitamins (especially vitamin C), minerals (like potassium), and dietary fiber.

Action and Pharmacology: White Grape and Grape are known for their antioxidant, anti-inflammatory, cardioprotective, neuroprotective, and anti-cancer properties. These pharmacological actions are attributed to the presence of polyphenols and other bioactive compounds in the fruits.

Method of Analysis: Analytical methods such as high-performance liquid chromatography (HPLC), spectrophotometry, and gas chromatography-mass spectrometry (GC-MS) are commonly used for the qualitative and quantitative analysis of bioactive compounds in White Grape and Grape products.

Health Benefits: White Grape and Grape products are associated with numerous health benefits including improving cardiovascular health, supporting cognitive function, promoting skin health, enhancing immune function, and reducing the risk of chronic diseases such as cancer and diabetes.

Indication and Usage: They are often consumed as dried fruits, fruit powders, concentrates, juices, or as ingredients in various food products and supplements. White Grape and Grape products are used to promote overall health and well-being, and are also incorporated into skincare products for their antioxidant properties.

Usual Constituents with Percentages: Typical constituents of dried powder or concentrate of Vitis alba (White Grape) and Vitis vinifera (Grape) include:

- Polyphenols (up to 5-10%)
- Flavonoids
- Anthocyanins (in Grape)
- Vitamins (especially vitamin C)
- Minerals (like potassium)
- Dietary fiber

Mechanism of Action: The health benefits of White Grape and Grape are attributed to their rich polyphenol content, particularly resveratrol, which exerts antioxidant, anti-inflammatory, and other bioactive effects. These compounds help neutralize free radicals, reduce inflammation, and support various physiological processes in the body.

Dosage: The dosage of White Grape and Grape products may vary depending on the form of consumption and individual health goals. Typical doses range from 500 mg to 2 grams of dried powder or concentrate per day, or as recommended by a healthcare professional.

Contraindications: Individuals with known allergies to grapes or specific components of White Grape and Grape products should avoid consumption to prevent allergic reactions. Grape products may also interact with certain medications, particularly blood-thinning medications, due to their anticoagulant properties.

Precautions: It is advisable to consult a healthcare practitioner before using White Grape and Grape products, especially if you have any underlying health conditions or are pregnant or breastfeeding. Grape products should not be used as a substitute for medical treatment of any condition without professional guidance.

Adverse Reactions: While White Grape and Grape products are generally well-tolerated, some individuals may experience mild gastrointestinal upset or allergic reactions, especially in those with sensitivities to grapes or dietary supplements.

Research Standing: White Grape and Grape products have been the subject of numerous studies investigating their potential health benefits and therapeutic applications. Research suggests promising effects in improving cardiovascular health, cognitive function, skin health, and reducing oxidative stress and inflammation.

Pharmacokinetics and Pharmacodynamics: The pharmacokinetics and pharmacodynamics of White Grape and Grape products have been studied to some extent, with research focusing on their absorption, distribution, metabolism, and excretion in humans. Their bioavailability and physiological effects may vary depending on factors such as the form of consumption and individual characteristics.

Overdosage: Excessive consumption of White Grape and Grape products may lead to gastrointestinal discomfort or allergic reactions in some individuals. It is important to adhere to recommended dosage guidelines and monitor for any adverse effects.

International Standing: White Grape and Grape products are widely recognized and consumed internationally for their potential health benefits. They are commonly used in food products, supplements, and skincare formulations.

Indian Standing: In India, White Grape and Grape products are gaining popularity as awareness of their health benefits grows. They are imported and can be found in specialty stores, supermarkets, and online platforms.

Research Summary: Research on White Grape and Grape products underscores their potential as functional foods with significant health-promoting properties. Numerous studies have demonstrated their antioxidant, anti-inflammatory, cardioprotective, and neuroprotective effects, supporting their traditional use and therapeutic applications. Further research is needed to elucidate their mechanisms of action and optimize their therapeutic potential.

112) WHEAT GERM

Introduction: Wheat germ refers to the embryo of the wheat kernel, which is the reproductive part of the wheat plant. It is rich in nutrients and bioactive compounds, making it a popular dietary supplement and functional food ingredient.

Synonym Name and Common Name: Synonym: None Common Name: Wheat Germ

Pharmacognosy/Chemistry: Wheat germ is a concentrated source of various nutrients including vitamins (such as vitamin E, vitamin B complex), minerals (like zinc, magnesium, and iron), proteins, healthy fats, fiber, and phytochemicals (such as phytosterols and polyphenols).

Action and Pharmacology: Wheat germ exhibits several pharmacological actions including antioxidant, anti-inflammatory, immunomodulatory, cardioprotective, and neuroprotective effects. These actions are attributed to its rich nutrient and bioactive compound content.

Method of Analysis: Analytical methods such as high-performance liquid chromatography (HPLC), gas chromatography-mass spectrometry (GC-MS), and spectrophotometry are commonly used for the qualitative and quantitative analysis of nutrients and bioactive compounds in wheat germ.

Health Benefits: Wheat germ is associated with numerous health benefits including supporting cardiovascular health, boosting immune function, improving skin health, promoting digestion, enhancing energy levels, and supporting overall vitality and well-being.

Indication and Usage: It is often consumed as a dietary supplement in various forms such as raw, toasted, or as an ingredient in cereals, smoothies, baked goods, and other culinary preparations. Wheat germ supplements are used to provide additional nutritional support.

Usual Constituents with Percentages: Typical constituents of wheat germ include:

- Vitamins (especially vitamin E)
- Vitamin B complex
- Minerals (like zinc, magnesium, iron)
- Proteins
- Healthy fats
- Fiber
- Phytochemicals (such as phytosterols and polyphenols)

Mechanism of Action: The health benefits of wheat germ are attributed to its rich nutrient and bioactive compound content, particularly vitamin E and other antioxidants, which help neutralize free radicals, reduce inflammation, and support various physiological processes in the body.

Dosage: The dosage of wheat germ supplements may vary depending on the form and intended use. Typical doses range from 1 to 3 tablespoons of raw or toasted wheat germ per day, or as recommended by a healthcare professional.

Contraindications: Individuals with wheat allergies or celiac disease should avoid wheat germ products to prevent allergic reactions or gluten-related symptoms. People with certain medical conditions or on medications should consult a healthcare provider before using wheat germ supplements.

Precautions: It is important to choose high-quality wheat germ products and store them properly to maintain their nutritional integrity. Individuals with digestive disorders or sensitivities should start with small doses of wheat germ to assess tolerance.

Adverse Reactions: While wheat germ is generally safe for most people, excessive consumption may lead to gastrointestinal discomfort such as bloating, gas, or diarrhea, especially in individuals with sensitive digestive systems.

Research Standing: Wheat germ has been the subject of various studies investigating its nutritional composition and potential health benefits. Research suggests promising effects in supporting cardiovascular health, enhancing immune function, and providing antioxidant protection.

Pharmacokinetics and Pharmacodynamics: The pharmacokinetics and pharmacodynamics of wheat germ have not been extensively studied. However, its bioavailability and physiological effects may vary depending on factors such as the form of consumption and individual characteristics.

Overdosage: Excessive consumption of wheat germ supplements may lead to an intake of nutrients beyond recommended levels, which could potentially cause adverse effects or interfere with certain medications. It is important to adhere to recommended dosage guidelines.

International Standing: Wheat germ is recognized and consumed internationally as a nutritious food ingredient and dietary supplement. It is commonly available in health food stores, supermarkets, and online platforms.

Indian Standing: In India, wheat germ is also recognized for its nutritional value and health benefits. It is used in various culinary preparations and is available in health food stores and supermarkets in urban areas.

Research Summary: Research on wheat germ highlights its potential as a nutrient-dense food source and dietary supplement. Studies have demonstrated its beneficial effects on cardiovascular health, immune function, and overall well-being. Further research is needed to elucidate its mechanisms of action and optimize its therapeutic applications.

113) Zingiber officinale - rhizome standardized extracts

Introduction: Zingiber officinale, commonly known as Ginger, is a flowering plant whose rhizome is widely used as a spice and traditional medicine. Ginger

Introduction: Zingiber officinale, commonly known as Ginger, is a flowering plant whose rhizome is widely used as a spice and traditional medicine. Ginger has a long history of culinary and medicinal use, especially in Asian cultures, and is prized for its unique flavor and potential health benefits.

Synonym Name and Common Name: Synonym: None Common Name: Ginger

Pharmacognosy/Chemistry: Ginger contains various bioactive compounds including gingerol, shogaol, paradol, zingerone, and volatile oils such as zingiberene. These compounds contribute to its characteristic flavor and aroma, as well as its medicinal properties.

Action and Pharmacology: Ginger exhibits several pharmacological actions including anti-inflammatory, antioxidant, antiemetic, analgesic, and digestive stimulant effects. These actions are attributed to its bioactive compounds, particularly gingerol, which exert various beneficial effects on the body.

Method of Analysis: Analytical methods such as high-performance liquid chromatography (HPLC), gas chromatography-mass spectrometry (GC-MS), and spectrophotometry are commonly used for the qualitative and quantitative analysis of bioactive compounds in ginger rhizome extracts.

Health Benefits: Ginger is associated with numerous health benefits including relieving nausea and vomiting, reducing inflammation and pain, improving digestion, boosting immune function, and supporting cardiovascular health.

Indication and Usage: It is used in various forms including fresh, dried, powdered, or as an extract in culinary dishes, teas, and supplements. Ginger is commonly used to alleviate symptoms of motion sickness, morning sickness during pregnancy, indigestion, and arthritis pain.

Usual Constituents with Percentages: Typical constituents of standardized ginger rhizome extracts include:

- Gingerols (up to 5-10%)
- Shogaols
- Paradols
- Zingerone
- Volatile oils (such as zingiberene)

Mechanism of Action: The health benefits of ginger are attributed to its bioactive compounds, particularly gingerol, which exert anti-inflammatory, antioxidant, and other pharmacological effects. Gingerol inhibits inflammatory pathways, scavenges free radicals, and modulates neurotransmitter activity to relieve symptoms such as nausea and pain.

Dosage: The dosage of standardized ginger rhizome extracts may vary depending on the formulation and intended use. Typical doses range from 250 mg to 1000 mg of extract per day, divided into multiple doses. It is best to follow the recommendations provided by healthcare professionals or product labels.

Contraindications: Individuals with gallstones, bleeding disorders, or who are on blood-thinning medications should use ginger with caution due to its potential anticoagulant effects. Ginger supplements are not recommended for pregnant women without consulting a healthcare provider.

Precautions: It is advisable to consult a healthcare practitioner before using ginger supplements, especially if you have any underlying health conditions or are taking medications. Ginger may interact with certain drugs, including anticoagulants, and should be used with caution.

Adverse Reactions: While ginger is generally well-tolerated, some individuals may experience mild gastrointestinal upset, heartburn, or allergic reactions, especially with high doses or prolonged use of ginger supplements.

Research Standing: Ginger has been extensively researched for its pharmacological properties and therapeutic applications. Numerous studies support its efficacy in alleviating nausea, reducing inflammation and pain, improving digestion, and supporting overall health and well-being.

Pharmacokinetics and Pharmacodynamics: The pharmacokinetics and pharmacodynamics of ginger have been studied to some extent, with research focusing on its absorption, distribution, metabolism, and excretion in humans. Ginger's bioavailability and physiological effects may vary depending on factors such as the form of consumption and individual characteristics.

Overdosage: Excessive consumption of ginger supplements may lead to gastrointestinal discomfort or allergic reactions in some individuals. It is important to adhere to recommended dosage guidelines and monitor for any adverse effects.

International Standing: Ginger is recognized and used internationally as a culinary spice and traditional medicine. Ginger supplements and extracts are widely available in health food stores, pharmacies, and online platforms worldwide.

Indian Standing: In India, ginger has a long history of use in Ayurvedic medicine and culinary traditions. It is commonly used in various dishes, teas, and remedies for its flavor and potential health benefits.

Research Summary: Research on ginger highlights its diverse pharmacological properties and therapeutic potential. Studies have demonstrated its efficacy in relieving nausea, reducing inflammation and pain, improving digestion, and supporting overall health. Further research is needed to fully elucidate its mechanisms of action and optimize its therapeutic applications.

Schedule IV
Prebiotics and Probiotic

Details on Prebiotic Compounds

1) POLYDEXTROSE

Introduction: Polydextrose is a soluble fiber compound commonly used as a food additive and dietary supplement. It is a synthetic polymer of glucose that is partially fermented in the colon, offering various health benefits.

Synonym Name and Common Name: Synonym Name: None Common Name: Polydextrose

Pharmacognosy/Chemistry: Polydextrose is a complex carbohydrate synthesized from dextrose (glucose) through condensation polymerization. It consists of randomly linked glucose units with various degrees of polymerization. Chemically, it is classified as a sugar alcohol and is soluble in water.

Action and Pharmacology: Polydextrose functions primarily as a soluble fiber in the digestive tract. It is not broken down by human digestive enzymes, so it passes through the small intestine intact and is partially fermented by gut bacteria in the colon. This fermentation produces short-chain fatty acids, which can provide energy to colonic cells and have beneficial effects on gut health.

Method of Analysis: Analysis of polydextrose typically involves methods such as high-performance liquid chromatography (HPLC) or gas chromatography (GC) to quantify its content in food products and dietary supplements. Other analytical techniques may be used to assess its purity, molecular weight distribution, and degree of polymerization.

Health Benefits: Polydextrose offers several health benefits, including improved digestive health, regulation of blood sugar levels, promotion of satiety and weight management, and support for healthy cholesterol levels. Additionally, it can help maintain regular bowel movements and may contribute to overall gut health.

Indication and Usage: Polydextrose is commonly used as a food additive to increase fiber content and improve the texture, mouthfeel, and shelf-life of various food products. It is also available as a dietary supplement for individuals looking to increase their fiber intake or support digestive health.

Usual Constituents with Percentages: Polydextrose is typically available as a powder or liquid and is composed entirely of polydextrose molecules. The percentage of polydextrose in a product can vary depending on the formulation and intended use, but it is often used in food products at concentrations ranging from 1% to 15%.

Mechanism of Action: The mechanism of action of polydextrose involves its role as a soluble fiber in the digestive tract. It passes through the small intestine without being digested and is fermented by gut bacteria in the colon, leading to the production of short-chain fatty acids and other metabolites that benefit gut health.

Dosage: The recommended dosage of polydextrose can vary depending on the individual's dietary needs and health goals. As a food additive, it is generally used in small amounts to achieve the desired texture and fiber content in food products. As a dietary supplement, typical doses range from 2 to 20 grams per day.

Contraindications: Polydextrose is generally considered safe for most people when consumed in appropriate amounts. However, individuals with certain digestive disorders or sensitivities to fiber may experience gastrointestinal discomfort or bloating when consuming large amounts of polydextrose.

Precautions: Consumption of polydextrose should be accompanied by adequate fluid intake to prevent dehydration and maintain bowel regularity. Individuals with pre-existing medical conditions or those taking medication should consult with a healthcare professional before using polydextrose supplements.

Adverse Reactions: While rare, some individuals may experience mild gastrointestinal side effects such as bloating, gas, or diarrhea when consuming polydextrose supplements, particularly at higher doses. These symptoms usually resolve on their own and can be minimized by gradually increasing intake.

Research Standing: Polydextrose has been extensively studied for its effects on digestive health, glycemic control, weight management, and cholesterol levels. Research indicates its potential to improve bowel regularity, promote satiety, and support overall gut health when consumed as part of a balanced diet.

Pharmacokinetics and Pharmacodynamics: Polydextrose is not absorbed in the small intestine and passes into the colon intact, where it is partially fermented by gut bacteria. The fermentation process produces short-chain fatty acids, which are absorbed and metabolized by colonic cells, providing energy and supporting gut health.

Overdosage: There is no established risk of overdosage with polydextrose, as it is not absorbed in the small intestine and excess amounts are excreted in the feces. However, consuming very large amounts of polydextrose may lead to gastrointestinal discomfort or diarrhea in some individuals.

International Standing: Polydextrose is approved for use as a food additive in many countries, including the United States, European Union, Canada, and Australia. It is recognized as safe by regulatory authorities such as the US Food and Drug Administration (FDA) and the European Food Safety Authority (EFSA).

Indian Standing: In India, polydextrose is also used as a food additive and dietary supplement, although regulatory approval and acceptance may vary. It is generally regarded as safe for consumption and is available in various food products and dietary supplements marketed for digestive health and weight management.

Research Summary: Research on polydextrose supports its role as a soluble fiber with various health benefits, including improved digestive health, blood sugar control, weight management, and cholesterol levels. While further studies are needed to fully elucidate its mechanisms of action and optimal dosage, existing research suggests its potential as a valuable dietary component for promoting overall well-being.

2) SOYA POLY-SACCHARIDES AND SOYA OLIGOSACCHARIDES

Introduction: Soya polysaccharides and soya oligosaccharides are carbohydrate compounds derived from soybeans, a legume known for its nutritional value and health benefits. These compounds offer various health-promoting properties and are often used as dietary supplements.

Synonym Name and Common Name: Synonym Name: Soy polysaccharides, soy oligosaccharides Common Name: Soya polysaccharides, soya oligosaccharides

Pharmacognosy/Chemistry: Soya polysaccharides are complex carbohydrates composed of long chains of monosaccharide units, while soya oligosaccharides consist of shorter chains of monosaccharides. They are derived from the cell walls of soybeans and contain various types of sugars, including glucose, galactose, and fructose.

Action and Pharmacology: Soya polysaccharides and oligosaccharides exert their effects primarily through their prebiotic properties. They serve as food for beneficial bacteria in the gut, promoting their growth and activity. Additionally, they may have anti-inflammatory and immunomodulatory effects, contributing to overall gut health and immune function.

Method of Analysis: Analysis of soya polysaccharides and oligosaccharides typically involves methods such as high-performance liquid chromatography (HPLC), gas chromatography (GC), or enzymatic assays to quantify their content in food products and dietary supplements. Structural characterization may also be performed using techniques such as mass spectrometry.

Health Benefits: Soya polysaccharides and oligosaccharides offer several health benefits, including improved digestive health, enhanced immune function, regulation of blood sugar levels, and maintenance of healthy cholesterol levels. They may also have anti-inflammatory and antioxidant properties.

Indication and Usage: Soya polysaccharides and oligosaccharides are commonly used as dietary supplements to support gut health, boost immune function, and promote overall well-being. They may be recommended for individuals with digestive issues, immune system deficiencies, or metabolic disorders.

Usual Constituents with Percentages: The usual constituents of soya polysaccharides and oligosaccharides can vary depending on the source and processing method. However, they typically contain a mixture of polysaccharides and oligosaccharides, with percentages varying based on the product formulation.

Mechanism of Action: The mechanism of action of soya polysaccharides and oligosaccharides involves their role as prebiotics. They selectively stimulate the growth and activity of beneficial bacteria in the gut, such as lactobacilli and bifidobacteria, while inhibiting the growth of harmful bacteria. This promotes a healthy gut microbiota and supports overall gut health and immune function.

Dosage: The recommended dosage of soya polysaccharides and oligosaccharides can vary depending on the specific product and intended use. Typical doses range from a few grams to several grams per day, taken orally as part of a balanced diet or as a dietary supplement.

Contraindications: Soya polysaccharides and oligosaccharides are generally considered safe for most people when consumed in appropriate amounts. However, individuals with soy allergies or sensitivities should avoid products containing these compounds.

Precautions: Individuals with underlying health conditions or those taking medications should consult a healthcare professional before using soya polysaccharides and oligosaccharides supplements. Careful monitoring may be necessary, especially in vulnerable populations.

Adverse Reactions: Adverse reactions to soya polysaccharides and oligosaccharides supplements are rare but may include gastrointestinal symptoms such as bloating, gas, or diarrhea, particularly with high intake. These symptoms usually resolve on their own and can be minimized by starting with lower doses and gradually increasing intake.

Research Standing: Soya polysaccharides and oligosaccharides have been the subject of numerous studies investigating their health benefits and mechanisms of action. Research indicates their potential to improve gut health, modulate immune function, and support metabolic health. However, more clinical trials are needed to fully elucidate their effects and optimal dosage.

Pharmacokinetics and Pharmacodynamics: The pharmacokinetics and pharmacodynamics of soya polysaccharides and oligosaccharides involve their selective fermentation by gut bacteria in the colon. They are not absorbed in the small intestine and reach the colon intact, where they serve as substrates for bacterial fermentation, producing short-chain fatty acids and other metabolites that benefit gut health and immune function.

Overdosage: While there is no established risk of overdosage with soya polysaccharides and oligosaccharides, excessive intake may lead to gastrointestinal discomfort or diarrhea, especially in individuals not accustomed to high-fiber diets. Adherence to recommended dosage guidelines is advisable.

International Standing: Soya polysaccharides and oligosaccharides are recognized internationally as safe and effective dietary supplements with potential health benefits. They are widely used in various food products and dietary supplements marketed for digestive health and overall well-being.

Indian Standing: In India, soya polysaccharides and oligosaccharides are also used in food products and dietary supplements, although regulatory approval and acceptance may vary. They are generally regarded as safe for consumption and are available in various forms for individuals seeking to improve their gut health and immune function.

Research Summary: Research on soya polysaccharides and oligosaccharides suggests their potential as prebiotics with various health benefits, including improved gut health, enhanced immune function, and regulation of metabolic parameters. While further clinical studies are needed to confirm their efficacy and optimal dosage, existing research supports their use as dietary supplements for promoting overall well-being

3) ISOMALTO-OLIGOSACCHARIDES

Introduction: Isomalto-oligosaccharides (IMO) are a type of carbohydrate commonly used as a food additive and dietary supplement. They are composed of short chains of glucose molecules linked together and have gained popularity due to their prebiotic properties and potential health benefits.

Synonym Name and Common Name: Synonym Name: Isomalto-oligosaccharides, IMO, Isomaltooligosaccharides Common Name: Isomalto-oligosaccharides

Pharmacognosy/Chemistry: Isomalto-oligosaccharides are derived from enzymatic hydrolysis of starch, resulting in a mixture of glucose oligomers with varying degrees of polymerization. They consist of α-(1→6) and α-(1→4) glycosidic bonds, giving them resistance to human digestive enzymes.

Action and Pharmacology: Isomalto-oligosaccharides act primarily as prebiotics in the gastrointestinal tract. They selectively stimulate the growth and activity of beneficial bacteria in the colon, such as bifidobacteria and lactobacilli, while inhibiting the growth of harmful bacteria. This promotes a healthy gut microbiota and supports digestive health and immune function.

Method of Analysis: Analysis of isomalto-oligosaccharides typically involves methods such as high-performance liquid chromatography (HPLC), gas chromatography (GC), or enzymatic assays to quantify their content in food products and dietary supplements. Structural characterization may also be performed using techniques such as mass spectrometry.

Health Benefits: Isomalto-oligosaccharides offer several health benefits, including improved digestive health, enhanced immune function, regulation of blood sugar levels, and maintenance of healthy cholesterol levels. They may also have potential anti-inflammatory and antioxidant properties.

Indication and Usage: Isomalto-oligosaccharides are commonly used as a food additive to increase fiber content, improve texture, and enhance sweetness in various food products. They are also available as dietary supplements for individuals seeking to support gut health, boost immune function, or regulate blood sugar levels.

Usual Constituents with Percentages: The usual constituents of isomalto-oligosaccharides consist of short chains of glucose molecules with varying degrees of polymerization. The percentage composition of specific oligomers can vary depending on the manufacturing process and product formulation.

Mechanism of Action: The mechanism of action of isomalto-oligosaccharides involves their role as prebiotics. They selectively stimulate the growth and activity of beneficial bacteria in the colon, leading to the production of short-chain fatty acids and other metabolites that support gut health and immune function.

Dosage: The recommended dosage of isomalto-oligosaccharides can vary depending on the specific product and intended use. Typical doses range from a few grams to several grams per day, taken orally as part of a balanced diet or as a dietary supplement.

Contraindications: Isomalto-oligosaccharides are generally considered safe for most people when consumed in appropriate amounts. However, individuals with sensitivities to fiber or prebiotics may experience gastrointestinal discomfort or bloating with high intake.

Precautions: Individuals with underlying health conditions or those taking medications should consult a healthcare professional before using isomalto-oligosaccharides supplements. Careful monitoring may be necessary, especially in vulnerable populations.

Adverse Reactions: Adverse reactions to isomalto-oligosaccharides supplements are rare but may include mild gastrointestinal symptoms such as bloating, gas, or diarrhea, particularly with high intake. These symptoms usually resolve on their own and can be minimized by starting with lower doses and gradually increasing intake.

Research Standing: Isomalto-oligosaccharides have been the subject of numerous studies investigating their health benefits and mechanisms of action. Research indicates their potential to improve gut health, modulate immune function, and support metabolic health. However, more clinical trials are needed to fully elucidate their effects and optimal dosage.

Pharmacokinetics and Pharmacodynamics: Isomalto-oligosaccharides are not absorbed in the small intestine and reach the colon intact, where they serve as substrates for bacterial fermentation. They are selectively metabolized by beneficial bacteria, leading to the production of short-chain fatty acids and other metabolites that contribute to various physiological effects.

Overdosage: While there is no established risk of overdosage with isomalto-oligosaccharides, excessive intake may lead to gastrointestinal discomfort or diarrhea, especially in individuals not accustomed to high-fiber diets. Adherence to recommended dosage guidelines is advisable.

International Standing: Isomalto-oligosaccharides are recognized internationally as safe and effective food additives and dietary supplements. They are widely used in various food products and dietary supplements marketed for digestive health and overall well-being.

Indian Standing: In India, isomalto-oligosaccharides are also used in food products and dietary supplements, although regulatory approval and acceptance may vary. They are generally regarded as safe for consumption and are available in various forms for individuals seeking to improve their gut health and immune function.

Research Summary: Research on isomalto-oligosaccharides suggests their potential as prebiotics with various health benefits, including improved gut health, enhanced immune function, and regulation of metabolic parameters. While further clinical studies are needed to confirm their efficacy and optimal dosage, existing research supports their use as dietary supplements for promoting overall well-being.

4) FRUCTO-OLIGOSACCHARIDES

Introduction: Fructo-oligosaccharides (FOS) are a type of carbohydrate composed of short chains of fructose molecules linked together. They occur naturally in various fruits, vegetables, and grains and are also produced commercially for use as dietary supplements and food additives.

Synonym Name and Common Name: Synonym Name: Fructo-oligosaccharides, FOS, Oligofructose Common Name: Fructo-oligosaccharides

Pharmacognosy/Chemistry: Fructo-oligosaccharides are composed of fructose units linked together by β-(2→1) glycosidic bonds. They are classified as soluble fibers and are resistant to digestion by human enzymes, reaching the colon intact where they serve as a substrate for fermentation by gut bacteria.

Action and Pharmacology: Fructo-oligosaccharides act primarily as prebiotics in the gastrointestinal tract. They selectively stimulate the growth and activity of beneficial bacteria in the colon, such as bifidobacteria and lactobacilli, while inhibiting the growth of harmful bacteria. This promotes a healthy gut microbiota and supports digestive health and immune function.

Method of Analysis: Analysis of fructo-oligosaccharides typically involves methods such as high-performance liquid chromatography (HPLC), gas chromatography (GC), or enzymatic assays to quantify their content in food products and dietary supplements. Structural characterization may also be performed using techniques such as mass spectrometry.

Health Benefits: Fructo-oligosaccharides offer several health benefits, including improved digestive health, enhanced immune function, regulation of blood sugar levels, and maintenance of healthy cholesterol levels. They may also have potential anti-inflammatory and antioxidant properties.

Indication and Usage: Fructo-oligosaccharides are commonly used as dietary supplements to support gut health, boost immune function, and promote overall well-being. They are also added to various food products as a prebiotic fiber to increase fiber content and improve nutritional value.

Usual Constituents with Percentages: The usual constituents of fructo-oligosaccharides consist of short chains of fructose molecules with varying degrees of polymerization. The percentage composition of specific oligomers can vary depending on the manufacturing process and product formulation.

Mechanism of Action: The mechanism of action of fructo-oligosaccharides involves their role as prebiotics. They selectively stimulate the growth and activity of beneficial bacteria in the colon, leading to the production of short-chain fatty acids and other metabolites that support gut health and immune function.

Dosage: The recommended dosage of fructo-oligosaccharides can vary depending on the specific product and intended use. Typical doses range from a few grams to several grams per day, taken orally as part of a balanced diet or as a dietary supplement.

Contraindications: Fructo-oligosaccharides are generally considered safe for most people when consumed in appropriate amounts. However, individuals with sensitivities to fiber or prebiotics may experience gastrointestinal discomfort or bloating with high intake.

Precautions: Individuals with underlying health conditions or those taking medications should consult a healthcare professional before using fructo-oligosaccharides supplements. Careful monitoring may be necessary, especially in vulnerable populations.

Adverse Reactions: Adverse reactions to fructo-oligosaccharides supplements are rare but may include mild gastrointestinal symptoms such as bloating, gas, or diarrhea, particularly with high intake. These symptoms usually resolve on their own and can be minimized by starting with lower doses and gradually increasing intake.

Research Standing: Fructo-oligosaccharides have been the subject of numerous studies investigating their health benefits and mechanisms of action. Research indicates their potential to improve gut health, modulate immune function, and support metabolic health. However, more clinical trials are needed to fully elucidate their effects and optimal dosage.

Pharmacokinetics and Pharmacodynamics: Fructo-oligosaccharides are not absorbed in the small intestine and reach the colon intact, where they serve as substrates for bacterial fermentation. They are selectively metabolized by beneficial bacteria, leading to the production of short-chain fatty acids and other metabolites that contribute to various physiological effects.

Overdosage: While there is no established risk of overdosage with fructo-oligosaccharides, excessive intake may lead to gastrointestinal discomfort or diarrhea, especially in individuals not accustomed to high-fiber diets. Adherence to recommended dosage guidelines is advisable.

International Standing: Fructo-oligosaccharides are recognized internationally as safe and effective food additives and dietary supplements. They are widely used in various food products and dietary supplements marketed for digestive health and overall well-being.

Indian Standing: In India, fructo-oligosaccharides are also used in food products and dietary supplements, although regulatory approval and acceptance may vary. They are generally regarded as safe for consumption and are available in various forms for individuals seeking to improve their gut health and immune function.

Research Summary: Research on fructo-oligosaccharides suggests their potential as prebiotics with various health benefits, including improved gut health, enhanced immune function, and regulation of metabolic parameters. While further clinical studies are needed to confirm their efficacy and optimal dosage, existing research supports their use as dietary supplements for promoting overall well-being.

5) GLUCO-OLIGOSACCHARIDES

Introduction: Gluco-oligosaccharides are a type of carbohydrate compound composed of short chains of glucose molecules linked together. They are widely used as food additives and dietary supplements due to their prebiotic properties and potential health benefits.

Synonym Name and Common Name: Synonym Name: Gluco-oligosaccharides, GOS Common Name: Gluco-oligosaccharides

Pharmacognosy/Chemistry: Gluco-oligosaccharides are oligosaccharides composed of glucose units linked together by α-(1→4) glycosidic bonds. They are soluble fibers and are resistant to digestion by human enzymes, reaching the colon intact where they serve as a substrate for fermentation by gut bacteria.

Action and Pharmacology: Gluco-oligosaccharides act primarily as prebiotics in the gastrointestinal tract. They selectively stimulate the growth and activity of beneficial bacteria in the colon, such as bifidobacteria and lactobacilli, while inhibiting the growth of harmful bacteria. This promotes a healthy gut microbiota and supports digestive health and immune function.

Method of Analysis: Analysis of gluco-oligosaccharides typically involves methods such as high-performance liquid chromatography (HPLC), gas chromatography (GC), or enzymatic assays to quantify their content in food products and dietary supplements. Structural characterization may also be performed using techniques such as mass spectrometry.

Health Benefits: Gluco-oligosaccharides offer several health benefits, including improved digestive health, enhanced immune function, regulation of blood sugar levels, and maintenance of healthy cholesterol levels. They may also have potential anti-inflammatory and antioxidant properties.

Indication and Usage: Gluco-oligosaccharides are commonly used as dietary supplements to support gut health, boost immune function, and promote overall well-being. They are also added to various food products as a prebiotic fiber to increase fiber content and improve nutritional value.

Usual Constituents with Percentages: The usual constituents of gluco-oligosaccharides consist of short chains of glucose molecules with varying degrees of polymerization. The percentage composition of specific oligomers can vary depending on the manufacturing process and product formulation.

Mechanism of Action: The mechanism of action of gluco-oligosaccharides involves their role as prebiotics. They selectively stimulate the growth and activity of beneficial bacteria in the colon, leading to the production of short-chain fatty acids and other metabolites that support gut health and immune function.

Dosage: The recommended dosage of gluco-oligosaccharides can vary depending on the specific product and intended use. Typical doses range from a few grams to several grams per day, taken orally as part of a balanced diet or as a dietary supplement.

Contraindications: Gluco-oligosaccharides are generally considered safe for most people when consumed in appropriate amounts. However, individuals with sensitivities to fiber or prebiotics may experience gastrointestinal discomfort or bloating with high intake.

Precautions: Individuals with underlying health conditions or those taking medications should consult a healthcare professional before using gluco-oligosaccharides supplements. Careful monitoring may be necessary, especially in vulnerable populations.

Adverse Reactions: Adverse reactions to gluco-oligosaccharides supplements are rare but may include mild gastrointestinal symptoms such as bloating, gas, or diarrhea, particularly with high intake. These symptoms usually resolve on their own and can be minimized by starting with lower doses and gradually increasing intake.

Research Standing: Gluco-oligosaccharides have been the subject of numerous studies investigating their health benefits and mechanisms of action. Research indicates their potential to improve gut health, modulate immune function, and support metabolic health. However, more clinical trials are needed to fully elucidate their effects and optimal dosage.

Pharmacokinetics and Pharmacodynamics: Gluco-oligosaccharides are not absorbed in the small intestine and reach the colon intact, where they serve as substrates for bacterial fermentation. They are selectively metabolized by beneficial bacteria, leading to the production of short-chain fatty acids and other metabolites that contribute to various physiological effects.

Overdosage: While there is no established risk of overdosage with gluco-oligosaccharides, excessive intake may lead to gastrointestinal discomfort or diarrhea, especially in individuals not accustomed to high-fiber diets. Adherence to recommended dosage guidelines is advisable.

International Standing: Gluco-oligosaccharides are recognized internationally as safe and effective food additives and dietary supplements. They are widely used in various food products and dietary supplements marketed for digestive health and overall well-being.

Indian Standing: In India, gluco-oligosaccharides are also used in food products and dietary supplements, although regulatory approval and acceptance may vary. They are generally regarded as safe for consumption and are available in various forms for individuals seeking to improve their gut health and immune function.

Research Summary: Research on gluco-oligosaccharides suggests their potential as prebiotics with various health benefits, including improved gut health, enhanced immune function, and regulation of metabolic parameters. While further clinical studies are needed to confirm their efficacy and optimal dosage, existing research supports their use as dietary supplements for promoting overall well-being.

6) XYLO-OLIGOSACCHARIDES

Introduction: Xylo-oligosaccharides (XOS) are a type of oligosaccharide composed of short chains of xylose molecules linked together. They are naturally found in certain plant materials and are also produced commercially for use as dietary supplements and food additives.

Synonym Name and Common Name: Synonym Name: Xylo-oligosaccharides, XOS Common Name: Xylo-oligosaccharides

Pharmacognosy/Chemistry: Xylo-oligosaccharides are oligosaccharides composed of xylose units linked together by β-(1→4) glycosidic bonds. They are classified as soluble fibers and are resistant to digestion by human enzymes, reaching the colon intact where they serve as a substrate for fermentation by gut bacteria.

Action and Pharmacology: Xylo-oligosaccharides act primarily as prebiotics in the gastrointestinal tract. They selectively stimulate the growth and activity of beneficial bacteria in the colon, such as bifidobacteria and lactobacilli, while inhibiting the growth of harmful bacteria. This promotes a healthy gut microbiota and supports digestive health and immune function.

Method of Analysis: Analysis of xylo-oligosaccharides typically involves methods such as high-performance liquid chromatography (HPLC), gas chromatography (GC), or enzymatic assays to quantify their content in food products and dietary supplements. Structural characterization may also be performed using techniques such as mass spectrometry.

Health Benefits: Xylo-oligosaccharides offer several health benefits, including improved digestive health, enhanced immune function, regulation of blood sugar levels, and maintenance of healthy cholesterol levels. They may also have potential anti-inflammatory and antioxidant properties.

Indication and Usage: Xylo-oligosaccharides are commonly used as dietary supplements to support gut health, boost immune function, and promote overall well-being. They are also added to various food products as a prebiotic fiber to increase fiber content and improve nutritional value.

Usual Constituents with Percentages: The usual constituents of xylo-oligosaccharides consist of short chains of xylose molecules with varying degrees of polymerization. The percentage composition of specific oligomers can vary depending on the manufacturing process and product formulation.

Mechanism of Action: The mechanism of action of xylo-oligosaccharides involves their role as prebiotics. They selectively stimulate the growth and activity of beneficial bacteria in the colon, leading to the production of short-chain fatty acids and other metabolites that support gut health and immune function.

Dosage: The recommended dosage of xylo-oligosaccharides can vary depending on the specific product and intended use. Typical doses range from a few grams to several grams per day, taken orally as part of a balanced diet or as a dietary supplement.

Contraindications: Xylo-oligosaccharides are generally considered safe for most people when consumed in appropriate amounts. However, individuals with sensitivities to fiber or prebiotics may experience gastrointestinal discomfort or bloating with high intake.

Precautions: Individuals with underlying health conditions or those taking medications should consult a healthcare professional before using xylo-oligosaccharides supplements. Careful monitoring may be necessary, especially in vulnerable populations.

Adverse Reactions: Adverse reactions to xylo-oligosaccharides supplements are rare but may include mild gastrointestinal symptoms such as bloating, gas, or diarrhea, particularly with high intake. These symptoms usually resolve on their own and can be minimized by starting with lower doses and gradually increasing intake.

Research Standing: Xylo-oligosaccharides have been the subject of numerous studies investigating their health benefits and mechanisms of action. Research indicates their potential to improve gut health, modulate immune function, and support metabolic health. However, more clinical trials are needed to fully elucidate their effects and optimal dosage.

Pharmacokinetics and Pharmacodynamics: Xylo-oligosaccharides are not absorbed in the small intestine and reach the colon intact, where they serve as substrates for bacterial fermentation. They are selectively metabolized by beneficial bacteria, leading to the production of short-chain fatty acids and other metabolites that contribute to various physiological effects.

Overdosage: While there is no established risk of overdosage with xylo-oligosaccharides, excessive intake may lead to gastrointestinal discomfort or diarrhea, especially in individuals not accustomed to high-fiber diets. Adherence to recommended dosage guidelines is advisable.

International Standing: Xylo-oligosaccharides are recognized internationally as safe and effective food additives and dietary supplements. They are widely used in various food products and dietary supplements marketed for digestive health and overall well-being.

Indian Standing: In India, xylo-oligosaccharides are also used in food products and dietary supplements, although regulatory approval and acceptance may vary. They are generally regarded as safe for consumption and are available in various forms for individuals seeking to improve their gut health and immune function.

Research Summary: Research on xylo-oligosaccharides suggests their potential as prebiotics with various health benefits, including improved gut health, enhanced immune function, and regulation of metabolic parameters. While further clinical studies are needed to confirm their efficacy and optimal dosage, existing research supports their use as dietary supplements for promoting overall well-being.

7) XYLO-OLIGOSACCHARIDES

Introduction: Xylo-oligosaccharides (XOS) are a type of oligosaccharide composed of short chains of xylose molecules linked together. They are naturally found in certain plant materials and are also produced commercially for use as dietary supplements and food additives.

Synonym Name and Common Name: Synonym Name: Xylo-oligosaccharides, XOS Common Name: Xylo-oligosaccharides

Pharmacognosy/Chemistry: Xylo-oligosaccharides are oligosaccharides composed of xylose units linked together by β-(1→4) glycosidic bonds. They are classified as soluble fibers and are resistant to digestion by human enzymes, reaching the colon intact where they serve as a substrate for fermentation by gut bacteria.

Action and Pharmacology: Xylo-oligosaccharides act primarily as prebiotics in the gastrointestinal tract. They selectively stimulate the growth and activity of beneficial bacteria in the colon, such as bifidobacteria and lactobacilli, while inhibiting the growth of harmful bacteria. This promotes a healthy gut microbiota and supports digestive health and immune function.

Method of Analysis: Analysis of xylo-oligosaccharides typically involves methods such as high-performance liquid chromatography (HPLC), gas chromatography (GC), or enzymatic assays to quantify their content in food products and dietary supplements. Structural characterization may also be performed using techniques such as mass spectrometry.

Health Benefits: Xylo-oligosaccharides offer several health benefits, including improved digestive health, enhanced immune function, regulation of blood sugar levels, and maintenance of healthy cholesterol levels. They may also have potential anti-inflammatory and antioxidant properties.

Indication and Usage: Xylo-oligosaccharides are commonly used as dietary supplements to support gut health, boost immune function, and promote overall well-being. They are also added to various food products as a prebiotic fiber to increase fiber content and improve nutritional value.

Usual Constituents with Percentages: The usual constituents of xylo-oligosaccharides consist of short chains of xylose molecules with varying degrees of polymerization. The percentage composition of specific oligomers can vary depending on the manufacturing process and product formulation.

Mechanism of Action: The mechanism of action of xylo-oligosaccharides involves their role as prebiotics. They selectively stimulate the growth and activity of beneficial bacteria in the colon, leading to the production of short-chain fatty acids and other metabolites that support gut health and immune function.

Dosage: The recommended dosage of xylo-oligosaccharides can vary depending on the specific product and intended use. Typical doses range from a few grams to several grams per day, taken orally as part of a balanced diet or as a dietary supplement.

Contraindications: Xylo-oligosaccharides are generally considered safe for most people when consumed in appropriate amounts. However, individuals with sensitivities to fiber or prebiotics may experience gastrointestinal discomfort or bloating with high intake.

Precautions: Individuals with underlying health conditions or those taking medications should consult a healthcare professional before using xylo-oligosaccharides supplements. Careful monitoring may be necessary, especially in vulnerable populations.

Adverse Reactions: Adverse reactions to xylo-oligosaccharides supplements are rare but may include mild gastrointestinal symptoms such as bloating, gas, or diarrhea, particularly with high intake. These symptoms usually resolve on their own and can be minimized by starting with lower doses and gradually increasing intake.

Research Standing: Xylo-oligosaccharides have been the subject of numerous studies investigating their health benefits and mechanisms of action. Research indicates their potential to improve gut health, modulate immune function, and support metabolic health. However, more clinical trials are needed to fully elucidate their effects and optimal dosage.

Pharmacokinetics and Pharmacodynamics: Xylo-oligosaccharides are not absorbed in the small intestine and reach the colon intact, where they serve as substrates for bacterial fermentation. They are selectively metabolized by beneficial bacteria, leading to the production of short-chain fatty acids and other metabolites that contribute to various physiological effects.

Overdosage: While there is no established risk of overdosage with xylo-oligosaccharides, excessive intake may lead to gastrointestinal discomfort or diarrhea, especially in individuals not accustomed to high-fiber diets. Adherence to recommended dosage guidelines is advisable.

International Standing: Xylo-oligosaccharides are recognized internationally as safe and effective food additives and dietary supplements. They are widely used in various food products and dietary supplements marketed for digestive health and overall well-being.

Indian Standing: In India, xylo-oligosaccharides are also used in food products and dietary supplements, although regulatory approval and acceptance may vary. They are generally regarded as safe for consumption and are available in various forms for individuals seeking to improve their gut health and immune function.

Research Summary: Research on xylo-oligosaccharides suggests their potential as prebiotics with various health benefits, including improved gut health, enhanced immune function, and regulation of metabolic parameters. While further clinical studies are needed to confirm their efficacy and optimal dosage, existing research supports their use as dietary supplements for promoting overall well-being.

8) INULIN

Introduction: Inulin is a type of dietary fiber that belongs to the fructan group. It occurs naturally in various plants, such as chicory root, Jerusalem artichoke, and dandelion. Inulin is widely used in food products and dietary supplements due to its prebiotic properties and potential health benefits.

Synonym Name and Common Name: Synonym Name: Inulin, fructan Common Name: Inulin

Pharmacognosy/Chemistry: Inulin is a polysaccharide composed of fructose units linked together by β-(2→1) glycosidic bonds. It is a soluble fiber that is resistant to digestion by human enzymes, reaching the colon intact where it serves as a substrate for fermentation by gut bacteria.

Action and Pharmacology: Inulin acts primarily as a prebiotic in the gastrointestinal tract. It selectively stimulates the growth and activity of beneficial bacteria in the colon, such as bifidobacteria and lactobacilli, while inhibiting the growth of harmful bacteria. This promotes a healthy gut microbiota and supports digestive health and immune function.

Method of Analysis: Analysis of inulin typically involves methods such as high-performance liquid chromatography (HPLC), enzymatic assays, or spectrophotometry to quantify its content in food products and dietary supplements. Structural characterization may also be performed using techniques such as nuclear magnetic resonance (NMR) spectroscopy.

Health Benefits: Inulin offers several health benefits, including improved digestive health, enhanced immune function, regulation of blood sugar levels, and maintenance of healthy cholesterol levels. It may also help with weight management by promoting satiety and reducing calorie absorption.

Indication and Usage: Inulin is commonly used as a dietary supplement to support gut health, boost immune function, and promote overall well-being. It is also added to various food products as a prebiotic fiber to increase fiber content and improve nutritional value.

Usual Constituents with Percentages: The usual constituents of inulin consist of fructose units linked together in chains of varying lengths. The percentage composition of specific chain lengths can vary depending on the source and processing method used to extract the inulin.

Mechanism of Action: The mechanism of action of inulin involves its role as a prebiotic fiber. It selectively stimulates the growth and activity of beneficial bacteria in the colon, leading to the production of short-chain fatty acids and other metabolites that support gut health and immune function.

Dosage: The recommended dosage of inulin can vary depending on the specific product and intended use. Typical doses range from a few grams to several grams per day, taken orally as part of a balanced diet or as a dietary supplement.

Contraindications: Inulin is generally considered safe for most people when consumed in appropriate amounts. However, individuals with sensitivities to fiber or prebiotics may experience gastrointestinal discomfort or bloating with high intake.

Precautions: Individuals with underlying health conditions or those taking medications should consult a healthcare professional before using inulin supplements. Careful monitoring may be necessary, especially in vulnerable populations.

Adverse Reactions: Adverse reactions to inulin supplements are rare but may include mild gastrointestinal symptoms such as bloating, gas, or diarrhea, particularly with high intake. These symptoms usually resolve on their own and can be minimized by starting with lower doses and gradually increasing intake.

Research Standing: Inulin has been the subject of numerous studies investigating its health benefits and mechanisms of action. Research indicates its potential to improve gut health, modulate immune function, and support metabolic health. However, more clinical trials are needed to fully elucidate its effects and optimal dosage.

Pharmacokinetics and Pharmacodynamics: Inulin is not absorbed in the small intestine and reaches the colon intact, where it serves as a substrate for bacterial fermentation. It is selectively metabolized by beneficial bacteria, leading to the production of short-chain fatty acids and other metabolites that contribute to various physiological effects.

Overdosage: While there is no established risk of overdosage with inulin, excessive intake may lead to gastrointestinal discomfort or diarrhea, especially in individuals not accustomed to high-fiber diets. Adherence to recommended dosage guidelines is advisable.

International Standing: Inulin is recognized internationally as safe and effective food additives and dietary supplements. It is widely used in various food products and dietary supplements marketed for digestive health and overall well-being.

Indian Standing: In India, inulin is also used in food products and dietary supplements, although regulatory approval and acceptance may vary. It is generally regarded as safe for consumption and is available in various forms for individuals seeking to improve their gut health and immune function.

Research Summary: Research on inulin suggests its potential as a prebiotic with various health benefits, including improved gut health, enhanced immune function, and regulation of metabolic parameters. While further clinical studies are needed to confirm its efficacy and optimal dosage, existing research supports its use as a dietary supplement for promoting overall well-being.

9) ISOMALTULOSE

Introduction: Isomaltulose, also known as palatinose, is a disaccharide carbohydrate composed of glucose and fructose. It is a naturally occurring sugar found in honey and sugar cane extract. Isomaltulose is known for its slow-release energy properties, making it a popular alternative sweetener in various food and beverage products.

Synonym Name and Common Name: Synonym Name: Palatinose Common Name: Isomaltulose

Pharmacognosy/Chemistry: Isomaltulose is a disaccharide composed of glucose and fructose units linked together by an α-1,6-glycosidic bond. Chemically, it is classified as a reducing sugar and has a molecular formula of $C12H22O11$.

Action and Pharmacology: Isomaltulose is metabolized slowly in the body due to its unique glycosidic bond structure. This slow-release property results in a gradual increase in blood glucose levels, providing sustained energy without causing rapid spikes or crashes in blood sugar levels.

Method of Analysis: Analytical methods for quantifying isomaltulose typically involve chromatographic techniques such as high-performance liquid chromatography (HPLC) or gas chromatography (GC). These methods allow for the accurate determination of isomaltulose content in food and beverage products.

Health Benefits: Isomaltulose offers several potential health benefits, including sustained energy release, improved glycemic control, and reduced risk of dental caries. Its slow-release properties make it suitable for individuals seeking a more stable source of energy throughout the day.

Indication and Usage: Isomaltulose is commonly used as a low-glycemic sweetener in various food and beverage products, including sports drinks, energy bars, and meal replacement shakes. It can also be used as a sugar substitute for individuals looking to manage their blood sugar levels.

Usual Constituents with Percentages: Isomaltulose is typically used in its pure form as a food ingredient or sweetener. It is composed entirely of glucose and fructose, with each molecule containing one molecule of each sugar unit.

Mechanism of Action: The slow-release mechanism of isomaltulose is attributed to its unique α-1,6-glycosidic bond structure, which slows down the enzymatic hydrolysis of the disaccharide in the small intestine. This results in a gradual release of glucose and fructose into the bloodstream, providing sustained energy over time.

Dosage: The dosage of isomaltulose varies depending on the specific product and intended use. As a sweetener, it is typically used in concentrations similar to sucrose. As a dietary supplement for sustained energy, recommended doses may range from a few grams to several grams per serving.

Contraindications: Isomaltulose is generally regarded as safe for consumption and does not have any specific contraindications. However, individuals with known allergies or sensitivities to carbohydrates should exercise caution when consuming products containing isomaltulose.

Precautions: Although rare, some individuals may experience gastrointestinal discomfort, bloating, or diarrhea when consuming large amounts of isomaltulose. It is recommended to start with small doses and gradually increase intake to assess tolerance.

Adverse Reactions: Adverse reactions to isomaltulose are uncommon but may include gastrointestinal symptoms such as bloating, gas, or diarrhea in sensitive individuals. These symptoms are typically mild and transient.

Research Standing: Research on isomaltulose has demonstrated its potential as a low-glycemic sweetener and source of sustained energy. Clinical studies have shown that isomaltulose consumption leads to a slower increase in blood glucose levels compared to sucrose, making it beneficial for individuals with diabetes or those seeking to manage their blood sugar levels.

Pharmacokinetics and Pharmacodynamics: Isomaltulose is absorbed slowly in the small intestine and undergoes gradual enzymatic hydrolysis to release glucose and fructose into the bloodstream. This slow-release property results in a sustained increase in blood glucose levels and provides prolonged energy without causing rapid spikes or crashes.

Overdosage: There is no established risk of overdosage with isomaltulose when consumed in typical dietary amounts. However, excessive intake may lead to gastrointestinal discomfort or other mild adverse effects.

International Standing: Isomaltulose is approved for use as a food ingredient and sweetener in many countries worldwide, including the United States, European Union, Japan, and Australia. It is considered safe for human consumption and has a generally recognized as safe (GRAS) status.

Indian Standing: In India, isomaltulose is also approved for use as a food ingredient and sweetener. It is commonly used in various food and beverage products marketed to health-conscious consumers and individuals with diabetes or other metabolic conditions.

Research Summary: Research on isomaltulose supports its role as a low-glycemic sweetener and source of sustained energy. Clinical studies have shown that isomaltulose consumption leads to a slower increase in blood glucose levels compared to sucrose, making it beneficial for individuals seeking to manage their blood sugar levels or maintain energy levels throughout the day. Overall, isomaltulose is considered a safe and effective alternative sweetener with potential health benefits.

10) GENTIO-OLOGSACCHARIDES

Introduction: Gentio-oligosaccharides (GOS) are a type of prebiotic carbohydrate that consist of short chains of galactose molecules linked by β-glycosidic bonds. They are naturally found in certain plants and are also produced commercially for use in food products and dietary supplements.

Synonym Name and Common Name: Synonym Name: GOS Common Name: Gentio-oligosaccharides

Pharmacognosy/Chemistry: Gentio-oligosaccharides are oligosaccharides composed of galactose molecules linked together by β-glycosidic bonds. They are classified as non-digestible carbohydrates due to their resistance to enzymatic hydrolysis in the human digestive tract.

Action and Pharmacology: Gentio-oligosaccharides act as prebiotics, selectively promoting the growth and activity of beneficial bacteria in the gut, such as bifidobacteria and lactobacilli. They serve as a substrate for fermentation by these bacteria, leading to the production of short-chain fatty acids and other metabolites that support gut health and immune function.

Method of Analysis: Analysis of gentio-oligosaccharides typically involves chromatographic techniques such as high-performance liquid chromatography (HPLC) or gas chromatography (GC). These methods allow for the quantification and characterization of GOS in food products and dietary supplements.

Health Benefits: Gentio-oligosaccharides offer several health benefits, including improved digestive health, enhanced immune function, and modulation of gut microbiota composition. They may also help alleviate symptoms of gastrointestinal disorders such as irritable bowel syndrome (IBS) and reduce the risk of colorectal cancer.

Indication and Usage: Gentio-oligosaccharides are commonly used as dietary supplements to support gut health and overall well-being. They are also added to various food products, including infant formula, dairy products, and functional foods, to enhance their prebiotic content.

Usual Constituents with Percentages: The usual constituents of gentio-oligosaccharides consist primarily of short chains of galactose molecules, typically containing 2 to 6 galactose units. The exact composition and percentage of GOS can vary depending on the source and processing method used.

Mechanism of Action: The mechanism of action of gentio-oligosaccharides involves their fermentation by beneficial bacteria in the colon. This fermentation process produces short-chain fatty acids such as acetate, propionate, and butyrate, which provide energy for colonocytes and help maintain intestinal barrier function.

Dosage: The recommended dosage of gentio-oligosaccharides varies depending on the specific product and intended use. Typical doses range from a few grams to several grams per day, taken orally as part of a balanced diet or as a dietary supplement.

Contraindications: Gentio-oligosaccharides are generally considered safe for most people when consumed in appropriate amounts. However, individuals with underlying health conditions or those taking medications should consult a healthcare professional before using GOS supplements.

Precautions: Individuals with known allergies or sensitivities to galactose or other carbohydrates should exercise caution when consuming products containing gentio-oligosaccharides. It is advisable to start with small doses and gradually increase intake to assess tolerance.

Adverse Reactions: Adverse reactions to gentio-oligosaccharides are rare but may include gastrointestinal symptoms such as bloating, gas, or diarrhea, especially with high intake. These symptoms are usually mild and transient and can be minimized by starting with lower doses.

Research Standing: Research on gentio-oligosaccharides has demonstrated their potential as prebiotics with various health benefits. Clinical studies have shown that GOS supplementation can improve gut health, modulate immune function, and alleviate symptoms of gastrointestinal disorders. However, more research is needed to fully elucidate their effects and optimal dosage.

Pharmacokinetics and Pharmacodynamics: Gentio-oligosaccharides are not digested in the small intestine and reach the colon intact, where they are fermented by gut bacteria. The fermentation process produces short-chain fatty acids and other metabolites that exert beneficial effects on gut health and immune function.

Overdosage: While there is no established risk of overdosage with gentio-oligosaccharides, excessive intake may lead to gastrointestinal discomfort or diarrhea, especially in individuals not accustomed to high-fiber diets. Adherence to recommended dosage guidelines is advisable.

International Standing: Gentio-oligosaccharides are recognized internationally as safe and effective prebiotics with potential health benefits. They are widely used in various food products and dietary supplements marketed for digestive health and overall well-being.

Indian Standing: In India, gentio-oligosaccharides are also used in food products and dietary supplements, although regulatory approval and acceptance may vary. They are generally regarded as safe for consumption and are available in various forms for individuals seeking to improve their gut health and immune function.

Research Summary: Research on gentio-oligosaccharides supports their role as prebiotics with various health benefits, including improved gut health, enhanced immune function, and modulation of gut microbiota composition. While further clinical studies are needed to fully elucidate their effects and optimal dosage, existing research suggests that GOS supplementation can be beneficial for overall well-being.

11) LACTULOSE

Introduction: Lactulose is a synthetic disaccharide sugar composed of galactose and fructose molecules. It is widely used as a laxative and prebiotic agent due to its ability to increase the water content and volume of stool, facilitating bowel movements and promoting the growth of beneficial gut bacteria.

Synonym Name and Common Name: Synonym Name: 4-O-β-D-Galactopyranosyl-D-fructose Common Name: Lactulose

Pharmacognosy/Chemistry: Lactulose is a non-absorbable sugar that remains intact in the gastrointestinal tract. It is a synthetic derivative of lactose, consisting of a β-galactose molecule linked to a fructose molecule through a β-glycosidic bond.

Action and Pharmacology: Lactulose acts primarily as an osmotic laxative by drawing water into the colon, which softens stools and increases bowel movements. Additionally, it serves as a prebiotic, promoting the growth of beneficial gut bacteria such as bifidobacteria, which ferment lactulose into short-chain fatty acids.

Method of Analysis: Analytical methods for lactulose typically involve chromatographic techniques such as high-performance liquid chromatography (HPLC) or gas chromatography (GC). These methods allow for the accurate quantification of lactulose in pharmaceutical formulations and biological samples.

Health Benefits: Lactulose offers several health benefits, including the relief of constipation by softening stools and promoting regular bowel movements. Additionally, it may help improve gut health by supporting the growth of beneficial bacteria and facilitating the absorption of essential nutrients.

Indication and Usage: Lactulose is indicated for the treatment of constipation and hepatic encephalopathy. It is commonly used orally as a syrup or solution for constipation relief and is also administered rectally as an enema for hepatic encephalopathy.

Usual Constituents with Percentages: Lactulose is typically used as a pure compound in pharmaceutical formulations and laxative products. It is composed entirely of galactose and fructose molecules, with specific percentages depending on the formulation.

Mechanism of Action: The osmotic action of lactulose draws water into the colon, softening stools and increasing stool volume. This stimulates bowel movements and helps alleviate constipation. Additionally, lactulose fermentation by gut bacteria produces short-chain fatty acids, which promote gut health.

Dosage: The dosage of lactulose varies depending on the indication and individual response. For constipation, typical oral doses range from 15 to 30 mL daily, while doses for hepatic encephalopathy may be higher. Dosage adjustments may be necessary based on patient tolerance and response.

Contraindications: Lactulose is contraindicated in patients with galactosemia, a rare genetic disorder characterized by the inability to metabolize galactose. It should also be used with caution in patients with diabetes mellitus due to its sugar content.

Precautions: Patients using lactulose should ensure an adequate fluid intake to prevent dehydration. It may take several days for the full laxative effect to occur, so patients should be advised to continue treatment as directed by their healthcare provider.

Adverse Reactions: Common adverse reactions to lactulose include abdominal cramps, flatulence, and diarrhea, especially with high doses. These symptoms are usually mild and transient but may require dosage adjustments or discontinuation of treatment in some cases.

Research Standing: Lactulose has been extensively studied for its efficacy and safety in the treatment of constipation and hepatic encephalopathy. Clinical trials have demonstrated its effectiveness in relieving constipation and reducing ammonia levels in patients with hepatic encephalopathy.

Pharmacokinetics and Pharmacodynamics: Lactulose is minimally absorbed in the small intestine and reaches the colon intact, where it exerts its osmotic and prebiotic effects. It is fermented by gut bacteria into short-chain fatty acids, which contribute to its laxative and gut health-promoting properties.

Overdosage: Overdosage of lactulose may lead to severe diarrhea, electrolyte imbalances, and dehydration. In case of overdose, supportive measures such as fluid replacement and electrolyte monitoring should be instituted.

International Standing: Lactulose is approved for medical use in many countries worldwide and is available in various formulations, including oral syrups and rectal enemas. It is considered an essential medication by the World

Health Organization (WHO) for its role in treating constipation and hepatic encephalopathy.

Indian Standing: In India, lactulose is widely available as a prescription and over-the-counter medication for the treatment of constipation and hepatic encephalopathy. It is regulated by the Drugs Controller General of India (DCGI) and is commonly prescribed by healthcare professionals.

Research Summary: Research on lactulose supports its efficacy and safety in the treatment of constipation and hepatic encephalopathy. Clinical studies have demonstrated its ability to relieve constipation, soften stools, and improve bowel function. Additionally, lactulose has been shown to reduce ammonia levels and improve mental status in patients with hepatic encephalopathy. Overall, lactulose is considered a valuable medication for managing gastrointestinal disorders and promoting gut health.

12) LACTOFERRIN

Introduction: Lactoferrin is a glycoprotein found in milk and other bodily fluids, such as saliva, tears, and nasal secretions. It plays a crucial role in the innate immune response and has various health-promoting properties.

Synonym Name and Common Name: Synonym Name: Lactotransferrin Common Name: Lactoferrin

Pharmacognosy/Chemistry: Lactoferrin is a multifunctional protein belonging to the transferrin family. It is characterized by its high affinity for iron and its ability to bind to cell surface receptors. Structurally, lactoferrin consists of a single polypeptide chain folded into two globular lobes, each containing an iron-binding site.

Action and Pharmacology: Lactoferrin exhibits multiple biological activities, including antimicrobial, anti-inflammatory, antioxidant, and immunomodulatory effects. It helps regulate iron homeostasis, sequesters iron to inhibit microbial growth, modulates immune responses, and promotes tissue repair and wound healing.

Method of Analysis: Analytical methods for lactoferrin often involve immunoassays such as enzyme-linked immunosorbent assay (ELISA) or western blotting. These techniques allow for the detection and quantification of lactoferrin in various biological samples and food products.

Health Benefits: Lactoferrin offers a range of health benefits, including immune support, gastrointestinal health promotion, anti-inflammatory effects, antioxidant activity, and wound healing properties. It may also have potential applications in the prevention and treatment of infections, cancer, and inflammatory disorders.

Indication and Usage: Lactoferrin is used as a dietary supplement and functional ingredient in various food products, infant formulas, and pharmaceutical preparations. It is also investigated for its therapeutic potential in conditions such as infections, inflammatory diseases, and cancer.

Usual Constituents with Percentages: Lactoferrin is typically present in milk and colostrum at concentrations ranging from 1 to 5 grams per liter. The exact percentage of lactoferrin in milk can vary depending on factors such as species, lactation stage, and individual variation.

Mechanism of Action: The mechanism of action of lactoferrin involves its ability to bind and sequester iron, which is essential for microbial growth and virulence. By limiting the availability of iron, lactoferrin inhibits the growth and proliferation of bacteria, fungi, and viruses. Additionally, lactoferrin interacts with cell surface receptors to modulate immune responses and promote tissue repair and regeneration.

Dosage: The dosage of lactoferrin supplements varies depending on the specific product and intended use. Typical doses range from 100 to 1,000 milligrams per day, taken orally with meals. Dosage recommendations may vary based on individual factors such as age, health status, and the reason for supplementation.

Contraindications: Lactoferrin is generally considered safe for most people when consumed in recommended amounts. However, individuals with lactoferrin allergies or hypersensitivity should avoid lactoferrin supplements. Additionally, caution is advised in individuals with iron overload disorders or hemochromatosis, as lactoferrin may exacerbate iron accumulation.

Precautions: Individuals with underlying health conditions or those taking medications should consult a healthcare professional before using lactoferrin supplements. Pregnant and breastfeeding women should also exercise caution and seek medical advice before supplementation.

Adverse Reactions: Adverse reactions to lactoferrin supplements are rare but may include gastrointestinal symptoms such as nausea, abdominal discomfort, or diarrhea, especially with high doses. Allergic reactions to lactoferrin are possible but uncommon.

Research Standing: Lactoferrin has been extensively studied for its health-promoting properties and therapeutic potential. Clinical research has investigated its efficacy in various conditions, including infections, inflammatory diseases, gastrointestinal disorders, and cancer. While some studies have shown promising results, further research is needed to elucidate the optimal dosage, safety profile, and long-term effects of lactoferrin supplementation.

Pharmacokinetics and Pharmacodynamics: Lactoferrin is well-absorbed in the gastrointestinal tract, with peak plasma concentrations reached within a few hours after oral administration. It undergoes rapid distribution to various tissues and organs, where it exerts its biological effects. Lactoferrin is metabolized in the liver and excreted primarily in the urine and feces.

Overdosage: There is limited information available on the potential effects of lactoferrin overdose. However, excessive intake of lactoferrin supplements may lead to gastrointestinal symptoms or allergic reactions. Adherence to recommended dosage guidelines is advisable to minimize the risk of adverse effects.

International Standing: Lactoferrin is widely recognized internationally for its health benefits and therapeutic potential. It is approved for use as a dietary supplement and functional ingredient in various countries worldwide. Lactoferrin supplements are available over-the-counter and through healthcare providers in many regions.

Indian Standing: In India, lactoferrin supplements are also available and used for their health-promoting properties. They are regulated by the Food Safety and Standards Authority of India (FSSAI) and may be found in pharmacies, health food stores, and online retailers. Lactoferrin is included in various food products and dietary supplements marketed for immune support, gastrointestinal health, and overall well-being.

Research Summary: Research on lactoferrin continues to expand, with numerous studies investigating its mechanisms of action, therapeutic applications, and potential health benefits. While existing evidence supports the immune-modulating, antimicrobial, anti-inflammatory, and wound healing properties of lactoferrin, further research is warranted to elucidate its full therapeutic potential and clinical efficacy in various health conditions.

13) SUGAR ALCOHOLS SUCH AS LACTITOL, SORBITOL, MALTITOL, INOSITOL, ISOMALT

Introduction: Sugar alcohols are a group of low-calorie sweeteners derived from carbohydrates. They are often used as sugar substitutes in food and pharmaceutical products due to their reduced calorie content and minimal impact on blood sugar levels.

Synonym Name and Common Name: Synonym Names: Polyols, Polyhydric alcohols Common Names: Lactitol, Sorbitol, Maltitol, Inositol, Isomalt

Pharmacognosy/Chemistry: Sugar alcohols are polyhydric alcohols derived from the reduction of sugars. They have a similar chemical structure to both sugars and alcohols, containing multiple hydroxyl groups. Each sugar alcohol has its own specific chemical structure and properties.

Action and Pharmacology: Sugar alcohols are incompletely absorbed in the small intestine, leading to minimal increases in blood glucose levels and insulin secretion. They are partially fermented by gut bacteria in the colon, producing short-chain fatty acids and gases. This fermentation process can cause osmotic effects, leading to laxative effects in some individuals.

Method of Analysis: Analytical methods for sugar alcohols typically involve chromatographic techniques such as high-performance liquid chromatography (HPLC) or gas chromatography (GC). These methods allow for the accurate quantification of sugar alcohols in food products, pharmaceutical formulations, and biological samples.

Health Benefits: Sugar alcohols offer several health benefits, including their low glycemic index, reduced calorie content, and tooth-friendly properties. They can be used as sugar substitutes for individuals with diabetes or those following a low-calorie diet. Additionally, some sugar alcohols, such as sorbitol and xylitol, have been shown to have prebiotic effects and may promote gut health.

Indication and Usage: Sugar alcohols are used as sweeteners and bulking agents in a wide range of food and beverage products, including sugar-free candies, chewing gum, desserts, and beverages. They are also used in pharmaceutical formulations as excipients and in oral hygiene products such as toothpaste and mouthwash.

Usual Constituents with Percentages: The usual constituents and percentages of sugar alcohols vary depending on the specific product and formulation. In food products, sugar alcohols are typically added in concentrations ranging from 5% to 70%, depending on the desired sweetness level and texture.

Mechanism of Action: The mechanism of action of sugar alcohols involves their incomplete absorption in the small intestine and subsequent fermentation by gut bacteria in the colon. This fermentation process produces short-chain fatty acids, gases, and osmotic effects, which can lead to laxative effects and changes in gut microbiota composition.

Dosage: The dosage of sugar alcohols depends on the specific product and intended use. In food products and dietary supplements, sugar alcohols are typically used in amounts sufficient to achieve the desired sweetness level or texture. As sugar substitutes, they are generally considered safe when consumed in moderation.

Contraindications: Sugar alcohols may cause gastrointestinal discomfort, bloating, and diarrhea in some individuals, particularly when consumed in large amounts. Individuals with irritable bowel syndrome (IBS) or fructose intolerance may be more sensitive to the laxative effects of certain sugar alcohols and should limit their intake accordingly.

Precautions: Consumption of sugar alcohols should be moderated, especially for individuals prone to gastrointestinal symptoms or those following a low FODMAP (fermentable oligosaccharides, disaccharides, monosaccharides, and polyols) diet. Excessive intake of sugar alcohols may lead to gastrointestinal discomfort and laxative effects.

Adverse Reactions: Adverse reactions to sugar alcohols may include gastrointestinal symptoms such as bloating, flatulence, abdominal pain, and diarrhea, especially when consumed in large amounts. Some individuals may be more sensitive to the laxative effects of certain sugar alcohols and may experience symptoms even at lower doses.

Research Standing: Sugar alcohols have been extensively studied for their safety, efficacy, and physiological effects. Clinical research has investigated their impact on blood sugar levels, dental health, gastrointestinal tolerance, and overall health outcomes. While sugar alcohols are generally recognized as safe (GRAS) by regulatory authorities, further research is ongoing to explore their potential health benefits and limitations.

Pharmacokinetics and Pharmacodynamics: Sugar alcohols are incompletely absorbed in the small intestine and undergo fermentation by gut bacteria in the colon. They have minimal effects on blood glucose levels and insulin secretion, making them suitable for individuals with diabetes or those seeking to reduce their sugar intake. The pharmacokinetics of sugar alcohols vary depending on factors such as molecular weight, solubility, and absorption rate.

Overdosage: Overconsumption of sugar alcohols may lead to gastrointestinal symptoms such as bloating, cramping, and diarrhea, particularly in sensitive individuals. Moderation is key to avoiding adverse effects, and individuals should be mindful of their sugar alcohol intake, especially when consuming products labeled as “sugar-free” or “low-calorie.”

14) GALACTO-OLIGOSACCHARIDES

Introduction: Galacto-oligosaccharides (GOS) are prebiotic carbohydrates composed of galactose molecules linked together. They are naturally found in various plant-based foods and dairy products and are also produced commercially for use as dietary supplements and functional ingredients.

Synonym Name and Common Name: Synonym Name: Galactooligosaccharides Common Name: GOS

Pharmacognosy/Chemistry: Galacto-oligosaccharides are oligosaccharides composed of short chains of galactose molecules linked by β-glycosidic bonds. They are typically derived from lactose through enzymatic hydrolysis or transgalactosylation reactions.

Action and Pharmacology: Galacto-oligosaccharides serve as prebiotics, selectively stimulating the growth and activity of beneficial bacteria in the colon, such as Bifidobacteria and Lactobacilli. They are fermented by gut microbiota, producing short-chain fatty acids (SCFAs) and promoting a healthy gut microbiome balance. GOS also have osmotic properties, which can help regulate bowel movements and improve stool consistency.

Method of Analysis: Analytical methods for galacto-oligosaccharides typically involve chromatographic techniques such as high-performance liquid chromatography (HPLC) or gas chromatography (GC). These methods allow for the accurate quantification and characterization of GOS in food products, dietary supplements, and biological samples.

Health Benefits: Galacto-oligosaccharides offer several health benefits, including promoting digestive health by selectively stimulating the growth of beneficial gut bacteria, improving gut barrier function, enhancing mineral absorption, and modulating immune function. They may also have potential protective effects against intestinal infections and inflammation.

Indication and Usage: Galacto-oligosaccharides are used as dietary supplements and functional ingredients in various food products, including infant formulas, dairy products, cereals, baked goods, and nutritional supplements. They are also used in pharmaceutical formulations and oral hygiene products.

Usual Constituents with Percentages: The usual constituents and percentages of galacto-oligosaccharides in food products and supplements vary depending on the specific product and formulation. GOS are typically added in concentrations ranging from 1% to 10%, depending on the desired prebiotic effect and application.

Mechanism of Action: Galacto-oligosaccharides exert their effects primarily through their prebiotic activity in the gut. They are selectively fermented by beneficial gut bacteria, leading to the production of SCFAs, which help maintain intestinal health and modulate immune function. GOS also have osmotic properties, which can help regulate bowel movements and improve stool consistency.

Dosage: The dosage of galacto-oligosaccharides depends on the specific product and intended use. Typical doses range from 2 to 10 grams per day for adults and may vary for children and infants. Dosage recommendations may also vary based on factors such as age, health status, and dietary needs.

Contraindications: Galacto-oligosaccharides are generally considered safe for most individuals when consumed in recommended amounts. However, individuals with lactose intolerance or sensitivity to GOS may experience gastrointestinal symptoms such as bloating, gas, and diarrhea. In such cases, intake should be limited or avoided.

Precautions: Individuals with underlying gastrointestinal disorders or conditions such as irritable bowel syndrome (IBS) should exercise caution when consuming galacto-oligosaccharides and may benefit from starting with lower doses to assess tolerance. Pregnant and breastfeeding women should consult healthcare professionals before using GOS supplements.

Adverse Reactions: Adverse reactions to galacto-oligosaccharides may include gastrointestinal symptoms such as bloating, gas, abdominal discomfort, and diarrhea, particularly in individuals with lactose intolerance or sensitivity to GOS. These symptoms are usually mild and transient and may resolve with continued use or dosage adjustment.

Research Standing: Galacto-oligosaccharides have been extensively studied for their health-promoting effects and safety profile. Clinical research has investigated their impact on gut health, immune function, and overall well-being. While most studies have reported beneficial effects, further research is ongoing to explore their mechanisms of action, optimal dosage, and long-term health outcomes.

Pharmacokinetics and Pharmacodynamics: Galacto-oligosaccharides are not absorbed intact in the small intestine but reach the colon where they are fermented by gut bacteria. This fermentation process produces SCFAs and gases, contributing to their prebiotic effects and osmotic properties. The pharmacokinetics of GOS vary depending on factors such as molecular weight, structure, and dosage form.

Overdosage: Overconsumption of galacto-oligosaccharides may lead to gastrointestinal symptoms such as bloating, gas, and diarrhea, especially in sensitive individuals. Adherence to recommended dosage guidelines is important to minimize the risk of adverse effects.

15) PARTIALLY HYDROLYZED GUAR GUM

Introduction: Partially Hydrolyzed Guar Gum (PHGG) is a dietary fiber derived from the guar plant's endosperm. It is a water-soluble fiber that has been enzymatically processed to reduce its viscosity and improve its solubility, making it easier to incorporate into food and beverages.

Synonym Name and Common Name: Synonym Name: Hydrolyzed guar gum, Galactomannan Common Name: PHGG

Pharmacognosy/Chemistry: Partially Hydrolyzed Guar Gum is derived from the endosperm of the guar plant (Cyamopsis tetragonoloba). It consists of galactomannan, a polysaccharide composed of galactose and mannose units linked by β-glycosidic bonds. The hydrolysis process breaks down the long chains of guar gum into shorter oligosaccharides, resulting in improved solubility and digestibility.

Action and Pharmacology: Partially Hydrolyzed Guar Gum acts as a soluble dietary fiber in the gastrointestinal tract. It forms a viscous gel in the stomach and intestines, which helps slow down digestion and absorption of nutrients. PHGG is fermented by gut bacteria in the colon, producing short-chain fatty acids (SCFAs) and promoting a healthy gut microbiota balance. It also helps increase fecal bulk and improve bowel regularity.

Method of Analysis: Analytical methods for Partially Hydrolyzed Guar Gum typically involve techniques such as high-performance liquid chromatography (HPLC) or enzymatic assays to quantify the oligosaccharide content. These methods allow for the accurate determination of PHGG concentration in food products, dietary supplements, and biological samples.

Health Benefits: Partially Hydrolyzed Guar Gum offers several health benefits, including promoting digestive health, supporting weight management, and improving glycemic control. It helps regulate bowel movements, alleviate constipation, and reduce symptoms of irritable bowel syndrome (IBS). PHGG also contributes to satiety, which may aid in appetite control and weight loss.

Indication and Usage: Partially Hydrolyzed Guar Gum is used as a dietary supplement and functional ingredient in various food products, including beverages, dairy products, baked goods, and dietary fiber supplements. It is also used in medical nutrition products and pharmaceutical formulations to support digestive health and manage gastrointestinal disorders.

Usual Constituents with Percentages: Partially Hydrolyzed Guar Gum typically contains oligosaccharides derived from guar gum, with varying degrees of hydrolysis. The percentage of oligosaccharides in PHGG products may range from 85% to 95%, depending on the processing method and product specifications.

Mechanism of Action: Partially Hydrolyzed Guar Gum forms a viscous gel in the gastrointestinal tract, which slows down the digestion and absorption of nutrients, including carbohydrates and fats. This delayed gastric emptying helps regulate blood sugar levels and promotes satiety, making it beneficial for weight management and glycemic control. In the colon, PHGG is fermented by gut bacteria, leading to the production of SCFAs and promoting gut health.

Dosage: The dosage of Partially Hydrolyzed Guar Gum depends on the specific product and intended use. Typical doses range from 5 to 15 grams per day for adults, divided into multiple doses with adequate fluid intake. Dosage recommendations may vary based on individual health status, dietary needs, and treatment goals.

Contraindications: Partially Hydrolyzed Guar Gum is generally well-tolerated, but individuals with gastrointestinal disorders such as intestinal obstruction, esophageal stenosis, or severe motility disorders should avoid its use. Individuals with allergies to guar gum or galactomannans should also exercise caution when using PHGG supplements.

Precautions: Individuals with a history of allergic reactions to guar gum or other legume-derived products should consult healthcare professionals before using Partially Hydrolyzed Guar Gum supplements. Adequate fluid intake is important when consuming PHGG to prevent potential gastrointestinal discomfort and ensure optimal fiber benefits.

Adverse Reactions: Adverse reactions to Partially Hydrolyzed Guar Gum may include gastrointestinal symptoms such as bloating, gas, abdominal discomfort, and diarrhea, especially when consumed in high doses or by individuals with sensitive digestive systems. These symptoms are usually mild and transient and may improve with continued use or dosage adjustment.

Research Standing: Partially Hydrolyzed Guar Gum has been extensively studied for its health benefits and safety profile. Clinical research has demonstrated its efficacy in improving digestive health, supporting weight management, and managing gastrointestinal disorders such as constipation and IBS. PHGG is generally recognized as safe (GRAS) by regulatory authorities and has a strong scientific basis supporting its use as a dietary fiber supplement.

Pharmacokinetics and Pharmacodynamics: Partially Hydrolyzed Guar Gum is partially digested and absorbed in the small intestine, with the remaining undigested fibers reaching the colon where they are fermented by gut bacteria. This fermentation process produces SCFAs, which contribute to the health-promoting effects of PHGG on gut microbiota and overall digestive health. The pharmacokinetics of PHGG depend on factors such as molecular weight, degree of hydrolysis, and individual variations in gastrointestinal transit time.

Overdosage: Overconsumption of Partially Hydrolyzed Guar Gum may lead to gastrointestinal symptoms such as bloating, gas, abdominal discomfort, and diarrhea, especially in individuals with sensitive digestive systems. Adherence to recommended dosage guidelines and gradual titration of intake can help minimize the risk of adverse effects.

16) PECTIN

Introduction: Pectin is a naturally occurring complex polysaccharide found in the cell walls of fruits, particularly in citrus fruits, apples, and berries. It is widely used as a gelling agent, thickener, and stabilizer in food and pharmaceutical industries due to its unique gel-forming properties.

Synonym Name and Common Name: Synonym Name: Fruit pectin Common Name: Pectin

Pharmacognosy/Chemistry: Pectin is a heteropolysaccharide composed mainly of α-(1-4)-linked D-galacturonic acid units. It may also contain variable amounts of other monosaccharides such as D-glucose, D-mannose, and L-rhamnose, depending on the plant source and extraction method.

Action and Pharmacology: Pectin acts as a soluble dietary fiber in the gastrointestinal tract. When consumed, it forms a gel-like substance in the presence of water, which helps to increase stool bulk and promote regular bowel movements. Pectin also binds to cholesterol and bile acids in the intestine, aiding in their excretion and potentially lowering cholesterol levels.

Method of Analysis: Analytical methods for pectin typically involve spectrophotometric techniques to quantify the galacturonic acid content, which is a marker for pectin concentration. Other methods include high-performance liquid chromatography (HPLC) and gel permeation chromatography (GPC) for molecular weight determination.

Health Benefits: Pectin offers several health benefits, including promoting digestive health, lowering cholesterol levels, and aiding in weight management. It helps regulate bowel movements, alleviates constipation, and may reduce the risk of colorectal cancer. Pectin's ability to bind to cholesterol may also have cardiovascular benefits.

Indication and Usage: Pectin is commonly used as a food additive in the manufacturing of jams, jellies, fruit preserves, and confectionery products to improve texture and stability. It is also used in pharmaceutical formulations as a binder in tablet production and as a demulcent in oral suspensions.

Usual Constituents with Percentages: The composition of pectin varies depending on the plant source and extraction method. Generally, pectin consists of approximately 65-85% galacturonic acid units, with the remaining content comprising neutral sugars such as glucose, mannose, and rhamnose.

Mechanism of Action: Pectin forms a gel-like structure in the gastrointestinal tract, which increases stool bulk and promotes regular bowel movements. It also binds to cholesterol and bile acids in the intestine, preventing their reabsorption and facilitating their excretion, which may contribute to cholesterol-lowering effects.

Dosage: The dosage of pectin depends on the specific product and intended use. In food products, pectin is typically used in concentrations ranging from 0.5% to 2% by weight. As a dietary supplement, recommended doses may vary, but typical ranges are 5-10 grams per day for adults.

Contraindications: Pectin is generally safe for consumption and is well-tolerated by most individuals. However, individuals with allergies to citrus fruits or other sources of pectin should avoid its use. Pectin may also interfere with the absorption of certain medications, so caution should be exercised when taken concurrently with other drugs.

Precautions: Individuals with gastrointestinal disorders such as gastroesophageal reflux disease (GERD) or peptic ulcers should use pectin-containing products with caution, as they may exacerbate symptoms. Adequate fluid intake is important when consuming pectin supplements to prevent potential gastrointestinal discomfort.

Adverse Reactions: Adverse reactions to pectin are rare but may include gastrointestinal symptoms such as bloating, gas, abdominal discomfort, and diarrhea, especially when consumed in large amounts. These symptoms are usually mild and transient and may resolve with discontinuation of pectin intake.

Research Standing: Pectin has been extensively studied for its health benefits and safety profile. Clinical research has demonstrated its efficacy in promoting digestive health, lowering cholesterol levels, and aiding in weight management. Pectin is generally recognized as safe (GRAS) by regulatory authorities and is widely used in food and pharmaceutical industries.

Pharmacokinetics and Pharmacodynamics: Pectin is not absorbed intact in the gastrointestinal tract but passes through the digestive system intact, contributing to its bulking and cholesterol-lowering effects. It binds to water and forms a gel, which slows down digestion and promotes satiety. Pectin's pharmacokinetics and pharmacodynamics may vary depending on factors such as molecular weight, dosage form, and individual gastrointestinal transit time.

Overdosage: Overconsumption of pectin may lead to gastrointestinal symptoms such as bloating, gas, abdominal discomfort, and diarrhea, especially in individuals with sensitive digestive systems. Adherence to recommended dosage guidelines is important to minimize the risk of adverse effects

17) RESISTANT DEXTRIN

Introduction: Resistant dextrin, also known as resistant maltodextrin or resistant starch, is a type of soluble fiber derived from the enzymatic hydrolysis of starch. It is characterized by its resistance to digestion in the small intestine and its fermentation by gut bacteria in the large intestine.

Synonym Name and Common Name: Synonym Name: Resistant maltodextrin, Resistant starch Common Name: Resistant dextrin

Pharmacognosy/Chemistry: Resistant dextrin is a complex carbohydrate composed of glucose units linked together by alpha (α)-glycosidic bonds. It is produced through the partial hydrolysis of starch using enzymes, resulting in a mixture of short-chain oligosaccharides that resist digestion by human enzymes.

Action and Pharmacology: Resistant dextrin acts primarily as a prebiotic fiber in the gastrointestinal tract. It reaches the colon intact, where it serves as a substrate for fermentation by beneficial gut bacteria. This fermentation process produces short-chain fatty acids (SCFAs), such as acetate, propionate, and butyrate, which have various physiological effects, including promoting gut health and metabolic function.

Method of Analysis: Analytical methods for the analysis of resistant dextrin include enzymatic assays, high-performance liquid chromatography (HPLC), and total dietary fiber analysis. These methods allow for the quantification of resistant dextrin content in food products, dietary supplements, and biological samples.

Health Benefits: Resistant dextrin offers several health benefits, including promoting digestive health, supporting weight management, improving glycemic control, and enhancing satiety. It acts as a prebiotic, stimulating the growth of beneficial gut bacteria and improving gut microbiota balance. Resistant dextrin may also help reduce cholesterol levels and inflammation.

Indication and Usage: Resistant dextrin is commonly used as a functional ingredient in various food products, including beverages, baked goods, dairy products, and dietary supplements. It is often added to low-calorie and high-fiber foods to enhance their nutritional value and provide health benefits related to digestion and metabolism.

Usual Constituents with Percentages: The composition of resistant dextrin varies depending on factors such as the source of starch and the degree of hydrolysis. Typically, it consists of short-chain oligosaccharides, with a molecular weight ranging from 2,000 to 10,000 Da. Resistant dextrin may contain approximately 85-95% dietary fiber by weight.

Mechanism of Action: Resistant dextrin functions primarily as a fermentable fiber in the colon. It resists digestion in the small intestine and reaches the colon intact, where it is fermented by colonic bacteria. This fermentation process produces SCFAs, which contribute to the maintenance of gut health, modulation of immune function, and regulation of metabolism.

Dosage: The recommended dosage of resistant dextrin varies depending on the specific product and intended health benefits. Typical doses range from 5 to 15 grams per day for adults, although higher doses may be used in some clinical applications. It is important to follow the dosage instructions provided by the manufacturer or healthcare provider.

Contraindications: Resistant dextrin is generally well-tolerated, but individuals with gastrointestinal disorders such as irritable bowel syndrome (IBS) or inflammatory bowel disease (IBD) may experience digestive discomfort when consuming high doses. People with allergies to corn or wheat should avoid products containing resistant dextrin derived from these sources.

Precautions: Individuals using resistant dextrin supplements should ensure adequate fluid intake to prevent potential gastrointestinal discomfort and promote optimal digestion. It is advisable to start with low doses and gradually increase intake to minimize the risk of adverse effects.

Adverse Reactions: Adverse reactions to resistant dextrin are rare but may include gastrointestinal symptoms such as bloating, gas, abdominal discomfort, and diarrhea, especially when consumed in high doses or by individuals with sensitive digestive systems. These symptoms are usually mild and transient.

Research Standing: Resistant dextrin has been extensively studied for its health benefits and safety profile. Clinical research supports its efficacy in promoting digestive health, modulating metabolism, and improving markers of metabolic syndrome. Resistant dextrin is generally recognized as safe (GRAS) by regulatory authorities and is widely used in food and dietary supplement industries.

Pharmacokinetics and Pharmacodynamics: Resistant dextrin is not digested in the small intestine but reaches the colon intact, where it undergoes fermentation by colonic bacteria. The fermentation process produces SCFAs, which are absorbed and metabolized by the host, contributing to various physiological effects such as energy production, immune modulation, and gut health.

Overdosage: Overconsumption of resistant dextrin may lead to gastrointestinal symptoms such as bloating, gas, abdominal discomfort, and diarrhea, especially in individuals with sensitive digestive systems. Adherence to recommended dosage guidelines is important to minimize the risk of adverse effects.

Details on Strains of Probiotics

1) LACTOBACIILUS ACIDOPHILUS

Introduction

Lactobacillus acidophilus is a species of Gram-positive bacteria in the genus Lactobacillus. It is a commonly used probiotic, or "friendly" bacteria, which is naturally found in the human and animal gastrointestinal tract, mouth, and vagina.

Synonym and Common Names

Synonym: None widely recognized.

Common Names: Acidophilus, L. acidophilus.

Pharmacognosy/Chemistry

L. acidophilus is a homofermentative, microaerophilic species, producing lactic acid from carbohydrate fermentation. It is part of the normal flora of the human and animal gastrointestinal tract and a common probiotic ingredient in yogurt and dietary supplements.

Action and Pharmacology

Action: It acts primarily by colonizing the gut, outcompeting potentially harmful bacteria, and promoting gut health.

Pharmacology: L. acidophilus helps maintain the integrity of intestinal mucosa and supports the immune function.

Method of Analysis

The analysis of L. acidophilus typically involves microbial enumeration techniques such as plate counts on selective media and molecular methods like PCR for species-specific identification.

Health Benefits

- Enhances gut health and digestion
- Supports the immune system
- Helps in the management of diarrhea
- May aid in reducing lactose intolerance symptoms
- Potentially beneficial in managing and preventing atopic dermatitis

Indications and Usage

L. acidophilus is used as a probiotic supplement for maintaining and restoring gut flora. It is indicated for digestive disturbances, diarrhea, and as a supplement during antibiotic treatment to prevent antibiotic-associated diarrhea.

Usual Constituents

L. acidophilus is used in concentrations ranging from one to ten billion colony-forming units (CFU) per dose in various supplements.

Mechanism of Action

L. acidophilus functions by adhering to the gut epithelium, competing with pathogenic bacteria for adhesion sites, producing antimicrobial substances, and modulating the immune system.

Dosage

Typical dosages of L. acidophilus range from 1 billion to 10 billion CFU per day, depending on the formulation and intended use.

Contraindications

Contraindicated in individuals with known hypersensitivity to Lactobacillus preparations or components of the growth media.

Precautions

- Immunocompromised individuals should use with caution.
- Potential for infection in vulnerable populations.

Adverse Reactions

Generally well tolerated, but can occasionally cause gas, bloating, or diarrhea.

Research Standing

Numerous clinical trials have assessed the benefits of L. acidophilus in various health conditions, confirming its safety and efficacy for specific uses.

Pharmacokinetics

Being a live bacterium, L. acidophilus primarily acts locally in the gut and does not undergo the typical pharmacokinetic phases of absorption, distribution, metabolism, and excretion.

Pharmacodynamics

Its effects are exerted through interactions with gut flora and the immune system.

Overdosage

There have been no reported adverse effects specifically linked to overdosage of L. acidophilus.

International Standing

L. acidophilus is widely used globally as a probiotic supplement and is included in many health products.

Indian Standing

In India, L. acidophilus is included in various probiotic preparations marketed for gut health and improving digestion.

Research Summary

Research has extensively documented the benefits of L. acidophilus in promoting gut health and supporting the immune system. Continuous studies aim to elucidate its role in various other health conditions and its potential therapeutic applications.

2) LACTIPLANTIBACILLUS PLANTARUM

Introduction

Lactiplantibacillus plantarum (formerly known as Lactobacillus plantarum) is a versatile, lactic acid-producing bacteria found in many fermented food products as well as human and animal gastrointestinal tracts. It is widely used as a probiotic, which contributes to the health of the host.

Synonym and Common Names

Synonym: Lactobacillus plantarum

Common Names: L. plantarum, plantarum

Pharmacognosy/Chemistry

L. plantarum is facultatively heterofermentative and is capable of producing both lactic acid and acetic acid. This bacterium can survive at a wide range of pH levels and temperatures, making it highly adaptable and capable of colonization in various environments.

Action and Pharmacology

Action: L. plantarum can improve gut health, modulate the immune system, and help in the absorption of nutrients.

Pharmacology: It exerts beneficial effects through mechanisms such as competitive exclusion of pathogens, enhancement of the intestinal barrier, and modulation of local and systemic immune responses.

Method of Analysis

The typical analysis involves plating on selective media for bacterial count and identification through DNA sequencing techniques like PCR to confirm its strain specificity.

Health Benefits

- Promotes a healthy digestive system
- Supports the immune system
- Reduces symptoms of bloating and gas in IBS patients
- Could reduce the frequency of colds and flu
- Helps in managing allergies

Indications and Usage

L. plantarum is recommended for improving gastrointestinal health, enhancing immune response, and as an adjunct in the treatment and prevention of specific allergic reactions. It is also used in managing symptoms of IBS.

Usual Constituents

In probiotic formulations, L. plantarum is typically included at levels ranging from about 1 billion to 20 billion CFU per dose.

Mechanism of Action

L. plantarum acts by adhering to the mucosa and colonizing the gut, thereby inhibiting the growth of pathogenic bacteria through competitive exclusion and antimicrobial compound production. It also influences local immune responses.

Dosage

The recommended dosage for L. plantarum varies, typically around 1-20 billion CFUs per day, depending on the intended health benefit.

Contraindications

Avoid use in individuals with known hypersensitivity to any components of plantarum probiotic formulations.

Precautions

- Use cautiously in immunocompromised patients due to the risk of bacterial translocation.
- Should be used carefully in patients with short bowel syndrome.

Adverse Reactions

Generally well tolerated; however, some users may experience digestive disturbances such as gas or bloating, especially at high doses.

Research Standing

There is extensive research supporting the use of L. plantarum in health improvement, particularly in digestive health and immune modulation.

Pharmacokinetics

The pharmacokinetics of L. plantarum is not like traditional drugs since it is a live bacterium; it primarily acts in the gastrointestinal tract without systemic absorption.

Pharmacodynamics

The beneficial effects are primarily localized to the gut but can also affect systemic immunity and inflammation through interaction with gut-associated lymphoid tissue.

Overdosage

No serious outcomes are associated with the overdosage of L. plantarum, though excessive consumption may lead to digestive discomfort.

International Standing

L. plantarum is recognized and utilized worldwide in the production of fermented foods and as a probiotic supplement.

Indian Standing

In India, L. plantarum is widely incorporated in various probiotic formulations intended to promote gut health and prevent gastrointestinal disorders.

Research Summary

Research has consistently shown that L. plantarum can help maintain intestinal health and balance the immune system. Studies have also explored its potential in treating allergies and improving the symptoms of irritable bowel syndrome (IBS). Ongoing research continues to investigate broader applications and mechanisms of action.

3) LIMOSILACTOBACILLUS REUTERI

Introduction

Limosilactobacillusreuteri (formerly known as Lactobacillus reuteri) is a Gram-positive bacterium that naturally inhabits the gut of humans and other mammals. It is recognized for its health-promoting properties and is commonly used as a probiotic in various supplements and food products.

Synonym and Common Names

Synonym: Lactobacillus reuteri

Common Names: L. reuteri, Reuteri

Pharmacognosy/Chemistry

L. reuteri is a heterofermentative bacterium that produces reuterin, a broad-spectrum antimicrobial substance, during glycerol fermentation. This capability plays a crucial role in its probiotic effects, contributing to its ability to inhibit the growth of harmful bacteria.

Action and Pharmacology

Action: L. reuteri promotes gastrointestinal health, enhances immune function, and can improve oral health.

Pharmacology: Its probiotic effects are due to its ability to produce antimicrobial substances, compete with pathogens for adhesion sites, and modulate immune responses.

Method of Analysis

The identification and quantification of L. reuteri are typically performed using selective culture media and molecular techniques such as quantitative PCR for accurate strain differentiation and counting.

Health Benefits

- Enhances gut health and digestion
- Reduces gastrointestinal discomfort in infants and adults
- Boosts the immune system
- May help in managing oral health by reducing the prevalence of harmful oral bacteria

Indications and Usage

L. reuteri is indicated for the improvement of gut health, enhancement of the immune system, management of colic in infants, and as an adjunct in oral health regimens.

Usual Constituents

Probiotic formulations containing L. reuteri typically include doses ranging from 100 million to 10 billion CFU per serving, depending on the product and target audience.

Mechanism of Action

L. reuteri adheres to mucosal surfaces in the gastrointestinal tract, competes with pathogens, and modulates immune system activity through its metabolic products like reuterin, which inhibits the growth of pathogenic bacteria.

Dosage

- The recommended dosage of L. reuteri can vary:
- For gastrointestinal health: 100 million to 1 billion CFU daily.
- For oral health: 200 million to 1 billion CFU daily.

Contraindications

Known hypersensitivity to L. reuteri or any components of the formulation in which it is contained.

Precautions

- Caution is advised for use in immunocompromised individuals due to the potential for systemic infection.
- Consultation with a healthcare provider is recommended before starting any new probiotic supplementation.

Adverse Reactions

L. reuteri is generally well tolerated, but side effects can include gas and bloating, particularly during the initial days of treatment.

Research Standing

Numerous clinical trials and research studies have validated the health benefits of L. reuteri, particularly in areas related to gastrointestinal and oral health.

Pharmacokinetics

As a live bacterium, L. reuteri primarily acts locally in the gut and is not absorbed into the bloodstream, thus it does not follow traditional pharmacokinetic patterns.

Pharmacodynamics

The effects of L. reuteri are exerted through its interactions with gut flora and the immune system, as well as through the production of antimicrobial substances like reuterin.

Overdosage

No adverse effects are generally associated with the overdosage of L. reuteri; however, excessive intake may lead to digestive symptoms like bloating or gas.

International Standing

L. reuteri enjoys widespread use internationally both as a dietary supplement and as an additive in foods and beverages aimed at improving health.

Indian Standing

In India, L. reuteri is increasingly popular in the burgeoning probiotic market, featured in supplements aimed at improving digestive health and enhancing immunity.

Research Summary

L. reuteri has been the subject of extensive research, showing positive effects on health, particularly in improving gastrointestinal function and oral health, reducing infant colic, and enhancing immune responses. Ongoing research continues to explore its broader health impacts.

4) LACTICASEIBACILLUS RHAMNOSUS

Introduction: Lacticaseibacillus rhamnosus, formerly known as Lactobacillus rhamnosus, is a gram-positive bacterium belonging to the Lactobacillus genus. It is a commonly studied probiotic bacterium due to its potential health benefits.

Synonym Name and Common Name: Synonym Name: Lactobacillus rhamnosus Common Name: L. rhamnosus

Pharmacognosy/Chemistry: L. rhamnosus is a rod-shaped bacterium that is non-spore forming and typically appears as a single cell or in pairs. It is characterized by its ability to produce lactic acid through the fermentation of various sugars.

Action and Pharmacology: L. rhamnosus exerts its effects primarily through its probiotic action. It colonizes the gut and helps maintain the balance of beneficial bacteria, which can positively influence digestion, immune function, and overall health.

Method of Analysis: Analysis of L. rhamnosus typically involves culturing techniques to quantify viable bacterial counts. Molecular methods such as PCR (Polymerase Chain Reaction) may also be employed for species identification and strain characterization.

Health Benefits: L. rhamnosus has been associated with various health benefits, including improved digestive health, enhanced immune function, prevention of antibiotic-associated diarrhea, and potential alleviation of symptoms related to conditions like irritable bowel syndrome (IBS).

Indication and Usage: L. rhamnosus is commonly used as a probiotic supplement to support gut health and overall well-being. It may be recommended for individuals experiencing digestive issues or those seeking to boost their immune system.

Usual Constituents with Percentages: L. rhamnosus contains various strains, each with its own unique composition. Common constituents include Lacticaseibacillus rhamnosus GG strain, which typically makes up a significant portion of probiotic supplements containing this bacterium.

Mechanism of Action: The exact mechanism of action of L. rhamnosus is not fully understood but is thought to involve modulation of the gut microbiota, reinforcement of the intestinal barrier, and interaction with the immune system.

Dosage: Dosage recommendations for L. rhamnosus can vary depending on the specific product and indication. Typical doses range from 1 to 10 billion CFUs (colony-forming units) per day, taken orally.

Contraindications: Individuals with compromised immune systems or those undergoing immunosuppressive therapy should consult a healthcare professional before taking L. rhamnosus or any probiotic supplement.

Precautions: While generally considered safe, precautions should be taken in individuals with severe underlying health conditions or those at risk of bacterial translocation.

Adverse Reactions: Adverse reactions to L. rhamnosus are rare but may include mild gastrointestinal symptoms such as bloating, gas, or diarrhea, particularly when first starting supplementation.

Research Standing: L. rhamnosus has been extensively studied in both clinical and preclinical research settings, with numerous studies supporting its beneficial effects on gut health and immunity. However, more research is needed to fully elucidate its mechanisms of action and potential therapeutic applications.

Pharmacokinetics and Pharmacodynamics: L. rhamnosus survives transit through the acidic environment of the stomach and reaches the intestines where it can colonize and exert its probiotic effects. Its pharmacodynamics involve interactions with the gut microbiota and the host immune system.

Overdosage: While there is no established upper limit for L. rhamnosus supplementation, exceeding recommended doses may lead to an imbalance in gut microbiota or potential adverse effects. It is advisable to follow dosage instructions provided by healthcare professionals or product labels.

International Standing: L. rhamnosus is recognized internationally as a safe and effective probiotic bacterium, commonly used in dietary supplements and functional foods.

Indian Standing: In India, L. rhamnosus is also utilized in probiotic formulations and is available as a dietary supplement for promoting digestive health and immunity.

Research Summary: Research on Lacticaseibacillus rhamnosus spans various fields including gastroenterology, immunology, and microbiology. Studies have demonstrated its potential to alleviate symptoms of gastrointestinal disorders, support immune function, and improve overall well-being. Further research is ongoing to explore its mechanisms of action and therapeutic applications in diverse health conditions.

5) LIGILACTOBACILLUS SALIVARIUS

Introduction: Ligilactobacillus salivarius, previously known as Lactobacillus salivarius, is a gram-positive bacterium belonging to the Lactobacillus genus. It is commonly found in the oral cavity, gastrointestinal tract, and other mucosal surfaces of humans and animals.

Synonym Name and Common Name: Synonym Name: Lactobacillus salivarius Common Name: L. salivarius

Pharmacognosy/Chemistry: L. salivarius is a rod-shaped bacterium that is non-spore forming and typically appears singly or in chains. It produces lactic acid as a metabolic byproduct through the fermentation of sugars.

Action and Pharmacology: L. salivarius exerts its effects primarily through its probiotic action. It colonizes mucosal surfaces, including the oral cavity and gastrointestinal tract, where it competes with pathogens for nutrients and space, modulates the immune system, and helps maintain microbial balance.

Method of Analysis: Analysis of L. salivarius involves culturing techniques to quantify viable bacterial counts. Molecular methods such as PCR may also be used for species identification and strain characterization.

Health Benefits: L. salivarius has been associated with various health benefits, including improved oral health, digestive health, immune function, and potential prevention or alleviation of conditions like irritable bowel syndrome (IBS), inflammatory bowel disease (IBD), and infections.

Indication and Usage: L. salivarius is commonly used as a probiotic supplement to support oral and gastrointestinal health. It may be recommended for individuals with oral health issues, digestive disturbances, or those seeking to boost their immune system.

Usual Constituents with Percentages: L. salivarius contains various strains, each with its own unique composition. Common constituents include Ligilactobacillus salivarius UCC118 strain, which is well-studied and often used in probiotic formulations.

Mechanism of Action: The exact mechanism of action of L. salivarius involves multiple factors, including competitive exclusion of pathogens, production of antimicrobial compounds, modulation of the immune response, and reinforcement of mucosal barriers.

Dosage: Dosage recommendations for L. salivarius can vary depending on the specific product and indication. Typical doses range from 1 to 10 billion CFUs (colony-forming units) per day, taken orally.

Contraindications: Individuals with compromised immune systems or those undergoing immunosuppressive therapy should consult a healthcare professional before taking L. salivarius or any probiotic supplement.

Precautions: While generally considered safe, precautions should be taken in individuals with severe underlying health conditions or those at risk of bacterial translocation.

Adverse Reactions: Adverse reactions to L. salivarius are rare but may include mild gastrointestinal symptoms such as bloating, gas, or diarrhea, particularly when first starting supplementation.

Research Standing: L. salivarius has been the subject of numerous studies investigating its potential health benefits and mechanisms of action. While much of the research is promising, more clinical trials are needed to fully establish its efficacy and safety in various health conditions.

Pharmacokinetics and Pharmacodynamics: L. salivarius survives transit through the acidic environment of the stomach and reaches the intestines where it can colonize and exert its probiotic effects. Its pharmacodynamics involve interactions with the gut microbiota, the immune system, and mucosal surfaces.

Overdosage: While there is no established upper limit for L. salivarius supplementation, exceeding recommended doses may lead to an imbalance in gut microbiota or potential adverse effects. It is advisable to follow dosage instructions provided by healthcare professionals or product labels.

International Standing: L. salivarius is recognized internationally as a safe and effective probiotic bacterium, commonly used in dietary supplements and functional foods.

Indian Standing: In India, L. salivarius is also utilized in probiotic formulations and is available as a dietary supplement for promoting oral and gastrointestinal health.

Research Summary: Research on Ligilactobacillus salivarius encompasses various fields including oral health, gastroenterology, immunology, and microbiology. Studies have demonstrated its potential to support oral hygiene, digestive health, and immune function, as well as its role in preventing or alleviating various gastrointestinal disorders. Further research is ongoing to explore its mechanisms of action and therapeutic applications in diverse health conditions.

6) LACTICASEIBACILLUS CASEI

Introduction: Lacticaseibacillus casei, formerly known as Lactobacillus casei, is a gram-positive bacterium belonging to the Lactobacillus genus. It is commonly found in the human gastrointestinal tract, dairy products, and fermented foods.

Synonym Name and Common Name: Synonym Name: Lactobacillus casei Common Name: L. casei

Pharmacognosy/Chemistry: L. casei is a rod-shaped bacterium that is non-spore forming and typically appears singly or in pairs. It produces lactic acid as a metabolic byproduct through the fermentation of sugars.

Action and Pharmacology: L. casei exerts its effects primarily through its probiotic action. It colonizes the gastrointestinal tract, where it competes with pathogens for nutrients and space, modulates the immune system, and helps maintain microbial balance.

Method of Analysis: Analysis of L. casei involves culturing techniques to quantify viable bacterial counts. Molecular methods such as PCR may also be used for species identification and strain characterization.

Health Benefits: L. casei has been associated with various health benefits, including improved digestive health, enhanced immune function, prevention of antibiotic-associated diarrhea, and potential alleviation of symptoms related to conditions like irritable bowel syndrome (IBS).

Indication and Usage: L. casei is commonly used as a probiotic supplement to support gut health and overall well-being. It may be recommended for individuals experiencing digestive issues or those seeking to boost their immune system.

Usual Constituents with Percentages: L. casei contains various strains, each with its own unique composition. Common constituents include Lacticaseibacillus casei Shirota strain, which is well-studied and often used in probiotic formulations.

Mechanism of Action: The exact mechanism of action of L. casei involves multiple factors, including competitive exclusion of pathogens, production of antimicrobial compounds, modulation of the immune response, and reinforcement of mucosal barriers.

Dosage: Dosage recommendations for L. casei can vary depending on the specific product and indication. Typical doses range from 1 to 10 billion CFUs (colony-forming units) per day, taken orally.

Contraindications: Individuals with compromised immune systems or those undergoing immunosuppressive therapy should consult a healthcare professional before taking L. casei or any probiotic supplement.

Precautions: While generally considered safe, precautions should be taken in individuals with severe underlying health conditions or those at risk of bacterial translocation.

Adverse Reactions: Adverse reactions to L. casei are rare but may include mild gastrointestinal symptoms such as bloating, gas, or diarrhea, particularly when first starting supplementation.

Research Standing: L. casei has been the subject of numerous studies investigating its potential health benefits and mechanisms of action. While much of the research is promising, more clinical trials are needed to fully establish its efficacy and safety in various health conditions.

Pharmacokinetics and Pharmacodynamics: L. casei survives transit through the acidic environment of the stomach and reaches the intestines where it can colonize and exert its probiotic effects. Its pharmacodynamics involve interactions with the gut microbiota, the immune system, and mucosal surfaces.

Overdosage: While there is no established upper limit for L. casei supplementation, exceeding recommended doses may lead to an imbalance in gut microbiota or potential adverse effects. It is advisable to follow dosage instructions provided by healthcare professionals or product labels.

International Standing: L. casei is recognized internationally as a safe and effective probiotic bacterium, commonly used in dietary supplements and functional foods.

Indian Standing: In India, L. casei is also utilized in probiotic formulations and is available as a dietary supplement for promoting gut health and immunity.

Research Summary: Research on Lacticaseibacillus casei spans various fields including gastroenterology, immunology, and microbiology. Studies have demonstrated its potential to alleviate symptoms of gastrointestinal disorders, support immune function, and improve overall well-being. Further research is ongoing to explore its mechanisms of action and therapeutic applications in diverse health conditions.

7) LEVILACTOBACILLUS BREVIS

Introduction: Levilactobacillus brevis, formerly known as Lactobacillus brevis, is a gram-positive bacterium belonging to the Lactobacillus genus. It is commonly found in fermented foods and beverages and has been studied for its potential health benefits.

Synonym Name and Common Name: Synonym Name: Lactobacillus brevis Common Name: L. brevis

Pharmacognosy/Chemistry: L. brevis is a rod-shaped bacterium that is non-spore forming and typically appears singly or in chains. It produces lactic acid as a metabolic byproduct through the fermentation of sugars.

Action and Pharmacology: L. brevis exerts its effects primarily through its probiotic action. It colonizes the gastrointestinal tract, where it competes with pathogens for nutrients and space, modulates the immune system, and helps maintain microbial balance.

Method of Analysis: Analysis of L. brevis involves culturing techniques to quantify viable bacterial counts. Molecular methods such as PCR may also be used for species identification and strain characterization.

Health Benefits: L. brevis has been associated with various health benefits, including improved digestive health, enhanced immune function, potential prevention of respiratory infections, and modulation of inflammatory responses.

Indication and Usage: L. brevis is commonly used as a probiotic supplement to support gut health and overall well-being. It may be recommended for individuals experiencing digestive issues, respiratory infections, or those seeking to boost their immune system.

Usual Constituents with Percentages: L. brevis contains various strains, each with its own unique composition. Common constituents include Levilactobacillus brevis KB290 strain, which is well-studied and often used in probiotic formulations.

Mechanism of Action: The exact mechanism of action of L. brevis involves multiple factors, including competitive exclusion of pathogens, production of antimicrobial compounds, modulation of the immune response, and reinforcement of mucosal barriers.

Dosage: Dosage recommendations for L. brevis can vary depending on the specific product and indication. Typical doses range from 1 to 10 billion CFUs (colony-forming units) per day, taken orally.

Contraindications: Individuals with compromised immune systems or those undergoing immunosuppressive therapy should consult a healthcare professional before taking L. brevis or any probiotic supplement.

Precautions: While generally considered safe, precautions should be taken in individuals with severe underlying health conditions or those at risk of bacterial translocation.

Adverse Reactions: Adverse reactions to L. brevis are rare but may include mild gastrointestinal symptoms such as bloating, gas, or diarrhea, particularly when first starting supplementation.

Research Standing: L. brevis has been the subject of numerous studies investigating its potential health benefits and mechanisms of action. While much of the research is promising, more clinical trials are needed to fully establish its efficacy and safety in various health conditions.

Pharmacokinetics and Pharmacodynamics: L. brevis survives transit through the acidic environment of the stomach and reaches the intestines where it can colonize and exert its probiotic effects. Its pharmacodynamics involve interactions with the gut microbiota, the immune system, and mucosal surfaces.

Overdosage: While there is no established upper limit for L. brevis supplementation, exceeding recommended doses may lead to an imbalance in gut microbiota or potential adverse effects. It is advisable to follow dosage instructions provided by healthcare professionals or product labels.

International Standing: L. brevis is recognized internationally as a safe and effective probiotic bacterium, commonly used in dietary supplements and functional foods.

Indian Standing: In India, L. brevis is also utilized in probiotic formulations and is available as a dietary supplement for promoting gut health and immunity.

Research Summary: Research on Levilactobacillus brevis encompasses various fields including gastroenterology, immunology, and microbiology. Studies have demonstrated its potential to alleviate symptoms of gastrointestinal disorders, support immune function, and improve overall well-being. Further research is ongoing to explore its mechanisms of action and therapeutic applications in diverse health conditions.

8) LACTOBACILLUS JOHNSONII

Introduction: Lactobacillus johnsonii is a gram-positive bacterium belonging to the Lactobacillus genus. It is a commensal microorganism commonly found in the human gastrointestinal tract, where it plays a crucial role in maintaining gut health and overall well-being.

Synonym Name and Common Name: Synonym Name: None Common Name: L. johnsonii

Pharmacognosy/Chemistry: L. johnsonii is a rod-shaped bacterium with a complex cell wall structure. It produces lactic acid as a metabolic byproduct through the fermentation of carbohydrates. The composition of its cell wall and metabolic byproducts contribute to its pharmacological properties.

Action and Pharmacology: L. johnsonii exerts its effects primarily through its probiotic action. It colonizes the gastrointestinal tract, where it helps maintain a healthy balance of gut microbiota, modulates the immune system, and promotes overall digestive health.

Method of Analysis: Analysis of L. johnsonii involves culturing techniques to quantify viable bacterial counts. Molecular methods such as PCR (Polymerase Chain Reaction) may also be used for species identification and strain characterization.

Health Benefits: L. johnsonii has been associated with various health benefits, including improved digestive function, enhanced immune response, reduction of inflammation, prevention of gastrointestinal infections, and potential alleviation of symptoms related to conditions like irritable bowel syndrome (IBS).

Indication and Usage: L. johnsonii is commonly used as a probiotic supplement to support gut health and overall immune function. It may be recommended for individuals experiencing digestive discomfort, those seeking to strengthen their immune system, or as an adjunct therapy for certain gastrointestinal conditions.

Usual Constituents with Percentages: L. johnsonii contains various strains, each with its own unique composition. Common constituents include Lactobacillus johnsonii NCC 533, which is well-studied and often used in probiotic formulations.

Mechanism of Action: The exact mechanism of action of L. johnsonii involves multiple factors, including competitive exclusion of pathogenic bacteria, production of antimicrobial compounds, modulation of the host immune response, and reinforcement of the gut barrier function.

Dosage: Dosage recommendations for L. johnsonii can vary depending on the specific product and indication. Typical doses range from 1 to 10 billion CFUs (colony-forming units) per day, taken orally.

Contraindications: Individuals with compromised immune systems or those undergoing immunosuppressive therapy should consult a healthcare professional before taking L. johnsonii or any probiotic supplement.

Precautions: While generally considered safe, precautions should be taken in individuals with severe underlying health conditions or those at risk of bacterial translocation.

Adverse Reactions: Adverse reactions to L. johnsonii are rare but may include mild gastrointestinal symptoms such as bloating, gas, or diarrhea, particularly when first starting supplementation.

Research Standing: L. johnsonii has been the subject of numerous studies investigating its potential health benefits and mechanisms of action. While much of the research is promising, more clinical trials are needed to fully establish its efficacy and safety in various health conditions.

Pharmacokinetics and Pharmacodynamics: L. johnsonii survives transit through the acidic environment of the stomach and reaches the intestines where it can colonize and exert its probiotic effects. Its pharmacodynamics involve interactions with the gut microbiota, the immune system, and mucosal surfaces.

Overdosage: While there is no established upper limit for L. johnsonii supplementation, exceeding recommended doses may lead to an imbalance in gut microbiota or potential adverse effects. It is advisable to follow dosage instructions provided by healthcare professionals or product labels.

International Standing: L. johnsonii is recognized internationally as a safe and effective probiotic bacterium, commonly used in dietary supplements and functional foods.

Indian Standing: In India, L. johnsonii is also utilized in probiotic formulations and is available as a dietary supplement for promoting gut health and immunity.

Research Summary: Research on Lactobacillus johnsonii encompasses various fields including gastroenterology, immunology, and microbiology. Studies have demonstrated its potential to alleviate symptoms of gastrointestinal disorders, support immune function, and improve overall well-being. Further research is ongoing to explore its mechanisms of action and therapeutic applications in diverse health conditions.

9) LACTOBACILLUS DELBRUECKII SUB- SP. BULGARICUS

Introduction: Lactobacillus delbrueckii subsp. bulgaricus is a gram-positive bacterium widely used in the production of yogurt and other fermented dairy products. It is known for its probiotic properties and has been studied for its potential health benefits.

Synonym Name and Common Name: Synonym Name: None Common Name: L. bulgaricus

Pharmacognosy/Chemistry: L. bulgaricus is a rod-shaped bacterium with a complex cell wall structure. It produces lactic acid as a metabolic byproduct through the fermentation of lactose. The composition of its cell wall and metabolic byproducts contribute to its pharmacological properties.

Action and Pharmacology: L. bulgaricus exerts its effects primarily through its probiotic action. It colonizes the gastrointestinal tract, where it helps maintain a healthy balance of gut microbiota, aids in digestion, and may contribute to overall gut health.

Method of Analysis: Analysis of L. bulgaricus involves culturing techniques to quantify viable bacterial counts. Molecular methods such as PCR (Polymerase Chain Reaction) may also be used for species identification and strain characterization.

Health Benefits: L. bulgaricus has been associated with various health benefits, including improved digestion, enhanced immune function, reduction of lactose intolerance symptoms, and potential prevention of gastrointestinal infections.

Indication and Usage: L. bulgaricus is commonly used in the production of yogurt and other fermented dairy products. It may also be used as a probiotic supplement to support gut health and digestion.

Usual Constituents with Percentages: L. bulgaricus contains various strains, each with its own unique composition. Common constituents include Lactobacillus delbrueckii subsp. bulgaricus, which typically makes up a significant portion of yogurt cultures.

Mechanism of Action: The exact mechanism of action of L. bulgaricus involves multiple factors, including production of lactic acid, competition with pathogenic bacteria for nutrients and adhesion sites, and modulation of the gut microbiota.

Dosage: Dosage recommendations for L. bulgaricus can vary depending on the specific product and indication. When consumed as part of yogurt or other fermented dairy products, there is no specific dosage, as it is typically consumed in amounts sufficient to provide probiotic benefits.

Contraindications: Individuals with compromised immune systems or those undergoing immunosuppressive therapy should consult a healthcare professional before consuming L. bulgaricus or any probiotic supplement.

Precautions: While generally considered safe, precautions should be taken in individuals with severe underlying health conditions or those at risk of bacterial translocation.

Adverse Reactions: Adverse reactions to L. bulgaricus are rare but may include mild gastrointestinal symptoms such as bloating, gas, or diarrhea, particularly in individuals with lactose intolerance.

Research Standing: L. bulgaricus has been studied extensively for its role in fermentation and its potential health benefits. While much of the research has focused on its use in dairy products, more studies are needed to fully elucidate its mechanisms of action and therapeutic applications as a probiotic supplement.

Pharmacokinetics and Pharmacodynamics: L. bulgaricus survives transit through the acidic environment of the stomach and reaches the intestines where it can colonize and exert its probiotic effects. Its pharmacodynamics involve interactions with the gut microbiota and the host immune system.

Overdosage: There is no established risk of overdosage with L. bulgaricus when consumed as part of fermented dairy products. However, excessive consumption may lead to gastrointestinal discomfort in sensitive individuals.

International Standing: L. bulgaricus is recognized internationally as a safe and effective probiotic bacterium, commonly used in the production of yogurt and other fermented dairy products.

Indian Standing: In India, L. bulgaricus is also widely used in the production of yogurt and other fermented dairy products. It is recognized for its role in promoting digestive health and is commonly consumed as part of the diet.

Research Summary: Research on Lactobacillus delbrueckii subsp. bulgaricus has primarily focused on its use in fermentation and its potential health benefits when consumed as part of yogurt and other fermented dairy products. While it is generally regarded as safe and beneficial, further research is needed to explore its specific mechanisms of action and potential therapeutic applications as a probiotic supplement.

10) BACILLUS COAGULANS

Introduction: Bacillus coagulans is a gram-positive, spore-forming bacterium that belongs to the Bacillus genus. It is commonly used as a probiotic supplement due to its ability to survive harsh conditions and its potential health benefits.

Synonym Name and Common Name: Synonym Name: Lactobacillus sporogenes Common Name: B. coagulans

Pharmacognosy/Chemistry: B. coagulans is characterized by its spore-forming ability, which allows it to survive in a dormant state until conditions become favorable for growth. It produces lactic acid and other beneficial compounds through fermentation.

Action and Pharmacology: B. coagulans exerts its effects primarily through its probiotic action. It colonizes the gastrointestinal tract, where it helps maintain a healthy balance of gut microbiota, aids in digestion, and may contribute to overall gut health and immune function.

Method of Analysis: Analysis of B. coagulans typically involves culturing techniques to quantify viable bacterial counts. Molecular methods such as PCR may also be used for species identification and strain characterization.

Health Benefits: B. coagulans has been associated with various health benefits, including improved digestive function, enhanced immune response, reduction of gastrointestinal discomfort, and potential prevention of antibiotic-associated diarrhea.

Indication and Usage: B. coagulans is commonly used as a probiotic supplement to support gut health and overall well-being. It may be recommended for individuals experiencing digestive issues, those seeking to boost their immune system, or those taking antibiotics to prevent diarrhea.

Usual Constituents with Percentages: B. coagulans contains various strains, each with its own unique composition. Common constituents include Bacillus coagulans MTCC 5856, which is well-studied and often used in probiotic formulations.

Mechanism of Action: The exact mechanism of action of B. coagulans involves multiple factors, including production of lactic acid and other antimicrobial compounds, competition with pathogenic bacteria for nutrients and adhesion sites, and modulation of the gut microbiota and immune system.

Dosage: Dosage recommendations for B. coagulans can vary depending on the specific product and indication. Typical doses range from 1 to 10 billion CFUs (colony-forming units) per day, taken orally.

Contraindications: Individuals with compromised immune systems, those undergoing immunosuppressive therapy, or those with severe underlying health conditions should consult a healthcare professional before taking B. coagulans or any probiotic supplement.

Precautions: While generally considered safe, precautions should be taken in individuals with severe underlying health conditions or those at risk of bacterial translocation.

Adverse Reactions: Adverse reactions to B. coagulans are rare but may include mild gastrointestinal symptoms such as bloating, gas, or diarrhea, particularly when first starting supplementation.

Research Standing: B. coagulans has been the subject of numerous studies investigating its potential health benefits and mechanisms of action. While much of the research is promising, more clinical trials are needed to fully establish its efficacy and safety in various health conditions.

Pharmacokinetics and Pharmacodynamics: B. coagulans survives transit through the acidic environment of the stomach and reaches the intestines where it can germinate and exert its probiotic effects. Its pharmacodynamics involve interactions with the gut microbiota and the host immune system.

Overdosage: While there is no established risk of overdosage with B. coagulans, exceeding recommended doses may lead to an imbalance in gut microbiota or potential adverse effects. It is advisable to follow dosage instructions provided by healthcare professionals or product labels.

International Standing: B. coagulans is recognized internationally as a safe and effective probiotic bacterium, commonly used in dietary supplements and functional foods.

Indian Standing: In India, B. coagulans is also utilized in probiotic formulations and is available as a dietary supplement for promoting gut health and immunity.

Research Summary: Research on Bacillus coagulans has primarily focused on its potential health benefits as a probiotic supplement, particularly in promoting digestive health and immune function. While more studies are needed to fully elucidate its mechanisms of action and therapeutic applications, existing research suggests promising outcomes in various health conditions.

11) LIMOSILACTOBACILLUS FERMENT

Introduction: Limosilactobacillus fermentum, formerly known as Lactobacillus fermentum, is a gram-positive bacterium belonging to the Lactobacillus genus. It is commonly found in fermented foods and has been studied for its potential health benefits as a probiotic.

Synonym Name and Common Name: Synonym Name: Lactobacillus fermentum Common Name: L. fermentum

Pharmacognosy/Chemistry: L. fermentum is a rod-shaped bacterium with a complex cell wall structure. It produces lactic acid as a metabolic byproduct through the fermentation of sugars. Its chemical composition includes various metabolites and proteins.

Action and Pharmacology: L. fermentum exerts its effects primarily through its probiotic action. It colonizes the gastrointestinal tract, where it helps maintain a healthy balance of gut microbiota, supports digestion, modulates the immune system, and may contribute to overall gut health.

Method of Analysis: Analysis of L. fermentum involves culturing techniques to quantify viable bacterial counts. Molecular methods such as PCR may also be used for species identification and strain characterization.

Health Benefits: L. fermentum has been associated with various health benefits, including improved digestive function, enhanced immune response, reduction of gastrointestinal discomfort, prevention of antibiotic-associated diarrhea, and potential alleviation of symptoms related to conditions like irritable bowel syndrome (IBS).

Indication and Usage: L. fermentum is commonly used as a probiotic supplement to support gut health and overall well-being. It may be recommended for individuals experiencing digestive issues, those seeking to boost their immune system, or thōse taking antibiotics to prevent diarrhea.

Usual Constituents with Percentages: L. fermentum contains various strains, each with its own unique composition. Common constituents include Limosilactobacillus fermentum ME-3 strain, which is well-studied and often used in probiotic formulations.

Mechanism of Action: The exact mechanism of action of L. fermentum involves multiple factors, including production of lactic acid and other antimicrobial compounds, competition with pathogenic bacteria for nutrients and adhesion sites, and modulation of the gut microbiota and immune system.

Dosage: Dosage recommendations for L. fermentum can vary depending on the specific product and indication. Typical doses range from 1 to 10 billion CFUs (colony-forming units) per day, taken orally.

Contraindications: Individuals with compromised immune systems, those undergoing immunosuppressive therapy, or those with severe underlying health conditions should consult a healthcare professional before taking L. fermentum or any probiotic supplement.

Precautions: While generally considered safe, precautions should be taken in individuals with severe underlying health conditions or those at risk of bacterial translocation.

Adverse Reactions: Adverse reactions to L. fermentum are rare but may include mild gastrointestinal symptoms such as bloating, gas, or diarrhea, particularly when first starting supplementation.

Research Standing: L. fermentum has been the subject of numerous studies investigating its potential health benefits and mechanisms of action. While much of the research is promising, more clinical trials are needed to fully establish its efficacy and safety in various health conditions.

Pharmacokinetics and Pharmacodynamics: L. fermentum survives transit through the acidic environment of the stomach and reaches the intestines where it can colonize and exert its probiotic effects. Its pharmacodynamics involve interactions with the gut microbiota and the host immune system.

Overdosage: While there is no established risk of overdosage with L. fermentum, exceeding recommended doses may lead to an imbalance in gut microbiota or potential adverse effects. It is advisable to follow dosage instructions provided by healthcare professionals or product labels.

International Standing: L. fermentum is recognized internationally as a safe and effective probiotic bacterium, commonly used in dietary supplements and functional foods.

Indian Standing: In India, L. fermentum is also utilized in probiotic formulations and is available as a dietary supplement for promoting gut health and immunity.

Research Summary: Research on Limosilactobacillus fermentum has primarily focused on its potential health benefits as a probiotic supplement, particularly in promoting digestive health, immune function, and overall well-being. While more studies are needed to fully elucidate its mechanisms of action and therapeutic applications, existing research suggests promising outcomes in various health conditions.

12) LACTOBACILLUS CAUCASICUS

Introduction: Lactobacillus caucasicus is a gram-positive bacterium belonging to the Lactobacillus genus. It is commonly found in fermented foods and has gained attention for its potential health benefits as a probiotic.

Synonym Name and Common Name: Synonym Name: None Common Name: L. caucasicus

Pharmacognosy/Chemistry: L. caucasicus is a rod-shaped bacterium with a complex cell wall structure. It produces lactic acid as a metabolic byproduct through the fermentation of sugars. Its chemical composition includes various metabolites, proteins, and cell wall components.

Action and Pharmacology: L. caucasicus exerts its effects primarily through its probiotic action. It colonizes the gastrointestinal tract, where it helps maintain a healthy balance of gut microbiota, aids in digestion, modulates the immune system, and may contribute to overall gut health.

Method of Analysis: Analysis of L. caucasicus involves culturing techniques to quantify viable bacterial counts. Molecular methods such as PCR may also be used for species identification and strain characterization.

Health Benefits: L. caucasicus has been associated with various health benefits, including improved digestive function, enhanced immune response, reduction of gastrointestinal discomfort, prevention of antibiotic-associated diarrhea, and potential alleviation of symptoms related to conditions like irritable bowel syndrome (IBS).

Indication and Usage: L. caucasicus is commonly used as a probiotic supplement to support gut health and overall well-being. It may be recommended for individuals experiencing digestive issues, those seeking to boost their immune system, or those taking antibiotics to prevent diarrhea.

Usual Constituents with Percentages: L. caucasicus contains various strains, each with its own unique composition. Common constituents include Lactobacillus caucasicus DSM 2653 strain, which is well-studied and often used in probiotic formulations.

Mechanism of Action: The exact mechanism of action of L. caucasicus involves multiple factors, including production of lactic acid and other antimicrobial compounds, competition with pathogenic bacteria for nutrients and adhesion sites, and modulation of the gut microbiota and immune system.

Dosage: Dosage recommendations for L. caucasicus can vary depending on the specific product and indication. Typical doses range from 1 to 10 billion CFUs (colony-forming units) per day, taken orally.

Contraindications: Individuals with compromised immune systems, those undergoing immunosuppressive therapy, or those with severe underlying health conditions should consult a healthcare professional before taking L. caucasicus or any probiotic supplement.

Precautions: While generally considered safe, precautions should be taken in individuals with severe underlying health conditions or those at risk of bacterial translocation.

Adverse Reactions: Adverse reactions to L. caucasicus are rare but may include mild gastrointestinal symptoms such as bloating, gas, or diarrhea, particularly when first starting supplementation.

Research Standing: L. caucasicus has been the subject of numerous studies investigating its potential health benefits and mechanisms of action. While much of the research is promising, more clinical trials are needed to fully establish its efficacy and safety in various health conditions.

Pharmacokinetics and Pharmacodynamics: L. caucasicus survives transit through the acidic environment of the stomach and reaches the intestines where it can colonize and exert its probiotic effects. Its pharmacodynamics involve interactions with the gut microbiota and the host immune system.

Overdosage: While there is no established risk of overdosage with L. caucasicus, exceeding recommended doses may lead to an imbalance in gut microbiota or potential adverse effects. It is advisable to follow dosage instructions provided by healthcare professionals or product labels.

International Standing: L. caucasicus is recognized internationally as a safe and effective probiotic bacterium, commonly used in dietary supplements and functional foods.

Indian Standing: In India, L. caucasicus is also utilized in probiotic formulations and is available as a dietary supplement for promoting gut health and immunity.

Research Summary: Research on Lactobacillus caucasicus has primarily focused on its potential health benefits as a probiotic supplement, particularly in promoting digestive health, immune function, and overall well-being. While more studies are needed to fully elucidate its mechanisms of action and therapeutic applications, existing research suggests promising outcomes in various health conditions.

13) LACTOBACILLUS HELVETICUS

Introduction: Lactobacillus helveticus is a gram-positive bacterium belonging to the Lactobacillus genus. It is commonly found in various fermented dairy products and has gained attention for its potential health benefits as a probiotic.

Synonym Name and Common Name: Synonym Name: None Common Name: L. helveticus

Pharmacognosy/Chemistry: L. helveticus is a rod-shaped bacterium with a complex cell wall structure. It produces lactic acid as a metabolic byproduct through the fermentation of lactose. Its chemical composition includes various metabolites, proteins, and cell wall components.

Action and Pharmacology: L. helveticus exerts its effects primarily through its probiotic action. It colonizes the gastrointestinal tract, where it helps maintain a healthy balance of gut microbiota, aids in digestion, modulates the immune system, and may contribute to overall gut health.

Method of Analysis: Analysis of L. helveticus involves culturing techniques to quantify viable bacterial counts. Molecular methods such as PCR may also be used for species identification and strain characterization.

Health Benefits: L. helveticus has been associated with various health benefits, including improved digestive function, enhanced immune response, reduction of gastrointestinal discomfort, prevention of antibiotic-associated diarrhea, and potential alleviation of symptoms related to conditions like irritable bowel syndrome (IBS).

Indication and Usage: L. helveticus is commonly used as a probiotic supplement to support gut health and overall well-being. It may be recommended for individuals experiencing digestive issues, those seeking to boost their immune system, or those looking to improve their overall gut health.

Usual Constituents with Percentages: L. helveticus contains various strains, each with its own unique composition. Common constituents include Lactobacillus helveticus R0052 and Lactobacillus helveticus R0065, which are well-studied and often used in probiotic formulations.

Mechanism of Action: The exact mechanism of action of L. helveticus involves multiple factors, including production of lactic acid and other antimicrobial compounds, competition with pathogenic bacteria for nutrients and adhesion sites, and modulation of the gut microbiota and immune system.

Dosage: Dosage recommendations for L. helveticus can vary depending on the specific product and indication. Typical doses range from 1 to 10 billion CFUs (colony-forming units) per day, taken orally.

Contraindications: Individuals with compromised immune systems, those undergoing immunosuppressive therapy, or those with severe underlying health conditions should consult a healthcare professional before taking L. helveticus or any probiotic supplement.

Precautions: While generally considered safe, precautions should be taken in individuals with severe underlying health conditions or those at risk of bacterial translocation.

Adverse Reactions: Adverse reactions to L. helveticus are rare but may include mild gastrointestinal symptoms such as bloating, gas, or diarrhea, particularly when first starting supplementation.

Research Standing: L. helveticus has been the subject of numerous studies investigating its potential health benefits and mechanisms of action. While much of the research is promising, more clinical trials are needed to fully establish its efficacy and safety in various health conditions.

Pharmacokinetics and Pharmacodynamics: L. helveticus survives transit through the acidic environment of the stomach and reaches the intestines where it can colonize and exert its probiotic effects. Its pharmacodynamics involve interactions with the gut microbiota and the host immune system.

Overdosage: While there is no established risk of overdosage with L. helveticus, exceeding recommended doses may lead to an imbalance in gut microbiota or potential adverse effects. It is advisable to follow dosage instructions provided by healthcare professionals or product labels.

International Standing: L. helveticus is recognized internationally as a safe and effective probiotic bacterium, commonly used in dietary supplements and functional foods.

Indian Standing: In India, L. helveticus is also utilized in probiotic formulations and is available as a dietary supplement for promoting gut health and immunity.

Research Summary: Research on Lactobacillus helveticus has primarily focused on its potential health benefits as a probiotic supplement, particularly in promoting digestive health, immune function, and overall well-being. While more studies are needed to fully elucidate its mechanisms of action and therapeutic applications, existing research suggests promising outcomes in various health conditions.

14) LACTOBACILLUS LACTIS

Introduction: Lactobacillus lactis is a gram-positive bacterium belonging to the Lactobacillus genus. It is commonly found in various fermented foods and has been extensively studied for its probiotic properties.

Synonym Name and Common Name: Synonym Name: Lactobacillus lactis subsp. lactis Common Name: L. lactis

Pharmacognosy/Chemistry: L. lactis is a rod-shaped bacterium with a complex cell wall structure. It produces lactic acid as a metabolic byproduct through the fermentation of sugars. Its chemical composition includes various metabolites, proteins, and cell wall components.

Action and Pharmacology: L. lactis exerts its effects primarily through its probiotic action. It colonizes the gastrointestinal tract, where it helps maintain a healthy balance of gut microbiota, aids in digestion, modulates the immune system, and may contribute to overall gut health.

Method of Analysis: Analysis of L. lactis involves culturing techniques to quantify viable bacterial counts. Molecular methods such as PCR may also be used for species identification and strain characterization.

Health Benefits: L. lactis has been associated with various health benefits, including improved digestive function, enhanced immune response, reduction of gastrointestinal discomfort, prevention of antibiotic-associated diarrhea, and potential alleviation of symptoms related to conditions like irritable bowel syndrome (IBS).

Indication and Usage: L. lactis is commonly used as a probiotic supplement to support gut health and overall well-being. It may be recommended for individuals experiencing digestive issues, those seeking to boost their immune system, or those looking to improve their overall gut health.

Usual Constituents with Percentages: L. lactis contains various strains, each with its own unique composition. Common constituents include Lactobacillus lactis subsp. lactis DSM 20481 and Lactobacillus lactis subsp. lactis ATCC 11454, which are well-studied and often used in probiotic formulations.

Mechanism of Action: The exact mechanism of action of L. lactis involves multiple factors, including production of lactic acid and other antimicrobial compounds, competition with pathogenic bacteria for nutrients and adhesion sites, and modulation of the gut microbiota and immune system.

Dosage: Dosage recommendations for L. lactis can vary depending on the specific product and indication. Typical doses range from 1 to 10 billion CFUs (colony-forming units) per day, taken orally.

Contraindications: Individuals with compromised immune systems, those undergoing immunosuppressive therapy, or those with severe underlying health conditions should consult a healthcare professional before taking L. lactis or any probiotic supplement.

Precautions: While generally considered safe, precautions should be taken in individuals with severe underlying health conditions or those at risk of bacterial translocation.

Adverse Reactions: Adverse reactions to L. lactis are rare but may include mild gastrointestinal symptoms such as bloating, gas, or diarrhea, particularly when first starting supplementation.

Research Standing: L. lactis has been the subject of numerous studies investigating its potential health benefits and mechanisms of action. While much of the research is promising, more clinical trials are needed to fully establish its efficacy and safety in various health conditions.

Pharmacokinetics and Pharmacodynamics: L. lactis survives transit through the acidic environment of the stomach and reaches the intestines where it can colonize and exert its probiotic effects. Its pharmacodynamics involve interactions with the gut microbiota and the host immune system.

Overdosage: While there is no established risk of overdosage with L. lactis, exceeding recommended doses may lead to an imbalance in gut microbiota or potential adverse effects. It is advisable to follow dosage instructions provided by healthcare professionals or product labels.

International Standing: L. lactis is recognized internationally as a safe and effective probiotic bacterium, commonly used in dietary supplements and functional foods.

Indian Standing: In India, L. lactis is also utilized in probiotic formulations and is available as a dietary supplement for promoting gut health and immunity.

Research Summary: Research on Lactobacillus lactis has primarily focused on its potential health benefits as a probiotic supplement, particularly in promoting digestive health, immune function, and overall well-being. While more studies are needed to fully elucidate its mechanisms of action and therapeutic applications, existing research suggests promising outcomes in various health conditions.

15) LACTOBACILLUS AMYLOVORUS

Introduction: Lactobacillus amylovorus is a gram-positive bacterium belonging to the Lactobacillus genus. It is commonly found in various fermented foods and has been studied for its potential health benefits as a probiotic.

Synonym Name and Common Name: Synonym Name: None Common Name: L. amylovorus

Pharmacognosy/Chemistry: L. amylovorus is a rod-shaped bacterium with a complex cell wall structure. It produces lactic acid as a metabolic byproduct through the fermentation of carbohydrates. Its chemical composition includes various metabolites, proteins, and cell wall components.

Action and Pharmacology: L. amylovorus exerts its effects primarily through its probiotic action. It colonizes the gastrointestinal tract, where it helps maintain a healthy balance of gut microbiota, aids in digestion, modulates the immune system, and may contribute to overall gut health.

Method of Analysis: Analysis of L. amylovorus involves culturing techniques to quantify viable bacterial counts. Molecular methods such as PCR may also be used for species identification and strain characterization.

Health Benefits: L. amylovorus has been associated with various health benefits, including improved digestive function, enhanced immune response, reduction of gastrointestinal discomfort, prevention of antibiotic-associated diarrhea, and potential alleviation of symptoms related to conditions like irritable bowel syndrome (IBS).

Indication and Usage: L. amylovorus is commonly used as a probiotic supplement to support gut health and overall well-being. It may be recommended for individuals experiencing digestive issues, those seeking to boost their immune system, or those looking to improve their overall gut health.

Usual Constituents with Percentages: L. amylovorus contains various strains, each with its own unique composition. Common constituents include Lactobacillus amylovorus DSM 20531 and Lactobacillus amylovorus DSM 19280, which are well-studied and often used in probiotic formulations.

Mechanism of Action: The exact mechanism of action of L. amylovorus involves multiple factors, including production of lactic acid and other antimicrobial compounds, competition with pathogenic bacteria for nutrients and adhesion sites, and modulation of the gut microbiota and immune system.

Dosage: Dosage recommendations for L. amylovorus can vary depending on the specific product and indication. Typical doses range from 1 to 10 billion CFUs (colony-forming units) per day, taken orally.

Contraindications: Individuals with compromised immune systems, those undergoing immunosuppressive therapy, or those with severe underlying health conditions should consult a healthcare professional before taking L. amylovorus or any probiotic supplement.

Precautions: While generally considered safe, precautions should be taken in individuals with severe underlying health conditions or those at risk of bacterial translocation.

Adverse Reactions: Adverse reactions to L. amylovorus are rare but may include mild gastrointestinal symptoms such as bloating, gas, or diarrhea, particularly when first starting supplementation.

Research Standing: L. amylovorus has been the subject of numerous studies investigating its potential health benefits and mechanisms of action. While much of the research is promising, more clinical trials are needed to fully establish its efficacy and safety in various health conditions.

Pharmacokinetics and Pharmacodynamics: L. amylovorus survives transit through the acidic environment of the stomach and reaches the intestines where it can colonize and exert its probiotic effects. Its pharmacodynamics involve interactions with the gut microbiota and the host immune system.

Overdosage: While there is no established risk of overdosage with L. amylovorus, exceeding recommended doses may lead to an imbalance in gut microbiota or potential adverse effects. It is advisable to follow dosage instructions provided by healthcare professionals or product labels.

International Standing: L. amylovorus is recognized internationally as a safe and effective probiotic bacterium, commonly used in dietary supplements and functional foods.

Indian Standing: In India, L. amylovorus is also utilized in probiotic formulations and is available as a dietary supplement for promoting gut health and immunity.

Research Summary: Research on Lactobacillus amylovorus has primarily focused on its potential health benefits as a probiotic supplement, particularly in promoting digestive health, immune function, and overall well-being. While more studies are needed to fully elucidate its mechanisms of action and therapeutic applications, existing research suggests promising outcomes in various health conditions.

16) LACTOBACILLUS GALLINARUM

Introduction: Lactobacillus gallinarum is a gram-positive bacterium belonging to the Lactobacillus genus. It is commonly found in the gastrointestinal tract of poultry and other birds. While less studied compared to some other lactobacilli species, L. gallinarum shows promise as a potential probiotic.

Synonym Name and Common Name: Synonym Name: None Common Name: L. gallinarum

Pharmacognosy/Chemistry: L. gallinarum is a rod-shaped bacterium with a complex cell wall structure. It produces lactic acid as a metabolic byproduct through the fermentation of carbohydrates. Its chemical composition includes various metabolites, proteins, and cell wall components.

Action and Pharmacology: L. gallinarum exerts its effects primarily through its probiotic action. It may colonize the gastrointestinal tract, where it helps maintain a healthy balance of gut microbiota, aids in digestion, and may contribute to overall gut health. However, further research is needed to fully elucidate its pharmacology.

Method of Analysis: Analysis of L. gallinarum involves culturing techniques to quantify viable bacterial counts. Molecular methods such as PCR may also be used for species identification and strain characterization.

Health Benefits: Limited research suggests that L. gallinarum may offer potential health benefits similar to other probiotic bacteria, including improved digestive function, enhanced immune response, and overall gut health. However, more studies are needed to confirm these effects in humans.

Indication and Usage: Due to limited research, specific indications and usage guidelines for L. gallinarum have not been established. However, it may be considered for individuals seeking to support gut health, digestion, and immune function.

Usual Constituents with Percentages: The usual constituents and percentages of L. gallinarum have not been extensively studied and may vary depending on the source and strain. Further research is needed to determine the typical composition of this bacterium.

Mechanism of Action: The exact mechanism of action of L. gallinarum is not fully understood. However, it is hypothesized to exert its probiotic effects through interactions with the gut microbiota, production of beneficial metabolites such as lactic acid, and modulation of the host immune response.

Dosage: Due to limited research, specific dosage recommendations for L. gallinarum are not available. Dosage may vary depending on the formulation and intended use. It is advisable to consult a healthcare professional for personalized guidance.

Contraindications: Contraindications for L. gallinarum have not been well-established. However, individuals with compromised immune systems or those undergoing immunosuppressive therapy should exercise caution when using probiotic supplements, including L. gallinarum.

Precautions: As with any probiotic supplement, individuals should be cautious when using L. gallinarum, especially if they have underlying health conditions or are taking medications. It is advisable to consult a healthcare professional before starting any new supplement regimen.

Adverse Reactions: Adverse reactions to L. gallinarum are rare but may include mild gastrointestinal symptoms such as bloating, gas, or diarrhea, particularly when first starting supplementation. Individuals experiencing persistent or severe adverse reactions should discontinue use and consult a healthcare professional.

Research Standing: Research on Lactobacillus gallinarum is limited compared to other lactobacilli species. While some studies suggest potential health benefits, more research is needed to fully understand its effects, mechanisms of action, and safety profile in humans.

Pharmacokinetics and Pharmacodynamics: The pharmacokinetics and pharmacodynamics of L. gallinarum have not been extensively studied in humans. Further research is needed to determine its survival, colonization, and interactions within the gastrointestinal tract.

Overdosage: Due to limited research, the risk of overdosage with L. gallinarum is not well-defined. However, exceeding recommended dosages of probiotic supplements may disrupt the balance of gut microbiota and lead to adverse effects. It is advisable to follow recommended dosage guidelines.

International Standing: L. gallinarum is not widely recognized as a probiotic species in international regulatory agencies or scientific literature. Further research is needed to establish its international standing and potential use as a probiotic supplement.

Indian Standing: Information regarding the Indian standing of L. gallinarum, including its regulatory status and usage in dietary supplements, is not readily available. Further research and regulatory evaluation may be necessary to determine its standing in the Indian market.

Research Summary: Overall, research on Lactobacillus gallinarum is limited, and its potential health benefits, mechanism of action, and safety profile in humans require further investigation. While preliminary studies show promise, more rigorous clinical trials are needed to establish its efficacy and safety as a probiotic supplement.

17) LACTOBACILLUS DELBRUECKII

Introduction: Lactobacillus delbrueckii is a gram-positive bacterium commonly found in various fermented foods and dairy products. It belongs to the Lactobacillus genus and is known for its probiotic properties.

Synonym Name and Common Name: Synonym Name: None Common Name: L. delbrueckii

Pharmacognosy/Chemistry: L. delbrueckii is a rod-shaped bacterium with a complex cell wall structure. It produces lactic acid as a metabolic byproduct through the fermentation of sugars. Its chemical composition includes various metabolites, proteins, carbohydrates, and cell wall components.

Action and Pharmacology: L. delbrueckii exerts its effects primarily through its probiotic action. It colonizes the gastrointestinal tract, where it helps maintain a healthy balance of gut microbiota, aids in digestion, modulates the immune system, and may contribute to overall gut health.

Method of Analysis: Analysis of L. delbrueckii involves culturing techniques to quantify viable bacterial counts. Molecular methods such as PCR may also be used for species identification and strain characterization. Additionally, biochemical assays and microscopy may be employed for further characterization.

Health Benefits: L. delbrueckii has been associated with various health benefits, including improved digestive function, enhanced immune response, reduction of gastrointestinal discomfort, prevention of antibiotic-associated diarrhea, and potential alleviation of symptoms related to conditions like irritable bowel syndrome (IBS).

Indication and Usage: L. delbrueckii is commonly used as a probiotic supplement to support gut health and overall well-being. It may be recommended for individuals experiencing digestive issues, those seeking to boost their immune system, or those looking to improve their overall gut health.

Usual Constituents with Percentages: The usual constituents and percentages of L. delbrueckii can vary depending on the strain and source. Common constituents include various strains of Lactobacillus delbrueckii, each with its own unique composition.

Mechanism of Action: The exact mechanism of action of L. delbrueckii involves multiple factors, including production of lactic acid and other antimicrobial compounds, competition with pathogenic bacteria for nutrients and adhesion sites, and modulation of the gut microbiota and immune system.

Dosage: Dosage recommendations for L. delbrueckii can vary depending on the specific product and indication. Typical doses range from 1 to 10 billion CFUs (colony-forming units) per day, taken orally.

Contraindications: Individuals with compromised immune systems, those undergoing immunosuppressive therapy, or those with severe underlying health conditions should consult a healthcare professional before taking L. delbrueckii or any probiotic supplement.

Precautions: While generally considered safe, precautions should be taken in individuals with severe underlying health conditions or those at risk of bacterial translocation. It is advisable to consult a healthcare professional before starting any new supplement regimen.

Adverse Reactions: Adverse reactions to L. delbrueckii are rare but may include mild gastrointestinal symptoms such as bloating, gas, or diarrhea, particularly when first starting supplementation.

Research Standing: L. delbrueckii has been the subject of numerous studies investigating its potential health benefits and mechanisms of action. While much of the research is promising, more clinical trials are needed to fully establish its efficacy and safety in various health conditions.

Pharmacokinetics and Pharmacodynamics: L. delbrueckii survives transit through the acidic environment of the stomach and reaches the intestines where it can colonize and exert its probiotic effects. Its pharmacodynamics involve interactions with the gut microbiota and the host immune system.

Overdosage: While there is no established risk of overdosage with L. delbrueckii, exceeding recommended doses may lead to an imbalance in gut microbiota or potential adverse effects. It is advisable to follow dosage instructions provided by healthcare professionals or product labels.

International Standing: L. delbrueckii is recognized internationally as a safe and effective probiotic bacterium, commonly used in dietary supplements and functional foods.

Indian Standing: In India, L. delbrueckii is also utilized in probiotic formulations and is available as a dietary supplement for promoting gut health and immunity.

Research Summary: Research on Lactobacillus delbrueckii has primarily focused on its potential health benefits as a probiotic supplement, particularly in promoting digestive health, immune function, and overall well-being. While more studies are needed to fully elucidate its mechanisms of action and therapeutic applications, existing research suggests promising outcomes in various health conditions.

18) BIFIDOBACTERIUM BIFIDUM

Introduction: Bifidobacterium bifidum is a gram-positive, anaerobic bacterium that is a common member of the human gut microbiota. It belongs to the Bifidobacterium genus, known for its probiotic properties.

Synonym Name and Common Name: Synonym Name: None Common Name: B. bifidum

Pharmacognosy/Chemistry: B. bifidum is a rod-shaped bacterium with a unique morphology and structure. It produces lactic acid and other beneficial metabolites through the fermentation of carbohydrates. Its chemical composition includes various proteins, carbohydrates, and cell wall components.

Action and Pharmacology: B. bifidum exerts its effects primarily through its probiotic action. It colonizes the gastrointestinal tract, where it helps maintain a healthy balance of gut microbiota, aids in digestion, modulates the immune system, and may contribute to overall gut health.

Method of Analysis: Analysis of B. bifidum involves culturing techniques to quantify viable bacterial counts. Molecular methods such as PCR may also be used for species identification and strain characterization. Additionally, biochemical assays and microscopy may be employed for further characterization.

Health Benefits: B. bifidum has been associated with various health benefits, including improved digestive function, enhanced immune response, reduction of gastrointestinal discomfort, prevention of antibiotic-associated diarrhea, and potential alleviation of symptoms related to conditions like irritable bowel syndrome (IBS).

Indication and Usage: B. bifidum is commonly used as a probiotic supplement to support gut health and overall well-being. It may be recommended for individuals experiencing digestive issues, those seeking to boost their immune system, or those looking to improve their overall gut health.

Usual Constituents with Percentages: The usual constituents and percentages of B. bifidum can vary depending on the strain and source. Common constituents include various strains of Bifidobacterium bifidum, each with its own unique composition.

Mechanism of Action: The exact mechanism of action of B. bifidum involves multiple factors, including production of lactic acid and other antimicrobial compounds, competition with pathogenic bacteria for nutrients and adhesion sites, and modulation of the gut microbiota and immune system.

Dosage: Dosage recommendations for B. bifidum can vary depending on the specific product and indication. Typical doses range from 1 to 10 billion CFUs (colony-forming units) per day, taken orally.

Contraindications: Individuals with compromised immune systems, those undergoing immunosuppressive therapy, or those with severe underlying health conditions should consult a healthcare professional before taking B. bifidum or any probiotic supplement.

Precautions: While generally considered safe, precautions should be taken in individuals with severe underlying health conditions or those at risk of bacterial translocation. It is advisable to consult a healthcare professional before starting any new supplement regimen.

Adverse Reactions: Adverse reactions to B. bifidum are rare but may include mild gastrointestinal symptoms such as bloating, gas, or diarrhea, particularly when first starting supplementation.

Research Standing: B. bifidum has been the subject of numerous studies investigating its potential health benefits and mechanisms of action. While much of the research is promising, more clinical trials are needed to fully establish its efficacy and safety in various health conditions.

Pharmacokinetics and Pharmacodynamics: B. bifidum survives transit through the acidic environment of the stomach and reaches the intestines where it can colonize and exert its probiotic effects. Its pharmacodynamics involve interactions with the gut microbiota and the host immune system.

Overdosage: While there is no established risk of overdosage with B. bifidum, exceeding recommended doses may lead to an imbalance in gut microbiota or potential adverse effects. It is advisable to follow dosage instructions provided by healthcare professionals or product labels.

International Standing: B. bifidum is recognized internationally as a safe and effective probiotic bacterium, commonly used in dietary supplements and functional foods.

Indian Standing: In India, B. bifidum is also utilized in probiotic formulations and is available as a dietary supplement for promoting gut health and immunity.

Research Summary: Research on Bifidobacterium bifidum has primarily focused on its potential health benefits as a probiotic supplement, particularly in promoting digestive health, immune function, and overall well-being. While more studies are needed to fully elucidate its mechanisms of action and therapeutic applications, existing research suggests promising outcomes in various health conditions.

19) BIFIDOBACTERIUM LACTIS

Introduction: Bifidobacterium lactis is a gram-positive, anaerobic bacterium that belongs to the Bifidobacterium genus, known for its probiotic properties. It is commonly found in the human gastrointestinal tract and is used in various probiotic supplements and fermented dairy products.

Synonym Name and Common Name: Synonym Name: None Common Name: B. lactis

Pharmacognosy/Chemistry: B. lactis is a rod-shaped bacterium with a unique cell wall structure. It produces lactic acid and other beneficial metabolites through the fermentation of carbohydrates. Its chemical composition includes various proteins, carbohydrates, and cell wall components.

Action and Pharmacology: B. lactis exerts its effects primarily through its probiotic action. It helps maintain a healthy balance of gut microbiota, aids in digestion, modulates the immune system, and may contribute to overall gut health. It also produces short-chain fatty acids that provide energy to colon cells.

Method of Analysis: Analysis of B. lactis involves culturing techniques to quantify viable bacterial counts. Molecular methods such as PCR may also be used for species identification and strain characterization. Additionally, biochemical assays and microscopy may be employed for further characterization.

Health Benefits: B. lactis has been associated with various health benefits, including improved digestive function, enhanced immune response, reduction of gastrointestinal discomfort, prevention of antibiotic-associated diarrhea, and potential alleviation of symptoms related to conditions like irritable bowel syndrome (IBS).

Indication and Usage: B. lactis is commonly used as a probiotic supplement to support gut health and overall well-being. It may be recommended for individuals experiencing digestive issues, those seeking to boost their immune system, or those looking to improve their overall gut health.

Usual Constituents with Percentages: The usual constituents and percentages of B. lactis can vary depending on the strain and source. Common constituents include various strains of Bifidobacterium lactis, each with its own unique composition.

Mechanism of Action: The exact mechanism of action of B. lactis involves multiple factors, including production of lactic acid and other antimicrobial compounds, competition with pathogenic bacteria for nutrients and adhesion sites, and modulation of the gut microbiota and immune system.

Dosage: Dosage recommendations for B. lactis can vary depending on the specific product and indication. Typical doses range from 1 to 10 billion CFUs (colony-forming units) per day, taken orally.

Contraindications: Individuals with compromised immune systems, those undergoing immunosuppressive therapy, or those with severe underlying health conditions should consult a healthcare professional before taking B. lactis or any probiotic supplement.

Precautions: While generally considered safe, precautions should be taken in individuals with severe underlying health conditions or those at risk of bacterial translocation. It is advisable to consult a healthcare professional before starting any new supplement regimen.

Adverse Reactions: Adverse reactions to B. lactis are rare but may include mild gastrointestinal symptoms such as bloating, gas, or diarrhea, particularly when first starting supplementation.

Research Standing: B. lactis has been the subject of numerous studies investigating its potential health benefits and mechanisms of action. While much of the research is promising, more clinical trials are needed to fully establish its efficacy and safety in various health conditions.

Pharmacokinetics and Pharmacodynamics: B. lactis survives transit through the acidic environment of the stomach and reaches the intestines where it can colonize and exert its probiotic effects. Its pharmacodynamics involve interactions with the gut microbiota and the host immune system.

Overdosage: While there is no established risk of overdosage with B. lactis, exceeding recommended doses may lead to an imbalance in gut microbiota or potential adverse effects. It is advisable to follow dosage instructions provided by healthcare professionals or product labels.

International Standing: B. lactis is recognized internationally as a safe and effective probiotic bacterium, commonly used in dietary supplements and functional foods.

Indian Standing: In India, B. lactis is also utilized in probiotic formulations and is available as a dietary supplement for promoting gut health and immunity.

Research Summary: Research on Bifidobacterium lactis has primarily focused on its potential health benefits as a probiotic supplement, particularly in promoting digestive health, immune function, and overall well-being. While more studies are needed to fully elucidate its mechanisms of action and therapeutic applications, existing research suggests promising outcomes in various health conditions.

20) BIFIDOBACTERIUM BREVE

Introduction: Bifidobacterium breve is a gram-positive, anaerobic bacterium belonging to the Bifidobacterium genus. It is commonly found in the gastrointestinal tract, particularly in breastfed infants, and is known for its probiotic properties.

Synonym Name and Common Name: Synonym Name: None Common Name: B. breve

Pharmacognosy/Chemistry: B. breve is a rod-shaped bacterium with a unique cell wall structure. It produces lactic acid and other beneficial metabolites through the fermentation of carbohydrates. Its chemical composition includes various proteins, carbohydrates, and cell wall components.

Action and Pharmacology: B. breve exerts its effects primarily through its probiotic action. It colonizes the gastrointestinal tract, where it helps maintain a healthy balance of gut microbiota, aids in digestion, modulates the immune system, and may contribute to overall gut health.

Method of Analysis: Analysis of B. breve involves culturing techniques to quantify viable bacterial counts. Molecular methods such as PCR may also be used for species identification and strain characterization. Additionally, biochemical assays and microscopy may be employed for further characterization.

Health Benefits: B. breve has been associated with various health benefits, including improved digestive function, enhanced immune response, reduction of gastrointestinal discomfort, prevention of antibiotic-associated diarrhea, and potential alleviation of symptoms related to conditions like irritable bowel syndrome (IBS).

Indication and Usage: B. breve is commonly used as a probiotic supplement to support gut health and overall well-being. It may be recommended for individuals experiencing digestive issues, those seeking to boost their immune system, or those looking to improve their overall gut health.

Usual Constituents with Percentages: The usual constituents and percentages of B. breve can vary depending on the strain and source. Common constituents include various strains of Bifidobacterium breve, each with its own unique composition.

Mechanism of Action: The exact mechanism of action of B. breve involves multiple factors, including production of lactic acid and other antimicrobial compounds, competition with pathogenic bacteria for nutrients and adhesion sites, and modulation of the gut microbiota and immune system.

Dosage: Dosage recommendations for B. breve can vary depending on the specific product and indication. Typical doses range from 1 to 10 billion CFUs (colony-forming units) per day, taken orally.

Contraindications: Individuals with compromised immune systems, those undergoing immunosuppressive therapy, or those with severe underlying health conditions should consult a healthcare professional before taking B. breve or any probiotic supplement.

Precautions: While generally considered safe, precautions should be taken in individuals with severe underlying health conditions or those at risk of bacterial translocation. It is advisable to consult a healthcare professional before starting any new supplement regimen.

Adverse Reactions: Adverse reactions to B. breve are rare but may include mild gastrointestinal symptoms such as bloating, gas, or diarrhea, particularly when first starting supplementation.

Research Standing: B. breve has been the subject of numerous studies investigating its potential health benefits and mechanisms of action. While much of the research is promising, more clinical trials are needed to fully establish its efficacy and safety in various health conditions.

Pharmacokinetics and Pharmacodynamics: B. breve survives transit through the acidic environment of the stomach and reaches the intestines where it can colonize and exert its probiotic effects. Its pharmacodynamics involve interactions with the gut microbiota and the host immune system.

Overdosage: While there is no established risk of overdosage with B. breve, exceeding recommended doses may lead to an imbalance in gut microbiota or potential adverse effects. It is advisable to follow dosage instructions provided by healthcare professionals or product labels.

International Standing: B. breve is recognized internationally as a safe and effective probiotic bacterium, commonly used in dietary supplements and functional foods.

Indian Standing: In India, B. breve is also utilized in probiotic formulations and is available as a dietary supplement for promoting gut health and immunity.

Research Summary: Research on Bifidobacterium breve has primarily focused on its potential health benefits as a probiotic supplement, particularly in promoting digestive health, immune function, and overall well-being. While more studies are needed to fully elucidate its mechanisms of action and therapeutic applications, existing research suggests promising outcomes in various health conditions.

21) BIFIDOBACTERIUM LONGUM

Introduction: Bifidobacterium longum is a gram-positive, anaerobic bacterium belonging to the Bifidobacterium genus. It is commonly found in the gastrointestinal tract and is known for its probiotic properties.

Synonym Name and Common Name: Synonym Name: None Common Name: B. longum

Pharmacognosy/Chemistry: B. longum is a rod-shaped bacterium with a unique cell wall structure. It produces lactic acid and other beneficial metabolites through the fermentation of carbohydrates. Its chemical composition includes various proteins, carbohydrates, and cell wall components.

Action and Pharmacology: B. longum exerts its effects primarily through its probiotic action. It colonizes the gastrointestinal tract, where it helps maintain a healthy balance of gut microbiota, aids in digestion, modulates the immune system, and may contribute to overall gut health.

Method of Analysis: Analysis of B. longum involves culturing techniques to quantify viable bacterial counts. Molecular methods such as PCR may also be used for species identification and strain characterization. Additionally, biochemical assays and microscopy may be employed for further characterization.

Health Benefits: B. longum has been associated with various health benefits, including improved digestive function, enhanced immune response, reduction of gastrointestinal discomfort, prevention of antibiotic-associated diarrhea, and potential alleviation of symptoms related to conditions like irritable bowel syndrome (IBS).

Indication and Usage: B. longum is commonly used as a probiotic supplement to support gut health and overall well-being. It may be recommended for individuals experiencing digestive issues, those seeking to boost their immune system, or those looking to improve their overall gut health.

Usual Constituents with Percentages: The usual constituents and percentages of B. longum can vary depending on the strain and source. Common constituents include various strains of Bifidobacterium longum, each with its own unique composition.

Mechanism of Action: The exact mechanism of action of B. longum involves multiple factors, including production of lactic acid and other antimicrobial compounds, competition with pathogenic bacteria for nutrients and adhesion sites, and modulation of the gut microbiota and immune system.

Dosage: Dosage recommendations for B. longum can vary depending on the specific product and indication. Typical doses range from 1 to 10 billion CFUs (colony-forming units) per day, taken orally.

Contraindications: Individuals with compromised immune systems, those undergoing immunosuppressive therapy, or those with severe underlying health conditions should consult a healthcare professional before taking B. longum or any probiotic supplement.

Precautions: While generally considered safe, precautions should be taken in individuals with severe underlying health conditions or those at risk of bacterial translocation. It is advisable to consult a healthcare professional before starting any new supplement regimen.

Adverse Reactions: Adverse reactions to B. longum are rare but may include mild gastrointestinal symptoms such as bloating, gas, or diarrhea, particularly when first starting supplementation.

Research Standing: B. longum has been the subject of numerous studies investigating its potential health benefits and mechanisms of action. While much of the research is promising, more clinical trials are needed to fully establish its efficacy and safety in various health conditions.

Pharmacokinetics and Pharmacodynamics: B. longum survives transit through the acidic environment of the stomach and reaches the intestines where it can colonize and exert its probiotic effects. Its pharmacodynamics involve interactions with the gut microbiota and the host immune system.

Overdosage: While there is no established risk of overdosage with B. longum, exceeding recommended doses may lead to an imbalance in gut microbiota or potential adverse effects. It is advisable to follow dosage instructions provided by healthcare professionals or product labels.

International Standing: B. longum is recognized internationally as a safe and effective probiotic bacterium, commonly used in dietary supplements and functional foods.

Indian Standing: In India, B. longum is also utilized in probiotic formulations and is available as a dietary supplement for promoting gut health and immunity.

Research Summary: Research on Bifidobacterium longum has primarily focused on its potential health benefits as a probiotic supplement, particularly in promoting digestive health, immune function, and overall well-being. While more studies are needed to fully elucidate its mechanisms of action and therapeutic applications, existing research suggests promising outcomes in various health conditions.

22) BIFIDOBACTERIUM ANIMALIS

Introduction: Bifidobacterium animalis is a gram-positive, anaerobic bacterium belonging to the Bifidobacterium genus. It is commonly found in the gastrointestinal tract of humans and animals and is known for its probiotic properties.

Synonym Name and Common Name: Synonym Name: Bifidobacterium lactis subsp. animalis Common Name: B. animalis

Pharmacognosy/Chemistry: B. animalis is a rod-shaped bacterium with a unique cell wall structure. It produces lactic acid and other beneficial metabolites through the fermentation of carbohydrates. Its chemical composition includes various proteins, carbohydrates, and cell wall components.

Action and Pharmacology: B. animalis exerts its effects primarily through its probiotic action. It colonizes the gastrointestinal tract, where it helps maintain a healthy balance of gut microbiota, aids in digestion, modulates the immune system, and may contribute to overall gut health.

Method of Analysis: Analysis of B. animalis involves culturing techniques to quantify viable bacterial counts. Molecular methods such as PCR may also be used for species identification and strain characterization. Additionally, biochemical assays and microscopy may be employed for further characterization.

Health Benefits: B. animalis has been associated with various health benefits, including improved digestive function, enhanced immune response, reduction of gastrointestinal discomfort, prevention of antibiotic-associated diarrhea, and potential alleviation of symptoms related to conditions like irritable bowel syndrome (IBS).

Indication and Usage: B. animalis is commonly used as a probiotic supplement to support gut health and overall well-being. It may be recommended for individuals experiencing digestive issues, those seeking to boost their immune system, or those looking to improve their overall gut health.

Usual Constituents with Percentages: The usual constituents and percentages of B. animalis can vary depending on the strain and source. Common constituents include various strains of Bifidobacterium animalis, each with its own unique composition.

Mechanism of Action: The exact mechanism of action of B. animalis involves multiple factors, including production of lactic acid and other antimicrobial compounds, competition with pathogenic bacteria for nutrients and adhesion sites, and modulation of the gut microbiota and immune system.

Dosage: Dosage recommendations for B. animalis can vary depending on the specific product and indication. Typical doses range from 1 to 10 billion CFUs (colony-forming units) per day, taken orally.

Contraindications: Individuals with compromised immune systems, those undergoing immunosuppressive therapy, or those with severe underlying health conditions should consult a healthcare professional before taking B. animalis or any probiotic supplement.

Precautions: While generally considered safe, precautions should be taken in individuals with severe underlying health conditions or those at risk of bacterial translocation. It is advisable to consult a healthcare professional before starting any new supplement regimen.

Adverse Reactions: Adverse reactions to B. animalis are rare but may include mild gastrointestinal symptoms such as bloating, gas, or diarrhea, particularly when first starting supplementation.

Research Standing: B. animalis has been the subject of numerous studies investigating its potential health benefits and mechanisms of action. While much of the research is promising, more clinical trials are needed to fully establish its efficacy and safety in various health conditions.

Pharmacokinetics and Pharmacodynamics: B. animalis survives transit through the acidic environment of the stomach and reaches the intestines where it can colonize and exert its probiotic effects. Its pharmacodynamics involve interactions with the gut microbiota and the host immune system.

Overdosage: While there is no established risk of overdosage with B. animalis, exceeding recommended doses may lead to an imbalance in gut microbiota or potential adverse effects. It is advisable to follow dosage instructions provided by healthcare professionals or product labels.

International Standing: B. animalis is recognized internationally as a safe and effective probiotic bacterium, commonly used in dietary supplements and functional foods.

Indian Standing: In India, B. animalis is also utilized in probiotic formulations and is available as a dietary supplement for promoting gut health and immunity.

Research Summary: Research on Bifidobacterium animalis has primarily focused on its potential health benefits as a probiotic supplement, particularly in promoting digestive health, immune function, and overall well-being. While more studies are needed to fully elucidate its mechanisms of action and therapeutic applications, existing research suggests promising outcomes in various health conditions.

23) BIFIDOBACTERIUM INFANTIS

Introduction: Bifidobacterium infantis is a gram-positive, anaerobic bacterium belonging to the Bifidobacterium genus. It is commonly found in the gastrointestinal tract, particularly in infants, and is known for its probiotic properties.

Synonym Name and Common Name: Synonym Name: None Common Name: B. infantis

Pharmacognosy/Chemistry: B. infantis is a rod-shaped bacterium with a unique cell wall structure. It produces lactic acid and other beneficial metabolites through the fermentation of carbohydrates. Its chemical composition includes various proteins, carbohydrates, and cell wall components.

Action and Pharmacology: B. infantis exerts its effects primarily through its probiotic action. It colonizes the gastrointestinal tract, where it helps maintain a healthy balance of gut microbiota, aids in digestion, modulates the immune system, and may contribute to overall gut health.

Method of Analysis: Analysis of B. infantis involves culturing techniques to quantify viable bacterial counts. Molecular methods such as PCR may also be used for species identification and strain characterization. Additionally, biochemical assays and microscopy may be employed for further characterization.

Health Benefits: B. infantis has been associated with various health benefits, particularly in infants, including improved digestion, prevention of gastrointestinal discomfort, reduction of colic symptoms, and support of overall immune health.

Indication and Usage: B. infantis is commonly used as a probiotic supplement, especially in infants, to support gut health and overall well-being. It may be recommended for infants experiencing digestive issues, those with colic symptoms, or those at risk of developing allergies.

Usual Constituents with Percentages: The usual constituents and percentages of B. infantis can vary depending on the strain and source. Common constituents include various strains of Bifidobacterium infantis, each with its own unique composition.

Mechanism of Action: The exact mechanism of action of B. infantis involves multiple factors, including production of lactic acid and other antimicrobial compounds, competition with pathogenic bacteria for nutrients and adhesion sites, and modulation of the gut microbiota and immune system.

Dosage: Dosage recommendations for B. infantis can vary depending on the specific product and indication. Typical doses range from 1 to 10 billion CFUs (colony-forming units) per day, administered orally, especially in infants.

Contraindications: Individuals with compromised immune systems, those undergoing immunosuppressive therapy, or those with severe underlying health conditions should consult a healthcare professional before administering B. infantis or any probiotic supplement, particularly in infants.

Precautions: While generally considered safe, precautions should be taken, especially when administering B. infantis to infants. Careful monitoring for adverse reactions and consultation with a healthcare professional is advisable, particularly in vulnerable populations.

Adverse Reactions: Adverse reactions to B. infantis are rare but may include mild gastrointestinal symptoms such as bloating, gas, or diarrhea, particularly when first starting supplementation, especially in infants.

Research Standing: B. infantis has been the subject of numerous studies, especially in the context of infant health and development. Research indicates its potential role in supporting gut health, alleviating colic symptoms, and modulating the immune system in infants.

Pharmacokinetics and Pharmacodynamics: B. infantis survives transit through the acidic environment of the stomach and reaches the intestines where it can colonize and exert its probiotic effects, especially in infants. Its pharmacodynamics involve interactions with the developing gut microbiota and the nascent immune system in infants.

Overdosage: While there is no established risk of overdosage with B. infantis, exceeding recommended doses may lead to an imbalance in gut microbiota or potential adverse effects, especially in infants. Careful adherence to dosage recommendations is advisable.

International Standing: B. infantis is recognized internationally as a safe and effective probiotic bacterium, commonly used in dietary supplements and functional foods, especially for infant health.

Indian Standing: In India, B. infantis is also utilized in probiotic formulations, particularly for infant health and development, and is available as a dietary supplement.

Research Summary: Research on Bifidobacterium infantis has primarily focused on its role in supporting infant gut health, alleviating colic symptoms, and modulating the developing immune system. While more studies are needed to fully elucidate its mechanisms of action and therapeutic applications, existing research suggests promising outcomes in infant health and development.

24) STREPTOCOCCUS THERMOPHILUS

Introduction: Streptococcus thermophilus is a gram-positive, facultative anaerobic bacterium commonly used in the production of yogurt and other fermented dairy products. It belongs to the Streptococcus genus and is known for its probiotic properties.

Synonym Name and Common Name: Synonym Name: None Common Name: S. thermophilus

Pharmacognosy/Chemistry: S. thermophilus is a spherical bacterium that forms chains. It produces lactic acid and other metabolites during the fermentation of lactose. Its chemical composition includes various proteins, polysaccharides, and cell wall components.

Action and Pharmacology: S. thermophilus exerts its effects primarily through its probiotic action. It contributes to the fermentation process in the gut, helps maintain a healthy balance of gut microbiota, and may contribute to overall gut health.

Method of Analysis: Analysis of S. thermophilus involves culturing techniques to quantify viable bacterial counts. Molecular methods such as PCR may also be used for species identification and strain characterization. Additionally, biochemical assays and microscopy may be employed for further characterization.

Health Benefits: S. thermophilus has been associated with various health benefits, including improved digestion, lactose digestion in lactose-intolerant individuals, immune system modulation, and potential reduction of gastrointestinal discomfort.

Indication and Usage: S. thermophilus is commonly used in the production of yogurt and other fermented dairy products. It may also be consumed as a probiotic supplement to support gut health and overall well-being.

Usual Constituents with Percentages: The usual constituents and percentages of S. thermophilus in fermented dairy products can vary depending on the fermentation process and strain used. Generally, it is present in significant proportions alongside other lactic acid bacteria.

Mechanism of Action: The exact mechanism of action of S. thermophilus involves its ability to ferment lactose, produce lactic acid, and modulate the gut microbiota. It may also interact with the immune system and epithelial cells in the gut.

Dosage: Dosage recommendations for S. thermophilus consumption in fermented dairy products vary depending on individual dietary preferences. Probiotic supplements containing S. thermophilus may have specific dosage recommendations provided by the manufacturer.

Contraindications: Individuals with compromised immune systems, those undergoing immunosuppressive therapy, or those with severe underlying health conditions should consult a healthcare professional before consuming products containing S. thermophilus.

Precautions: While generally considered safe, precautions should be taken in individuals with severe underlying health conditions or those at risk of bacterial translocation. It is advisable to consume S. thermophilus-containing products as part of a balanced diet.

Adverse Reactions: Adverse reactions to S. thermophilus are rare but may include mild gastrointestinal symptoms such as bloating, gas, or diarrhea, particularly in individuals with lactose intolerance.

Research Standing: S. thermophilus has been extensively studied for its role in fermentation processes and its potential health benefits as a probiotic. However, more research is needed to fully elucidate its mechanisms of action and therapeutic applications.

Pharmacokinetics and Pharmacodynamics: S. thermophilus is able to survive transit through the acidic environment of the stomach and reach the intestines where it can exert its probiotic effects. Its pharmacodynamics involve interactions with the gut microbiota and the host immune system.

Overdosage: While there is no established risk of overdosage with S. thermophilus, excessive consumption of fermented dairy products containing high concentrations of this bacterium may lead to gastrointestinal discomfort.

International Standing: S. thermophilus is recognized internationally as a safe and widely used probiotic bacterium, particularly in the production of fermented dairy products.

Indian Standing: In India, S. thermophilus is commonly used in the production of yogurt and other fermented dairy products, and it is also available as a probiotic supplement.

Research Summary: Research on Streptococcus thermophilus has primarily focused on its role in fermentation processes and its potential health benefits as a probiotic. While it is generally recognized as safe and beneficial, further research is needed to fully understand its mechanisms of action and therapeutic potential.

25) SACCHAROMYCES BOULARDII

Introduction: Saccharomyces boulardii is a probiotic yeast species known for its beneficial effects on gut health. It is commonly used as a dietary supplement to support gastrointestinal function and alleviate symptoms of digestive disorders.

Synonym Name and Common Name: Synonym Name: None Common Name: S. boulardii

Pharmacognosy/Chemistry: S. boulardii is a non-pathogenic yeast species closely related to Saccharomyces cerevisiae. It is heat-resistant and survives passage through the acidic environment of the stomach. The cell wall of S. boulardii contains mannan and beta-glucan polysaccharides.

Action and Pharmacology: S. boulardii exerts its effects by multiple mechanisms, including competitive inhibition of pathogenic bacteria, enhancement of intestinal barrier function, modulation of the immune response, and production of factors that inhibit toxins produced by pathogens.

Method of Analysis: Analysis of S. boulardii involves culturing techniques to quantify viable yeast counts. Molecular methods such as PCR may also be used for species identification and strain characterization. Additionally, biochemical assays may be employed to assess metabolic activity.

Health Benefits: S. boulardii has been shown to have several health benefits, including the prevention and treatment of antibiotic-associated diarrhea, reduction of symptoms associated with irritable bowel syndrome (IBS), alleviation of acute infectious diarrhea, and maintenance of remission in inflammatory bowel disease (IBD).

Indication and Usage: S. boulardii is commonly used as a probiotic supplement for the prevention and treatment of various gastrointestinal disorders, including diarrhea, IBS, IBD, and traveler's diarrhea. It may also be used to support gut health during antibiotic therapy.

Usual Constituents with Percentages: The usual constituents of S. boulardii supplements typically include live and active yeast cells, with concentrations ranging from 5 to 10 billion CFUs (colony-forming units) per dose.

Mechanism of Action: The mechanism of action of S. boulardii involves several key pathways, including direct antimicrobial effects against pathogens, enhancement of the intestinal barrier function, modulation of the immune response, and production of factors that neutralize toxins produced by pathogens.

Dosage: The typical dosage of S. boulardii supplements ranges from 250 to 1000 milligrams per day, taken orally in divided doses. Dosage may vary depending on the specific indication and severity of symptoms.

Contraindications: Individuals with compromised immune function, those undergoing immunosuppressive therapy, and patients with central venous catheters should use caution when taking S. boulardii due to the risk of fungemia. It is contraindicated in patients with known yeast allergies.

Precautions: Patients with underlying health conditions or those taking medications should consult with a healthcare professional before using S. boulardii supplements. It is important to adhere to recommended dosage guidelines and monitor for adverse reactions.

Adverse Reactions: Adverse reactions to S. boulardii are rare but may include mild gastrointestinal symptoms such as bloating, gas, or constipation. Allergic reactions, including rash or itching, may occur in individuals with yeast allergies.

Research Standing: S. boulardii has been extensively studied in both clinical and preclinical settings, and numerous studies have demonstrated its efficacy and safety in the treatment and prevention of various gastrointestinal disorders. It is widely recognized as an effective probiotic therapy.

Pharmacokinetics and Pharmacodynamics: S. boulardii survives passage through the acidic environment of the stomach and reaches the intestines where it exerts its probiotic effects. Its pharmacodynamics involve interactions with the gut microbiota, modulation of immune responses, and inhibition of pathogen colonization.

Overdosage: While there is no established risk of overdosage with S. boulardii, exceeding recommended dosages may increase the risk of adverse reactions. It is important to follow dosage guidelines provided by healthcare professionals or product labels.

International Standing: S. boulardii is widely used and recognized as a safe and effective probiotic supplement internationally. It is available over-the-counter in many countries and is commonly prescribed by healthcare professionals.

Indian Standing: In India, S. boulardii is available as a dietary supplement and is commonly used for the prevention and treatment of gastrointestinal disorders. It is widely available in pharmacies and health food stores.

Research Summary: Research on Saccharomyces boulardii has consistently demonstrated its efficacy and safety in the prevention and treatment of various gastrointestinal disorders. Its mechanisms of action, including antimicrobial effects and immune modulation, have been well characterized. Overall, S. boulardii is considered a valuable probiotic therapy for maintaining gut health and alleviating symptoms of digestive disorders.

26)SACCHAROMYCES CEREVISIAE

Introduction: Saccharomyces cerevisiae, commonly known as baker's yeast or brewer's yeast, is a species of yeast widely used in food production and as a dietary supplement. It belongs to the Saccharomyces genus and has been extensively studied for its various health benefits.

Synonym Name and Common Name: Synonym Name: Brewer's yeast, baker's yeast Common Name: S. cerevisiae

Pharmacognosy/Chemistry: S. cerevisiae is a unicellular fungus with a spherical to ovoid shape. It reproduces asexually through budding and is capable of fermenting sugars into alcohol and carbon dioxide. Its chemical composition includes proteins, carbohydrates, lipids, vitamins, and minerals.

Action and Pharmacology: S. cerevisiae exerts its effects through multiple mechanisms, including its role as a probiotic, modulation of the immune system, production of antimicrobial compounds, and enhancement of nutrient absorption in the gut.

Method of Analysis: Analysis of S. cerevisiae involves culturing techniques to quantify viable yeast counts. Molecular methods such as PCR may also be used for species identification and strain characterization. Additionally, biochemical assays may be employed to assess metabolic activity and production of bioactive compounds.

Health Benefits: S. cerevisiae has been associated with various health benefits, including improved digestion, enhanced immune function, regulation of blood sugar levels, support of cardiovascular health, and promotion of overall well-being.

Indication and Usage: S. cerevisiae is commonly used as a dietary supplement for individuals seeking to support gut health, boost their immune system, regulate blood sugar levels, or improve their overall health and well-being.

Usual Constituents with Percentages: The usual constituents of S. cerevisiae supplements typically include live and active yeast cells, with concentrations ranging from 1 to 10 billion CFUs (colony-forming units) per dose.

Mechanism of Action: The mechanism of action of S. cerevisiae involves its ability to colonize the gastrointestinal tract, modulate the gut microbiota, stimulate the immune system, produce antimicrobial compounds, and enhance nutrient absorption.

Dosage: The typical dosage of S. cerevisiae supplements ranges from 500 milligrams to 5 grams per day, taken orally. Dosage may vary depending on the specific product and indication.

Contraindications: Individuals with known yeast allergies or compromised immune function should avoid taking S. cerevisiae supplements. It is contraindicated in patients with yeast infections or those undergoing immunosuppressive therapy.

Precautions: Patients with underlying health conditions or those taking medications should consult with a healthcare professional before using S. cerevisiae supplements. It is important to adhere to recommended dosage guidelines and monitor for adverse reactions.

Adverse Reactions: Adverse reactions to S. cerevisiae supplements are rare but may include mild gastrointestinal symptoms such as bloating, gas, or diarrhea. Allergic reactions, including rash or itching, may occur in individuals with yeast allergies.

Research Standing: S. cerevisiae has been extensively studied for its various health benefits and mechanisms of action. Numerous clinical trials and preclinical studies have demonstrated its efficacy and safety in supporting gut health, enhancing immune function, and promoting overall well-being.

Pharmacokinetics and Pharmacodynamics: S. cerevisiae survives passage through the acidic environment of the stomach and reaches the intestines where it exerts its probiotic effects. Its pharmacodynamics involve interactions with the gut microbiota, modulation of immune responses, and enhancement of nutrient absorption.

Overdosage: While there is no established risk of overdosage with S. cerevisiae, exceeding recommended dosages may increase the risk of adverse reactions. It is important to follow dosage guidelines provided by healthcare professionals or product labels.

International Standing: S. cerevisiae is widely recognized as a safe and effective dietary supplement internationally. It is available over-the-counter in many countries and is commonly used to promote gut health and overall well-being.

Indian Standing: In India, S. cerevisiae supplements are available in various forms and are commonly used for their health benefits. They are widely available in pharmacies and health food stores.

Research Summary: Research on Saccharomyces cerevisiae has demonstrated its diverse health benefits and mechanisms of action, including its role as a probiotic, immunomodulator, and nutrient enhancer. It is considered a valuable dietary supplement for supporting gut health, boosting immune function, and promoting overall well-being.

27) LACTICASEIBACILLUS PARACASEI

Introduction: Lacticaseibacillus paracasei is a gram-positive, facultatively anaerobic bacterium belonging to the Lacticaseibacillus genus. It is a probiotic microorganism known for its beneficial effects on gut health and overall well-being.

Synonym Name and Common Name: Synonym Name: None Common Name: L. paracasei

Pharmacognosy/Chemistry: L. paracasei is a rod-shaped bacterium with a unique cell wall structure. It produces lactic acid and other metabolites through the fermentation of carbohydrates. Its chemical composition includes proteins, carbohydrates, lipids, and various cell wall components.

Action and Pharmacology: L. paracasei exerts its effects primarily through its probiotic action. It colonizes the gastrointestinal tract, where it helps maintain a healthy balance of gut microbiota, supports digestion, modulates the immune system, and may contribute to overall gut health.

Method of Analysis: Analysis of L. paracasei involves culturing techniques to quantify viable bacterial counts. Molecular methods such as PCR may also be used for species identification and strain characterization. Additionally, biochemical assays may be employed for further characterization.

Health Benefits: L. paracasei has been associated with various health benefits, including improved digestion, prevention of gastrointestinal discomfort, support of immune function, reduction of allergies, and modulation of inflammatory responses.

Indication and Usage: L. paracasei is commonly used as a probiotic supplement to support gut health and overall well-being. It may be recommended for individuals experiencing digestive issues, those with compromised immune function, or those seeking to maintain a healthy balance of gut microbiota.

Usual Constituents with Percentages: The usual constituents and percentages of L. paracasei can vary depending on the formulation and dosage form. Commonly, probiotic supplements contain L. paracasei in concentrations ranging from millions to billions of CFUs (colony-forming units) per dose.

Mechanism of Action: The mechanism of action of L. paracasei involves multiple factors, including production of lactic acid and other antimicrobial compounds, competitive exclusion of pathogenic bacteria, modulation of the gut microbiota, and interaction with the host immune system.

Dosage: Dosage recommendations for L. paracasei can vary depending on the specific product and indication. Typical doses range from 1 to 10 billion CFUs per day, administered orally, either as a standalone supplement or as part of a probiotic blend.

Contraindications: Individuals with compromised immune systems, those undergoing immunosuppressive therapy, or those with severe underlying health conditions should consult a healthcare professional before using L. paracasei supplements.

Precautions: While generally considered safe, precautions should be taken when using L. paracasei supplements, especially in vulnerable populations.

Careful monitoring for adverse reactions and consultation with a healthcare professional is advisable.

Adverse Reactions: Adverse reactions to L. paracasei supplements are rare but may include mild gastrointestinal symptoms such as bloating, gas, or diarrhea, particularly when first starting supplementation or in individuals with sensitivities.

Research Standing: L. paracasei has been the subject of numerous studies investigating its health benefits and mechanisms of action. Research indicates its potential role in supporting gut health, modulating immune function, and alleviating gastrointestinal symptoms.

Pharmacokinetics and Pharmacodynamics: L. paracasei survives transit through the acidic environment of the stomach and reaches the intestines where it can colonize and exert its probiotic effects. Its pharmacodynamics involve interactions with the gut microbiota and the host immune system.

Overdosage: While there is no established risk of overdosage with L. paracasei, exceeding recommended doses may lead to an imbalance in gut microbiota or potential adverse effects, especially in susceptible individuals. Adherence to recommended dosage guidelines is advisable.

International Standing: L. paracasei is recognized internationally as a safe and effective probiotic bacterium, commonly used in dietary supplements and functional foods to promote gut health and overall well-being.

Indian Standing: In India, L. paracasei is also utilized in probiotic formulations, available in various dietary supplements and functional foods aimed at supporting gut health and immune function.

Research Summary: Research on Lacticaseibacillus paracasei suggests its potential as a probiotic for improving gut health, modulating immune function, and alleviating gastrointestinal symptoms. While more studies are needed to fully elucidate its mechanisms of action and therapeutic applications, existing research indicates promising outcomes in promoting overall well-being

28) LACTOBACILLUS GASSERI

Introduction: Lactobacillus gasseri is a gram-positive, rod-shaped bacterium that belongs to the Lactobacillus genus. It is considered a beneficial bacterium and is commonly found in the human gastrointestinal tract, as well as in certain fermented foods.

Synonym Name and Common Name: Synonym Name: None Common Name: L. gasseri

Pharmacognosy/Chemistry: L. gasseri is characterized by its rod-shaped morphology and gram-positive staining. It produces lactic acid as a metabolic byproduct and is known for its ability to ferment sugars. The chemical composition includes proteins, carbohydrates, lipids, and various cell wall components.

Action and Pharmacology: L. gasseri exerts its effects primarily through its probiotic action. It helps maintain a healthy balance of gut microbiota, supports digestion, modulates the immune system, and may have anti-inflammatory properties.

Method of Analysis: Analysis of L. gasseri involves culturing techniques to quantify viable bacterial counts. Molecular methods such as PCR may also be used for species identification and strain characterization. Additionally, biochemical assays may be employed to assess metabolic activity and production of bioactive compounds.

Health Benefits: L. gasseri has been associated with various health benefits, including improved digestion, prevention of gastrointestinal discomfort, support of immune function, regulation of blood sugar levels, and maintenance of vaginal health in women.

Indication and Usage: L. gasseri is commonly used as a probiotic supplement to support gut health, boost the immune system, and promote overall well-being. It may be recommended for individuals experiencing digestive issues, those with compromised immune function, or those seeking to maintain a healthy microbiota balance.

Usual Constituents with Percentages: The usual constituents of L. gasseri supplements typically include live and active bacterial cells, with concentrations ranging from millions to billions of CFUs (colony-forming units) per dose.

Mechanism of Action: The mechanism of action of L. gasseri involves multiple factors, including competitive exclusion of pathogenic bacteria, production of antimicrobial compounds, modulation of the gut microbiota composition, enhancement of intestinal barrier function, and interaction with the host immune system.

Dosage: Dosage recommendations for L. gasseri can vary depending on the specific product and indication. Typical doses range from 1 to 10 billion CFUs per day, administered orally, either as a standalone supplement or as part of a probiotic blend.

Contraindications: Individuals with compromised immune systems, those undergoing immunosuppressive therapy, or those with severe underlying health conditions should consult a healthcare professional before using L. gasseri supplements.

Precautions: While generally considered safe, precautions should be taken when using L. gasseri supplements, especially in vulnerable populations. Careful monitoring for adverse reactions and consultation with a healthcare professional is advisable.

Adverse Reactions: Adverse reactions to L. gasseri supplements are rare but may include mild gastrointestinal symptoms such as bloating, gas, or diarrhea. Allergic reactions, including rash or itching, may occur in individuals with sensitivities.

Research Standing: L. gasseri has been the subject of numerous studies investigating its health benefits and mechanisms of action. Research indicates its potential role in supporting gut health, modulating immune function, and alleviating gastrointestinal symptoms.

Pharmacokinetics and Pharmacodynamics: L. gasseri survives transit through the acidic environment of the stomach and reaches the intestines where it can colonize and exert its probiotic effects. Its pharmacodynamics involve interactions with the gut microbiota and the host immune system.

Overdosage: While there is no established risk of overdosage with L. gasseri, exceeding recommended doses may lead to an imbalance in gut microbiota or potential adverse effects, especially in susceptible individuals. Adherence to recommended dosage guidelines is advisable.

International Standing: L. gasseri is recognized internationally as a safe and effective probiotic bacterium, commonly used in dietary supplements and functional foods to promote gut health and overall well-being.

Indian Standing: In India, L. gasseri is also utilized in probiotic formulations, available in various dietary supplements and functional foods aimed at supporting gut health and immune function.

Research Summary: Research on Lactobacillus gasseri has demonstrated its diverse health benefits and mechanisms of action, including its role as a probiotic, immunomodulator, and gut health promoter. While more studies are needed to fully elucidate its mechanisms of action and therapeutic applications, existing research indicates promising outcomes in promoting overall well-being.

29) BACILLUS CLAUSII

Introduction: Bacillus clausii is a gram-positive, spore-forming bacterium that belongs to the Bacillus genus. It is known for its ability to survive harsh environmental conditions and colonize the human gastrointestinal tract, where it exhibits probiotic properties.

Synonym Name and Common Name: Synonym Name: None Common Name: B. clausii

Pharmacognosy/Chemistry: B. clausii is characterized by its rod-shaped morphology and ability to form spores. It produces a variety of metabolites, including enzymes, peptides, and antimicrobial substances. Its chemical composition includes proteins, carbohydrates, lipids, and various cell wall components.

Action and Pharmacology: B. clausii exerts its effects primarily through its probiotic action. It helps maintain a healthy balance of gut microbiota, supports digestion, modulates the immune system, and may have anti-inflammatory properties.

Method of Analysis: Analysis of B. clausii involves culturing techniques to quantify viable bacterial counts. Molecular methods such as PCR may also be used for species identification and strain characterization. Additionally, biochemical assays may be employed to assess metabolic activity and production of bioactive compounds.

Health Benefits: B. clausii has been associated with various health benefits, including improved digestion, prevention of gastrointestinal discomfort, support of immune function, reduction of antibiotic-associated diarrhea, and alleviation of symptoms associated with irritable bowel syndrome (IBS).

Indication and Usage: B. clausii is commonly used as a probiotic supplement to support gut health, boost the immune system, and promote overall well-being. It may be recommended for individuals experiencing digestive issues, those with compromised immune function, or those seeking to maintain a healthy microbiota balance.

Usual Constituents with Percentages: The usual constituents of B. clausii supplements typically include live and active bacterial cells, with concentrations ranging from millions to billions of CFUs (colony-forming units) per dose.

Mechanism of Action: The mechanism of action of B. clausii involves multiple factors, including competitive exclusion of pathogenic bacteria, production of antimicrobial compounds, modulation of the gut microbiota composition, enhancement of intestinal barrier function, and interaction with the host immune system.

Dosage: Dosage recommendations for B. clausii can vary depending on the specific product and indication. Typical doses range from 1 to 10 billion CFUs per day, administered orally, either as a standalone supplement or as part of a probiotic blend.

Contraindications: Individuals with compromised immune systems, those undergoing immunosuppressive therapy, or those with severe underlying health conditions should consult a healthcare professional before using B. clausii supplements.

Precautions: While generally considered safe, precautions should be taken when using B. clausii supplements, especially in vulnerable populations. Careful monitoring for adverse reactions and consultation with a healthcare professional is advisable.

Adverse Reactions: Adverse reactions to B. clausii supplements are rare but may include mild gastrointestinal symptoms such as bloating, gas, or diarrhea. Allergic reactions, including rash or itching, may occur in individuals with sensitivities.

Research Standing: B. clausii has been the subject of numerous studies investigating its health benefits and mechanisms of action. Research indicates its potential role in supporting gut health, modulating immune function, and alleviating gastrointestinal symptoms.

Pharmacokinetics and Pharmacodynamics: B. clausii survives transit through the acidic environment of the stomach and reaches the intestines where it can colonize and exert its probiotic effects. Its pharmacodynamics involve interactions with the gut microbiota and the host immune system.

Overdosage: While there is no established risk of overdosage with B. clausii, exceeding recommended doses may lead to an imbalance in gut microbiota or potential adverse effects, especially in susceptible individuals. Adherence to recommended dosage guidelines is advisable.

International Standing: B. clausii is recognized internationally as a safe and effective probiotic bacterium, commonly used in dietary supplements and functional foods to promote gut health and overall well-being.

Indian Standing: In India, B. clausii is also utilized in probiotic formulations, available in various dietary supplements and functional foods aimed at supporting gut health and immune function.

Research Summary: Research on Bacillus clausii has demonstrated its diverse health benefits and mechanisms of action, including its role as a probiotic, immunomodulator, and gut health promoter. While more studies are needed to fully elucidate its mechanisms of action and therapeutic applications, existing research indicates promising outcomes in promoting overall well-being.

30) ESTABLISHED PROBIOTIC STRAINS OF BACILLUS SUBTILIS

Introduction: Bacillus subtilis is a gram-positive, rod-shaped bacterium commonly found in soil and the gastrointestinal tract of humans and animals. It is known for its robustness and ability to form spores, making it suitable for various industrial and probiotic applications.

Synonym Name and Common Name: Synonym Name: None Common Name: B. subtilis

Pharmacognosy/Chemistry: B. subtilis exhibits a rod-shaped morphology and forms endospores under adverse conditions. Its chemical composition includes proteins, carbohydrates, lipids, and various cell wall components. It produces a wide range of enzymes and metabolites.

Action and Pharmacology: B. subtilis exerts its effects through various mechanisms, including competitive exclusion of pathogens, production of antimicrobial compounds, modulation of the gut microbiota, enhancement of intestinal barrier function, and stimulation of the immune system.

Method of Analysis: Analysis of B. subtilis involves culturing techniques to quantify viable bacterial counts. Molecular methods such as PCR may also be used for species identification and strain characterization. Additionally, biochemical assays may be employed to assess metabolic activity and production of bioactive compounds.

Health Benefits: B. subtilis has been associated with various health benefits, including improved digestion, prevention of gastrointestinal discomfort, support of immune function, reduction of antibiotic-associated diarrhea, and alleviation of symptoms associated with irritable bowel syndrome (IBS).

Indication and Usage: Established probiotic strains of B. subtilis are commonly used as dietary supplements to support gut health, boost the immune system, and promote overall well-being. They may be recommended for individuals experiencing digestive issues or seeking to maintain a healthy microbiota balance.

Usual Constituents with Percentages: The usual constituents of B. subtilis supplements typically include live and active bacterial cells, with concentrations ranging from millions to billions of CFUs (colony-forming units) per dose.

Mechanism of Action: The mechanism of action of established probiotic strains of B. subtilis involves multiple factors, including competitive exclusion of pathogenic bacteria, production of antimicrobial compounds, modulation of the gut microbiota composition, enhancement of intestinal barrier function, and interaction with the host immune system.

Dosage: Dosage recommendations for established probiotic strains of B. subtilis can vary depending on the specific product and indication. Typical doses range from 1 to 10 billion CFUs per day, administered orally, either as a standalone supplement or as part of a probiotic blend.

Contraindications: Individuals with compromised immune systems, those undergoing immunosuppressive therapy, or those with severe underlying health conditions should consult a healthcare professional before using B. subtilis supplements.

Precautions: While generally considered safe, precautions should be taken when using B. subtilis supplements, especially in vulnerable populations. Careful monitoring for adverse reactions and consultation with a healthcare professional is advisable.

Adverse Reactions: Adverse reactions to established probiotic strains of B. subtilis supplements are rare but may include mild gastrointestinal symptoms such as bloating, gas, or diarrhea. Allergic reactions, including rash or itching, may occur in individuals with sensitivities.

Research Standing: Established probiotic strains of B. subtilis have been the subject of numerous studies investigating their health benefits and mechanisms of action. Research indicates their potential role in supporting gut health, modulating immune function, and alleviating gastrointestinal symptoms.

Pharmacokinetics and Pharmacodynamics: Established probiotic strains of B. subtilis survive transit through the acidic environment of the stomach and reach the intestines where they can colonize and exert their probiotic effects. Their pharmacodynamics involve interactions with the gut microbiota and the host immune system.

Overdosage: While there is no established risk of overdosage with established probiotic strains of B. subtilis, exceeding recommended doses may lead to an imbalance in gut microbiota or potential adverse effects, especially in susceptible individuals. Adherence to recommended dosage guidelines is advisable.

International Standing: Established probiotic strains of B. subtilis are recognized internationally as safe and effective probiotic bacteria, commonly used in dietary supplements and functional foods to promote gut health and overall well-being.

Indian Standing: In India, established probiotic strains of B. subtilis are also utilized in probiotic formulations, available in various dietary supplements and functional foods aimed at supporting gut health and immune function.

Research Summary: Research on established probiotic strains of Bacillus subtilis suggests their potential as probiotics for improving gut health, modulating immune function, and alleviating gastrointestinal symptoms. While more studies are needed to fully elucidate their mechanisms of action and therapeutic applications, existing research indicates promising outcomes in promoting overall well-being.

31) BACILLUS INDICUS

Introduction: Bacillus indicus, also known as Bacillus coagulans, is a gram-positive, spore-forming bacterium belonging to the Bacillus genus. It is recognized for its potential health benefits and is commonly used as a probiotic supplement.

Synonym Name and Common Name: Synonym Name: Bacillus coagulans Common Name: B. indicus

Pharmacognosy/Chemistry: Bacillus indicus is characterized by its rod-shaped morphology and ability to form spores. Its chemical composition includes proteins, carbohydrates, lipids, and various cell wall components. It produces lactic acid as a metabolic byproduct.

Action and Pharmacology: B. indicus exerts its effects primarily through its probiotic action. It helps maintain a healthy balance of gut microbiota, supports digestion, modulates the immune system, and may have anti-inflammatory properties.

Method of Analysis: Analysis of Bacillus indicus involves culturing techniques to quantify viable bacterial counts. Molecular methods such as PCR may also be used for species identification and strain characterization. Additionally, biochemical assays may be employed to assess metabolic activity and production of bioactive compounds.

Health Benefits: Bacillus indicus has been associated with various health benefits, including improved digestion, prevention of gastrointestinal discomfort, support of immune function, reduction of antibiotic-associated diarrhea, and alleviation of symptoms associated with irritable bowel syndrome (IBS).

Indication and Usage: Bacillus indicus is commonly used as a probiotic supplement to support gut health, boost the immune system, and promote overall well-being. It may be recommended for individuals experiencing digestive issues or seeking to maintain a healthy microbiota balance.

Usual Constituents with Percentages: The usual constituents of Bacillus indicus supplements typically include live and active bacterial cells, with concentrations ranging from millions to billions of CFUs (colony-forming units) per dose.

Mechanism of Action: The mechanism of action of Bacillus indicus involves multiple factors, including competitive exclusion of pathogenic bacteria, production of antimicrobial compounds, modulation of the gut microbiota composition, enhancement of intestinal barrier function, and interaction with the host immune system.

Dosage: Dosage recommendations for Bacillus indicus can vary depending on the specific product and indication. Typical doses range from 1 to 10 billion CFUs per day, administered orally, either as a standalone supplement or as part of a probiotic blend.

Contraindications: Individuals with compromised immune systems, those undergoing immunosuppressive therapy, or those with severe underlying health conditions should consult a healthcare professional before using Bacillus indicus supplements.

Precautions: While generally considered safe, precautions should be taken when using Bacillus indicus supplements, especially in vulnerable populations. Careful monitoring for adverse reactions and consultation with a healthcare professional is advisable.

Adverse Reactions: Adverse reactions to Bacillus indicus supplements are rare but may include mild gastrointestinal symptoms such as bloating, gas, or diarrhea. Allergic reactions, including rash or itching, may occur in individuals with sensitivities.

Research Standing: Bacillus indicus has been the subject of numerous studies investigating its health benefits and mechanisms of action. Research indicates its potential role in supporting gut health, modulating immune function, and alleviating gastrointestinal symptoms.

Pharmacokinetics and Pharmacodynamics: Bacillus indicus survives transit through the acidic environment of the stomach and reaches the intestines where it can colonize and exert its probiotic effects. Its pharmacodynamics involve interactions with the gut microbiota and the host immune system.

Overdosage: While there is no established risk of overdosage with Bacillus indicus, exceeding recommended doses may lead to an imbalance in gut microbiota or potential adverse effects, especially in susceptible individuals. Adherence to recommended dosage guidelines is advisable.

International Standing: Bacillus indicus is recognized internationally as a safe and effective probiotic bacterium, commonly used in dietary supplements and functional foods to promote gut health and overall well-being.

Indian Standing: In India, Bacillus indicus is also utilized in probiotic formulations, available in various dietary supplements and functional foods aimed at supporting gut health and immune function.

Research Summary: Research on Bacillus indicus suggests its potential as a probiotic for improving gut health, modulating immune function, and alleviating gastrointestinal symptoms. While more studies are needed to fully elucidate its mechanisms of action and therapeutic applications, existing research indicates promising outcomes in promoting overall well-being.